NEUROSENSORY DISORDERS IN MILD TRAUMATIC BRAIN INJURY

NEUROSENSORY DISORDERS IN MILD TRAUMATIC BRAIN INJURY

Edited by

MICHAEL E. HOFFER
Department of Otolaryngology and Neurological Surgery,
University of Miami, Miller School of Medicine, Miami, FL, United States

CAREY D. BALABAN
Departments of Otolaryngology, Neurobiology, Communication Sciences & Disorders, and Bioengineering,
University of Pittsburgh, Pittsburgh, PA, United States

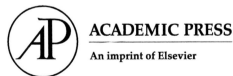

ACADEMIC PRESS
An imprint of Elsevier

Academic Press is an imprint of Elsevier
125 London Wall, London EC2Y 5AS, United Kingdom
525 B Street, Suite 1650, San Diego, CA 92101, United States
50 Hampshire Street, 5th Floor, Cambridge, MA 02139, United States
The Boulevard, Langford Lane, Kidlington, Oxford OX5 1GB, United Kingdom

Notices

Knowledge and best practice in this field are constantly changing. As new research and experience broaden our
understanding, changes in research methods, professional practices, or medical treatment may become necessary.

Practitioners and researchers must always rely on their own experience and knowledge in evaluating and using
any information, methods, compounds, or experiments described herein. In using such information or methods
they should be mindful of their own safety and the safety of others, including parties for whom they have a
professional responsibility.

To the fullest extent of the law, neither the Publisher nor the authors, contributors, or editors, assume any liability
for any injury and/or damage to persons or property as a matter of products liability, negligence or otherwise, or
from any use or operation of any methods, products, instructions, or ideas contained in the material herein.

British Library Cataloguing-in-Publication Data
A catalogue record for this book is available from the British Library

Library of Congress Cataloging-in-Publication Data
A catalog record for this book is available from the Library of Congress

ISBN: 978-0-12-812344-7

For Information on all Academic Press publications
visit our website at https://www.elsevier.com/books-and-journals

  Working together
to grow libraries in
developing countries

www.elsevier.com • www.bookaid.org

Publisher: Nikki Levy
Acquisition Editor: Melanie Tucker
Editorial Project Manager: Tracy Tufaga
Production Project Manager: Paul Prasad Chandramohan
Cover Designer: Christian Bilbow

Typeset by MPS Limited, Chennai, India

We would like to dedicate this book to the men and women of the United States Military where uncommon valor is always a common virtue.

We would like to thank our families for their unwavering support throughout the years.

Contents

III

NEUROSENSORY DISORDERS IN CLINICAL PRACTICE

13. Cognitive-Emotional-Vestibular Triad in Mild Traumatic Brain Injury

NIKHIL BANERJEE, SARAH J. GETZ
AND BONNIE E. LEVIN

14. Sleep Issues and Mild Traumatic Brain Injury

DAVID Y. GOLDRICH, B. TUCKER WOODSON, MD, FACS,
JASDEEP S. HUNDAL, PSYD, ABPP-CN AND P. ASHLEY
WACKYM, MD, FACS, FAAP

15. Vision Disorders in Mild Traumatic Brain Injury

ERIC SINGMAN, MD, PHD AND PATRICK QUAID,
OPTOMETRIST, MCOPTOM, FCOVD, PHD

IV

DIAGNOSIS AND TREATMENT

16. Diagnostic Approaches Techniques in Concussion/Mild Traumatic Brain Injury: Where are we?

REBECCA SMITH, MARIYA CHEPISHEVA,
THOMAS CRONIN, PHD AND BARRY M. SEEMUNGAL

List of Contributors

Abdulaziz A. Alkathiry, PT, PhD Department of Physical Therapy, Majmaah University, Al Majmaah, Saudi Arabia

Justine J. Allen, M.S., CCC-SLP Division of Speech Pathology, Department of Otolaryngology, University of Miami, Miller School of Medicine, Miami, FL, United States

Carey D. Balaban, PhD Departments of Otolaryngology, Neurobiology, Communication Sciences & Disorders, and Bioengineering, University of Pittsburgh, Pittsburgh, PA, United States

Nikhil Banerjee Department of Neurology, University of Miami, Miller School of Medicine, Miami, FL, United States

Russell M. Bauer, PhD, ABPP Department of Clinical & Health Psychology, University of Florida, Gainesville, FL, United States

Sara Bressler, BS Department of Otolaryngology, University of Miami, Miller School of Medicine, Miami, FL, United States

Sagar Buch, PhD The MRI Institute for Biomedical Research, Waterloo, ON, Canada

James K. Buskirk, MS Ed., PT, SCS, AIB-CON Department of Otolaryngology, Batchelor's Children's Research Institute, University of Miami, Miller School of Medicine, Miami, FL, United States

Mariya Chepisheva Department of Medicine, Imperial College, London, United Kingdom

David X. Cifu, MD Innovation and System Integration, Virginia Commonwealth University School of Medicine, Richmond, VA, United States; The Herman J. Flax, M.D. Professor and Chair, Department of PM&R, Virginia Commonwealth University School of Medicine, Richmond, VA, United States; Chronic Effects of Neurotrauma Consortium, US Department of Veterans Affairs, Richmond, VA, United States; Sports Sciences, NHL Florida Panthers, Sunrise, FL, United States

Bruce A. Citron Laboratory of Molecular Biology, Research and Development 151, Bay Pines VA Healthcare System, Bay Pines, FL, United States; Department of Molecular Medicine, USF Morsani College of Medicine, Tampa, FL, United States

Thomas Cronin, PhD Department of Medicine, Imperial College, London, United Kingdom

Blessen C. Eapen, MD Department of Rehabilitation Medicine, UT Health San Antonio, San Antonio, TX, United States; Polytrauma Rehabilitation Center, Polytrauma/TBI Fellowship Program, Physical Medicine and Rehabilitation Services PM&RS (MC 117), South Texas Veterans Health Care System, San Antonio, TX, United States

Laurel M. Fisher, PhD Caruso Department of Otolaryngology—Head and Neck Surgery, Keck School of Medicine of USC, Los Angeles, CA, United States

Joseph M. Furman, MD, PhD Department of Otolaryngology, University of Pittsburgh, Pittsburgh, PA, United States

Sarah J. Getz Miller School of Medicine, Department of Neurology, Division of Neuropsychology, University of Miami, FL, United States

Kiarash Ghassaban, MS Magnetic Resonance Innovations, Inc., Detroit, MI, United States

David Y. Goldrich Medical Student, Rutgers Robert Wood Johnson Medical School, New Brunswick, NJ, United States

Kim R. Gottshall, PhD, PT Naval Health Research Center, San Diego, CA, United States

Nigel H. Greig, PhD Drug Design & Development Section, Translational Gerontology Branch, Intramural Research Program, National Institute on Aging, National Institutes of Health, Baltimore, MD, United States

E. Mark Haacke, PhD Magnetic Resonance Innovations, Inc., Detroit, MI, United States; The MRI Institute for Biomedical Research, Detroit, MI, United States; The MRI Institute for Biomedical Research, Waterloo, ON, Canada; Department of Biomedical Engineering, Wayne State University College of Engineering, Detroit, MI, United States; Department of Radiology, Wayne State University School of Medicine, Detroit, MI, United States

Kendall Haven Story Consultant, Fulton, CA, United States

Barry J. Hoffer, MD, PhD Department of Neurosurgery, Case Western Reserve University School of Medicine, Cleveland, OH, United States

Michael E. Hoffer, MD Department of Otolaryngology and Neurological Surgery, University of Miami, Miller School of Medicine, Miami, FL, United States

Michael E. Hoffer, MD, FACS Department of Otolaryngology, University of Miami, Miami, FL, United States

S. Alan Hoffer, MD Department of Neurological Surgery, The Neurological Institute, University Hospitals Cleveland Medical Center, Cleveland, OH, United States

Gillian Hotz, PhD Sports Medicine Institute, Concussion Program and The Miami Project to Cure Paralysis, University of Miami, Miller School of Medicine, Miami, FL, United States

Jasdeep S. Hundal, PsyD, ABPP-Cn Departments of Medicine and Neurology, Rutgers Robert Wood Johnson Medical School, New Brunswick, NJ, United States; Cancer Institute of New Jersey, New Brunswick, NJ, United States

Michael S. Jaffee, MD Department of Neurology, University of Florida, Gainesville, FL, United States

Alexander Kiderman Chief Technology Officer, Neuro Kinetics, Inc., Pittsburgh, PA, United States

Anthony P. Kontos, PhD Department of Orthopedic Surgery, University of Pittsburgh, Pittsburgh, PA, United States

Ja-Won Koo, MD, PhD Department of Otorhinolaryngology-Head and Neck Surgery, Seoul National University Bundang Hospital, Seongnam, South Korea

Zhifeng Kou, PhD Department of Biomedical Engineering, Wayne State University College of Engineering, Detroit, MI, United States; Department of Radiology, Wayne State University School of Medicine, Detroit, MI, United States

Marta Kulich, BA Caruso Department of Otolaryngology—Head and Neck Surgery, Keck School of Medicine of USC, Los Angeles, CA, United States; Northwestern University Feinberg School of Medicine, Chicago, IL, United States

Bonnie Levin Department of Neurology, University of Miami, Miller School of Medicine, Miami, FL, United States

Nicola Maggio, MD, PhD Department of Neurology, The Chaim Sheba Medical Center, Tel Hashomer, Israel; Department of Neurology and Neurosurgery, Sackler Faculty of Medicine, Tel Aviv University, Tel Aviv, Israel; Talpiot Medical Leadership Program, The Chaim Sheba Medical Center, Tel Hashomer, Israel; Sagol School of Neuroscience, Tel Aviv University, Tel Aviv, Israel

Teshamae S. Monteith, MD Department of Neurology, Headache Division, University of Miami, Miller School of Medicine, Miami, FL, United States

Kester J. Nedd, DO Sports Medicine Institute, Concussion Program and The Miami Project to Cure Paralysis, University of Miami, Miller School of Medicine, Miami, FL, United States

Jonathan Pace, MD Department of Neurological Surgery, The Neurological Institute, University Hospitals Cleveland Medical Center, Cleveland, OH, United States

Joo Hyun Park, MD, PhD Department of Otorhinolaryngology-Head and Neck Surgery, Dongguk University Ilsan Hospital, Goyang, South Korea

Chaim G. Pick, PhD Sagol School of Neuroscience, Tel Aviv University, Tel Aviv, Israel; Department of Anatomy, Sackler Faculty of Medicine, Tel Aviv University, Tel Aviv, Israel; The Dr. Miriam and Sheldon G. Adelson Chair and Center for the Biology of Addictive Diseases, Tel Aviv University, Tel Aviv, Israel

Kyle Platek UF Health Fixel Center for Neurological Diseases, University of Florida, Gainesville, FL, United States

Matthew R. Powell, PhD, LP Department of Psychiatry and Psychology, Mayo Clinic, Rochester, MN, United States

Patrick Quaid, Optometrist, MCOptom, FCOVD, PhD Vue-Cubed Vision Therapy Network, Guelph and North York, ON, Canada; Adjunct Faculty, School of Optometry and Vision Science, University of Waterloo, Waterloo, ON, Canada; Consultant Optometrist, David L. MacIntosh Sports Medicine Clinic and Faculty of Kinesiology, University of Toronto, Toronto, ON, Canada

Vardit Rubovitch Department of Anatomy, Sackler Faculty of Medicine, Tel Aviv University, Tel Aviv, Israel

Barry M. Seemungal Department of Medicine, Imperial College, London, United Kingdom

Michael D. Seidman, MD, FACS Director Otologic/Neurotologic/Skull Base Surgery, Medical Director Wellness and Integrative Medicine, Advent Health (Celebration and South Campuses), Roslyn, NY, United States; Professor Otolaryngology Head and Neck Surgery, University of Central Florida College of Medicine, Orlando, FL, United States; Adjunct Professor Otolaryngology Head & Neck Surgery, University of South Florida College of Medicine, Tampa, FL, United States

Tad Seifert, MD Norton Sports Neurology, Norton Healthcare, University of Kentucky, Louisville, KY, United States

Berje Shammassian, MD Department of Neurological Surgery, The Neurological Institute, University Hospitals Cleveland Medical Center, Cleveland, OH, United States

Tanya Singh, MS Department of Medical Education, University of Central Florida College of Medicine, Orlando, FL, United States

Eric Singman, MD, PhD Milton & Muriel Shurr Division Chief, General Eye Services Clinic of the Wilmer Eye Institute, Johns Hopkins Hospital, Baltimore, MD, United States

Martin Slade, PhD Medicine and Public Health, Yale University, New Haven, CT, United States

Rebecca Smith Department of Medicine, Imperial College, London, United Kingdom

Patrick J. Sparto, PT, PhD Department of Physical Therapy, University of Pittsburgh, Pittsburgh, PA, United States

Jeffrey P. Staab, MD, MS Department of Psychiatry and Psychology, Mayo Clinic, Rochester, MN, United States

Molly Sullan, MS Department of Clinical & Health Psychology, University of Florida, Gainesville, FL, United States

Stephen Z. Sutton, PT, DPT UF Health Rehabilitation Center, University of Florida, Gainesville, FL, United States

Mikhaylo Szczupak, MD Department of Otolaryngology, University of Miami, Miami, FL, United States

Rebecca N. Tapia, MD Polytrauma Network Site, Physical Medicine and Rehabilitation Services PM&RS (MC 117), South Texas Veterans Health Care System, San Antonio, TX, United States; Department of Rehabilitation Medicine, UT Health San Antonio, San Antonio, TX, United States

David T. Utriainen, BS Magnetic Resonance Innovations, Inc., Detroit, MI, United States; The MRI Institute for Biomedical Research, Detroit, MI, United States

Courtney Voelker, MD, PhD Caruso Department of Otolaryngology—Head and Neck Surgery, Keck School of Medicine of USC, Los Angeles, CA, United States

P. Ashley Wackym, MD, FACS, FAAP Department of Otolaryngology—Head and Neck Surgery, Rutgers Robert Wood Johnson Medical School, New Brunswick, NJ, United States

Susan L. Whitney, DPT, PhD Department of Physical Therapy and Otolaryngology, University of Pittsburgh, Pittsburgh, PA, United States

Natalie M. Wiseman Department of Psychiatry and Behavioral Neurosciences, Wayne State University School of Medicine, Detroit, MI, United States

B. Tucker Woodson, MD, FACS Division of Sleep Medicine and Upper Airway Reconstructive Surgery, Department of Otolaryngology and Communication Sciences, Medical College Wisconsin, Milwaukee, WI, United States

Kurt D. Yankaskas Code 34, Office of Naval Research, Arlington, VA, United States

About the Editors

Dr. Michael E. Hoffer

Dr. Michael E. Hoffer, MD, FACS is Professor of Otolaryngology and Neurological Surgery at the University of Miami, Miller School of Medicine. He assumed these roles after an over 20-year military career in which he studied mild traumatic brain injury (mTBI) on active duty service members. He performs both basic and clinical research and has an active practice in neurotology. His lab focuses on traumatic damage to the inner ear and brain. He has authored or coauthored over 60 papers and has a particular expertise in dizziness and balance disorders as well as neurosensory consequences after mTBI. He and his collaborators have done pioneering work on pharmaceutical countermeasures for mTBI as well as optimized diagnosis and management of neurosensory disorders seen after mTBI.

Dr. Carey D. Balaban

Dr. Carey D. Balaban is Professor of Otolaryngology in the School of Medicine, with secondary appointments in Neurobiology, Communication Sciences and Disorders, and Bioengineering as well as being Director of the Center for National Preparedness. He earned his bachelor's degree in History at Michigan State University and his PhD degree in Anatomy from the University of Chicago. His research program has been supported with funding from a variety of sources including the National Institutes of Health (NIH), NASA, the Office of Naval Research and several other agencies and corporations. He has extensive experience in conducting multidisciplinary, cross-cutting research in biomedical sciences, engineering, and social sciences and has participated in the emerging fields of augmented cognition and neuroergonomics. His overriding interest has been formulation of mathematical models, heuristic models, and teleological approaches to interpret data from basic science experiments in terms of behavioral and clinical phenomena. Using this approach, he has examined the interplay between neurological and psychological features of comorbid aspects of balance disorders, migraines, and anxiety disorders. His recent work is extending the implications of these models to analogous features of mild traumatic brain injury, acoustic trauma, and posttraumatic stress disorder, including work in the nascent field of mass spectrometric histological imaging. He has also participated in developing new patented technologies to gauge situational awareness and cognitive engagement from postural orienting responses and decision support software for responses to mass casualty events. In addition to more than 170 peer-reviewed basic research and scholarly articles and two patents, He is an author of two books on 17th century medicine.

DEFINING MILD TBI

1

What Is Mild Traumatic Brain Injury? Translational Definitions to Guide Translational Research

Michael E. Hoffer, MD[1] and Carey D. Balaban, PhD[2]

[1]Department of Otolaryngology and Neurological Surgery, University of Miami, Miller School of Medicine, Miami, FL, United States [2]Departments of Otolaryngology, Neurobiology, Communication Sciences & Disorders, and Bioengineering, University of Pittsburgh, Pittsburgh, PA, United States

Mild traumatic brain injury (mTBI) is a common public health concern that has garnered increased attention in both the lay press and medical literature. mTBI/concussion is particularly common in the military where up to 20% of individuals deployed to Southwest Asia have been affected.[1–7] In the US Military, between 2000 and 2016, 361,092 active duty service members suffered from TBI, ranging from mild (82% of cases) to severe or penetrating.[2] However, the diagnosis is not restricted to the military; recent literature reports that the incidence and prevalence of TBI in the civilian population is increasing.[8] A number of reports that focused on selected populations, such as high school athletes[9] or emergency departments (EDs) over limited time frames[10,11] give estimates of the relative prevalence of mTBI in different populations. For example, Marin et al.[12] used the Nationwide Emergency Department Sample to investigate trends of visits to EDs for TBI between 2006 and 2010. The data, pooled from a sample of 950 hospitals, showed a sharp increase in the weighted rates of ED visits from 2006 to 2010. In 2006, there were 637 TBI visits per 100,000 ED visits and by 2010 this figure was up to 822 per 100,000, with a disproportionate increase in the number of reported mTBI or concussion visits.[13] It is noteworthy that there was a commensurate increase in the number of peer-viewed journal publications in the ISI Web of Science with "mild traumatic brain" as a term in the title, from 27 in 2006, to 44 in 2010, 49 in 2011, and 158 in 2017 (Fig. 1.1). One may suggest that the increased number of visits reflected an increased recognition of a common phenomenon rather than a sudden increase in prevalence of mTBI.

Despite the recent focus on the prevalence of this disorder in the media, the question of the establishment of precise, mechanistically anchored criteria for mTBI remains

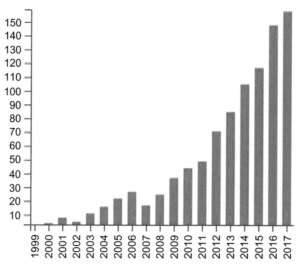

FIGURE 1.1   Peer reviewed research publications by year.

challenging because it requires that the signs and symptoms are linked temporally to a traumatic event as the proximate cause. The National Institute of Health (NIH) has a very straightforward definition: "Traumatic brain injury (TBI), a form of acquired brain injury, occurs when a sudden trauma causes damage to the brain."[14] While this seems straightforward, the definition of a "sudden trauma" can be the subject of debate as its causal linkage to acute, subacute, and chronic symptoms can be problematic. For the purposes of this book we will broadly define the "sudden trauma" as any force (or "directed energy") that causes the brain itself or the contents of the brain to be altered sufficiently to cause physiological dysfunction, biochemical dysfunction, or structural alterations. There is some evidence to suggest that there are significant differences in the mode of TBI presentation based on etiology, but these differences still produce effects that are within a spectrum of those that can be seen in TBI irrespective of the etiology.[15,16] Despite the debate, the NIH definition was crafted pragmatically to allow general acceptance.

Initially TBI was broadly divided into mild, moderate, and severe using the well-established Glasgow Coma Scale (GCS) as an acute metric.[15] While this method seems straightforward given the objective nature of the GCS, this criterion has three main shortcomings. Firstly, most of the individuals with GCS scores less than 13 have some form of severe TBI, meaning the remaining individuals are compressed into a fairly tight range of 13–15 with the vast majority of these being 15. As such the numerical value of the GCS seems ideally suited to distinguish severe from mild or moderate TBI, but this distinction is generally clinically apparent. Beyond that, the scale provides little value for individuals with mild TBI. Secondly, the vast majority of individuals with mTBI do not receive a GCS at the time of injury. Hence, the value of any subsequent or "retrospective" GCS, especially days later, is suspect at best. Finally, individuals with mTBI have a range of sequelae and different outcomes despite having a GCS of 14 or 15; as such, the value does little to distinguish patients on the basis of signs and symptoms that characterize the functional pathology.

THE NIH DEFINITION

A person with a mild TBI may remain conscious or may experience a loss of consciousness for a few seconds or minutes. Other symptoms of mild TBI include headache, confusion, lightheadedness, dizziness, blurred vision or tired eyes, ringing in the ears, bad taste in the mouth, fatigue or lethargy, a change in sleep patterns, behavioral or mood changes, and trouble with memory, concentration, attention, or thinking.

This description incorporates three generally accepted definitions of mTBI that have been published over time.[17] In 1993 the American Congress of Rehabilitation Medicine (ACRM) described mTBI as an alteration of brain function caused by an external force with one of more to the following: (1) loss of consciousness (LOC) of 0–30 minutes; (2) posttraumatic amnesia (PTA) lasting 0–24 hours; (3) focal neurologic deficits may or may not be transient; and (4) alteration of mental state at the time of the accident (confusion, disorientation, slow-thinking).[18] In 2003, the Centers for Disease Control and Prevention (CDC) offered a slightly less specific classification in which an individual must have any period of observed or self-reported transient confusion, disorientation, or impaired consciousness around the time of a head injury with LOC lasting 0–30 minutes.[19] In 2009, the Department of Defense (DoD) established guidelines similar to the ACRM guidelines, but added that the alteration of consciousness (AOC) lasts less than 24 hours.[20] The DoD updated this definition in 2016 and defined mTBI as: "traumatically induced structural or physiologic disruption of brain function as a result of an external force with new onset or worsening of at least one of the following: loss or decreased level of consciousness, (LOC < 30 minutes, AOC <24 hours), PTA (<1 day), alteration in mental status (e.g., confusion, disorientation, etc.), Neurological deficit (weakness, loss of balance, sensory losses, etc.)." They added that the GCS should be 13–15 and structural imaging should be normal.[21] To summarize colloquially, mild TBI is diagnosed by a documented directed energy event that results in the patient reporting symptoms or displaying nonlocalizing signs of being "not quite right."

Complicating these definitions of mTBI include the subcategories of "complicated mTBI" and concussion. Some investigators use the term "complicated mTBI" when the mTBI symptoms are accompanied by positive findings with radiologic imaging.[22–24] The difficulty with this diagnosis is that imaging changes over time. The original definition of "complicated mTBI" relied on CT scans that showed abnormalities; there is some evidence that these individuals followed a course more similar to moderate TBI.[23,24] Therefore, positive CT scan findings often shift diagnosis to the moderate TBI group. However, more modern imaging, including traditional MRI, fMRI, high Tesla MRI, and other scans, do detect abnormalities in some individuals and it is unclear whether these abnormalities have any longer term clinical or functional implications that distinguish them from symptomatic, but radiologically negative, patients.

The term concussion is often used synonymously with mTBI. It is likely the case that concussion is simply a type of mTBI. While it is usually on the milder side of the spectrum, the short-term and long-term consequences provide little basis for distinguishing between these terms. The diagnostic criteria for concussion in athletes has been examined by a group of experts meeting every other year who have published updated guidelines after each of these meetings.[25,26]

While the diagnosis of mTBI and concussion remain difficult to differentiate, postconcussion syndrome has an acceptable definition provide for the International Classification of Diseases 10th edition (ICD-10).[27] This World Health organization-accepted medical definition requires the following: (1) The syndrome follows a head trauma, and (2) The individual present with at least three of the following eight symptoms: headache, dizziness, fatigue, irritability, difficulty concentrating, memory impairment, insomnia, and intolerance to stress, emotion, or alcohol. Because this definition of concussion appears to be synonymous with mTBI, there seems to be little value in assigning this term only to the "mildest" cases until there is a more objective and precise way of making this determination.

We must acknowledge that: the diagnosis of mTBI or concussion requires the presumption of a causal link to a documented traumatic event. The dilemma becomes most evident when a patient appears for a workman's compensation examination, reporting a plethora of nonspecific symptoms that could indicate mTBI. The patient attributes the symptoms to an unwitnessed head-bump several weeks earlier. If one subjects the patient to a large battery of neurologic tests and advanced imaging, what is the likelihood that incidental chronic findings might be misattributed to an undocumented traumatic event? These considerations obviously mandate a healthy skepticism prior to asserting post hoc diagnoses from unknown cranially directed energy exposures. Although we can document signs and symptoms that appear after documented traumatic events, the observations of a similar clinical syndrome are insufficient to substantiate a causal claim regarding an unverified (or assumed) traumatic incident.

The structure of symptom complexes in acute mTBI suggests that integrative, objective diagnosis should be tractable. For example, principal component analysis of a standard 22-item symptom scale showed acute mTBI and control subjects differed by a posttraumatic migraine/headache symptom cluster, a dizziness/mild cognitive impairment symptom cluster, an emotional lability symptom cluster, a cervicogenic (neck pain—fatigue—malaise) symptom cluster, and nausea.[28] Unfortunately, attempts to devise integrative approaches to overall objective diagnosis of mTBI signs have been complicated by several issues. Firstly, the symptom clusters do not unambiguously point to localized injury. Secondly, concerns have been raised about the accuracy of symptom self-reports, which seem to be inherently unreliable and unstable in patients with mTBI.[29,30] For example, symptom reports may be exaggerated or understated (denial) for secondary gain, which can produce symptom complex component scores on both tails of the distributions in acute mTBI patients (Hoffer et al. PLoS One, symptom complex paper) Thirdly, the heterogeneous presentation of mTBI makes unified objective diagnostic criteria difficult to identify. The presentation can vary with small changes in the magnitude or direction of the force, by the subjects' past medical and particularly, past head injury, history, and by a variety of other factors including anatomic and genetic differences. Fourthly, the manifestations of the mTBI change over time, based on external environmental and epigenetic influences that are independent of the trauma and, again, affect every individual differently. Fifthly, mTBI in an individual case may involve a number of parallel, but very small injuries, in more than one location in the brain or intracranial sensory organs Sixthly, home remedies, spontaneous compensation, and variations in treatment regimens complicate the subacute and chronic presentations. These factors may contribute to the conclusion that the trend of attempts to classify the disorder in terms of common objective features has been fraught with difficulty.[15]

Currently, there is no definitive path to make a "ground-truth" diagnosis of a mTBI without a validated, temporally proximate acute application of external force. The problem obviously becomes exacerbated as the latency increases between a suspected event and presentation of the patient. Criteria have been established by a variety of organizations, but there remains debate as to how best to apply these criteria. Moreover, there remains debate over what constitutes an "external force" and the latency between the event and onset of signs and symptoms. Most investigators agree that classifying TBI into mild, moderate, and severe is a highly imprecise medical classification system.[15,31] These researchers and clinicians advocate a more deliberate and objective approach to diagnosis that takes into account temporal sequences of symptoms, objective neurological signs, the recovery trajectory, and long-term outcomes.

As a pragmatic matter, there is no justification for eliminating the diagnostic term mTBI until better alternatives for differentiated diagnosis are available. We believe a reasonable diagnostic criterion is very similar to the most recent criteria proposed by the DoD/VA.[21] Our "operational definition" is that an individual: (1) suffers an impact to the head; (2) has LOC (<30 minutes) or AOC (<24 hours); and (3) presents with one of the symptoms including, but not limited to, balance disorder, hearing disorder, headache, visual changes, alteration in mental status, and sleep disturbance. This diagnostic criterion seems to brings together the criteria proposed and listed above and is in concordance with general clinical practice.

The difficulty in developing a definition for mTBI is magnified when attempting to utilize this definition for translational research. Research on animal models is vitally important to both develop new diagnostic and treatment algorithms, as well as to translate basic science findings into human use. Unfortunately, most rodent animal models seek to create a very homogenous pattern of injury, but are attempting to model a disorder that is very heterogeneous in humans.[32] In addition, physical damage that would be termed severe in a humans produces only modest behavioral signs in rodent animal models. The ability to reproduce rodent analogues of human psychological and social impacts of mTBI are far from incontrovertible. This is certainly an area where a more precise definition based on the site of injury or neuropathological findings would be helpful. That being said, those set of conditions (site of injury, neuropathological findings, etc.) are likely to be just as heterogeneous in affected humans as the current symptom spectrum of mTBI, therefore, such precision may not allow for better translational research.

No matter how it is defined, we believe that the term mTBI in particular and TBI in general must be "destigmatized." Too often there is serious debate over whether an individual has "TBI" when it is clear that the individual had a blow to the head, suffered and AOC, and has symptoms. The individual clearly has a brain injury that should be labeled as "TBI." This label implies nothing about short-term or even long-term consequences, nor should it be reserved for only a particular type of brain injury or particular class of individuals.

References

1. https://www.rand.org/news/press/2008/04/17.html.
2. Defense Medical Surveillance System (DMMS)S. DoD numbers for traumatic brain injury—worldwide: defense and veterans brain injury center (DVBIC). 2017.

3. Hoffer ME, Balaban C, Gottshall K, Balough BJ, Maddox MR, et al. Blast exposure: vestibular consequences and associated characteristics. *Otol Neurotol* 2010;**31**:232−6.

4. Scherer MR, Burrows H, Pinto R, Littlefield P, French LM, Tarbett AK, et al. Evidence of central and peripheral vestibular pathology in blast-related traumatic brain injury. *Otol Neurotol* 2011;**24**.

5. Hoge CW, McGurk D, Thomas JL, Cox AL, Engel CC, Castro CA. Mild traumatic brain injury in U.S. Soldiers returning from Iraq. *N Engl J Med* 2008;**358**:453−63.

6. Terrio H, Brenner LA, Ivins BJ, Cho JM, Helmick K, et al. Traumatic brain injury screening: preliminary findings in a US Army Brigade Combat Team. *J Head Trauma Rehabil* 2009;**24**:14−23.

7. Hosek B. *How is deployment to Iraq and Afghanistan affecting U.S. service members and their families? An overview of early RAND research on the topic.* Santa Monica, CA: RAND Corporation; 2011.

8. http://www.cdc.gov/TraumaticBrainInjury/index.html.

9. Powell JW, Barber-Foss KD. Traumatic brain injury in high school athlete. *JAMA* 1999;**282**(10):958−63. Available from: https://doi.org/10.1001/jama.282.10.958.

10. Guerrero JL, Thurman DJ, Sniezek JE. Emergency department visits associated with traumatic brain injury: United States, 1995−1996. *Brain Inj* 2000;**14**(2):181−6.

11. Kerr ZY, Harmon KJ, Marshall SW, Proescholdbell SK, Waller AE. The epidemiology of traumatic brain injuries treated in emergency departments in North Carolina, 2010−2011. *N C Med J* 2014;**75**(1):8−14.

12. Marin JR, Weaver MD, Yealy DM, Mannix RC. Trends in visits for traumatic brain injury to emergency departments in the United States. *JAMA* 2014;**311**(18):1917−19. Available from: https://doi.org/10.1001/jama.2014.3979.

13. Lagbas C, Bazargan-Hejazi S, Shaheen M, Kermah D, Pan D. Traumatic brain injury related hospitalization and mortality in California. *Biomed Res Int* 2013;143092. Available from: https://doi.org/10.1155/2013/143092. Epub November 13, 2013.

14. https://www.ninds.nih.gov/Disorders/All-Disorders/Traumatic-Brain-Injury-Information-Page.

15. Hawryluk GW, Manley GT. Classification of traumatic brain injury: past, present, and future. *Handb Clin Neurol* 2015;**127**:15−21. Available from: https://doi.org/10.1016/B978-0-444-52892-6.00002-7. Review. PubMed PMID: 25702207.

16. Mendez MF, Owens EM, Reza Berenji G, Peppers DC, Liang LJ, Licht EA. Mild traumatic brain injury from primary blast vs. blunt forces: post-concussion consequences and functional neuroimaging. *NeuroRehabilitation* 2013;**32**(2):397−407. Available from: https://doi.org/10.3233/NRE-130861. PubMed PMID: 23535805.

17. Katz D, Sara IC, Michael PA. Chapter 9. Mild traumatic brain injury. *Handb Clin Neurol* 2015;**127**C:131−56. Available from: https://doi.org/10.1016/B978-0-444-52892-6.00009-X.

18. American Congress of Rehabilitation Medicine, Brain Injury Interdisciplinary Special Interest Group, Disorders of Consciousness Task Force. Definition of mild traumatic brain injury. *J Head Trauma Rehabil* 1993;**8**:86−7.

19. National Center for Injury Prevention and Control. *Report to congress on mild traumatic brain injury in the United States: steps to prevent a serious public health problem.* Atlanta, GA: Centers for Disease Control and Prevention; 2003.

20. Department of Veterans Affairs. *Clinical practice guideline: management of concussion/mild traumatic brain injury.* Washington, DC: Department of Veterans Affairs, DOD; 2009.

21. https://www.healthquality.va.gov/guidelines/Rehab/mtbi/mTBICPGFullCPG50821816.pdf.

22. Williams DH, Levin HS, Eisenberg HM. Mild head injury classification. *Neurosurgery* 1990;**27**:422−8.

23. Iverson GL. Complicated vs uncomplicated mild traumatic brain injury: acute neuropsychological outcome. *Brain Inj* 2006;**20**:1335−44.

24. Kashluba S, Hanks RA, Casey JE, et al. Neuropsychologic and functional outcome after complicated mild traumatic brain injury. *Arch Phys Med Rehabil* 2008;**89**:904−11.

25. McCrory P, Meeuwisse W, Johnston K, et al. Consensus statement on Concussion in Sport, 3rd International Conference on Concussion in Sport held in Zurich, November 2008. *Clin J Sport Med* 2009;**19**:185−200.

26. McCrory P, Meeuwisse W, Dvořák J, Aubry M, Bailes J, Broglio S, et al. Consensus statement on concussion in sport-the 5th international conference on concussion in sport held in Berlin, October 2016. *Br J Sports Med* 2017;**51**(11):838−47. Available from: https://doi.org/10.1136/bjsports-2017-097699. Epub 2017 Apr 26. PubMed PMID: 28446457.

27. http://www.who.int/classifications/icd/icdonlineversions/en/

28. Hoffer ME, Szczupak M, Kiderman A, Crawford J, Murphy S, Marshall K, Pelusso C, Balaban C. Neurosensory symptom complexes after acute mild traumatic brain injury. *PLoS One* 2016;**11**(1). Available from: https://doi.org/10.1371/journal.pone.0146039. < https:e0146039. >, eCollection 2016.

29. Spencer RJ, Drag LL, Walker SJ, Bieliauskas LA. Self-reported cognitive symptoms following mild traumatic brain injury are poorly associated with neuropsychological performance in OIF/OEF veterans. *J Rehabil Res Dev* 2010;**47**(6):521−30 PubMed PMID: 20848365.

30. Waddington GS. Self report balance status is not reliable post concussion. *J Sci Med Sport* 2017;**20**(11):963. Available from: https://doi.org/10.1016/j.jsams.2017.09.004. PubMedPMID: 28927553.

31. McCrory P, Feddermann-Demont N, Dvořák J, Cassidy JD, McIntosh A, Vos PE Echemendia RJ, et al. What is the definition of sports-related concussion: a systematic review. *Br J Sports Med* 2017;**51**(11):877−87. Available from: https://doi.org/10.1136/bjsports-2016-097393. Review. PubMed PMID: 29098981.

32. Bolouri H, Zetterberg H. Animal models for concussion: molecular and cognitive assessments—relevance to sport and military concussions. In: Kobeissy FH, editor. *Brain neurotrauma: molecular, neuropsychological, and rehabilitation aspects*. Boca Raton, FL: CRC Press/Taylor & Francis; 2015. Chapter 46. PubMed PMID: 26269898.

Clinical Trajectories of Mild Traumatic Brain Injury

Rebecca N. Tapia, MD[1,2], *Blessen C. Eapen, MD*[2,3] *and David X. Cifu, MD*[4,5,6,7]

[1]Polytrauma Network Site, Physical Medicine and Rehabilitation Services PM&RS (MC 117), South Texas Veterans Health Care System, San Antonio, TX, United States [2]Department of Rehabilitation Medicine, UT Health San Antonio, San Antonio, TX, United States [3]Polytrauma Rehabilitation Center, Polytrauma/TBI Fellowship Program, Physical Medicine and Rehabilitation Services PM&RS (MC 117), South Texas Veterans Health Care System, San Antonio, TX, United States [4]Innovation and System Integration, Virginia Commonwealth University School of Medicine, Richmond, VA, United States [5]The Herman J. Flax, M.D. Professor and Chair, Department of PM&R, Virginia Commonwealth University School of Medicine, Richmond, VA, United States [6]Chronic Effects of Neurotrauma Consortium, US Department of Veterans Affairs, Richmond, VA, United States [7]Sports Sciences, NHL Florida Panthers, Sunrise, FL, United States

INTRODUCTION

Whether it is an athlete looking forward to the next game or a service-member aiming to return to combat, the trajectories of recovery after mild traumatic brain injury (mTBI) (or concussion) are personally, professionally and clinically important. Prognosis and development of plans to return to prior activity level should be integrated into the initial assessment and revisited at each follow-up. There are multiple contributors that may delay recovery patterns, but the majority of the research demonstrates a rapid predictable resolution of postconcussive symptoms within days to weeks, and certainly by 3 months of injury.[1] The trajectories of recovery may be divided into four cohorts of individuals:

- Recovery ahead of expectation.
- Recovery in line with expectation.

- Prolonged recovery with return to baseline.
- Prolonged recovery without return to baseline.

Unlike the expectations made in individuals who sustain a moderate or severe brain injury, prolonged recovery (more than 3 months) patterns seen with mTBI are rarely secondary to the actual brain injury and associated alterations in neurophysiology, but rather manifestations of perimorbid or exacerbations of premorbid conditions.[2] While initial estimation of recovery based on past medical history, injury event details, and current clinical presentation in the context of specialized patterns in special populations (e.g., athletes, soldiers) is possible, it is more reliable to use close longitudinal follow-up and to identify early individual recovery patterns to both better anticipate later difficulties and inform the treatment plan.

WHO IS CONCERNED ABOUT CLINICAL TRAJECTORY?

Traumatic events have the potential to disrupt multiple, if not all, aspects of life. Outside of the acute medical issues that need attention following trauma, oftentimes these occurrences are accompanied by social, occupational, and financial disruptions particularly in the setting of job-loss or legal challenges. Lacerations can be sutured and heal, fractures mend and follow a relatively predictable recovery, but looming after even a mTBI, questions about return to productivity (e.g., work, school, combat) can be more challenging to predict. Immediate considerations, such as an upcoming exam at school or playoff game next week, can be at the front of the mind for individuals, families, employers, professors, and coaches. While one can never completely accurately predict health care outcomes, it is important to be able to give individuals a reasonable and realistic estimate early in the course of care. Educating providers with the available evidence and recommendations can assist in these conversations. Beyond the individual, mTBI exists also as a public health burden with rates of TBI-related emergency visits steadily increasing.[3] Additionally, simply facilitating quick recovery after mTBI by promoting a positive prognosis and encouraging an early and rapid return to normalcy can actually help avoid development of chronic symptoms and optimize outcomes.

WHY DO WE MONITOR CLINICAL TRAJECTORY?

While the majority of patients may follow a predictable and reassuring return to baseline and can be told this early after injury, it is equally important to recognize that even the remaining small minority can be identified through clinical monitoring, whether using a structured follow-up appointment or with patient instructions to return for care should symptoms not improve as expected. This early advice and education provided by a medical professional regarding expectations of recovery can be critical to long-term outcomes.[4]

For those who are returning to baseline as expected, monitoring of clinical trajectory helps expedite and individualize return to prior level of function, such as a determination as to when to engage with testing at school or when to return to sports practice or games. Monitoring during this stage also represents a platform to reinforce recovery, recognize gains, and educate about prevention of future injuries. Early identification of those falling behind expected recovery timelines provides an opportunity for further investigation (primarily for psychological factors), supports efforts to prevent development of new symptoms, and keeps the individual focused on moving toward a return to prior level of function despite some persistent issue. Cognitive behavioral therapy provided soon after mTBI is a well-tolerated and effective intervention to reduce the risk of developing chronic symptoms in slow-to-progress individuals after mTBI.[5] Patients who are slow to improve will benefit most from a comprehensive team approach using tailored treatment plans, regular follow-ups, and clear step-wise goals.

HOW DO WE MONITOR CLINICAL TRAJECTORY?

Unfortunately, as with many brain-related conditions, obtaining objective, reliable, individualized, and longitudinal data regarding recovery after mTBI are elusive. Athletes are particularly prone to underreporting symptoms or poorly estimating cognitive function, as are children and their parents.[6–8] There may also be gender differences in symptom reporting, which further complicates the overall picture.[9] There are many standardized protocols to assess multiple domains in concussion, including; Sport Concussion Assessment Tool (SCAT5), which has utility for acute evaluation, diagnosis and tracking recovery progress[10]; the Neurobehavioral Symptom Inventory (NSI), a self-report tool to track multiple symptoms over time (divided into somatic, cognitive, affective, and sensory domains)[11–13]; and Immediate Post-Concussion Assessment and Cognitive Testing (ImPACT) testing, which can be useful for diagnostic purposes, but may be less helpful for prognostication and confounded by reliability and effort.[14–16] There are also a multitude of assessments of individual symptoms that are not necessarily specific to mTBI, such as the Headache Impact Test (HIT-6TM), Balance Error Scoring System (BESS), and Brief Smell Identification Test (BSIT). Outside of these standardized protocols, a provider can develop individual functional metrics to assess clinical recovery, such as hours able to study or work, or exercise tolerance, compared to baseline. Combining standardized assessments with metrics personally meaningful to the patient can provide insight into the objective and subjective clinical trajectories, which are often divergent.

GENERAL PRINCIPLES OF RECOVERY

There is a growing body of mTBI literature, particularly in populations of athletes and service members during and after combat experiences. Of note is the contrasting trajectories of these two cohorts who are otherwise similar (mostly male, mostly younger) which underscores the importance of viewing mTBI recovery patterns in the context of individual factors. A study on the clinical course of concussion after sports-related, mTBI in high school and college student athletes demonstrates complete symptom resolution in 80%–90% of athletes after 2 weeks without medical intervention. Approximately 2.5% had no objective findings at 45 days post-injury, but continued to report symptoms related to their concussion.[17] Outside of athletes, mTBI recovery patterns appear similarly predictable, with most individuals experiencing full recovery without persistent sequelae in a matter of days, even in the absence of medical interventions. However, those with poor premorbid health conditions, have suffered significant psychological distress, or have experienced combat concussions tend to be at higher risk for development of persistent symptoms.[2]

The following is a brief overview of factors and timelines (where available) of individual clinical symptom recovery in MTBI.

Balance Disorders

Dizziness and balance impairments are among the most common complaints following mTBI and are thought to be a product of both central and peripheral dysfunction.[18] Balance impairments typically last 3–10 days following injury,[19] but as with other postconcussive symptoms there is a subset of patients who go on to experience chronic symptoms. Posttraumatic dizziness is an independent factor for return to work 6 months after injury.[20] The blast exposure mechanism of injury may be associated with a unique and more significant pattern of vestibular disorders, and may produce symptoms that progress over time, when compared to blunt trauma.[21] Medications usage for other symptoms, such as insomnia or headache, may prolong the experience of imbalance or dizziness due to associated side-effects.

Hearing Disorders

Hearing loss, sensitivity to noise, and tinnitus are typically self-limited after mTBI, as damage to central auditory acuity is rare in mTBI, although premorbid hearing loss is common.[22] Hearing loss in the setting of complex trauma is often associated with CN VII damage, which may stem from a temporal bone fracture, again extremely rare with mTBI. Unlike other combat-related or mTBI-associated sensory deficits, hearing disorders are likely to progress with age and blast exposure may produce a delayed-onset hearing loss.[23] TBI also contributes to risk for long-term hearing loss, particularly in patients with traffic-related mTBI.[24]

Headaches

Headaches are the most common symptom, over 90% in some studies, reported after mTBI and often resolve within 1–2 weeks after injury. On the other hand, studies of persistent symptoms after mTBI, more than 50% of mTBI patients continuing to report new or worsening headaches at 1 year post-injury.[25] The International Classification of Headache Disorders, third edition-beta (ICHDIII) defines posttraumatic headaches (PTH) as a secondary headache disorder attributed to head and/or neck trauma in close temporal relationship to the traumatic event (within 7 days of injury to the head or within 7 days of regaining consciousness after injury or of discontinuation of any medication that could impair perception or experience of the headache).[26] Recovery patterns may be broken down into resolved, worsening, improving, or chronic, with poorer outcomes related to younger age, premorbid headache conditions, and posttraumatic stress disorder (PTSD).[27] PTH severity is also related to success in returning to work; with one study demonstrating a 50% drop in return to work potential for every one unit increase of the Numerical Pain Rating Scale.[28]

Cognitive Issues

Cognitive impairments after mTBI can present in areas of attention, concentration, processing speed, memory, executive function, communication, and visuospatial abilities.[29] These conditions have many contributory and overlapping factors in the postconcussive period, with attention and working memory being among the most common complaints.[30] Cognitive deficits are common in the first 2 weeks, while a very small percentage may experience a prolonged recovery of up to 1 year.[31] The etiology of long-term cognitive sequelae following mTBI is multifactorial, and rarely is due to direct injury to brain structures (i.e., white matter tracts). Lower cognitive reserve may predict higher rates of chronic cognitive symptoms.[32] The effects of other symptom burdens, such as posttraumatic stress, must also be taken into account.[33] Although physical recovery and return to work seems to track well with non-TBI trauma control groups, patients who have sustained mTBI are more likely to continue reporting problems with memory and concentration in their daily activities.[34]

Sleep Issues

Changes to sleep patterns are a common subjective experience following mTBI; occurring in up to 92% of individuals.[35] One pilot study in young adults suggests an increase in both total sleep time and nighttime sleep duration for at least the first month following mTBI,[36] whereas a study in concussed athletes demonstrates increased subjective complaints, but no changes to polysomnographic variables.[37] The experiences of poor sleep and fatigue following mTBI are complex, with fatigue directly contributing to anxiety, depression, and daytime sleepiness.[38] Perceived sleep quality is heavily related to psychological symptoms, with sleep quantity being a unique contributor to memory performance.[39] Fatigue itself is also common following mTBI, occurring in up to 45% of individuals at 1 year after mTBI.[40] Similar to sleep disruption, fatigue is related to sleep disturbance, sleep hygiene, satisfaction with life, anxiety, and depression.[41]

Smell and Taste Disorders

Gustatory and olfactory dysfunction are rare with mTBI.[42] In individuals with these deficits initially, when recovery occurs, it is likely to be achieved within the first 6 months after injury.[43] There is evidence of possible continued deterioration of olfactory function after brain injury.[44]

Visual Processing Disorders

The visual consequences of mTBI are poorly understood and are thought to be related to oculo-motor dysfunction.[45–47] Complaints of photophobia, blurred vision, and eye fatigue may occur after a concussive event, which can manifest as difficulty reading or increased headaches. Vestibulo-ocular dysfunction following pediatric, sports-related mTBI is associated with prolonged recovery and is an independent risk factor for development of chronic postconcussive symptoms.[48] Vision examination in an adolescent, acute sports concussion management clinic showed convergence insufficiency in 49% of patients and accommodative dysfunction in 50% of patients, with occurrence rates decreasing from 1 to 3 months.[49] A blast mechanism of brain trauma may introduce additional variables, via direct damage to globe, afferent or efferent visual pathways, or cortical processing areas.[46]

Autonomic Nervous System

Dysfunction of the autonomic nervous system following mTBI is quite rare and not immediately obvious to the patient or clinician. There is growing evidence that may suggest transient changes in autonomic cardiovascular functions, which resolve within a few days of injury.[50,51] These changes may be noted in difficulty with heart rate increase during exercise.[52] Paroxysmal sympathetic hyperactivity does not appear to affect individuals with mTBI.

WHAT ARE RELEVANT FACTORS IN RECOVERY?

There may be a discrepancy between resolution of physiological dysfunction and improvement of clinical symptoms, with physiological dysfunction persisting longer than the physical or cognitive manifestations of injury. Factors that affect expected recovery timelines are listed in Table 2.1.

TABLE 2.1   Factors That Affect Expected Recovery Timelines

Factor	Impact
Initial injury severity	Worse initial severity may predict longer recovery from mTBI[53]
Psychological distress	Persistent symptoms more common with psychological distress, particularly in acute phase[54]
Prior history of head injury	Prior injuries, particularly those closer in time and not completely recovered, may lengthen time of recovery for subsequent injuries
Comorbid injuries	Dealing with pain, fractures, or other ailments may prolong recovery secondary to medications or other barriers to return to function
Premorbid mental health conditions	Patients with premorbid mental health conditions face higher likelihood of development of chronic symptoms[54]
Substance abuse	Whether a chronic issue or part of the injury itself, dealing with substance abuse may impair recovery
Motivation/secondary gain	Patients incentivized to be impaired, whether through avoidance of an unpleasant activity or financial, may demonstrate slower progress toward function
Cognitive reserve	Lower cognitive reserve results in 4.14 times more likely to suffer from PCS[32]
Demographics	Older adults and women may take longer to recover[55]

It can be challenging for both patients and providers when clinical recovery does not occur as expected. Identifying patients at risk for slower recovery is imperative to allow for early counseling on self-efficacy techniques and to ensure that modifiable risk factors, such as poor sleep and mood disorders, are addressed proactively. The complex of stalled or slow recovery following mTBI has been referred to as "Postconcussion Syndrome" (PCS). It remains difficult to link PCS fully to the actual concussion, as the symptoms related to PCS are fairly common in the normal population and the associated psychological difficulties that may be seen after trauma (e.g., PTSD, depression).[56] Meares found that PCS criteria were just as likely to be met in the nonbrain injured population as the brain-injured population.[57] Additionally, in another study, the base rate of PCS symptoms in a group of healthy university students was relatively high and had no correlation to neuropsychological dysfunction.[58] Of note, preinjury history of mental health issues and the development of subacute depression or headaches have been associated with higher risk of persistent symptoms.[59]

CLINICAL CAVEATS AND SPECIAL POPULATIONS

As with other topics in brain injury, it can be useful to distinguish various subpopulations to better understand the factors associated with recovery. There are multiple factors that preselect individuals into any one group, such as active duty service members being more likely to be male and have blast exposures or civilian trauma victims who are intoxicated at time of injury being more likely to have mechanisms related to falls or violence.[60] While no one person is destined to follow a particular recovery pattern, general knowledge of characteristics among the broader groups (Table 2.2) of those who sustain mTBI can be helpful to monitoring recovery and developing interventions.

TABLE 2.2   Characteristics Among Broader Groups of Those Who Sustain mTBI

Group	Common Mechanisms	Average Recovery Time Course	Factors for Slowed Recovery
Service Members and Veterans	Blast, blunt trauma, falls, motor vehicle collision	Highly variable, poorer outcomes for combat related mTBI[61] 63% continuing to report moderate disability at 6–12 months,[62] possible worsening 1–5 years out from injury[63] confounded by psychological health	PTSD, older age, poor sleep, lower premorbid IQ, female[62–65]
Athletes	Blunt trauma, mostly contact with another player[66]	Approximately 1–2 weeks	Younger age, prior history of TBI, prior history of mental health diagnoses, female sex[59,67]
Civilian Trauma Victims	Motor vehicle collision, assault, falls	Highly variable, 1 week to 3 months, 30% with physical symptoms resolved but ongoing cognitive complaints at 3 months[34]	Preinjury history of psychiatric illness, females, older adults, compensation seeking[68,69]

ADVISING ON RETURN TO ACTIVITY

There is a fine balance between activity and rest following mTBI. Too much activity too soon, or prolonged activity restriction, may both have negative consequences during the recovery period. An individualized plan for gradual return to activity guided by symptom resolution, in the context of individual factors, is recommended to promote optimal function. The following key bullets provide some of the available evidence-supported recommendations:

- One to 2 days of rest following acute mTBI is recommended.[70]
- Excessive, early cognitive activity may prolong recovery from mTBI.[71]
- Bedrest has not proven to be an effective strategy following mTBI.[72]
- Accommodations should be provided as indicated to minimize time lost from school or work.
- For chronic or persistent symptoms, engagement with regular aerobic exercise that does not cause symptom exacerbation is regarded as an effective method for reducing postconcussion symptoms and improving activity tolerance.[73]

PUTTING IT TOGETHER: APPROACH TO DETERMINING RECOVERY TRAJECTORY

Understanding the basic principles and factors in mTBI recovery can best inform the initial conversations and treatment plans stemming from a concussive injury.

- Inventory first: demographics, past medical and psychiatric history, injury event history, prior and current level of function, determining factors that promote or inhibit recovery, such as history of learning disabilities.
- Select the patient-centered definition of recovery: What symptoms are most bothersome and why? How would they define full recovery? Combine both subjective and objective metrics to follow up.
- Monitor clinical recovery at intervals.
  - Create a return to play, learn, and/or duty plan through established guidelines and symptom resolution targets.[70,74,75]
  - Full recovery: return to prior level of function, educate on avoiding additional head injuries, provide support for recurrent symptoms although these are unlikely to be related to mTBI without new injury.
  - Prolonged recovery: step back to review big picture, identify individual barriers, and consider the biopsychosocial approach.[53]
    - Judiciously obtain additional evaluations or consultations.
    - Regular updating of individualized treatment planning.
    - Use discrete, measurable goals.
    - Employ structured follow-up and support.

Examining the brain itself (i.e., neuroimaging) will not inform you when full recovery has occurred. Any given patient may defy expectations and recover more quickly or more slowly than expected. Regardless of risk factors or the actual progress of recovery, appropriate care can be delivered by continuing to seek relevant recovery metrics, adapting and updating treatment plans to the individual, and understanding the "big picture" of recovery and reintegration far beyond neurophysiology.

References

1. McCrea M, Iverson GL, McAllister TW, Hammeke TA, Powell MR, Barr WB, et al. An integrated review of recovery after mild traumatic brain injury (MTBI): implications for clinical management. *Clin Neuropsychol* 2009;**23**(8):1368–90.
2. Cassidy JD, Cancelliere C, Carroll LJ, Côté P, Hincapié CA, Holm LW, et al. Systematic review of self-reported prognosis in adults after mild traumatic brain injury: results of the International Collaboration on Mild Traumatic Brain Injury Prognosis. *Arch Phys Med Rehabil* 2014;**95**(3 Suppl):S132–51.
3. Rates of TBI-related Emergency Department Visits, Hospitalizations, and Deaths — United States, 2001–2010. Available from: https://www.cdc.gov/traumaticbraininjury/data/rates.html.
4. Nelson Sheese AL, Hammeke TA. Rehabilitation from postconcussion syndrome: nonpharmacological treatment. *Prog Neurol Surg* 2014;**28**:149–60.
5. Silverberg ND, Hallam BJ, Rose A, Underwood H, Whitfield K, Thornton AE, et al. Cognitive-behavioral prevention of postconcussion syndrome in at-risk patients: a pilot randomized controlled trial. *J Head Trauma Rehabil* 2013;**28**(4):313–22.
6. McDonald T, Burghart MA, Nazir N. Underreporting of concussions and concussion-like symptoms in female high school athletes. *J Trauma Nurs Off J Soc Trauma Nurses* 2016;**23**(5):241–6.
7. Wojtowicz M, Iverson GL, Silverberg ND, Mannix R, Zafonte R, Maxwell B, et al. Consistency of self-reported concussion history in adolescent athletes. *J Neurotrauma* 2017;**34**(2):322–7.
8. Rowhani-Rahbar A, Chrisman SPD, Drescher S, Schiff MA, Rivara FP. Agreement between high school athletes and their parents on reporting athletic events and concussion symptoms. *J Neurotrauma* 2016;**33**(8):784–91.
9. Brown DA, Elsass JA, Miller AJ, Reed LE, Reneker JC. Differences in symptom reporting between males and females at baseline and after a sports-related concussion: a systematic review and meta-analysis. *Sports Med Auckl NZ* 2015;**45**(7):1027–40.
10. Yengo-Kahn AM, Hale AT, Zalneraitis BH, Zuckerman SL, Sills AK, Solomon GS. The Sport Concussion Assessment Tool: a systematic review. *Neurosurg Focus* 2016;**40**(4):E6.
11. Dretsch M, Bleiberg J, Williams K, Caban J, Kelly J, Grammer G, et al. Three scoring approaches to the neurobehavioral symptom inventory for measuring clinical change in service members receiving intensive treatment for combat-related mTBI. *J Head Trauma Rehabil* 2016;**31**(1):23–9.
12. Soble JR, Silva MA, Vanderploeg RD, Curtiss G, Belanger HG, Donnell AJ, et al. Normative data for the neurobehavioral symptom inventory (NSI) and post-concussion symptom profiles among TBI, PTSD, and nonclinical samples. *Clin Neuropsychol* 2014;**28**(4):614–32.
13. Vanderploeg RD, Silva MA, Soble JR, Curtiss G, Belanger HG, Donnell AJ, et al. The structure of postconcussion symptoms on the Neurobehavioral Symptom Inventory: a comparison of alternative models. *J Head Trauma Rehabil* 2015;**30**(1):1–11.
14. Sufrinko A, McAllister-Deitrick J, Womble M, Kontos A. Do sideline concussion assessments predict subsequent neurocognitive impairment after sport-related concussion? *J Athl Train* 2017;**52**(7):676–81.
15. Alsalaheen B, Stockdale K, Pechumer D, Broglio SP. Measurement error in the immediate postconcussion assessment and cognitive testing (ImPACT): systematic review. *J Head Trauma Rehabil* 2016;**31**(4):242–51.
16. Higgins KL, Denney RL, Maerlender A. Sandbagging on the immediate post-concussion assessment and cognitive testing (ImPACT) in a high school athlete population. *Arch Clin Neuropsychol Off J Natl Acad Neuropsychol* 2017;**32**(3):259–66.
17. McCrea M, Guskiewicz K, Randolph C, Barr WB, Hammeke TA, Marshall SW, et al. Incidence, clinical course, and predictors of prolonged recovery time following sport-related concussion in high school and college athletes. *J Int Neuropsychol Soc* 2013;**19**(1):22–33.

18. Franke LM, Walker WC, Cifu DX, Ochs AL, Lew HL. Sensorintegrative dysfunction underlying vestibular disorders after traumatic brain injury: a review. *J Rehabil Res Dev* 2012;**49**(7):985–94.

19. Valovich McLeod TC, Hale TD. Vestibular and balance issues following sport-related concussion. *Brain Inj* 2015;**29**(2):175–84.

20. Chamelian L, Feinstein A. Outcome after mild to moderate traumatic brain injury: the role of dizziness. *Arch Phys Med Rehabil* 2004;**85**(10):1662–6.

21. Hoffer ME, Balaban C, Gottshall K, Balough BJ, Maddox MR, Penta JR. Blast exposure: vestibular consequences and associated characteristics. *Otol Neurotol Off Publ Am Otol Soc Am Neurotol Soc Eur Acad Otol Neurotol* 2010;**31**(2):232–6.

22. Management of Concussion-mild Traumatic Brain Injury (mTBI) (2016) VA/DoD Clinical Practice Guidelines [Internet]. [cited 2017 Jun 8]. Available from: http://www.healthquality.va.gov/guidelines/Rehab/mtbi/.

23. Karch SJ, Capó-Aponte JE, McIlwain DS, Lo M, Krishnamurti S, Staton RN, et al. Hearing loss and tinnitus in military personnel with deployment-related mild traumatic brain injury. *US Army Med Dep J* 2016;**3–16**:52–63.

24. Shangkuan W-C, Lin H-C, Shih C-P, Cheng C-A, Fan H-C, Chung C-H, et al. Increased long-term risk of hearing loss in patients with traumatic brain injury: a nationwide population-based study. *The Laryngoscope* 2017;**127**(11):2627–35.

25. Lucas S, Hoffman JM, Bell KR, Dikmen S. A prospective study of prevalence and characterization of headache following mild traumatic brain injury. *Cephalalgia Int J Headache* 2014;**34**(2):93–102.

26. Headache Classification Committee of the International Headache Society (IHS). The International Classification of Headache Disorders, 3rd edition (beta version). *Cephalalgia Int J Headache* 2013;**33** (9):629–808.

27. Sawyer K, Bell KR, Ehde DM, Temkin N, Dikmen S, Williams RM, et al. Longitudinal study of headache trajectories in the year after mild traumatic brain injury: relation to posttraumatic stress disorder symptoms. *Arch Phys Med Rehabil* 2015;**96**(11):2000–6.

28. Dumke HA. Posttraumatic headache and its impact on return to work after mild traumatic brain injury. *J Head Trauma Rehabil* 2017;**32**(2):E55–65.

29. Barth JT, Macciocchi SN, Giordani B, Rimel R, Jane JA, Boll TJ. Neuropsychological sequelae of minor head injury. *Neurosurgery* 1983;**13**(5):529–33.

30. McAllister TW, Flashman LA, Sparling MB, Saykin AJ. Working memory deficits after traumatic brain injury: catecholaminergic mechanisms and prospects for treatment—a review. *Brain Inj* 2004;**18**(4):331–50.

31. Carroll LJ, Cassidy JD, Cancelliere C, Côté P, Hincapié CA, Kristman VL, et al. Systematic review of the prognosis after mild traumatic brain injury in adults: cognitive, psychiatric, and mortality outcomes: results of the International Collaboration on Mild Traumatic Brain Injury Prognosis. *Arch Phys Med Rehabil* 2014;**95**(3 Suppl):S152–73.

32. Oldenburg C, Lundin A, Edman G, Nygren-de Boussard C, Bartfai A. Cognitive reserve and persistent postconcussion symptoms—a prospective mild traumatic brain injury (mTBI) cohort study. *Brain Inj* 2016;**30** (2):146–55.

33. Neipert L, Pastorek NJ, Troyanskaya M, Scheibel RS, Petersen NJ, Levin HS. Effect of clinical characteristics on cognitive performance in service members and veterans with histories of blast-related mild traumatic brain injury. *Brain Inj* 2014;**28**(13–14):1667–74.

34. Ponsford J, Cameron P, Fitzgerald M, Grant M, Mikocka-Walus A. Long-term outcomes after uncomplicated mild traumatic brain injury: a comparison with trauma controls. *J Neurotrauma* 2011;**28**(6):937–46.

35. Towns SJ, Silva MA, Belanger HG. Subjective sleep quality and postconcussion symptoms following mild traumatic brain injury. *Brain Inj* 2015;**29**(11):1337–41.

36. Raikes AC, Schaefer SY. Sleep quantity and quality during acute concussion: a pilot study. *Sleep* 2016;**39** (12):2141–7.

37. Gosselin N, Lassonde M, Petit D, Leclerc S, Mongrain V, Collie A, et al. Sleep following sport-related concussions. *Sleep Med* 2009;**10**(1):35–46.

38. Ponsford J, Schönberger M, Rajaratnam SMW. A model of fatigue following traumatic brain injury. *J Head Trauma Rehabil* 2015;**30**(4):277–82.

39. Waldron-Perrine B, McGuire AP, Spencer RJ, Drag LL, Pangilinan PH, Bieliauskas LA. The influence of sleep and mood on cognitive functioning among veterans being evaluated for mild traumatic brain injury. *Mil Med* 2012;**177**(11):1293–301.

40. van der Naalt J, van Zomeren AH, Sluiter WJ, Minderhoud JM. One year outcome in mild to moderate head injury: the predictive value of acute injury characteristics related to complaints and return to work. *J Neurol Neurosurg Psychiatry* 1999;**66**(2):207–13.

41. Ponsford JL, Ziino C, Parcell DL, Shekleton JA, Roper M, Redman JR, et al. Fatigue and sleep disturbance following traumatic brain injury—their nature, causes, and potential treatments. *J Head Trauma Rehabil* 2012;**27**(3):224–33.

42. Xydakis MS, Mulligan LP, Smith AB, Olsen CH, Lyon DM, Belluscio L. Olfactory impairment and traumatic brain injury in blast-injured combat troops: a cohort study. *Neurology* 2015;**84**(15):1559–67.

43. Gudziol V, Hoenck I, Landis B, Podlesek D, Bayn M, Hummel T. The impact and prospect of traumatic brain injury on olfactory function: a cross-sectional and prospective study. *Eur Arch Otorhinolaryngol* 2014;**271**(6):1533–40.

44. Charland-Verville V, Lassonde M, Frasnelli J. Olfaction in athletes with concussion. *Am J Rhinol Allergy* 2012;**26**(3):222–6.

45. Ciuffreda KJ, Kapoor N, Rutner D, Suchoff IB, Han ME, Craig S. Occurrence of oculomotor dysfunctions in acquired brain injury: a retrospective analysis. *Optom St Louis Mo* 2007;**78**(4):155–61.

46. Cockerham GC, Goodrich GL, Weichel LED, Orcutt JC, Rizzo JF, Bower CKS, et al. Eye and visual function in traumatic brain injury. *J Rehabil Res Dev* 2009;**46**(6):811.

47. Green W, Ciuffreda KJ, Thiagarajan P, Szymanowicz D, Ludlam DP, Kapoor N. Accommodation in mild traumatic brain injury. *J Rehabil Res Dev* 2010;**47**(3):183–99.

48. Ellis MJ, Cordingley DM, Vis S, Reimer KM, Leiter J, Russell K. Clinical predictors of vestibulo-ocular dysfunction in pediatric sports-related concussion. *J Neurosurg Pediatr* 2017;**19**(1):38–45.

49. Master CL, Scheiman M, Gallaway M, Goodman A, Robinson RL, Master SR, et al. Vision diagnoses are common after concussion in adolescents. *Clin Pediatr (Phila)* 2016;**55**(3):260–7.

50. Dobson JL, Yarbrough MB, Perez J, Evans K, Buckley T. Sport-related concussion induces transient cardiovascular autonomic dysfunction. *Am J Physiol Regul Integr Comp Physiol* 2017;**312**(4):R575–84.

51. Bishop S, Dech R, Baker T, Butz M, Aravinthan K, Neary JP. Parasympathetic baroreflexes and heart rate variability during acute stage of sport concussion recovery. *Brain Inj* 2017;**31**(2):247–59.

52. Hinds A, Leddy J, Freitas M, Czuczman N, Willer B. The effect of exertion on heart rate and rating of perceived exertion in acutely concussed individuals. *J Neurol Neurophysiol* 2016;**7**(4):388–50.

53. Wood RL. Understanding the "miserable minority": a diasthesis-stress paradigm for post-concussional syndrome. *Brain Inj* 2004;**18**(11):1135–53.

54. Silverberg ND, Gardner AJ, Brubacher JR, Panenka WJ, Li JJ, Iverson GL. Systematic review of multivariable prognostic models for mild traumatic brain injury. *J Neurotrauma* 2015;**32**(8):517–26.

55. Iverson GL. Complicated vs uncomplicated mild traumatic brain injury: acute neuropsychological outcome. *Brain Inj* 2006;**20**(13–14):1335–44.

56. Iverson GL, Lange RT. Examination of "postconcussion-like" symptoms in a healthy sample. *Appl Neuropsychol* 2003;**10**(3):137–44.

57. Meares S, Shores EA, Taylor AJ, Batchelor J, Bryant RA, Baguley IJ, et al. Mild traumatic brain injury does not predict acute postconcussion syndrome. *J Neurol Neurosurg Psychiatry* 2008;**79**(3):300–6.

58. Wang Y, Chan RCK, Deng Y. Examination of postconcussion-like symptoms in healthy university students: relationships to subjective and objective neuropsychological function performance. *Arch Clin Neuropsychol Off J Natl Acad Neuropsychol* 2006;**21**(4):339–47.

59. Iverson GL, Gardner AJ, Terry DP, Ponsford JL, Sills AK, Broshek DK, et al. Predictors of clinical recovery from concussion: a systematic review. *Br J Sports Med* 2017;**51**(12):941–8.

60. Scheenen ME, de Koning ME, van der Horn HJ, Roks G, Yilmaz T, van der Naalt J, et al. Acute alcohol intoxication in patients with mild traumatic brain injury: characteristics, recovery, and outcome. *J Neurotrauma* 2016;**33**(4):339–45.

61. Mac Donald CL, Johnson AM, Wierzechowski L, Kassner E, Stewart T, Nelson EC, et al. Outcome trends after US military concussive traumatic brain injury. *J Neurotrauma* 2017;**134**(14):2206–19.

62. Mac Donald CL, Adam OR, Johnson AM, Nelson EC, Werner NJ, Rivet DJ, et al. Acute post-traumatic stress symptoms and age predict outcome in military blast concussion. *Brain J Neurol* 2015;**138**(Pt 5):1314–26.

63. Mac Donald CL, Barber J, Jordan M, Johnson AM, Dikmen S, Fann JR, et al. Early clinical predictors of 5-year outcome after concussive blast traumatic brain injury. *JAMA Neurol* 2017;**74**(7):821–9.

I. DEFINING MILD TBI

64. Stewart-Willis JJ, Heyanka D, Proctor-Weber Z, England H, Bruhns M, Premorbid IQ. Predicts postconcussive symptoms in OEF/OIF/OND veterans with mTBI. *Arch Clin Neuropsychol Off J Natl Acad Neuropsychol* 2018;**33** (2):206−15.

65. Brickell TA, Lippa SM, French LM, Kennedy JE, Bailie JM, Lange RT. Female service members and symptom reporting after combat and non-combat-related mild traumatic brain injury. *J Neurotrauma* 2017;**34**(2):300−12.

66. Lynall RC, Campbell KR, Wasserman EB, Dompier TP, Kerr Z. Concussion mechanisms and activities in youth, high school, and college football. *J Neurotrauma* 2017;**34**(19):2684−90.

67. Thomas DJ, Coxe K, Li H, Pommering TL, Young JA, Smith GA, et al. Length of recovery from sports-related concussions in pediatric patients treated at concussion clinics. *Clin J Sport Med Off J Can Acad Sport Med* 2018;**28**(1):56−63.

68. Ponsford J, Cameron P, Fitzgerald M, Grant M, Mikocka-Walus A, Schönberger M. Predictors of postconcussive symptoms 3 months after mild traumatic brain injury. *Neuropsychology* 2012;**26**(3):304−13.

69. Ponsford J, Willmott C, Rothwell A, Cameron P, Kelly AM, Nelms R, et al. Factors influencing outcome following mild traumatic brain injury in adults. *J Int Neuropsychol Soc* 2000;**6**(5):568−79.

70. McCrory P, Meeuwisse W, Dvorak J, Aubry M, Bailes J, Broglio S, et al. Consensus statement on concussion in sport-the 5(th) international conference on concussion in sport held in Berlin, October 2016. *Br J Sports Med* 2017;**51**:828−47.

71. Brown NJ, Mannix RC, O'Brien MJ, Gostine D, Collins MW, Meehan WP. Effect of cognitive activity level on duration of post-concussion symptoms. *Pediatrics* 2014;**133**(2):e299−304.

72. de Kruijk JR, Leffers P, Meerhoff S, Rutten J, Twijnstra A. Effectiveness of bed rest after mild traumatic brain injury: a randomised trial of no versus six days of bed rest. *J Neurol Neurosurg Psychiatry* 2002;**73**(2):167−72.

73. Howell DR, Mannix RC, Quinn B, Taylor JA, Tan CO, Meehan WP. Physical activity level and symptom duration are not associated after concussion. *Am J Sports Med* 2016;**44**(4):1040−6.

74. McNeal L, Selekmen J. Guidance for return to learn after a concussion. NASN Sch Nurse Print. 2017 May 1;1942602X17698487.

75. Progressive Return to Activity Following Acute Concussion/Mild TBI Clinical Suite. Available from: https:// dvbic.dcoe.mil/material/progressive-return-activity-following-acute-concussionmild-tbi-clinical-suite.

3

Imaging Findings in Mild Traumatic Brain Injury

Marta Kulich, BA[1,2], Laurel M. Fisher, PhD[1] and Courtney Voelker, MD, PhD[1]

[1]Caruso Department of Otolaryngology—Head and Neck Surgery, Keck School of Medicine of USC, Los Angeles, CA, United States [2]Northwestern University Feinberg School of Medicine, Chicago, IL, United States

INTRODUCTION

Traumatic brain injury (TBI) is one of the most common neurological disorders. The Centers for Disease Control estimate that TBI results in 2.5 million emergency department visits per year.[1] Among treated brain injuries, 70%—90% are classified as mild (mTBI), with a population-based rate of 100—300/100,000.[2] Often times, patients do not seek medical care for mTBI, so the actual incidence is estimated to be over 600/100,000.[2] TBI can occur in all age groups, and the most common mechanisms include falls, being struck by or against an object (such as in sports), and motor vehicle accidents.[1] The effects of TBI vary in length and severity of symptoms, and in overall health burden. The majority of patients with mTBI recover within weeks, however, approximately 15% remain symptomatic 1 year after injury.[3]

Concussion and mTBI are often used interchangeably. A discussion of these entities warrants working definitions. Diagnosis of mTBI is based on a history of head trauma (either blunt impact or acceleration/deceleration forces) and a Glasgow Coma Score (GCS) of 13—15. Other classification criteria for mTBI include normal structural imaging, loss of consciousness less than 30 minutes, and posttraumatic amnesia not lasting longer than 24 hours.[4] In contrast, concussion is a clinical syndrome in which biomechanical forces disrupt brain function causing neurocognitive signs and symptoms; it can coincide with mild, moderate, or severe TBI.[5] The most common symptoms of concussion are headache, dizziness, difficulty concentrating, photophobia, nausea, and drowsiness.[5] Patients who remain symptomatic after some time are diagnosed with postconcussive syndrome (PCS). Lack of a uniform definition for PCS makes comparing results across studies difficult; definitions used in research usually include three or more symptoms from a set list which last 1 month,[6] 3 months,[7] or for no specified duration.[8] Biomarkers for concussion and predictive factors for PCS are prominent areas of research.

Diagnosis and management of mTBI is based on clinical evaluation, with neuroimaging playing only a small role. The Canadian Computed Tomography (CT) Head Rule (CCHR) is a validated clinical decision tool to limit CT use to mTBI patients who meet criteria such as GCS <15 at 2 hours post-injury, suspicion for skull fracture, and vomiting.[9] CT allows diagnosis of structural abnormalities requiring neurosurgical intervention[9]; a positive finding would exclude the patient from the mild category of TBI. Likewise, most conventional structural magnetic resonance imaging (sMRI) methods, although more sensitive than CT, also provide information about macrostructural changes.[10] The pathophysiology of mTBI involves diffuse microenvironment alterations to axons, vasculature, and the blood—brain barrier which are not adequately evaluated by traditional methods.[11] Advanced neuroimaging techniques offer exciting potential for improved evaluation and management of mTBI and PCS. This chapter will review imaging findings in mTBI using several advanced modalities.

We will begin with a summary of traditional MRI use in mTBI. Our discussion of structural imagining will include susceptibility-weighted and diffusion-weighted imaging (DWI). The following sections will describe functional and then metabolic imaging. Each section will give an overview of common findings in each imaging modality at various time points. Longitudinal changes are important to consider for a better understanding of the natural history of the disease and symptomatology. We will highlight any differences between adult and pediatric patient populations. For any modality, there is substantially less data in children. This is a noteworthy area for future research as trauma can have distinct effects on the developing brain. Furthermore, we will review the links between imaging abnormalities and neurocognitive and behavioral functioning. Table 3.1 and the figures are provided as useful summaries of the findings.

This chapter will not include an independent discussion of CT findings. Clinically, CT remains the standard of care in acute evaluation of mTBI due to its speed, availability, and low cost. MRI is recommended in cases with a normal CT and persistent or worsening symptoms.[12] Many studies focus on the superiority of MRI over CT in identifying structural abnormalities.[13] Data from the prospective multicenter TRACK-TBI study showed early (average 12 days post-injury) MRI abnormalities in 27% of mTBI patients with unremarkable CT scans.[14] It is worthwhile to explore both traditional and advanced MRI techniques in subacute and chronic mTBI.

STRUCTURAL IMAGING

Structural Magnetic Resonance Imaging

Traditional MRI sequences include T_1, T_2-weighted, and FLAIR (Fluid Attenuated Inversion Recovery). These sequences can detect contusions and structural changes. Common specific findings include white matter (WM) hyperintensities [suggesting reactive change in glial cells associated with diffuse axonal injury (DAI)] and hypointense signals

TABLE 3.1 Comparison of Imaging Modalities in mTBI

Imaging Modality	Description	Pros	Cons	Findings
sMRI	• Traditional MRI sequences: T_1, T_2, and FLAIR • Detects contusions and structural changes	• Widely available • Good spatial resolution • More sensitive than CT for structural lesions • Noninvasive	• Not sensitive for DAI • WM hyperintensities not mTBI-specific	• Early sMRI abnormalities linked to poor 3-month outcomes • Use in the acute setting does not change management
SWI	• Gradient-echo technique with enhanced detection of blood byproducts • Can detect hypointense lesions indicative of hemorrhage • Can quantify iron accumulation	• Widely available • Good spatial resolution • Noninvasive • Microhemorrhage lesions seem to be TBI-specific	• No clear link between areas of hypointensity and patient's functional status	• Microbleeds present in 22%–75% mTBI patients; higher prevalence in PCS • Frontal and temporal lobes most common sites • mTBI group increased iron signal correlated with poorer scores on Mini Mental Status exam
DTI	• Measures magnitude and direction of water molecule diffusion to generate information about WM fibers	• Noninvasive • More sensitive than sMRI for WM lesions and DAI	• Acquisition protocol and analytical tool variation complicates study results comparison	• Decreased FA in CC, frontal lobes connecting tracks, and tracks traveling from the thalamus • DTI metric abnormalities linked to PCS, lower scores on neuropsychiatric testing, and poorer outcomes
BOLD-fMRI	• Measures change in ratio of oxyhemoglobin to deoxyhemoglobin • Change in ratio marker for neuronal activity • Task-based or resting-state	• Noninvasive • Widely available • Greater signal-to-noise ratio than ASL • Good spatial resolution	• Cannot quantify absolute values for CBF • Motor tasks limited by scanner	• mTBI-altered activation patterns in DLPFC and parietal lobe during working memory tasks • Altered BOLD signals linked to PCS • mTBI differences in resting network connectivity
ASL	• Measures CBF using radiofrequency pulse to tag blood water molecules	• Noninvasive • No intravenous contrast • Can quantify absolute values for CBF	• Weaker correlates between tasks and signal than BOLD-fMRI	• Hypoperfusion detected in several brain areas at rest • CBF alterations may be related to PCS

(Continued)

TABLE 3.1 (Continued)

Imaging Modality	Description	Pros	Cons	Findings
fNIRS	• Measures ratio of oxyhemoglobin to deoxyhemoglobin by detecting reflected photons of specific wavelengths • Change in signal marker for neuronal activity	• Relatively affordable • Portable • Noninvasive • Patient position vary by task • Sedation not needed for young children	• Poor spatial resolution • Cannot visualize subcortical structures • Cannot quantify absolute values for CBF • Nonprecise mapping of brain anatomy and external detector location	• Lower oxygenation levels in prefrontal cortex found in symptomatic mTBI patients
SPECT	• Measures CBF with decay in radioactive tracer	• More sensitive than standard CT for detecting abnormalities • Quantify absolute values for CBF	• Radiation exposure • Administration of intravenous tracer	• mTBI hypoperfusion in frontal and temporal lobes • Perfusion deficits in frontal lobe correlated with poorer outcomes and poorer executive function
PET	• Radioactive isotope measures glucose uptake and neuronal metabolic activity • Detects aggregates of neurodegenerative proteins	• Can quantify absolute cerebral metabolic rate of glucose use • Can be used to detect tau and amyloid aggregates	• Radiation exposure • Administration of intravenous tracer • Expensive	• mTBI reduced glucose metabolism • Glucose metabolism abnormalities (task-based and at rest) associated with symptoms and poor performance on cognitive tasks
MRS	• Measures resonant frequency peaks corresponding to specific brain metabolites	• Metabolic information not detectable by other modalities • Noninvasive • Widely available	• Variation in acquisition protocols and analytical tools make comparison of results across studies more difficult	• mTBI lower NAA in WM and lower Glx in gray matter

sMRI, structural magnetic resonance imaging; SWI, susceptibility-weighted imaging; DTI, diffusion tensor imaging; BOLD-fMRI, blood-oxygen level-dependent functional magnetic resonance imaging; ASL, arterial spin labeling; fNIRS, functional near-infrared spectroscopy; SPECT, single-photon emission computed tomography; PET, positron emission tomography; MRS, magnetic resonance spectroscopy; FLAIR, fluid attenuated inversion recovery; CBF, cerebral blood flow; PCS, postconcussive syndrome; FA, fractional anisotropy; DLPFC, dorsolateral prefrontal cortex; NAA, N-acetylaspartate; Glx, glutamine/glutamate.

(indicative of prior hemorrhage).[15] WM hyperintensities (Fig. 3.1A) are common and not specific to mTBI patients[16,17]; although when present, they have been linked to poor cognitive performance chronically.[17] Likewise, TRACK-TBI data showed a connection between early MRI abnormalities and poor 3-month outcomes.[14] MRI abnormalities in mTBI patients are weakly correlated with poor performance on neuropsychological tests acutely; however, the MRI findings are not predictive of PCS or return to work status at 6 months.[18]

Standard MRI protocols can be used for precise measurements of cortical thickness and volume for estimation of global or regional atrophy or edema after TBI. Brain volume reduction has been frequently associated with moderate and severe TBI.[13] The volumetric changes in mTBI are harder to parse out due to lack of mTBI-focused studies and the natural variation in brain volumes. Current evidence for volumetric changes in mTBI is conflicting. Cohen et al.[19] found volumetric reduction in the gray matter (GM) of mTBI subjects. Another study showed no significant changes in volume; however, surface area measurements indicated dilatation of accumbens and left caudate, and atrophy of the left

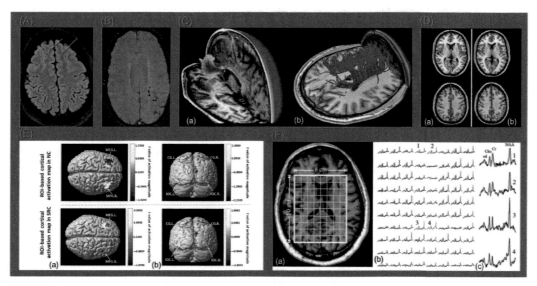

FIGURE 3.1 Examples of imaging findings in mTBI patients. (A) WM hyperintensities (red arrows) on FLAIR MRI in 34-year-old female with traumatic fall injury. (B) SWI image showing three parietal microhemorrhages (red arrow). (C) DTI fiber tractography of commonly damaged tracts in mTBI: (a) anterior corona radiata and genu of CC and (b) cingulum bundle in green and body of CC in red. (D) rs-fMRI. Between group contrast maps for chronic mTBI versus control. (a) DMN. (b) Task Positive network. Warm colors represent increased functional connectivity and cool colors represent reduced functional connectivity in the mTBI group. (E) fNIRS. Cortical activation maps in six regions of interest for subject and control groups during a visual attention task. NC, normal control; SRC, sports-related concussion; MFG.L., left middle frontal gyrus; MFG.R., right middle frontal gyrus; CG.L., left calcarine gyrus; CG.R., right calcarine gyrus; IOC.L., left inferior occipital cortex; IOC.R., right inferior occipital cortex. (F) MRS. (a) T_1 MRI of mTBI patient, with the $8 \times 10 \times 4.5$ volume of interest (thick white frame) and $16 \times 16 \times 6$ field of view (thin white grid) superimposed. The genu and the splenium of the CC outlined in red. MR spectra (b) corresponding to grid with detailed view including labels (c) of CC spectra. *Source: (A) Modified from Tate et al.[17] (B) Modified from de Haan et al.[25] (C) Modified from Niogi and Mukherjee.[33] (D) Modified from Sours et al.[78] (E) Modified from Wu et al.[154] (F) Modified from Grossman et al.[139]*

I. DEFINING MILD TBI

thalamus in a mTBI group compared to orthopedic injury control.[20] Zhou et al.[21] found both global and regional changes (anterior cingulate WM bilaterally and left cingulate gyrus isthmus) at 1 year after injury. In these mTBI subjects, reduced volumetric measurements correlated with postconcussive symptoms and neuropsychiatric testing. Volume data in pediatric mTBI patients is lacking. In a group of adults who sustained mTBI's years earlier as adolescent football players, there were no significant volumetric differences.[22] Volume measurements are an interesting application of sMRI images, yet they do not provide adequate insight into the pathological microchanges characterizing mTBI.

Susceptibility-Weighted Imaging

Susceptibility-weighted imaging (SWI) is a gradient-echo MR technique incorporating phase information to emphasize magnetic differences in tissues and enhance detection of blood byproducts.[23] Visualization and quantification of iron-containing molecules can indicate microhemorrhages from DAI, a well-studied pathological finding in TBI.[24] Small hypointense lesions on SWI (Fig. 3.1B) signify microhemorrhages. SWI is more sensitive than T_2*-weighted gradient-recalled-echo imaging in detecting microbleeds.[25,26] At various time points after injury, abnormalities on SWI are present in 22%–75% of mTBI patients.[17,26,27] Specifically, Liu et al.[26] cited a significantly higher prevalence of microbleeds in mTBI patients with PCS. Unlike WM hyperintensities on traditional imaging, SWI lesions seem to be specific to mTBI subjects and are not found in controls.[17,27]

There is conflicting evidence for the relationship between SWI findings and outcome. Tate et al.[17] did not find a significant association between SWI lesions and functional status of mTBI patients. Likewise, frontal lobe lesions are not associated with symptoms at 1 month post-injury[27] or functional outcome at 3 months.[25] However, de Haan et al.[25] noted poorer outcomes associated with temporal lobe lesions. Frontal and temporal lobes are the most common areas for microhemorrhagic lesions.[25] Location of the lesions is likely an important factor underlying impairment after mTBI.

In addition to localizing lesions, SWI can be used to quantify accumulation of iron. At intervals greater than 6 months after injury, mTBI patients had increased iron deposits in various regions of the basal ganglia. A robust iron signal in the right substantia nigra was correlated with poor Mini Mental State Examination (MMSE) performance.[16] These authors suggest that iron can be injurious to the brain via oxidative stress, and damage in susceptible areas can cause deficits.

To date, there are very few studies evaluating SWI findings in children. At 2 days post-injury, Babcock et al.[28] did not find any microhemorrhages in their pediatric mTBI population. The presence of microbleeds and utilization of SWI in the pediatric mTBI population is a compelling area for future research. Overall, SWI shows much promise in identifying abnormalities specific to mTBI adults and playing a role in clinical evaluation. Future research should focus on elucidating the effect of microhemorrhage on outcome, and the utility of SWI-detected lesions for prognosis and management.

Diffusion Tensor Imaging

Diffusion tensor imaging (DTI), an application of DWI, computes the orientation of WM fibers. It has been widely studied as a tool for detecting WM pathology, such as DAI in mTBI. DWI measures displacement of water molecules, a motion which is more rapid along axonal fibers than perpendicular to them.[29] DTI quantifies diffusion in multiple directions to generate information about WM fibers within a voxel. Diffusion data yields a set of measures frequently used in TBI research, the most common being fractional anisotropy (FA). FA, recorded from 0 to 1, denotes directionality of diffusion. A value of 1 signifies that all of the displacement occurs in one direction, as though along a WM fiber tract. An FA of 0 means that diffusion is occurring equally in all directions, such as in GM or CSF.[13] FA is nonspecific and can be reduced with edema, demyelination, gliosis and inflammation.[29] An increased FA may occur with cytotoxic edema.[30] Additional DTI measures include mean diffusivity (MD), radial diffusivity (RD), and axial diffusivity (AD). MD is based on the magnitude of diffusion within a voxel; RD and AD are perpendicular and parallel components of displacement.[31] Furthermore, DTI can be applied to track neuronal fibers and enhance visualization and study connections between brain regions.[32]

DTI is a valuable neuroimaging tool for mTBI due to its sensitivity in detecting WM lesions. Abnormalities on DTI can be identified in mTBI patients with unremarkable CT and sMRI scans.[33] However, some studies have found no differences in DTI metrics between uncomplicated mTBI patients and healthy controls.[34,35] There is substantial variability in DTI studies with respect to strength of manufacturer's magnet, brain regions observed, time since injury, and analytical tools used to analyze the data. There are two general approaches to analyze diffusion data: whole-brain analysis (WBA) and region of interest (ROI). WBA includes a voxel-based approach and tract-based spatial statistics (TBSS) to explore significant differences between groups. An ROI approach forgoes the potential for global analysis for greater within-region sensitivity.[36] Lipton et al.[37] developed Enhanced Z-score Microstructural Assessment for Pathology (EZ-MAP), a standardized whole-brain approach for DTI assessment of individual patients based on regional FA abnormalities. EZ-MAP was validated by Kim et al.[38] and determined to have both a sensitivity and specificity of 71% for differentiating mTBI patients from controls.

The location of neuronal injury depends on the mechanism of trauma; however, certain WM tracks may be more susceptible to shearing forces due to their length and anatomical relationships. The most commonly reported areas of abnormality on DTI are corpus callosum (CC), frontal lobe, internal capsule (IC), and cingulum[36] (Fig. 3.1C). These studies vary in type of analysis used, so additional areas may be implicated. A meta-analysis of ROI studies found a significant FA reduction in the CC,[39] but not in the IC or corona radiata. Subgroup analysis revealed that the posterior portion of the CC was most susceptible to injury from mTBI. A subsequent meta-analysis of TBSS (a whole-brain approach) noted decreased FA in mTBI subjects compared to controls in three clusters: thalamus extending to the splenium of the CC, forceps minor, and the right superior longitudinal fasciculus.[40] Interhemispheric connections, and those involving the thalamus and prefrontal cortex, seem to be most commonly implicated in mild head trauma.

Among DTI studies, there is substantial variability in the time since injury of mTBI subjects. A small portion of studies imaged patients longitudinally to gain more insight into temporal changes in WM. Understanding the trajectory of repair after DAI is important for clinical management. Unfortunately, the current literature does not provide clear longitudinal information. DTI differences between subjects and controls can be seen within days of injury, specifically higher MD and RD and lower FA[41–43] in mTBI groups. Acute elevations in FA and decreases in RD in the genu of the CC have also been reported.[44] Multiple studies observed temporal decreases in FA across multiple brain regions ranging from the acute period to subacute (3–6 months).[43–45] Veeramuthu et al.[43] also measured a reduction in MD longitudinally in mTBI patients. Conversely, Narayana et al.[42] did not observe any changes between baseline DTI and at 3 months post-injury. The indeterminate trends of longitudinal DTI data are further demonstrated by a study of concussed athletes who had lower FA and higher RD compared to controls at 2 days and 2 months post-injury; however, the interim imaging at 2 weeks did not show a difference.[41] Perhaps current DTI metrics are not sensitive enough to differentiate injury from the reparative milieu. Conflicting measurements of FA in the acute period warrant further investigation. Additional longitudinal studies with homogenous analyses are needed to elucidate this topic.

The significance of WM lesion relation to symptoms and functional outcomes is a prominent research area. Diffuse axonal damage, as detected with DTI, is assumed to contribute to the cognitive and behavioral symptoms that constitute PCS. A 2016 systematic review[46] found seven studies looking at DTI parameters as biomarkers for PCS; another three studies were prospectively studying the predictive value of DTI measures. When compared to controls, PCS patients had FA WM reductions in 7 out of 10 studies, MD elevations in four out of seven studies, and RD increases in three out of five studies. The CC was the most common region of study. Messe et al.[47] found significantly higher MD values in mTBI patients who went on to develop PCS compared to those with good outcomes; there were no differences between good outcome mTBI patients and healthy controls. Furthermore, regions of reduced FA are modestly predictive of poor outcome at 3 and 6 months measured by the Extended Glasgow Outcome Scale (GOS-E), a common assessment tool for global functioning after mTBI.[35] Significant correlations were found between DTI metrics and neuropsychological assessment scores in the domains of attention, language, and spatial and executive functioning.[43]

Additional considerations include the effects of age and sex on DTI measures. In a study of gender differences, male subjects with mTBI had significantly lower FA values in the bilateral uncinate fasciculus (UF).[48] Damage to the UF was determined to be an independent risk factor for PCS, and its sparing in females is thought to be related to progesterone receptor expression in these tracts.[48] In the pediatric population, WM changes are identified on DTI as early as 2 days after mild head trauma.[28] Babcock et al.[28] reported acutely higher FA in mTBI youths compared to orthopedic injury controls in eight WM regions, including left temporal gyrus, bilateral corona radiata, and right superior longitudinal fasciculus. The researchers also found higher AD and lower MD and RD in 4, 3, and 11 regions, respectively. Approximately 1 month after injury, Van Beek et al.[49] measured higher FA in the CC splenium and lower RD and MD in the CC genu compared to matched controls, which tended to resolve after 6–8 months.[50]

The evidence for mTBI-related cortical changes seen on DTI is growing, but is not yet strong enough to recommend for routine clinical use.[51] There is clearly some detectable alteration of WM, supporting the hypothesis of microstructural changes of DAI, and a link between DTI abnormalities and outcomes. Although there is great potential for DTI use in mTBI, the findings are not consistent enough to inform prognosis and management.

Diffusion Kurtosis Imaging

Diffusion Kurtosis Imaging (DKI) is an emerging neuroimaging tool providing distinct information beyond traditional diffusion measures. This technique is useful for exploring different brain pathologies, including mTBI. Kurtosis describes deviation from the normative pattern of diffusion. DKI parameters increase when there are divergences from the typical displacement distribution of water molecules.[52] The links between DKI metrics and pathology have not been fleshed out, but reductions in mean kurtosis (MK) suggest loss of cellular structure.[52]

Over any time point, mTBI patients been found to have lower MK in the IC, thalamus, CC, cingulum, and optic radiations when compared to controls.[53–55] Between-group differences varied in significance for each ROI among studies. Longitudinal studies have reported no significant change, worsening, or normalization in DKI measures.[54,55] On an individual basis, improvements in MK in the thalamus, IC, and CC have been correlated with better scores on cognitive tests.[55] MK in the thalamus in particular has been linked to performance on tests of attention, concentration, and information processing.[54] Overall, DKI use alongside traditional DTI measures may provide more insight into mTBI pathology and aid in improving specificity of diffusion imaging findings for function.

FUNCTIONAL IMAGING

Functional Magnetic Resonance Imaging

Functional magnetic resonance imaging (fMRI) measures cerebral blood flow (CBF) patterns during real-time neuronal activation for a task or at resting-state. The most common fMRI technique is blood oxygenation level-dependent (BOLD) imaging. BOLD-fMRI relies on the differences in magnetic properties between oxygenated and deoxygenated hemoglobin. Neuronal activity accumulation at the synapse triggers a local hemodynamic response leading to an oxyhemoglobin influx,[56] which is identified on MRI. This technique can determine the effects of diffuse microstructural pathology on brain activation. Additionally, arterial spin labeling (ASL) marks water molecules in blood with a radiofrequency pulse and then quantifies CBF[57] for functional information; it can be applied in a similar manner as BOLD-fMRI. In general, BOLD imaging yields stronger correlates between tasks and signal changes, whereas ASL can provide an absolute CBF quantification.[58] BOLD is considerably more common in mTBI research, and we begin our discussion of fMRI findings with this modality.

Blood Oxygenation Level-Dependent Functional Magnetic Resonance Imaging

There are two main types of BOLD-fMRI studies: task-based and resting-state (rs-fMRI). In the former, the specific tasks used include memory, working memory (a primary focus), executive function, and attention, often subjectively impaired in mTBI. BOLD changes are evident in brain regions involved in working memory, including dorsolateral prefrontal cortex (DLPFC) and parietal regions.[59] Researchers have reported areas of hypoactivation,[60,61] hyperactivation,[62–65] or both[66,67] when comparing mTBI patients to controls. A meta-analysis [59] of working memory fMRI studies suggested two explanations for the diverging results: task classification and task load. Hyperactivation was reported during continuous working memory tasks and at higher task loads. In contrast, hypoactivation was observed when the tasks had discrete trials or during low task load. The greater neuronal response needed for demanding exercises may explain some of the functional cognitive difficulties reported by mTBI patients.

BOLD signal changes detect perturbations in functional connectivity in mTBI. These patients often score within the normal limits on traditional neurocognitive tests,[60] resulting in a "normal" clinical assessment even in the presence of subjective complaints. mTBI subjects were found to have alterations in brain activation patterns even when task performance was no different than controls.[65–68] The data suggest that mTBI patients perform with matching accuracy and speed as their healthy peers on cognitively demanding tasks, but they have difficulty doing so due to their overall symptoms. Notably, evoked BOLD signal patterns have been correlated with symptomatology and scores on PCS assessments.[61,65,67,68] fMRI may be used as a sensitive biomarker for concussion or mTBI, as it is related to subjective impairments which are not detected by other means of testing.

Longitudinal task-based fMRI data is limited. Studies have reported abnormalities in BOLD signals as early as several days[65,69] to 1 year after mTBI injury.[70] Trends toward brain activation normalization have been observed longitudinally both subacutely[69] and chronically.[68] Apparent recovery from alterations in fMRI measures coincides with remission of symptoms. Lovell et al.[64] found that fMRI hyperactivation at the initial visit was predictive of delayed recovery at 1 month. Better understanding of longitudinal fMRI changes will aid transformation of the BOLD technique into a diagnostic and prognostic tool.

In contrast to task-based functional imaging, rs-fMRI measures spontaneous fluctuations in BOLD signal in an inactive state. The brain is assumed to be comprised of multiple large-scale networks, theoretically facilitating the integration of discrete processes into larger wholes. A concentration of neurons form the network nodes, which are therefore structurally and functionally linked.[71] It has been hypothesized that the diffuse mTBI micropathology disrupts those linkages between and/or within nodes and would be observed as changes in the BOLD signal.

The default mode network (DMN) is the most widely studied in mTBI using BOLD imaging (Fig. 3.1D). The principal nodes of the DMN include the medial prefrontal cortex and posterior cingulate cortex,[72] shown to be active at rest and playing a role in intrinsic mentation.[72] Compared to healthy controls, mTBI patients were found to have reduced connections within the DMN,[73–75] and the amount of connections decreased as the number of injuries accumulated.[73] Conflicting results were reported by Abbas et al.,[76] who noted DMN hyperconnectivity during a football season in which athletes sustained multiple subconcussive impacts. Alternatively, Zhang et al.[77] did not find DMN rs-fMRI differences until mTBI subjects underwent a physical stressor. Studies have reported increased connectivity between DMN nodes and other brain regions such as the task-related networks (involved in transferring attention from intrinsic to extrinsic stimuli), suggesting a disruption in network equilibrium which may cause greater distractibility.[74,78]

Altered DMN functional consequences have not been elucidated, although, impairments would likely occur in autobiographical memory, processing of social interactions, and future planning.[72] These cognitive impairments may be subclinical, paralleling DMN rs-fMRI abnormalities observed in asymptomatic mTBI patients.[73,76] Nonetheless, there does seem to be a relationship between DMN integrity and emotional, cognitive, and somatic symptoms. Acute changes in DMN connections predict patient complaints at a 3—5 month follow up.[74] Mayer et al.[74] reported that DMN alterations may differentiate mTBI patients from controls with 81% sensitivity and 88% specificity.

Brain networks other than the DMN and internetwork connections are likely perturbed in mTBI as well. Stevens et al.[79] used independent component analysis of rs-fMRI data to identify 12 separate brain networks which were all abnormal in mTBI. Postconcussive symptom severity was related to abnormal connections in five out of 12 networks. As in previous studies, there is both hypoconnectivity and hyperconnectivity between networks, suggesting a balance of functional deficits and compensation by other domains. Moreover, abnormalities of the executive and salience networks were found to be related to symptoms and depression scores in mTBI.[80] Shumskaya et al.[81] linked abnormalities in the motor-striatal network to lower scores on tests of psychomotor speed. The thalamus is also implicated in mTBI; Tang et al.[82] reported an increase in both thalamic connectivity and asymmetry of thalamic connections. Aberrations of thalamic connections are correlated with self-reported fatigue,[83] PCS symptoms,[82,84] and poor scores on neurocognitive tests.[82]

Studies have observed longitudinal changes in resting-state functional connectivity which may shed light on mTBI recovery. Researchers report partial recovery of networks at 4 months[84] and at 1 year[85] after head trauma. There is evidence that normalization of rs-fMRI data is related to clinical improvements.[84,85] Conversely, other studies found no significant longitudinal change in mTBI average resting-state functional data.[74,78] Perhaps it is worthwhile to subdivide mTBI populations based status of PCS and examine networks independently. PCS patients specifically had subacute alterations in the thalamus and temporal areas, but chronically the frontal lobe was most affected.[86] Thalamic connections normalized within 4 months among multiple networks, except with DMN.[84] Network recovery profiles may differ, but changes likely persist for a long time. Abbas et al.[76] found differences in rs-fMRI data between healthy controls and football players starting their season, suggesting that alterations of functional connectivity persist months after the preceding season ends.

Few investigators used fMRI in the pediatric population to study the effects of mTBI. Keightley et al.[87] performed evoked fMRI in concussed (9—90 days after injury) and healthy youths during working memory tasks. In contrast to adults, the pediatric mTBI group had poorer task performance, suggesting that the cortical networks may be too immature to compensate for insults. During the task, concussed children had hypoactivation in the DLPFC, premotor cortex, and superior parietal lobule. Task accuracy was strongly correlated to activation in the DLPFC. Westfall et al.[88] imaged a pediatric mTBI group an average of 7.5 months after injury and found no significant difference in working memory task performance, but the mTBI group showed overall hyperactivation during the task. Symptomatically concussed youths had greater cerebellar activation during an inhibitory task of executive control, which was correlated with their complaints.[89] Additionally, Yang et al.[90] reported hypoactivation across subcortical structures in mTBI youth, although neuropsychological testing did not differ from controls. Further investigation of functional connections both at rest and during tasks in children with mTBI is warranted. Networks responsible for attention, working memory, and executive control are thought to be particularly susceptible to concussive injury. Proper functioning of these networks is important for development, especially learning and school performance. BOLD-fMRI is a sensitive method of detecting injury which may not be detected by traditional imaging and may complement neuropsychological testing.

BOLD signals provide valuable information about the consequences of mTBI, extending beyond structural alterations to detecting altered functional processes. A methodological issue involves a potential mismatch between neural vasoactive signals and BOLD-fMRI-measured CBF from mTBI brain architecture disruption. Ellis et al.[91] reviewed the evidence for altered cerebrovascular reactivity in mTBI, and found it inconclusive. The relationship between functional and structural lesions has yet to be better understood. Several studies have investigated DTI and fMRI lesions in the same subjects,[74,92] but there were few definitive correlations. Nonetheless, task-based and resting-state fMRI shows potential for clinical relevance in mTBI management.

Arterial Spin Labeling

As described previously, specific measurements of CBF can be acquired using ASL MRI. This technique detects magnetized water flow in blood, in contrast to BOLD-fMRI oxyhemoglobin to deoxyhemoglobin ratio. Further studies have applied ASL to quantify CBF changes in mTBI. Compared to controls, mTBI adults had decreased CBF in the thalamus,[93] frontal,[94] occipital,[94] superior temporal,[95] and insular cortices.[95] However, two studies did not find any changes in resting CBF,[96,97] and one study found increased CBF in the left striatum and occipital and frontal lobes of the mTBI group.[98] Meier et al.[95] longitudinally followed concussed collegiate athletes and found that perfusion was lower acutely after injury, but normalized within 1 month. CBF differences 2 years after mTBI injury were reported by Ge et al.,[93] suggesting that perfusion alterations can last much longer than expected and may not normalize.

CBF measurements have been linked to neuropsychological performance[93] and postconcussive symptoms.[94,97,99] Interestingly, Lin et al.[94] found symptom severity correlated with increased frontal and occipital lobe CBF, areas which were hypoperfused in mTBI. Symptoms were also correlated with increased blood flow in posterior cortical areas[97] and anterior cingulate cortex.[100] Self-reported fatigue, in particular, was linked to increased CBF in the cingulate gyrus and decreased CBF in the frontal/thalamic network.[99]

ASL imaging has shown that, compared to healthy controls, mTBI youths, an average of 7 months post-injury, had decreased CBF in the fronto-temporal areas.[101] Barlow et al.[102] categorized pediatric mTBI subjects (40 days post-injury) into PCS and asymptomatic groups. The PCS subset had significantly higher CBF in multiple areas when compared to healthy controls, and the asymptomatic mTBI group had lower CBF.

Researchers also used dynamic susceptibility contrast (DSC) MRI to study perfusion in mTBI. Similar to work with ASL, a DSC study found hypoperfusion areas which were correlated with verbal memory, reaction time, and stress symptoms.[103] As intravenous contrast is not needed for ASL, this technique provides a noninvasive advantage over other types of perfusion imaging. The small number of ASL studies have demonstrated that there are hemodynamic disruptions in both children and adults as a result of micro-pathology associated with mTBI. Additional research is needed to clarify the changes in perfusion as current designs and inclusion criteria is quite variable. There seems to be a relationship between CBF alterations and postconcussive symptoms, and the changes may persist even when symptoms resolve. Future research should focus on the relevance of perfusion disruptions to behavioral functioning and prognostication after mTBI.

Functional Near-Infrared Spectroscopy

Functional Near-Infrared Spectroscopy (fNIRS) is an emerging method for characterizing real-time brain oxygenation, similar to fMRI. This technique takes advantage of the optical differences between oxygenated and deoxygenated hemoglobin. Photons near-infrared wavelengths are emitted from a headpiece, and the reflected wavelengths from two forms of brain vasculature hemoglobin are identified by a photodetector.[104] Brain regions receiving an increased ratio of oxygenated blood can be presumed to be activated (Fig. 3.1E). This paradigm is similar to the BOLD response, but has poorer spatial resolution and cannot be used to visualize subcortical structures. The advantages of fNIRS include irrelevance of motion artifact, affordability, and flexibility in location and patient positioning.[104]

Kontos et al.[105] used fNIRS to demonstrate decreased brain activation during working memory, spatial memory, and word memory tasks in symptomatic concussed adults. Similarly, Helmich et al.[106] reported that patients with persistent PCS had lower oxygenation in the prefrontal regions during working memory tasks. Oxygenation differences in the prefrontal cortex are seen between acute mTBI and control groups during a hypercapnic state.[107] In a pediatric mTBI sample, investigators found reduced coherence in the contralateral motor cortex during a finger tapping task, suggesting that interhemispheric communication is impaired. Overall, this limited evidence suggests that fNIRS may be sensitive to detecting cerebral hemodynamic perturbations in mTBI. The technology has the potential to be a convenient diagnostic and monitoring tool for the clinic, particularly for younger children who cannot tolerate lying motionless in an MRI without sedation.

Single-Photon Emission Computed Tomography

Single-photon emission computed tomography (SPECT) provides an additional way of visualizing cerebral perfusion by injecting the patient with a radioactive tracer, such as technetium-Tc99m-labeled hexamethylpropyleneamine oxime (Tc99m-HMPAO) or Tc99m-ethyl cysteinate dimer, which are administered intravenously.[108] Radioactive decay of these compounds gives off a photon indicating the tracer amount and location, providing three-dimensional CBF information.[109] Masdeu et al.[110] described two types of SPECT lesions in mTBI: (1) sharply demarcated areas of hypoperfusion surrounded by a ring of relative hyperperfusion, indicative of contusion; and (2) diffuse areas of hypoperfusion concentrated in the occipitotemporal lobes. When mTBI subjects were compared to controls at rest, studies reported hypoperfusion in the frontal and temporal areas.[111–113]

Gowda et al.[112] included children in their sample and noted a temporal lobe predominance in hypoperfusion changes. Overall there were no areas of hyperperfusion at rest.

SPECT is appropriate for evaluating both acute and chronic mTBI; abnormalities have been observed within 12 hours of injury[112] to over a year after the trauma.[109,114,115] A longitudinal study of mTBI patients undergoing SPECT at 4 weeks and then again at 3, 6, and 12 months reported a decrease in CBF abnormalities over time.[109] Amen et al.[113] applied SPECT imaging in National Football League players, a sample which accumulated multiple concussions. Hypoperfusion was noted in the temporal and frontal areas, in addition to the hippocampus, cerebellar vermis, and insula, suggesting that alterations from concussions are additive, and cerebrovascular profiles can be created to accurately classify football players and controls.

Exploring clinical relevance is the next step to assessing SPECT imaging findings. Jacobs et al.[109] noted that perfusion deficits in the frontal lobe are predictive of poor outcomes. Frontal area perfusion, both acutely and chronically, was associated with executive function (Stroop color naming task) in mTBI.[116] Hattori et al.[114] used SPECT during a task of attention and working memory, and found higher activation in the prefrontal cortex and decreased activation in the cerebellum relative to controls. The authors suggest a frontocerebellar dissociation resulting from diffuse damage to axonal tracts. Overall, there is some evidence that SPECT may be used for prognostication and monitoring recovery, however, the literature is not sufficient to recommend for routine use. Some drawbacks of SPECT include radiation exposure and necessity for intravenous tracer, further limiting use.

METABOLIC IMAGING

Positron Emission Tomography

Similar to SPECT, positron emission tomography (PET) is a technique using a radioactive tracer to detect signs of altered brain metabolism due to injury and neurodegeneration. The radioactive isotope in PET emits two photons traveling in opposite directions which interact with tomographic detectors. A three-dimensional image is rendered, localizing the accumulation of tracer in the body. The most common isotope used is [18F]fluorodeoxyglucose (FDG), an altered glucose molecule; the amount of neural uptake can be quantified, proportional to glucose use or neuronal metabolic activity.[117] A decrease of FDG-PET signal may indicate a diminished number of neurons or reduced activity. Similar to fMRI, PET scans can be conducted with the patient at rest or doing a task. Investigators also use PET to detect aggregation of tau and amyloid in patients with repetitive concussive impact histories. PET images can be analyzed via ROI or whole-brain voxel-based methods, and are limited by relatively poor spatial resolution.[118]

Researchers have measured changes to the cerebral metabolic rate of glucose after mTBI. With the exception of one case study which reported normal FDG uptake 2 days after injury,[119] all studies enrolled subjects months to years after the trauma. Subjects were often military veterans and/or experiencing persistent symptoms. Investigators found decreased rate of glucose metabolism at rest in chronic mTBI patients compared to controls in the amygdala, hippocampus, parahippocampal gyrus, thalamus, insula, parietal, somatosensory, and visual cortices.[120,121] Cortical FDG uptake differences were observed even when the same individuals' DTI showed structural damage limited to the genu of the CC.[120] A third group, however, did not find any FDG differences at rest.[122] Ruff et al.[123] reported decreased, task-based FDG uptake in the frontal and anteroparietal areas linked to impaired scores on neuropsychiatric tests. Likewise, abnormal metabolism in frontal, temporal, and parietal areas were associated with complaints of inattention, social withdrawal, irritability, along with poor outcomes on cognitive tasks.[124] While most studies cited an average decrease in FDG uptake in mTBI, Gross et al.[124] recorded abnormalities in signal corresponding to large divergences (>2 standard deviations) in either direction from normalized values. Buchsbaum et al.[125] noted that clusters of low FDG uptake are irregularly shaped in mTBI subjects, which may be caused by the mechanical shearing forces from trauma.

Other studies use different PET tracers to obtain information on injury/repair process and protein aggregation in subjects with histories of one or multiple mTBI's. In a group of retired football players with mood and cognitive symptoms or suspected chronic traumatic encephalopathy (CTE), researchers found increased uptake of [F-18]FDDNP in the amygdala, medial temporal lobe, and multiple subcortical structures.[126,127] These studies used [F-18]FDDNP as a marker of Tau aggregates and beta-amyloid plaques, proteins involved in Alzheimer's disease. Barrio et al.[127] noted that ex-football players had a distinct deposition pattern of FDDP, different from the Alzheimer group and controls, thus possibly linked to CTE. Coughlin et al.[128,129] used [11C]DPA-713 as a marker of a protein which may signify injury and repair processes in the brains of former NFL athletes. The researchers reported a higher distribution of [11C]DPA-713 in eight out of 12 regions, including the hippocampus, parahippocampal cortex, and supramarginal gyrus; however, their subjects did not differ from controls on neuropsychiatric testing. The data suggests that there are lasting changes from a history of repetitive concussions, and their role is yet to be fully elucidated.

PET offers in vivo visualization of brain metabolic processes which seem to be altered in mTBI. The data is limited by small sample numbers of symptomatic, military, or retired football athletes and is not readily generalizable. Considerations include the price tag and safety concerns of the radioactive tracers, in addition to the radiation exposure from the scan. Another question arises as to whether the diffusion and binding properties of these novel radioisotopes give an accurate representation of brain proteins. If so, the relevance for patient outcomes and possibility for early diagnosis of CTE should be explored.

Magnetic Resonance Spectroscopy

Magnetic resonance spectroscopy (MRS) is a technique which quantifies the amounts of distinct metabolites in tissue. 1-Hydrogen MRS detects differences in magnetic properties of protons specific to the compound's chemical structure. Resonant peak frequencies correspond to metabolites in a ROI (Fig. 3.1F). Common metabolites detected by MRS include N-acetylaspartate (NAA), creatine (Cr), choline (Cho), myoinositol (mI), and glutamine/glutamate (Glx). NAA is exclusive to the nervous system and is normally the highest peak; lower levels indicate neuronal loss. Cr is a marker of cell metabolism; its concentration is thought to remain relatively stable. Cho is a nonspecific marker of cell membrane turnover. Elevated mI signifies glial cell proliferation, such as in inflammation. Glx is directly involved in excitatory neurotransmission.[130] Head trauma may alter the levels of these metabolites, potentially impairing function.

MRS studies of mTBI differ in selection of voxel size and approach to metabolite localization, which affect the signal-to-noise ratio. Echo time can influence water suppression, peak appearance, and metabolite detection.[131] Metabolites can be reported as ratios or as absolute values. Ratios may require smaller sample sizes to show statistical significance, especially when both numerator and denominator shift in opposite directions. However, it is not always clear which shift (numerator or denominator) results in the observed difference. Absolute quantification may be preferable, although it requires additional steps and calibration.[132]

NAA is the most commonly reported metabolite in MRS studies. Many researchers have found a decrease in NAA/Cr ratio[133–137] and absolute NAA concentration[19,138,139] in mTBI. The size of decreased concentrations were as much as 18% for NAA/Cr[133,137] and 12% for whole-brain absolute NAA.[19] Lower NAA was reported globally and in WM regions of the frontal lobe, parietal lobe, prefrontal area, and genu of CC. The global NAA decrease reported by Kirov et al.[138] resulted completely from the WM and not GM pathology, suggesting metabolite perturbation from DAI. Several studies did not find significant differences in NAA levels between mTBI patients and controls.[140–144] A meta-analysis of TBI MRS data concluded that there is no significant change in NAA/Cr or Cho/Cr ratios in mTBI, although a decrease and increase, in both ratios respectively, was observed in severe TBI.[145] Moreover, researchers reported a higher Cr in mTBI compared to controls, specifically in WM.[146,147] Other metabolite concentrations are frequently reported as a ratio relative to Cr, and the stability of this metabolite as the reference denominator can be called into question. Other findings in mTBI include lower Glx in GM,[134,146,147] higher mI/Cr,[134,142] and both an increase[135] and decrease[140] in Cho/Cr.

Time since injury is an important consideration when comparing MRS results in the light of longitudinal metabolite changes. Vagnozzi et al.[133] measured a lower NAA/Cr in the mTBI group at 3 days with slight recovery at 15 days; at 30 days, the mTBI group was indistinguishable from controls, a result replicated with a larger sample.[137] Another group reported alterations in Cr and Glx at 15 days after injury, with normalization at 4 months.[147] In contrast, Henry et al.[134] does not show longitudinal normalization for all; NAA/Cr was lower in the mTBI group both acutely and chronically, Glx/Cr normalized in the primary motor region with time, and mI/Cr increased at the chronic time point. Nonetheless, there appears to be some variation with time, so caution must be used when creating study inclusion criteria for subjects with a wide range of injury onset times.

The link between metabolite perturbations and outcomes is not clear. Dean et al.[148] did not find an association between MRS findings and PCS, while Kirov et al.[149] did observe NAA disturbance in the PCS group which was absent in mTBI patients without PCS. Sivak et al.[150] found a correlation between frontal lobe NAA and performance on digit span backwards and Stroop color naming. Another group using Phosphorus-31 MRS noted lower nucleoside triphosphate (NTP) in mTBI.[151] Level of NTP, a substance involved in cell bioenergetics, was positively correlated with performance on neuropsychiatric testing.

A few studies examined metabolic changes after concussion in children. Maugans et al.[143] did not find any NAA differences over three time periods in youths with concussion compared to age-matched controls. A concussed pediatric group was found to have higher GABA/Cr, an inhibitory neurotransmitter.[152] Poole et al.[153] used a helmet tracking device in high school football players, and determined that number of subconcussive hits was correlated positively with Cr and negatively with Glx. The consequences of metabolic disturbances in these young brains is not yet clear.

MRS provides a fascinating window into mTBI-altered brain metabolism. Changes in metabolite concentrations potentially give insight into function on a cellular level—such as neuronal membrane stability, energetics, glial cell activation, and neurotransmission, but need to expand the effects on global function. Additional studies are needed with larger samples at distinct time points using homogenous acquisition and image processing protocols.

SUMMARY AND CONCLUSION

Advanced neuroimaging techniques have provided great insight into a neurological disease previously thought to be undetectable by standard diagnostic tools. The surge of research in the past two decades has documented an alteration in brain structure, functional connectivity, and metabolic processes, both in children and adults, even in milder forms. There are ample reports of advanced neuroimaging differences between mTBI subjects and controls, with uncertain relevance to mechanistic theories and low reproducibility of the findings. Consistencies in results support DAI, such as decreased FA in the CC, thalamic fibers, and in frontal lobe connections, as well as lower NAA levels in WM (Fig. 3.2).

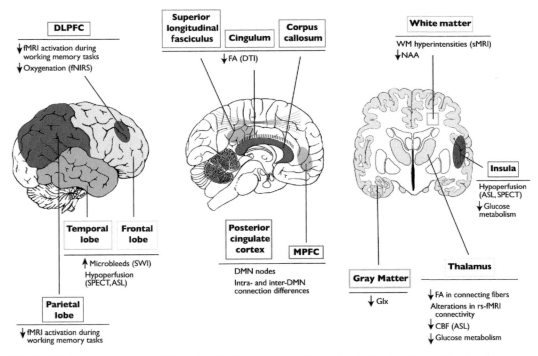

FIGURE 3.2 Summary of mTBI imaging findings, organized by anatomical region. See text for details.

Additionally, vasculature and CBF seem to be altered, as evidenced by microhemorrhages visualized on SWI and areas of hypoperfusion detected by ASL and SPECT. Metabolic and functional alterations include decreased level of neurotransmitter Glx in GM and altered task-based and resting-state connectivity as assessed by fMRI and fNIRS. Overall group level neuroimaging abnormalities across various modalities have been linked to worse outcomes, greater symptom severity, and poorer performance on neurocognitive tasks.

Perhaps the next step should explore how visualization of microlevel changes in cell and vascular architecture, along with cellular metabolism and integrity of neuronal networks, correspond to overall function and behavioral outcomes for patients. The location and nature of neural changes detected on imaging may indicate disruption of discrete processes, and the sum of which affect the whole in an unclear way. A patient-centered understanding of how and when a lesion leads to impairment is a worthwhile undertaking. Another goal of neuroimaging research may include a better understanding of disease course and affected structures, which will aid in prognostication and medical decision-making. The handful of longitudinal studies lend evidence to the evolving nature of this disease. It would be worthwhile to define biomarkers of damage, repair, and resolution (or lack thereof) in mTBI. This framework could be expanded to track deviations which may explain, and eventually predict, development of a more permanent and disabling disease. Evaluation of disease course with advanced neuroimaging may be applied holistically, including lifestyle counseling, focusing on return to school, work, or sport.

To achieve these goals, research should address inconsistencies in experimental design to expand on the promising, but not yet convincing, results. Comparison of studies is made difficult by heterogeneity of mTBI subjects, small sample sizes, and variation in data acquisition and analysis. The research will benefit from larger samples (including a subset of pediatric patients) tested at multiple discrete time points with standardized protocols, with clear functional measures consistently used. Choice of imaging modality must be carefully weighed against the hypothesis to be tested with risks and costs of imaging. A multimodal approach may be valuable, as an interplay of structure, metabolism, and function likely exists. Solid links between lesions and relevant functional outcomes will guide mTBI research toward meaningful findings for patients.

Acknowledgment

The authors thank Amy Martinez, MA, for designing and creating Fig. 3.2.

References

1. Centers for Disease Control and Prevention. *Report to Congress on traumatic brain injury in the United States: epidemiology and rehabilitation.* Atlanta, GA: National Center for Injury Prevention and Control; Division of Unintentional Injury Prevention; 2015.
2. Cassidy JD, Carroll LJ, Peloso PM, et al. Incidence, risk factors and prevention of mild traumatic brain injury: results of the WHO Collaborating Centre Task Force on Mild Traumatic Brain Injury. *J Rehabil Med* 2004;**36** (Suppl. 43):S28–60.
3. Rutherford WH, Merrett JD, McDonald JR. Symptoms at one year following concussion from minor head injuries. *Injury* 1979;**10**:225–30.

4. Management of Concussion-mild Traumatic Brain Injury Working Group. *VA/DoD clinical practice guideline for the management of concussion-mild traumatic brain injury.* Washington, D.C.: Department of Vetarans Affairs; Department of Defense, (Version 2.0), 2016, 1-133.

5. Kamins J, Giza CC. Concussion-mild traumatic brain injury: recoverable injury with potential for serious sequelae. *Neurosurg Clin North Am* 2016;**27**:441−52.

6. Tator CH, Davis HS, Dufort PA, et al. Postconcussion syndrome: demographics and predictors in 221 patients. *J Neurosurg* 2016;**125**:1206−16.

7. American Psychiatric Association. *Diagnostic and statistical manual of mental disorders.* 4th ed. Washington: American Psychiatric Association; 1994.

8. World Health Organization. *ICD-10 classification of mental and behavioural disorders: clinical descriptions and diagnostic guidelines.* Geneva: World Health Organization; 1992.

9. Stiell IG, Wells GA, Vandemheen K, et al. The Canadian CT Head Rule for patients with minor head injury. *Lancet (London, England)* 2001;**357**:1391−6.

10. Honce JM, Nyberg E, Jones I, Nagae L. Neuroimaging of concussion. *Phys. Med Rehabil Clin North Am* 2016;**27**:411−28.

11. Kan EM, Ling EA, Lu J. Microenvironment changes in mild traumatic brain injury. *Brain Res Bull* 2012;**87**:359−72.

12. Wintermark M, Sanelli PC, Anzai Y, Tsiouris AJ, Whitlow CT. Imaging evidence and recommendations for traumatic brain injury: conventional neuroimaging techniques. *J Am College Radiol* 2015;**12**:e1−e14.

13. Shenton ME, Hamoda HM, Schneiderman JS, et al. A review of magnetic resonance imaging and diffusion tensor imaging findings in mild traumatic brain injury. *Brain Imag Behav* 2012;**6**:137−92.

14. Yuh EL, Mukherjee P, Lingsma HF, et al. Magnetic resonance imaging improves 3-month outcome prediction in mild traumatic brain injury. *Ann Neurol* 2013;**73**:224−35.

15. Bigler ED, Abildskov TJ, Goodrich-Hunsaker NJ, et al. Structural neuroimaging findings in mild traumatic brain injury. *Sports Med Arthrosc Rev* 2016;**24**:e42−52.

16. Lu L, Cao H, Wei X, Li Y, Li W. Iron deposition is positively related to cognitive impairment in patients with chronic mild traumatic brain injury: assessment with susceptibility weighted imaging. *BioMed Res Int* 2015;**2015**:470676.

17. Tate DF, Gusman M, Kini J, et al. Susceptibility weighted imaging and white matter abnormality findings in service members with persistent cognitive symptoms following mild traumatic brain injury. *Military Med* 2017;**182**:e1651−8.

18. Hughes DG, Jackson A, Mason DL, Berry E, Hollis S, Yates DW. Abnormalities on magnetic resonance imaging seen acutely following mild traumatic brain injury: correlation with neuropsychological tests and delayed recovery. *Neuroradiology* 2004;**46**:550−8.

19. Cohen BA, Inglese M, Rusinek H, Babb JS, Grossman RI, Gonen O. Proton MR spectroscopy and MRI-volumetry in mild traumatic brain injury. *Am J Neuroradiol* 2007;**28**:907−13.

20. Tate DF, Wade BS, Velez CS, et al. Volumetric and shape analyses of subcortical structures in United States service members with mild traumatic brain injury. *J Neurol* 2016;**263**:2065−79.

21. Zhou Y, Kierans A, Kenul D, et al. Mild traumatic brain injury: longitudinal regional brain volume changes. *Radiology* 2013;**267**:880−90.

22. Terry DP, Miller LS. Repeated mild traumatic brain injuries is not associated with volumetric differences in former high school football players. *Brain Imag Behav* 2018;**12**:631-39.

23. Haacke EM, Mittal S, Wu Z, Neelavalli J, Cheng Y-CN. Susceptibility-weighted imaging: technical aspects and clinical applications, part 1. *Am J Neuroradiol* 2009;**30**:19−30.

24. Adams JH, Doyle D, Ford I, Gennarelli TA, Graham DI, McLellan DR. Diffuse axonal injury in head injury: definition, diagnosis and grading. *Histopathology* 1989;**15**:49−59.

25. de Haan S, de Groot JC, Jacobs B, van der Naalt J. The association between microhaemorrhages and post-traumatic functional outcome in the chronic phase after mild traumatic brain injury. *Neuroradiology* 2017;**59**(10):963−9.

26. Liu G, Ghimire P, Pang H, Wu G, Shi H. Improved sensitivity of 3.0 Tesla susceptibility-weighted imaging in detecting traumatic bleeds and its use in predicting outcomes in patients with mild traumatic brain injury. *Acta Radiol (Stockholm, Sweden: 1987)* 2015;**56**:1256−63.

27. van der Horn HJ, de Haan S, Spikman JM, de Groot JC, van der Naalt J. Clinical relevance of microhemorrhagic lesions in subacute mild traumatic brain injury. *Brain Imag Behav* 2018;**12**(3):912−16.

I. DEFINING MILD TBI

28. Babcock L, Yuan W, Leach J, Nash T, Wade S. White matter alterations in youth with acute mild traumatic brain injury. *J Pediatr Rehabil Med* 2015;**8**:285–96.

29. Assaf Y, Pasternak O. Diffusion tensor imaging (DTI)-based white matter mapping in brain research: a review. *J Molec Neurosci: MN* 2008;**34**:51–61.

30. Kou Z, Wu Z, Tong KA, et al. The role of advanced MR imaging findings as biomarkers of traumatic brain injury. *J Head Trauma Rehabil* 2010;**25**:267–82.

31. Alexander AL, Lee JE, Lazar M, Field AS. Diffusion tensor imaging of the brain. *Neurotherap: J Am Soc Exp NeuroTherapeut* 2007;**4**:316–29.

32. Conturo TE, Lori NF, Cull TS, et al. Tracking neuronal fiber pathways in the living human brain. *Proc Natl Acad Sci USA* 1999;**96**:10422–7.

33. Niogi SN, Mukherjee P. Diffusion tensor imaging of mild traumatic brain injury. *J Head Trauma Rehabil* 2010;**25**:241–55.

34. Panenka WJ, Lange RT, Bouix S, et al. Neuropsychological outcome and diffusion tensor imaging in complicated versus uncomplicated mild traumatic brain injury. *PLoS One* 2015;**10**:e0122746.

35. Yuh EL, Cooper SR, Mukherjee P, et al. Diffusion tensor imaging for outcome prediction in mild traumatic brain injury: a TRACK-TBI study. *J Neurotrauma* 2014;**31**:1457–77.

36. Hulkower MB, Poliak DB, Rosenbaum SB, Zimmerman ME, Lipton ML. A decade of DTI in traumatic brain injury: 10 years and 100 articles later. *Am J Neuroradiol* 2013;**34**:2064–74.

37. Lipton ML, Kim N, Park YK, et al. Robust detection of traumatic axonal injury in individual mild traumatic brain injury patients: intersubject variation, change over time and bidirectional changes in anisotropy. *Brain Imaging Behav* 2012;**6**:329–42.

38. Kim N, Branch CA, Kim M, Lipton ML. Whole brain approaches for identification of microstructural abnormalities in individual patients: comparison of techniques applied to mild traumatic brain injury. *PLoS One* 2013;**8**:e59382.

39. Angeli SI, Bared A, Ouyang X, Du LL, Yan D, Zhong Liu X. Audioprofiles and antioxidant enzyme genotypes in presbycusis. *The Laryngoscope* 2012;**122**:2539–42.

40. Aoki Y, Inokuchi R. A voxel-based meta-analysis of diffusion tensor imaging in mild traumatic brain injury. *Neurosci Biobehav Rev* 2016;**66**:119–26.

41. Murugavel M, Cubon V, Putukian M, et al. A longitudinal diffusion tensor imaging study assessing white matter fiber tracts after sports-related concussion. *J Neurotrauma* 2014;**31**:1860–71.

42. Narayana PA, Yu X, Hasan KM, et al. Multi-modal MRI of mild traumatic brain injury. *NeuroImage Clin* 2015;**7**:87–97.

43. Veeramuthu V, Narayanan V, Kuo TL, et al. Diffusion tensor imaging parameters in mild traumatic brain injury and its correlation with early neuropsychological impairment: a longitudinal study. *J Neurotrauma* 2015;**32**:1497–509.

44. Ling JM, Pena A, Yeo RA, et al. Biomarkers of increased diffusion anisotropy in semi-acute mild traumatic brain injury: a longitudinal perspective. *Brain: J Neurol* 2012;**135**:1281–92.

45. Mayer AR, Ling J, Mannell MV, et al. A prospective diffusion tensor imaging study in mild traumatic brain injury. *Neurology* 2010;**74**:643–50.

46. Khong E, Odenwald N, Hashim E, Cusimano MD. Diffusion tensor imaging findings in post-concussion syndrome patients after mild traumatic brain injury: a systematic review. *Front Neurol* 2016;**7**:156.

47. Messe A, Caplain S, Paradot G, et al. Diffusion tensor imaging and white matter lesions at the subacute stage in mild traumatic brain injury with persistent neurobehavioral impairment. *Human Brain Map* 2011;**32**:999–1011.

48. Fakhran S, Yaeger K, Collins M, Alhilali L. Sex differences in white matter abnormalities after mild traumatic brain injury: localization and correlation with outcome. *Radiology* 2014;**272**:815–23.

49. Van Beek L, Ghesquiere P, Lagae L, De Smedt B. Mathematical difficulties and white matter abnormalities in subacute pediatric mild traumatic brain injury. *J Neurotrauma* 2015;**32**:1567–78.

50. Van Beek L, Vanderauwera J, Ghesquiere P, Lagae L, De Smedt B. Longitudinal changes in mathematical abilities and white matter following paediatric mild traumatic brain injury. *Brain Injury* 2015;**29**:1701–10.

51. Wintermark M, Sanelli PC, Anzai Y, Tsiouris AJ, Whitlow CT. Imaging evidence and recommendations for traumatic brain injury: advanced neuro- and neurovascular imaging techniques. *Am J Neuroradiol* 2015;**36**:E1–e11.

52. Steven AJ, Zhuo J, Melhem ER. Diffusion kurtosis imaging: an emerging technique for evaluating the microstructural environment of the brain. *Am J Roentgenol* 2014;**202**:W26–33.

53. Grossman EJ, Ge Y, Jensen JH, et al. Thalamus and cognitive impairment in mild traumatic brain injury: a diffusional kurtosis imaging study. *J Neurotrauma* 2012;**29**:2318−27.

54. Grossman EJ, Jensen JH, Babb JS, et al. Cognitive impairment in mild traumatic brain injury: a longitudinal diffusional kurtosis and perfusion imaging study. *Am J Neuroradiol* 2013;**34** 951-7, s1-3.

55. Stokum JA, Sours C, Zhuo J, Kane R, Shanmuganathan K, Gullapalli RP. A longitudinal evaluation of diffusion kurtosis imaging in patients with mild traumatic brain injury. *Brain Injury* 2015;**29**:47−57.

56. Arthurs OJ, Boniface S. How well do we understand the neural origins of the fMRI BOLD signal? *Trends Neurosci* 2002;**25**:27−31.

57. Detre JA, Leigh JS, Williams DS, Koretsky AP. Perfusion imaging. *Magn Reson Med* 1992;**23**:37−45.

58. Detre JA, Rao H, Wang DJ, Chen YF, Wang Z. Applications of arterial spin labeled MRI in the brain. *J Magn Reson Imaging* 2012;**35**:1026−37.

59. Bryer EJ, Medaglia JD, Rostami S, Hillary FG. Neural recruitment after mild traumatic brain injury is task dependent: a meta-analysis. *J Int Neuropsychol Soc* 2013;**19**:751−62.

60. Mayer AR, Mannell MV, Ling J, et al. Auditory orienting and inhibition of return in mild traumatic brain injury: a FMRI study. *Human Brain Map* 2009;**30**:4152−66.

61. Gosselin N, Bottari C, Chen JK, et al. Electrophysiology and functional MRI in post-acute mild traumatic brain injury. *J Neurotrauma* 2011;**28**:329−41.

62. McAllister TW, Saykin AJ, Flashman LA, et al. Brain activation during working memory 1 month after mild traumatic brain injury: a functional MRI study. *Neurology* 1999;**53**:1300−8.

63. Zhang K, Johnson B, Pennell D, Ray W, Sebastianelli W, Slobounov S. Are functional deficits in concussed individuals consistent with white matter structural alterations: combined FMRI & DTI study. *Exp Brain Res* 2010;**204**:57−70.

64. Lovell MR, Pardini JE, Welling J, et al. Functional brain abnormalities are related to clinical recovery and time to return-to-play in athletes. *Neurosurgery* 2007;**61**:352−9 discussion 9−60.

65. Jantzen KJ, Anderson B, Steinberg FL, Kelso JA. A prospective functional MR imaging study of mild traumatic brain injury in college football players. *Am J Neuroradiol* 2004;**25**:738−45.

66. Witt ST, Lovejoy DW, Pearlson GD, Stevens MC. Decreased prefrontal cortex activity in mild traumatic brain injury during performance of an auditory oddball task. *Brain Imaging Behav* 2010;**4**:232−47.

67. Pardini JE, Pardini DA, Becker JT, et al. Postconcussive symptoms are associated with compensatory cortical recruitment during a working memory task. *Neurosurgery* 2010;**67**:1020−7 discussion 7−8.

68. Chen JK, Johnston KM, Petrides M, Ptito A. Recovery from mild head injury in sports: evidence from serial functional magnetic resonance imaging studies in male athletes. *Clin J Sport Med: Offic J Canadian Acad Sport Med* 2008;**18**:241−7.

69. Wylie GR, Freeman K, Thomas A, et al. Cognitive improvement after mild traumatic brain injury measured with functional neuroimaging during the acute period. *PLoS One* 2015;**10**:e0126110.

70. McAllister TW, Flashman LA, McDonald BC, Saykin AJ. Mechanisms of working memory dysfunction after mild and moderate TBI: evidence from functional MRI and neurogenetics. *J Neurotrauma* 2006;**23**:1450−67.

71. Park HJ, Friston K. Structural and functional brain networks: from connections to cognition. *Science (New York, NY)*. 2013;**342**:1238411.

72. Buckner RL, Andrews-Hanna JR, Schacter DL. The brain's default network: anatomy, function, and relevance to disease. *Ann NY Acad Sci* 2008;**1124**:1−38.

73. Johnson B, Zhang K, Gay M, et al. Alteration of brain default network in subacute phase of injury in concussed individuals: resting-state fMRI study. *NeuroImage* 2012;**59**:511−18.

74. Mayer AR, Mannell MV, Ling J, Gasparovic C, Yeo RA. Functional connectivity in mild traumatic brain injury. *Human Brain Map* 2011;**32**:1825−35.

75. Zhou Y, Milham MP, Lui YW, et al. Default-mode network disruption in mild traumatic brain injury. *Radiology* 2012;**265**:882−92.

76. Abbas K, Shenk TE, Poole VN, et al. Alteration of default mode network in high school football athletes due to repetitive subconcussive mild traumatic brain injury: a resting-state functional magnetic resonance imaging study. *Brain Connect* 2015;**5**:91−101.

77. Zhang K, Johnson B, Gay M, et al. Default mode network in concussed individuals in response to the YMCA physical stress test. *J Neurotrauma* 2012;**29**:756−65.

78. Sours C, Zhuo J, Roys S, Shanmuganathan K, Gullapalli RP. Disruptions in resting state functional connectivity and cerebral blood flow in mild traumatic brain injury patients. *PLoS One* 2015;**10**:e0134019.

I. DEFINING MILD TBI

79. Stevens MC, Lovejoy D, Kim J, Oakes H, Kureshi I, Witt ST. Multiple resting state network functional connectivity abnormalities in mild traumatic brain injury. *Brain Imaging Behav* 2012;**6**:293–318.
80. van der Horn HJ, Liemburg EJ, Scheenen ME, et al. Brain network dysregulation, emotion, and complaints after mild traumatic brain injury. *Human Brain Map* 2016;**37**:1645–54.
81. Shumskaya E, Andriessen TM, Norris DG, Vos PE. Abnormal whole-brain functional networks in homogeneous acute mild traumatic brain injury. *Neurology* 2012;**79**:175–82.
82. Tang L, Ge Y, Sodickson DK, et al. Thalamic resting-state functional networks: disruption in patients with mild traumatic brain injury. *Radiology* 2011;**260**:831–40.
83. Nordin LE, Moller MC, Julin P, Bartfai A, Hashim F, Li TQ. Post mTBI fatigue is associated with abnormal brain functional connectivity. *Sci Reports* 2016;**6**:21183.
84. Banks SD, Coronado RA, Clemons LR, et al. Thalamic functional connectivity in mild traumatic brain injury: longitudinal associations with patient-reported outcomes and neuropsychological tests. *Arch Phys Med Rehabil* 2016;**97**:1254–61.
85. Dall'Acqua P, Johannes S, Mica L, et al. Functional and structural network recovery after mild traumatic brain injury: a 1-year longitudinal study. *Front Human Neurosci* 2017;**11**:280.
86. Messe A, Caplain S, Pelegrini-Issac M, et al. Specific and evolving resting-state network alterations in post-concussion syndrome following mild traumatic brain injury. *PLoS One* 2013;**8**:e65470.
87. Keightley ML, Saluja RS, Chen JK, et al. A functional magnetic resonance imaging study of working memory in youth after sports-related concussion: is it still working? *J Neurotrauma* 2014;**31**:437–51.
88. Westfall DR, West JD, Bailey JN, et al. Increased brain activation during working memory processing after pediatric mild traumatic brain injury (mTBI). *J Pediatr Rehabil Med* 2015;**8**:297–308.
89. Krivitzky LS, Roebuck-Spencer TM, Roth RM, Blackstone K, Johnson CP, Gioia G. Functional magnetic resonance imaging of working memory and response inhibition in children with mild traumatic brain injury. *J Int Neuropsychol Soc* 2011;**17**:1143–52.
90. Yang Z, Yeo RA, Pena A, et al. An FMRI study of auditory orienting and inhibition of return in pediatric mild traumatic brain injury. *J Neurotrauma* 2012;**29**:2124–36.
91. Ellis MJ, Ryner LN, Sobczyk O, et al. Neuroimaging assessment of cerebrovascular reactivity in concussion: current concepts, methodological considerations, and review of the literature. *Front Neurol* 2016;**7**:61.
92. Astafiev SV, Shulman GL, Metcalf NV, et al. Abnormal white matter blood-oxygen-level-dependent signals in chronic mild traumatic brain injury. *J Neurotrauma* 2015;**32**:1254–71.
93. Ge Y, Patel MB, Chen Q, et al. Assessment of thalamic perfusion in patients with mild traumatic brain injury by true FISP arterial spin labelling MR imaging at 3T. *Brain Injury* 2009;**23**:666–74.
94. Lin CM, Tseng YC, Hsu HL, et al. Arterial spin labeling perfusion study in the patients with subacute mild traumatic brain injury. *PLoS One* 2016;**11**:e0149109.
95. Meier TB, Bellgowan PS, Singh R, Kuplicki R, Polanski DW, Mayer AR. Recovery of cerebral blood flow following sports-related concussion. *JAMA Neurol* 2015;**72**:530–8.
96. Militana AR, Donahue MJ, Sills AK, et al. Alterations in default-mode network connectivity may be influenced by cerebrovascular changes within 1 week of sports related concussion in college varsity athletes: a pilot study. *Brain Imaging Behav* 2016;**10**:559–68.
97. Churchill NW, Hutchison MG, Graham SJ, Schweizer TA. Symptom correlates of cerebral blood flow following acute concussion. *NeuroImage Clin* 2017;**16**:234–9.
98. Doshi H, Wiseman N, Liu J, et al. Cerebral hemodynamic changes of mild traumatic brain injury at the acute stage. *PLoS One* 2015;**10**:e0118061.
99. Moller MC, Nordin LE, Bartfai A, Julin P, Li TQ. Fatigue and cognitive fatigability in mild traumatic brain injury are correlated with altered neural activity during vigilance test performance. *Front Neurol* 2017;**8**:496.
100. Stephens JA, Liu P, Lu H, Suskauer SJ. Cerebral blood flow after mild traumatic brain injury: associations between symptoms and post-injury perfusion. *J Neurotrauma* 2018;**35**(2):241–8.
101. Wang Y, West JD, Bailey JN, et al. Decreased cerebral blood flow in chronic pediatric mild TBI: an MRI perfusion study. *Dev Neuropsychol* 2015;**40**:40–4.
102. Barlow KM, Marcil LD, Dewey D, et al. Cerebral perfusion changes in post-concussion syndrome: a prospective controlled cohort study. *J Neurotrauma* 2017;**34**:996–1004.
103. Liu W, Wang B, Wolfowitz R, et al. Perfusion deficits in patients with mild traumatic brain injury characterized by dynamic susceptibility contrast MRI. *NMR Biomed* 2013;**26**:651–63.

104. Irani F, Platek SM, Bunce S, Ruocco AC, Chute D. Functional near infrared spectroscopy (fNIRS): an emerging neuroimaging technology with important applications for the study of brain disorders. *Clin Neuropsychol* 2007;**21**:9−37.

105. Kontos AP, Huppert TJ, Beluk NH, et al. Brain activation during neurocognitive testing using functional near-infrared spectroscopy in patients following concussion compared to healthy controls. *Brain Imaging Behav* 2014;**8**:621−34.

106. Helmich I, Saluja RS, Lausberg H, et al. Persistent postconcussive symptoms are accompanied by decreased functional brain oxygenation. *J Neuropsychiatry Clin Neurosci* 2015;**27**:287−98.

107. Bishop SA, Neary JP. Assessing prefrontal cortex oxygenation after sport concussion with near-infrared spectroscopy. *Clin Physiol Function Imaging* 2018;**38**(4):573−85.

108. Accorsi R, Brain Single-Photon Emission CT. Physics principles. *Am J Neuroradiol* 2008;**29**:1247−56.

109. Jacobs A, Put E, Ingels M, Put T, Bossuyt A. One-year follow-up of technetium-99m-HMPAO SPECT in mild head injury. *J Nuclear Med: Offic Publicat Soc Nuclear Med* 1996;**37**:1605−9.

110. Masdeu JC, Van Heertum RL, Kleiman A, et al. Early single-photon emission computed tomography in mild head trauma. A controlled study. *J Neuroimaging: Offic J Am Soc Neuroimaging* 1994;**4**:177−81.

111. Bonne O, Gilboa A, Louzoun Y, et al. Cerebral blood flow in chronic symptomatic mild traumatic brain injury. *Psychiatry Res* 2003;**124**:141−52.

112. Gowda NK, Agrawal D, Bal C, et al. Technetium Tc-99m ethyl cysteinate dimer brain single-photon emission CT in mild traumatic brain injury: a prospective study. *Am J Neuroradiol* 2006;**27**:447−51.

113. Amen DG, Willeumier K, Omalu B, Newberg A, Raghavendra C, Raji CA. Perfusion neuroimaging abnormalities alone distinguish national football league players from a healthy population. *J Alzheimer's Disease* 2016;**53**:237−41.

114. Hattori N, Swan M, Stobbe GA, et al. Differential SPECT activation patterns associated with PASAT performance may indicate frontocerebellar functional dissociation in chronic mild traumatic brain injury. *J Nuclear Med: Offic Publicat Soc Nuclear Med* 2009;**50**:1054−61.

115. Lewine JD, Davis JT, Bigler ED, et al. Objective documentation of traumatic brain injury subsequent to mild head trauma: multimodal brain imaging with MEG, SPECT, and MRI. *J Head Trauma Rehabil* 2007;**22**:141−55.

116. Romero K, Lobaugh NJ, Black SE, Ehrlich L, Feinstein A. Old wine in new bottles: validating the clinical utility of SPECT in predicting cognitive performance in mild traumatic brain injury. *Psychiatry Res* 2015;**231**:15−24.

117. Reivich M, Kuhl D, Wolf A, et al. The [18F]fluorodeoxyglucose method for the measurement of local cerebral glucose utilization in man. *Circulat Res* 1979;**44**:127−37.

118. Byrnes KR, Wilson CM, Brabazon F, et al. FDG-PET imaging in mild traumatic brain injury: a critical review. *Front Neuroenerg* 2014;**5**:13.

119. Abu-Judeh HH, Singh M, Masdeu JC, Abdel-Dayem HM. Discordance between FDG uptake and technetium-99m-HMPAO brain perfusion in acute traumatic brain injury. *J Nuclear Med: Offic Publicat Soc Nuclear Med* 1998;**39**:1357−9.

120. Petrie EC, Cross DJ, Yarnykh VL, et al. Neuroimaging, behavioral, and psychological sequelae of repetitive combined blast/impact mild traumatic brain injury in Iraq and Afghanistan war veterans. *J Neurotrauma* 2014;**31**:425−36.

121. Stocker RP, Cieply MA, Paul B, et al. Combat-related blast exposure and traumatic brain injury influence brain glucose metabolism during REM sleep in military veterans. *NeuroImage* 2014;**99**:207−14.

122. Chen SH, Kareken DA, Fastenau PS, Trexler LE, Hutchins GD. A study of persistent post-concussion symptoms in mild head trauma using positron emission tomography. *J Neurol Neurosurg Psychiatry* 2003;**74**:326−32.

123. Ruff RM, Crouch JA, Troster AI, et al. Selected cases of poor outcome following a minor brain trauma: comparing neuropsychological and positron emission tomography assessment. *Brain Injury* 1994;**8**:297−308.

124. Gross H, Kling A, Henry G, Herndon C, Lavretsky H. Local cerebral glucose metabolism in patients with long-term behavioral and cognitive deficits following mild traumatic brain injury. *J Neuropsychiatry Clin Neurosci* 1996;**8**:324−34.

125. Buchsbaum MS, Simmons AN, DeCastro A, Farid N, Matthews SC. Clusters of Low (18)F-fluorodeoxyglucose uptake voxels in combat veterans with traumatic brain injury and post-traumatic stress disorder. *J Neurotrauma* 2015;**32**:1736−50.

126. Small GW, Kepe V, Siddarth P, et al. PET scanning of brain tau in retired national football league players: preliminary findings. *Am J Geriatric Psychiatry: Offic J Am Assoc Geriatric Psychiatry* 2013;**21**:138−44.

127. Barrio JR, Small GW, Wong KP, et al. In vivo characterization of chronic traumatic encephalopathy using [F-18]FDDNP PET brain imaging. *Proc Natl Acad Sci USA* 2015;**112**:E2039–47.
128. Coughlin JM, Wang Y, Minn I, et al. Imaging of glial cell activation and white matter integrity in brains of active and recently retired national football league players. *JAMA Neurol* 2017;**74**:67–74.
129. Coughlin JM, Wang Y, Munro CA, et al. Neuroinflammation and brain atrophy in former NFL players: an in vivo multimodal imaging pilot study. *Neurobiol Disease* 2015;**74**:58–65.
130. Bertholdo D, Watcharakorn A, Castillo M. Brain proton magnetic resonance spectroscopy: introduction and overview. *Neuroimaging Clin North Am* 2013;**23**:359–80.
131. Gardner A, Iverson GL, Stanwell P. A systematic review of proton magnetic resonance spectroscopy findings in sport-related concussion. *J Neurotrauma* 2014;**31**:1–18.
132. Hoch SE, Kirov II, Tal A. When are metabolic ratios superior to absolute quantification? A statistical analysis. *NMR Biomed* 2017;**30**.
133. Vagnozzi R, Signoretti S, Tavazzi B, et al. Temporal window of metabolic brain vulnerability to concussion: a pilot 1H-magnetic resonance spectroscopic study in concussed athletes--part III. *Neurosurgery* 2008;**62**: 1286–95 discussion95-6.
134. Henry LC, Tremblay S, Leclerc S, et al. Metabolic changes in concussed American football players during the acute and chronic post-injury phases. *BMC Neurol* 2011;**11**:105.
135. Govindaraju V, Gauger GE, Manley GT, Ebel A, Meeker M, Maudsley AA. Volumetric proton spectroscopic imaging of mild traumatic brain injury. *Am J Neuroradiol* 2004;**25**:730–7.
136. Johnson B, Gay M, Zhang K, et al. The use of magnetic resonance spectroscopy in the subacute evaluation of athletes recovering from single and multiple mild traumatic brain injury. *J Neurotrauma* 2012;**29**:2297–304.
137. Vagnozzi R, Signoretti S, Cristofori L, et al. Assessment of metabolic brain damage and recovery following mild traumatic brain injury: a multicentre, proton magnetic resonance spectroscopic study in concussed patients. *Brain: J Neurol* 2010;**133**:3232–42.
138. Kirov II, Tal A, Babb JS, Lui YW, Grossman RI, Gonen O. Diffuse axonal injury in mild traumatic brain injury: a 3D multivoxel proton MR spectroscopy study. *J Neurol* 2013;**260**:242–52.
139. Grossman EJ, Kirov II, Gonen O, et al. N-Acetyl-aspartate levels correlate with intra-axonal compartment parameters from diffusion MRI. *NeuroImage* 2015;**118**:334–43.
140. George EO, Roys S, Sours C, et al. Longitudinal and prognostic evaluation of mild traumatic brain injury: a 1H-magnetic resonance spectroscopy study. *J Neurotrauma* 2014;**31**:1018–28.
141. Kirov I, Fleysher L, Babb JS, Silver JM, Grossman RI, Gonen O. Characterizing 'mild' in traumatic brain injury with proton MR spectroscopy in the thalamus: initial findings. *Brain Injury* 2007;**21**:1147–54.
142. Kierans AS, Kirov II, Gonen O, et al. Myoinositol and glutamate complex neurometabolite abnormality after mild traumatic brain injury. *Neurology* 2014;**82**:521–8.
143. Maugans TA, Farley C, Altaye M, Leach J, Cecil KM. Pediatric sports-related concussion produces cerebral blood flow alterations. *Pediatrics* 2012;**129**:28–37.
144. Chamard E, Lassonde M, Henry L, et al. Neurometabolic and microstructural alterations following a sports-related concussion in female athletes. *Brain Injury* 2013;**27**:1038–46.
145. Brown M, Baradaran H, Christos PJ, Wright D, Gupta A, Tsiouris AJ. Magnetic resonance spectroscopy abnormalities in traumatic brain injury: a meta-analysis. *J Neuroradiol* 2018;**45**(2):123–9.
146. Gasparovic C, Yeo R, Mannell M, et al. Neurometabolite concentrations in gray and white matter in mild traumatic brain injury: an 1H-magnetic resonance spectroscopy study. *J Neurotrauma* 2009;**26**:1635–43.
147. Yeo RA, Gasparovic C, Merideth F, Ruhl D, Doezema D, Mayer AR. A longitudinal proton magnetic resonance spectroscopy study of mild traumatic brain injury. *J Neurotrauma* 2011;**28**:1–11.
148. Dean PJ, Otaduy MC, Harris LM, McNamara A, Seiss E, Sterr A. Monitoring long-term effects of mild traumatic brain injury with magnetic resonance spectroscopy: a pilot study. *Neuroreport* 2013;**24**:677–81.
149. Kirov II, Tal A, Babb JS, et al. Proton MR spectroscopy correlates diffuse axonal abnormalities with post-concussive symptoms in mild traumatic brain injury. *J Neurotrauma* 2013;**30**:1200–4.
150. Sivak S, Bittsansky M, Grossmann J, et al. Clinical correlations of proton magnetic resonance spectroscopy findings in acute phase after mild traumatic brain injury. *Brain Injury* 2014;**28**:341–6.
151. Sikoglu EM, Liso Navarro AA, Czerniak SM, et al. Effects of recent concussion on brain bioenergetics: a phosphorus-31 magnetic resonance spectroscopy study. *Cognit behav Neurol: Offic J Soc Behav Cognit Neurol* 2015;**28**:181–7.

152. Friedman SD, Poliakov AV, Budech C, et al. GABA alterations in pediatric sport concussion. *Neurology* 2017;**89**:2151−6.

153. Poole VN, Breedlove EL, Shenk TE, et al. Sub-concussive hit characteristics predict deviant brain metabolism in football athletes. *Dev Neuropsychol* 2015;**40**:12−17.

154. Wu Z, Mazzola CA, Catania L, et al. Altered cortical activation and connectivity patterns for visual attention processing in young adults post-traumatic brain injury: A functional near infrared spectroscopy study. *CNS neuroscience & therapeutics* 2018;**24**:539−48.

Defining Cure

Martin Slade, PhD[1] and Michael E. Hoffer, MD[2]

[1]Medicine and Public Health, Yale University, New Haven, CT, United States [2]Department of Otolaryngology and Neurological Surgery, University of Miami, Miller School of Medicine, Miami, FL, United States

Merriam-Webster defines cure as "a complete or permanent solution or remedy."[1] In practice, the notion of cure is much less tangible. For some diseases, cure is fairly straightforward and is used only when the disease is absent and has not recurred for a sufficient period of time. This is particularly true in oncology where cancer cures are well defined and the period of time necessary to be free from disease has been established. However, for most diseases, being free of symptoms can be considered being cured and this is where the notion of cure becomes more difficult to establish. This is particularly true when the disorder is poorly understood or the pathophysiology difficult to monitor in an exact fashion. Consider a migraine patient who is free of migraine headaches for the past 5 years. The individual might consider themselves cured, but it is difficult to say that the migraines are actually cured since tracking the pathologies of migraines and establishing that the particular pathology no longer exists is difficult to establish given current medical science. It might be more accurate to refer to this individual as controlled, but in modern usage many individuals use the term controlled to refer to conditions that are being managed with some type of therapeutic option. Consider, as well, a variety of musculoskeletal injuries. A broken bone can be mended and after the cast is removed and therapy is conducted the individual who suffered the break may be free from any symptoms, but is that broken bone truly "cured." Even plain film X-rays will show evidence of the old fracture throughout the person's lifetime.

In addition to being difficult to define, the notion of "cure" is temporal and related only to the current time because almost every disease entity once cured can be "uncured." Consider the three examples above; the cancer can recur, the migraines can begin again, and the once-broken bone can become a source of arthritis or a weak spot for a future facture. Even the most simple of cures where a bacterial infection is eradicated with antibiotics can leave the affected area of the body at risk for future infections and complications many years later.

So, if the notion of cure is difficult to fully describe and temporal in nature, applying such a concept to mild traumatic brain injury is an even more difficult challenge. Mild traumatic brain injury is a heterogeneous disorder that can be associated with a variety of sequelae. Describing resolution of these sequelae may be difficult to achieve but very possible. The individual may report no more headaches or dizziness and objective tests of vestibular function may largely normalize. However, symptom resolution alone is not entirely indicative or even necessary for a cure. In one scenario the symptoms may be relieved, but the injury to the brain itself may still persist.[2] In another scenario an individual could, theoretically, have a persistence of symptoms from a pathology that arose due to the brain injury or associated with the injury itself, but the brain itself may be totally healed.[3] An individual might, for instance, have a neck injury at the same time as a head injury and have a persistent headache due to the neck injury even after the brain has "entirely" healed.

The cure of mTBI involves brain healing which has been difficult to achieve or document. Most of the work in the area to date has been aimed at reducing or treating injury sequelae rather than addressing the primary pathophysiology of the disorder. Current strategies and developments in this area will be examined in this book. However, there have been a variety of strategies that have been utilized to address the issue of brain healing by reducing the volume or degree of injury in the first place. Some of these strategies have also been advocated to treat the sequelae of mTBI. Pharmaceutical countermeasures designed to limit the area of damage have included medicines with antioxidant, antiinflammatory, and antiapoptotic properties.[4–6] Other strategies to induce brain repair include limiting the volume of injury and inducing repair through blood flow and gene changes utilizing hypothermia or factors that directly affect nitric oxide metabolism.[7–10] Many investigators have begun to capitalize on successful trials in spinal cord injury and have examined stem cells use as a method for repopulating lost neurons.[11] This area of research holds tremendous promise and likely will be one of the most important advances in head injury treatment in the next several years. Finally, hyperbaric oxygen has been tried with mixed results.[12]

Whether or not mTBI can be truly cured, the most important question is when is it safe and appropriate for an individual to return to work, school, or play. For some individuals this may be simply based on symptoms and the ability to tolerate and perform job duties while symptom-free. But for other individuals, especially those engaged in activities like sports or the military, where the possibility of another injury is very real, determining when it is safe for that individual to return to work or play is a much more challenging issue. The impact of subsequent concussions has been a challenge for investigators. This is in part due to nomenclature of the so called "Second Impact Syndrome."[13] This nosology issue aside, there is solid scientific evidence demonstrating that the physiologic changes seen in initial injury are intensified and longer lasting with subsequent injury.[14,15] This work, as well as observations from the field, has resulted in most individuals concluding that subsequent impacts are potentially more harmful than a single impact.[16] The exact consequences are probably related to a great number of variables including the intensity and type of the impacts, the amount of time between the impacts, and the number of previous impacts. There is clearly a great deal of work to do in this area.

Almost as important as defining when an individual is clear to return to work is providing accurate prognostic estimates. This step is a critical component of caring for individuals with this disorder. Unfortunately, due to the heterogeneity of the disorder, the variable effects of the disorder on different individuals, a host of social issues, and the variability in medical care, predicting when a patient will be suitable to return to activities is very difficult. Tests designed to diagnose the disorder often do not have prognostic value[17,18] or have a variety of variables which can place a patient into a response category, but do not provide even remotely accurate prediction of response time.[19,20] Work is underway in our laboratory to examine novel test findings in the early and subacute periods to provide prognostic information to individuals, their work, their school, or their team.

Clearly there is a great deal of work to be done in evaluating the elements of cure in mTBI. Basic science work must continue to examine biomarkers, imaging, and functional tests that can truly determine when symptoms have resolved and when the brain has healed. Studies have to be done to evaluate the impact of subsequent concussions in the context of frequency, type, and force. Work must continue on developing tests and evaluations that not only provide information on when it is safe to return to work or play, but can estimate that day in advance. As health care advances we believe that the term "cure" will be made more clear and enabling learning how to best apply a range of test and treatment options that are specific to the affected individual and to the injury they experienced. It is incumbent on science and medicine to take the steps necessary to make this a reality.

References

1. https://www.merriam-webster.com/dictionary/cure.
2. Kamins J, Bigler E, Covassin T, Henry L, Kemp S, Leddy JJ, et al. What is the physiological time to recovery after concussion? A systematic review. *Br J Sports Med* 2017;**51**(12):935−40. Available from: https://doi.org/10.1136/bjsports-2016-097464. Epub 2017 Apr 28. Review. PubMed PMID: 28455363.
3. Kennedy E, Quinn D, Tumilty S, Chapple CM. Clinical characteristics and outcomes of treatment of the cervical spine in patients with persistent post-concussion symptoms: a retrospective analysis. *Musculoskelet Sci Pract* 2017;**29**:91−8. Available from: https://doi.org/10.1016/j.msksp.2017.03.002. Epub 2017 Mar 14. PubMed PMID: 28347935.
4. Hoffer ME, Balaban C, Slade MD, Tsao JW, Hoffer B. Amelioration of acute sequelae of blast induced mild traumatic brain injury by N-acetyl cysteine: a double-blind, placebo controlled study. *PLoS One* 2013;**8**(1): e54163. Available from: https://doi.org/10.1371/journal.pone.0054163.
5. Eakin K, Baratz-Goldstein R, Pick CG, Zindel O, Balaban CD, Hoffer ME, et al. Efficacy of N-acetyl cysteine in traumatic brain injury. *PLoS One* 2014;**9**(4):e90617. Available from: https://doi.org/10.1371/journal.pone.0090617.
6. Mei Z, Qiu J, Alcon S, Hashim J, Rotenberg A, Sun Y, et al. Memantine improves outcomes after repetitive traumatic brain injury. *Behav Brain Res* 2017. pii: S0166-4328(17)30621-6. doi: 10.1016/j.bbr.2017.04.017. [Epub ahead of print] PubMed PMID: 28412305.
7. Dietrich WD, Alonso O, Busto R, Globus MY, Ginsberg MD. Post-traumatic brain hypothermia reduces histopathological damage following concussive brain injury in the rat. *Acta Neuropathol* 1994;**87**(3):250−8 PubMed PMID: 8009957.
8. Koizumi H, Fujisawa H, Ito H, Maekawa T, Di X, Bullock R. Effects of mild hypothermia on cerebral blood flow-independent changes in cortical extracellular levels of amino acids following contusion trauma in the rat. *Brain Res* 1997;**747**(2):304−12 PubMed PMID: 9046006.

9. Matsushita M, Yonemori F, Furukawa N, Ohta A, Toide K, Uchida I, et al. Effects of the novel thyrotropin-releasing hormone analogue Na-((1S,2R)-2-methyl-4-oxocyclopentylcarbonyl)-L-histidyl-L-prol ina mide monohydrate on the central nervous system in mice and rats. *Arzneimittelforschung* 1993;**43**(8):813−17 PubMed PMID: 8216433.

10. Khan M, Khan H, Singh I, Singh AK. Hypoxia inducible factor-1 alpha stabilization for regenerative therapy in traumatic brain injury. *Neural Regen Res* 2017;**12**(5):696−701. Available from: https://doi.org/10.4103/1673-5374.206632. Review. PubMed PMID: 28616019; PubMed Central PMCID: PMC5461600.

11. Torper O, Götz M. Brain repair from intrinsic cell sources: turning reactive glia into neurons. *Prog Brain Res* 2017;**230**:69−97. Available from: https://doi.org/10.1016/bs.pbr.2016.12.010. Epub 2017 Feb 7. PubMed PMID: 28552236.

12. Figueroa XA, Wright JK. Hyperbaric oxygen: B-level evidence in mild traumatic brain injury clinical trials. *Neurology* 2016;**87**(13):1400−6. Available from: https://doi.org/10.1212/WNL.0000000000003146. Epub2016 Aug 31. Review. PubMed PMID: 27581219.

13. Stovitz SD, Weseman JD, Hooks MC, Schmidt RJ, Koffel JB, Patricios JS. What definition is used to describe second impact syndrome in sports? A systematic and critical review. *Curr Sports Med Rep* 2017;**16**(1):50−5. Available from: https://doi.org/10.1249/JSR.0000000000000326. Review. PubMed PMID: 28067742.

14. Mountney A, Boutté AM, Cartagena CM, Flerlage WF, Johnson WD, Rho C, et al. Functional and molecular correlates after single and repeated rat closed-head concussion: indices of vulnerability after brain injury. *J Neurotrauma* 2017. Available from: https://doi.org/10.1089/neu.2016.4679 [Epub ahead of print] PubMed PMID: 28326890.

15. Fidan E, Lewis J, Kline AE, Garman RH, Alexander H, Cheng JP, et al. Repetitive mild traumatic brain injury in the developing brain: effects on long-term functional outcome and neuropathology. *J Neurotrauma* 2016;**33**(7):641−51. Available from: https://doi.org/10.1089/neu.2015.3958. Epub 2015 Dec 1. PubMed PMID: 26214116; PubMed Central PMCID: PMC4827290.

16. Guskiewicz KM, Broglio SP. Acute sports-related traumatic brain injury and repetitive concussion. *Handb Clin Neurol* 2015;**127**:157−72. Available from: https://doi.org/10.1016/B978-0-444-52892-6.00010-6. Review. PubMed PMID: 25702215.

17. Sufrinko AM, Marchetti GF, Cohen PE, Elbin RJ, Re V, Kontos AP. Using acute performance on a comprehensive neurocognitive, vestibular, and ocular motor assessment battery to predict recovery duration after sport-related concussions. *Am J Sports Med* 2017;**45**(5):1187−94. Available from: https://doi.org/10.1177/0363546516685061. Epub 2017 Feb 13. PubMed PMID: 28192036.

18. Peters ME, Rao V, Bechtold KT, Roy D, Sair HI, Leoutsakos JM, et al. Head injury serum markers for assessing response to trauma: design of the HeadSMART study. *Brain Inj* 2017;**31**(3):370−8. Available from: https://doi.org/10.1080/02699052.2016.1231344. Epub 2017 Jan 31. PubMed PMID: 28140672.

19. Anzalone AJ, Blueitt D, Case T, McGuffin T, Pollard K, Garrison JC, et al. A positive vestibular/ocular motor screening (VOMS) is associated with increased recovery time after sports-related concussion in youth and adolescent athletes. *Am J Sports Med* 2017;**45**(2):474−9. Available from: https://doi.org/10.1177/0363546516668624. Epub 2016 Oct 28. PubMed PMID: 27789472.

20. Schwed AC, Boggs MM, Watanabe D, Plurad DS, Putnam BA, Kim DY. Admission variables associated with a favorable outcome after mild traumatic brain injury. *Am Surg* 2016;**82**(10):898−902 PubMed PMID: 27779969.

Concussion Center Dynamics for Diagnosis and Treatment

Gillian Hotz, PhD and Kester J. Nedd, DO

Sports Medicine Institute, Concussion Program and The Miami Project to Cure Paralysis, University of Miami, Miller School of Medicine, Miami, FL, United States

With the significant increase in attention in concussion in sports, there has been also an increase in the funding of research from the professional and college sports (NFL and NCAA) and other stakeholders trying to figure out how to make contact sports safer. From youth-level of play through to the pros, there has been significantly more attention given to setting up concussion protocols resulting in an increase in concussion treatment clinics and centers throughout the United States.

Every State in the United States has passed some kind of Youth Concussion Legislation which started with the Zack Lystedt Law[1] and with most state legislation including these basic elements: concussion education provided to coaches, parents, and players; if there is any sign of symptoms during play or practice, the player must be removed from play and not return that same day; players need to be evaluated by a medical professional and cleared before returning to play. Some States have defined who a medical professional is and others have included a return to school plan and baseline testing. The legislation has also assisted with encouraging high school and youth athletic programs to develop concussion management plans.

On the international scene, a group of concussion experts get together every 4 years to develop and update guidelines for the Consensus Statement on Concussion in Sports. The most recent and fifth international meeting was held in Berlin, Germany, in October 2016.[2]

There are many definitions of concussion; however, we will refer to the latest evidence-based one from a Berlin expert panel, which modified the previous CISG definition:

Sport-related concussion (SRC) is a traumatic brain injury (TBI) induced by biomechanical forces. Several common features that may be utilized in clinically defining the nature of a concussive head injury include:

53

- SRC may be caused either by a direct blow to the head, face, neck or elsewhere on the body with an impulsive force transmitted to the head.
- SRC typically results in the rapid onset of short-lived impairment of neurological function that resolves spontaneously. However, in some cases, signs and symptoms evolve over a number of minutes to hours.
- SRC may result in neuropathological changes, but the acute clinical signs and symptoms largely reflect a functional disturbance rather than a structural injury and, as such, no abnormality is seen on standard structural neuroimaging studies.
- SRC results in a range of clinical signs and symptoms that may or may not involve loss of consciousness. Resolution of the clinical and cognitive features typically follows a sequential course. However, in some cases, symptoms may be prolonged. The clinical signs and symptoms cannot be explained by drug, alcohol, medication use, or other injuries.

THE SPORTS CONCUSSION PROGRAM AT THE SPORTS MEDICINE INSTITUTE AT THE UNIVERSITY OF MIAMI MILLER SCHOOL OF MEDICINE

The aim of our program is to provide a solution to the growing concern about SRC in youth, high school, college, and professional sports. The State of Florida Youth Concussion Legislation was passed at the beginning of 2012. At this time, the Miami Dade County (MDC) Public School Athletic Director and Director of the Sports Concussion Program met and, with support from other stakeholders, developed the 6 Steps to Play Safe Protocol for a Countywide Concussion Care Program.[3] The program is an acute neurological focused program and implemented by a multidisciplinary team of experts.

Prior to implementing the first step of the protocol, education, and training of SRC is provided to all county high school athletic trainers and coaches. An annual training workshop was organized in 2012 and has continued annually.

EDUCATION AND TRAINING WORKSHOP

The workshop was designed to educate all athletic trainers on the six steps of the protocol and also importance of completing an online, concussion-injury surveillance form. Every year all ATCs (certified athletic trainers) that are employed by the MDC Public School Board are educated on the signs and symptoms of concussion, removal from play, gradual return to play (GRTP), and the importance and significance of the baseline neuropsychological testing which includes: ImPACT™,[4] balance error scoring system (BESS),[5] the Sport Concussion Assessment Tool, SCAT3,[6] and the King Devick[7] sideline test. Also, the use of classroom accommodation forms for athletes returning to school after a concussion is included in the training. Additionally, each ATC receives instructions to immediately remove any athlete from play or practice in the event of a suspected concussive event. The protocol is also made available online for reference when an athlete is suspected of having a head injury. The workshop incorporates core components for concussion training, injury prevention, heat and hydration, medical consultation, and performance evaluation. The protocol aligns with best practices and the latest Consensus Statement on SRC.[2]

The Concussion Center not only provides up-front training and education, but also ongoing support throughout the year. For the past couple of years we have educated the principals and physical education teachers of high schools in MDC. Additionally, our team has provided education to high school football players. We have tried using a 30-minute power point presentation during preseason by a retired NFL player and also a 15-minute educational video presented by a retired NFL player.[8-10] The shorter video presentation was shown to have more of an impact and was better accepted by the players

The Concussion Center staff provide a number of important support programs to ATCs.

1. Injury assessment: The ATCs employed by the MDC Public School Board are the first to evaluate and assess an athlete suspected of a concussion or any other injury. Emphasis is placed on collecting data pertinent to recognition and reporting of identified concussions.
2. Instruction: All ATCs are trained during the annual workshop held before the football season begins. Prior to each season, each ATC is contacted by email, phone, or personal instruction about how to access the surveillance form and complete each data point. ATCs are provided with an email address and phone number for the Concussion Center if they need a program coordinator to assist with technical support.
3. Clinic appointments and weekly reminders: Once an ATC suspects an athlete has sustained a concussion, the athlete is then evaluated at the Concussion Center. Regardless of which physician or concussion clinic they are referred to for follow-up, a surveillance form must be completed.

The Concussion Center utilizes a patient-centered approach. In 2001, The Institute of Medicine (IOM) defined patient-centered care as "providing care that is respectful of and responsive to individual patient preferences, needs, and values and ensuring that patient values guide all clinical decisions."[11] Patient-centered care is a method of care that relies on effective communication, empathy, and a feeling of partnership between doctor and patient to improve patient care outcomes and satisfaction, to lessen the patient's symptoms and to reduce unnecessary costs. The program at each step provides the patient, in this case the athlete, with experts along each stop of management starting with a trained ATC and coaches in concussion management. Then, in order to maximize the concussion center visit, a prescreening is completed by a trained clinical coordinator who receives information about the athlete from the ATC and the parent over the phone. Then a clinic appointment is made.

MULTIDISCIPLINARY TEAM APPROACH

The model we have developed and implemented since 2012 has grown significantly. A multidisciplinary approach has been effective in managing SRC. From a single neurologist and a behavioral neuroscientist, both with extensive neuro rehab experience in TBI, we have added other experts to the team, including a neuropsychologist, neuroophthalmologist, otolaryngologist, sports psychologist, neuroradiologist, and sports medicine physicians.

This multidisciplinary (or multifocal team) approach, also recommended by the Berlin meeting,[2] lends itself to diagnosing concussion with the variety of symptoms that may be reported. Common symptoms of SRC may include headache, dizziness, confusion, fatigue, nausea, vomiting, sensitivity to light and/or noise, memory, attention problems, depression, anxiety, etc.[12] Symptoms may be transient or last for days, weeks, or even months. The different team members share interest in treating concussions and are committed to adding their expertise in the assessment and treatment. It is best to evaluate and treat SRC as early as possible, and experts together at one place and at the same time is advantageous because athletes want to return to play as soon as possible and our job is to make sure they are asymptomatic, have returned to their baseline, and cleared before they return to play.

6 Steps to Play Safe

Preseason Baseline Testing

Two baseline tests are administered annually to athletes during the preseason. The Immediate Post Concussion Assessment and Cognitive Test (ImPACT)[4] measures verbal and visual memory, reaction time, processing speed, and potential symptoms. Also, the King Devick[7] screening test measures eye movement and neurological functions (see Fig. 5.1). Both can be administered by trained ATCs to high school athletes, and college athletes during preseason.

Sideline Evaluation

Once SRC is suspected, sideline evaluation is the first step to diagnosis and treatment. For college and professional sports, there are trained physicians and athletic trainers that conduct this sideline evaluation. Once an athlete demonstrates any signs or symptoms of concussion they should be immediately removed from play and evaluated by the ATC. The SCAT 3[13] and King Devick[7] are typically administered at this time. If the injury is serious, 911 is called and the athlete is transported to the closest ER. In youth and high school sports more programs have developed concussion management protocols and even without medical professionals or athletic trainers, coaches are required to be certified in concussion management and able to provide appropriate assistance.

ImPACT Retesting

Post-injury testing is recommended 24—72 hours post-injury so that any cognitive issues can be demonstrated and symptoms reported. This should be done by a trained ATC, neuropsychologist, or speech pathologist. This early testing also may assist in determining appropriate management, typically for assisting in return to school accommodations.[2,14−17] Once the athlete is asymptomatic, testing again may assist with return-to-play decisions.

Countywide Concussion Care Program

FIGURE 5.1 6 Steps to Play Safe Protocol.

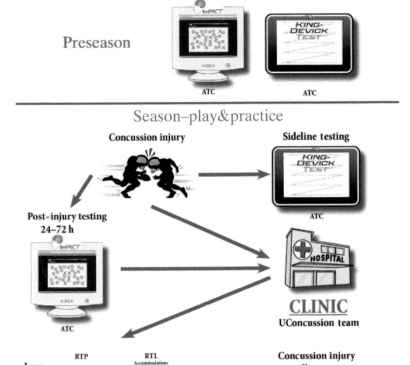

Concussion Clinic

Concussion is a clinical diagnosis that is made by a medical professional, usually a physician. Following a comprehensive evaluation or assessment by a single provider or a multidisciplinary team of experts, treatment recommendations are made depending on symptoms reported and findings from the evaluation. Most athletes that sustain SRC are seen in a clinic setting for evaluation and have to be cleared to return to play. Medical providers typically managing these cases include neurologists, pediatricians, family medicine physicians, neurosurgeons, or sports medicine physicians.

The key features of the clinical examination performed by a trained physician in SRC should entail a medical assessment including a comprehensive history and comprehensive neurological examination through a thorough assessment of mental status, sensorimotor, cognitive and behavioral functioning, sleep/wake disturbance, ocular function, vestibular function, gait, and balance.

The Sports Concussion Clinic at the University of Miami is an acute and neuro-based concussion clinic. The medical director, a neurologist with many years of experience in Neurotrauma and neurorehabilitation, performs a neurological examination each time the patient is seen at the clinic. The neurological evaluation includes the review of many systems: mental status, cranial nerves, vestibular, motor sensory, deep tendon reflex, cerebellar testing, provocative testing (Dix-Hallpike, spin, head shake), balance testing including tandem walk, etc.[18] This evaluation should also incorporate any information from coaches, ATCs, and parents, etc. In some cases, neuroimaging (CT or MRI) may be recommended for further evaluation of the injury. During the clinic visit, neuropsychological screening or a use of a computerized neurocognitive evaluation tool like ImPACT should be included and reviewed. The core clinical team providing care at our sports concussion clinic has been working together for many years and in this chapter, we share our experience and success of treating thousands of patients over the years.

Cognitive recovery largely overlaps with the time course of symptom recovery; cognitive recovery may occasionally precede or lag behind clinical symptom resolution, suggesting that the assessment of cognitive function should be an important component in the overall assessment of SRC and, in particular, any return-to-play protocol.[19,20] All high school athletes that play contact sports are required to take a baseline ImPACT test.[4] At our center, in cases where cognitive symptoms persist or are reported in the first visit, a neurocognitive screening performed by a neuropsychologist is recommended. The neuropsychological assessment should not be the sole basis of management decisions and should provide an aid to the clinical decision-making process in conjunction with a range of assessments of different clinical domains and investigational results. Neuropsychological testing may be helpful by adding useful information and provides an additional opportunity for the healthcare provider to discuss the significance of the concussion with the athletes and their families.[2]

The concussion clinic is a place where the different team members have the opportunity to evaluate the athlete and then, following a brief discussion, consensus is reached about a management plan for the athlete and appropriate recommendations are made. Athletes then return to clinic on a weekly basis so that they can be monitored and we can track their recovery until cleared to return to play.

THE TREATMENT PLAN

Physical rest is commonly recommended as part of the treatment plan.[21,22] Most consensus and agreement statements for managing SRC recommends that athletes rest until they become symptom-free.[2] The basis for recommending physical and cognitive rest is that rest may ease discomfort during the acute recovery period by mitigating postconcussion symptoms and/or that rest may promote recovery by minimizing brain energy demands following concussion.[2] To date, there is insufficient evidence recommending complete rest.[23] Most commonly following a brief time of rest during the acute phase (24–48 hours) post-injury, GRTP from low to higher exertional activities is encouraged if the athlete remains symptom-free. However, the exact amount and duration of rest is not yet well defined in the literature and requires further study.[24] The experience of the clinical team helps in making appropriate GRTP recommendations.[21]

Even though SRC treatment is currently managed by the treatment of symptoms, we have observed different recovery trajectories. The spectrum of symptoms may include headaches presented as musculoskeletal/vascular/migraine, vestibular issues, cognitive impairment, sleep issues, and changes in personality, etc.[24,25] To date, there is no standard treatment so, again, the experience of clinicians plays an important role in the choice for treatment.[26,27]

The use of neuroimaging or head CT scans or MRIs are not routinely recommended, but ordered if there is a clinical suspicion of skull fracture, focal neurological deficits, contusion, intracranial hemorrhage, prolonged period of posttraumatic amnesia, or loss of consciousness.[28]

Depending on the clinical experience and discipline of the clinician, a range of treatments depending on the severity of symptoms and circumstances of the patient are recommended. With SRC, most athletes want to return to play and class as soon as possible, so there is a need to balance out what pharmacological treatment, if any, would be beneficial, how much rest is needed, and accommodations recommended to assist with academic performance.

There are no clear, evidence-based guidelines of neuropharmacological treatment following SRC. However, concussion can be treated. The principles used by our clinical team include:

1. The importance of early intervention to mitigate effects of physical symptoms and cognitive impairments that often leads to negative neurobehavioral outcomes. Conditions such as dizziness, vertigo, headaches, decreased attention can lead to anxiety, panic attacks, anger management issues and, at times, obsessive compulsive disorder tendencies.
2. Focusing on the treatment of physical symptoms from the patient's results over findings from family or others. There is a tendency to treat what we see, as opposed to what the patient reports.
3. Choice of medication is significantly dependent on the stage, severity, and time dimensions of an injury. As a result, initial and ongoing accurate diagnosis and categorization of the patient's conditions will go a long way toward a proper treatment plan and neuropharmacological intervention. Due to the state of the brain at any point in time in the recovery process, various medications can have either a positive or negative effect on brain recovery. Clinicians must understand the stage of recovery and timing of treatment based on the state of the brain.
4. Neuropsychological and psychosocial factors help shape the patient's recovery and enhance the choice of medication. Factors such as self-esteem, prior life experience, family and team support, and substance abuse influence the choice of medication.
5. Choice of neuropharmacological agents are not only based on the mechanism of the action of those medications, but also the physician's ability to determine how such medication impacts on specific targeted symptom profiles.

Most patients following SRC do not require pharmacological treatment. However, clinicians must be knowledgeable about the positive and negative effects of medications prescribed. Our success has been demonstrated by first treating physical symptoms that are reported by the patients; those that are most bothersome to the patient, including vestibular function that is aggravated by motion in the environment. Vestibular dysfunction can be treated with benzodiazepines and some literature recommends longer-acting agents for sustained relief, such as clonazepam. Shorter-acting benzodiazepines are often utilized by physicians. However, in these cases, the patient will often report a return of symptoms as the medication wears off which can cause increased anxiety. While vestibular therapy is appropriate in the early stages, clinicians should understand that therapy could also increase symptoms as vestibular therapy may involve motion exercises.[26]

Headaches most commonly reported are musculoskeletal and vascular. Headaches are often triggered by vestibular function (motion in environment) or are due to visual convergence or divergence defects. For the most part, headaches reported are mostly musculoskeletal. These headaches can also resolve with proper management of vestibular issues, however nonsteroidal (ibuprofen, naproxen, Celebrex, etc.) and antiinflammatory agents and various muscle relaxants can be effective in managing these headaches.[29] In some cases, musculoskeletal headaches result from cervical and cervical occipital injuries. Various physical therapy modalities can be effective in managing these headaches.[30] The vitamin/mineral route that has proved to be beneficial is Riboflavin and Magnesium.

Musculoskeletal headaches, when severe, can trigger vascular headaches. In these cases, treatment of musculoskeletal headaches represent the most effective way of preventing vascular headaches from occurring. Failure of treatment of vascular/migraine headaches often result when clinicians ignore the impact of musculoskeletal headaches. Prior history of migraines and family history of migraines should be considered when treating postconcussion headaches as such headaches tend to increase following injury. Less common, but advantageous to keep in mind, is that the presence of a small amount of intracranial hemorrhage in the meninges or subarachnoid space not visible on CT or MRI can also result in severe vascular headaches. Medications such as Topamax and Lamotrigine can be effective in treating these types of headaches. Caution is urged in using agents such as Amitriptyline as they can increase physical symptoms of vertigo and dizziness due to the anticholinergic affects. Beta blockers can also be utilized, but can result in depression and other cognitive effects. Calcium channel blockers are effective and are best used over a longer term.

Also reported by patients are issues in cyclic phenomenon, such as sleep/wake cycle and energy/mood cycles, which are often impaired due to the disruption of brain hierarchical control.[31] The negative impact of such conditions on body systems and functioning of the patient can be quite severe. Early management of these conditions are critical to the recovery process. Generally speaking, patients in the acute phase of recovery sleep for longer periods. As the brain recovers, disruption in sleep initiation and restful sleep become an issue. Patients often experience ruminating thoughts that keep them awake for prolonged periods of time resulting in anxiety and frustration. In addition, these patients have limited restorative REM sleep and upon awakening, report that they are not feeling refreshed. The use of Melatonin or agents such as Lamotrigine, Oxcarbazepine, Depakote, Valproic acid, and some SSRIs can facilitate improvement of these conditions.

Neurocognitive issues are commonly reported postconcussion. Issues of attention are usually at the top of the list of reported issues. Proper classification of attentional dysfunction is necessary to determine which agents would be most effective. Attention dysfunction can be caused by pain, lack of sleep, and other physical and cognitive behavioral issues. Treatment of these conditions should be considered before using stimulate agents, such as Adderall, Vyvanse, Concerta, caffeine, etc. It should be noted that early use of stimulants can have negative effects such as headaches, seizures, anxiety, cardiovascular dysfunction, and arrhythmias. Stimulants are generally more effective for the longer term after some structural and physiological reorganization has occurred, and are better suited to subacute and chronic stages of recovery.

Neurobehavioral symptoms, such as depression, anxiety, and panic attacks, are generally the result of cognitive, physical, and emotional factors. A clear understanding of the major contributing cause of such conditions is necessary before treatment modalities are considered. Experienced clinicians, through a line of questioning and observation in the clinic and reported by other family members, must be able to determine the nature of the condition as these are often multifactorial. Neuropsychological testing or screening can be helpful in delineating cognitive from emotional factors.[32] There is, however, significant subjectively in the interpretation of such studies. Cognitive behavioral therapy and psychotherapy are critical in managing these conditions. The choices of medication intervention are often tied to the direct effects of agents that are selected due to less side effects on a neuropharmacological basis. SSRIS and SNRIs can provide relief from depression and anxiety and may act as a stimulant for attention and processing. Benzodiazepines are generally helpful in the acute stage in the management of anxiety and is a longer-acting agent. In our practice, Klonopin is preferred. Other agents, such as Buspar because of its dopaminergic affects, can also assist in providing relief to the patient who then can experience pleasure and euphoria without anxiety.

The use of atypical antipsychotics in the management of TBI and concussion has been excessive and, while they do have a place, these agents have more negative effects on recovery and may result in cognitive impairment in attention and motor recovery. Whatever medication is recommended by the physician, it is critical that ongoing close monitoring of the recovery process be performed given the shifts and changes that occur in brain recovery over time. As such, the appropriate changes in medication and dosing becomes necessary to match the stage, time, and state of brain recovery.

It is important to treat each SRC case individually. Concussions that are treated acutely with proper education and management, result in these athletes experiencing a full recovery and return to play. The appropriate neuropharmacological management and associated treatment modalities is important in preventing long-term conditions and delayed recovery.

Return to Play

Athletes must be completely free of symptoms and started on a gradual return-to-play protocol that typically begins with low exertional activities to moderate and heavy activities with contact drills. The ultimate return-to-play decision should remain a medical one in which a multidisciplinary approach, when possible, is taken.[33] Return to learn should also be monitored by any complaints of cognitive or academic issues. Return to learn must be managed in a step-wise program that fits the academic needs of the individual.[34] Our program found that most high school athletes return to play within 12—14 days, which is in agreement with other research.[8,35]

Concussion-Injury Surveillance System

Once the athlete has returned to full contact and competitive activities, the ATC will submit a 30 data-point online concussion-injury surveillance form. This information is prepared into quarterly reports and shared with the MDC Public School Board so that the information will help improve and monitor the Countywide Concussion Management Program and help to prevent future injuries.[8]

A RESEARCH OPPORTUNITY

Concussion Centers that treat many patients with a multifocal approach are the best places to conduct clinical research. Having a large population of athletes with concussion diagnosis, research should be included as part of their program. Expertise from these centers, whether studying biomarkers, MRIs, symptomatology or even helmet type injuries, are all important and will add to the existing literature. More funding is becoming available from the military, the NFL, and other key stakeholders, the study of mTBI/concussion is just at the beginning stages, and findings are rapidly evolving. However, evidence needs to be presented in order for current assessment and management to improve.

References

1. Zackery Lystedt Law. *Youth sports—concussion and head injury guidelines—injured athlete restrictions—short title.* <http://apps.leg.wa.gov/rcw/default.aspx?cite = 28a.600.190.>; 2017 [Accessed October 4].
2. McCroy P, Meeuwisse W, Dvorak J, Aubry M, Bailes J, Broglio S, et al. Consensus statement on concussion in sport—the 5th international conference in sport held in Berlin. *Br J Sport Med (Clin J Sports Med)* 2017;1—10.
3. Hotz G, Quintero A, Crittenden R, Baker L, Goldstein D, Nedd K. *A coutnywide program to manage concsussions in high school sports.* thesportjournal.org. <http://thesportjournal.org/article/a-countywide-program-to-manage-concussions-in-high-school-sports/>; 2014 [Accessed October 4].
4. Schatz P, Pardini JE, Lovell MR, Collins MW, Podell K. Sensitivity and specificity of the of the ImPACT Test battery for concussion in athletes. *Arch Clin Neuropsychol* 2006;91—9.
5. University of North Carolina Sports Medicine Research Laboratory. *Balance error scoring system.* <https://www.carolinashealthcare.org/documents/carolinasrehab/bess_manual_.pdf>; 2017 [Accessed October 4].
6. Dvorak J, McCory P, Aubry M, Molloy M, Engebretsen L. *Concussion sans frontieres.* http://bjsm.bmj.com. October 5. <http://bjsm.bmj.com/content/47/5/259.citation-tools>; 2017.
7. Galetta KM, Brandes LE, Maki K, et al. The King Devick test and sports-related concussion: study of a rapid visual tool in a collegiate cohort. *J Neurol Sci* 2011;34—9.
8. Hotz G, Crittenden R, Baker L, Hurley E, Duerr E, Golden C, et al. Countywide concussion injury surveillance system. *Curr Res: Concussion* 2015;2(X):11—16.
9. Hotz G, Crittenden R, Siegel J, Duerr E, Hurley E, Pagan E, et al. The challenges of providing concussion education to high school fotball players. *Curr Res Concussion* 2015;1—6.
10. Hotz G, Crittenden R, Siegel J, Pomares B. *Concussion: video education program for high school football players (pending publication).* Current Research: Concussion.
11. Institute of Medicine. Crossing the quality chasm: A new health system for the 21st century. *Inst Med* 2001;1—8.
12. Babikian T, Satz P, Zaucha K, Light R, Lewis RS, Asarnow RF. The UCLA longitutinal study of neurocognitive outcomes following mld pediatric traumatic brain injury. *J Int Neuropsychol Soc* 2011;886—95.

13. Giza CC, Jeffrey SK, Ashwal S, Barth J, Getchius TSD, Gioia GA, et al. Summary of evidence-based guideline update: evaluation and managment of concussion in sports. *Neurology* 2013;2250−7.

14. Broglio SP, Macciocchi SN, Ferrara MS. Neuroognitive performance of concussed athletes when symptom free. *J Athletic Train* 2007;504−8.

15. Broglio SP, Macciocchi SN, Ferrara MS. Sensitivity of the concussion assessment battery. *Neurosurgery* 2007;1050−8.

16. Gioia G, Janusz J, Gilstein K, et al. Neuropsychological management of concussion in children and adolescents: effects of age and gender on impact. *Br J Sports Med* 2004;657.

17. McCrory P, Collie A, Anderson V, et al. Can we manage sport related concsussion in children the same in adults? *Br J Sports Med* 2004;514−19.

18. Hoffer ME, Szczupak M, Kiderman A, Crawford J, Murphy S, Marshall K, et al. Neurosensory symptom complexes after acute mild traumatic brain injury. *PLoS One* 2016;**11**(1).

19. Bleidberg J, Cernich AN, Cameron K, et al. Duration of cognitive impairment after sports concussion. *Neurosurgery* 2004;1073−80.

20. Bleiberg J, Warden D. Duration of cognitive impairment in sports concussion. *Neurosurgery* 2005;E1166.

21. Harmon KG, Drezner JA, Gammons M, Guskiewicz KM, Halstead M, Herring SA, et al. American Medical Society for Sports Medicine position statement: concussion in sport. *Br J Sports Med* 2013;**47**(1):15−26.

22. Collins MW, Kontos AP, Okonkwo DO, Almquist J, Bailes J, Barisa M. Statments of agreement from the targeted evealuation and active managment (TEAM) approaches to treating concussion meeting held in Pittsburg, October 15−16, 2015. *Neurosurgery* 2016;912−29.

23. Schneider KJ, Leddy JJ, Guskiewicz KM, Seifert T, McCrea M, Silverberg ND, et al. Rest and treatment/rehabilitation following sport-related concussion: a systematic review. *BR J Sports Med* 2017;**51**(12):930−4.

24. Silverberg ND, Iverson GL. Is rest after concussion "the best medicine?": recommendations for activity resumption following concussion in athletes, civilians, and military service members. *J Head Trauma Rehabil* 2013;**28**(4):250−9.

25. Gibson S, Nigrovic LE, O'Brien M, Meehan 3rd WP. The effect of recommending cognitive rest on recovery from sport-related concussion. *Brain Injury* 2013;**27**(7−8):839−42.

26. Broglio SP, Collins MW, Williams RM, Mucha A, Kontos AP. Current and emerging rehabilitation for concussion: a review of the evidence. *Clin Sports Med* 2015;**34**(2):213−31.

27. Collins MW, Kontos AP, Okonkwo DO, Almquist J, Bailes J, Barisa M, et al. Statements of agreement from the targeted evaluation and active management (TEAM) approaches to treating concussion meeting held in Pittsburgh. *Neurosurgery* 2015;**79**(6):912−29.

28. Lee B, Newberg A. Neuroimaging in traumatic brain imaging. *NeuroRx* 2005;**2**(2):372−83.

29. Hadanny A, Efrati S. Treatment of persistent post-concussion syndrome due to mild traumatic brain injury: current status and future directions. *Expert Rev Neurother* 2016;**16**(8):875−87.

30. Zasler ND. Sports concussion headache. *Brain Injury* 2015;**29**:207−20.

31. Jaffee MS, Winter WC, Jones CC, Ling G. Sleep disturbances in athletic concussion. *Brain Injury* 2015;**29**(2):221−7.

32. Tsushima WT, Shirakawa N, Geling O. Neurocognitive functioning and symptom reporting of high school athletes following a single concussion. *Appl Neuropsychol Child* 2013;**2**(1):13−16.

33. Moser G, Schatz P. Efficacy of immediate and delayed cognitive and physical for treatment of sports-related concsussion. *J Pediatr* 2012;922−6.

34. Centers for Disease Control and Prevention: Returning to school after a concussion: a fact sheet for school professionals. *Heads UP schools.* CDC.gov. <https://www.cdc.gov/headsup/pdfs/schools/tbi_returning_to_school-a.pdf>; 2017 [Accessed October 4].

35. Hastead ME, McAvoy K, Devore CD, et al. Returning to learning following a concussion. *Pediatrics* 2013;948−57.

OVERVIEW OF NEUROSENSORY CONSEQUENCES

Neuronal Hyperexcitability Following mTBI: Cellular Molecular Mechanisms and Therapeutical Implications

Nicola Maggio, MD, PhD[1,2,3,4], *Vardit Rubovitch*[5], *Barry J. Hoffer, MD, PhD*[6], *Bruce A. Citron*[7,8], *Nigel H. Greig, PhD*[9] *and Chaim G. Pick, PhD*[4,5,10]

[1]Department of Neurology, The Chaim Sheba Medical Center, Tel Hashomer, Israel [2]Department of Neurology and Neurosurgery, Sackler Faculty of Medicine, Tel Aviv University, Tel Aviv, Israel [3]Talpiot Medical Leadership Program, The Chaim Sheba Medical Center, Tel Hashomer, Israel [4]Sagol School of Neuroscience, Tel Aviv University, Tel Aviv, Israel [5]Department of Anatomy, Sackler Faculty of Medicine, Tel Aviv University, Tel Aviv, Israel [6]Department of Neurosurgery, Case Western Reserve University School of Medicine, Cleveland, OH, United States [7]Laboratory of Molecular Biology, Research and Development 151, Bay Pines VA Healthcare System, Bay Pines, FL, United States [8]Department of Molecular Medicine, USF Morsani College of Medicine, Tampa, FL, United States [9]Drug Design & Development Section, Translational Gerontology Branch, Intramural Research Program, National Institute on Aging, National Institutes of Health, Baltimore, MD, United States [10]The Dr. Miriam and Sheldon G. Adelson Chair and Center for the Biology of Addictive Diseases, Tel Aviv University, Tel Aviv, Israel

MTBI: CELLULAR AND MOLECULAR MECHANISMS

There is rising alarm about traumatic brain injury (TBI) concerns associated with contemporary military deployments, contact sport athletes, motor vehicle accidents, and the aging population. To date, an estimated 1.7 million people sustain a TBI in the United States annually, not including those who seek care outside of the hospital Emergency Room setting or do not seek care at all . Of all incurred TBIs, 80%−90% fall under the classification of mild TBI (mTBI). Although the least severe classification, the term "mild" refers to the severity of the initial injury and not to the severity of the injury's consequences, which can include cognitive and behavioral deficits lasting from months to many years (Brain Injury Association of America).[1] Additionally, mTBI has been linked to an increased risk of developing a number of neurodegenerative conditions, such as Alzheimer's disease and Parkinson's disease, later in life,[2] and repetitive mTBI is a conduit to the development of chronic traumatic encephalopathy (CTE).[3]

TBI has two separate, but connected injury components. First, an externally derived mechanical force injures the head and second, an internal cascade of molecular mechanisms is instigated that is responsible for further neurological damage. Mechanisms underpinning this secondary injury continue to be elucidated, and include inflammatory, excitotoxic, and apoptotic processes.[4] In the case of mTBI where the primary injury is substantial but far less severe than other forms of TBI, it is the secondary injury that likely is responsible for most of the ensuing damage. Fortunately, it is also the secondary injury that may prove treatable, should an experimental treatment option be both effective against components that drive the secondary phase and administered early enough to inhibit it. As secondary injury spans minutes to days after the immediate insult, this creates a valuable window of opportunity for mTBI treatment once the time-dependent molecular mechanisms are understood. If effective treatments are identified to minimize the dysregulation resulting from mTBI, then cell death can be minimized to positively impact patient outcomes.

CTE is a progressive neurodegenerative disease resulting as a long-term consequence of single or repetitive closed head injuries.[5,6] Among others, it is known to affect US military veterans[6] and currently neither a treatment nor tools pertinent to screen predisposed individuals are available. A major factor for such a trend is the poor understanding of the mechanisms underlying the pathophysiology of the disorder. Recently, it has been reported that post-mortem brains of US military veterans exposed to blast concussive injuries showed marked signs of neurodegeneration that, in particular, included multifocal perivascular foci of neurofibrillary and glial tangles immunoreactive for tau epitopes.[5] Interestingly, this blast-associated CTE-linked tau neuropathology was indistinguishable from the tau neuropathology, neuroinflammation, and neurodegeneration observed in the brains of young-adult athletes with histories of repetitive concussive injuries.[5] In parallel, mice exposed to a single controlled blast injury revealed similar hystopathological findings 2 weeks after the trauma.[5] These findings are correlated with persistent hippocampal-dependent memory deficits and defective activity-dependent long-term potentiation (LTP) of synaptic transmission.[5] This study, notably, reveals that head trauma is the general initiator of the brain damage in CTE, yet data on a specific molecular mechanism of injury are lacking. Current theories have proposed that the trauma may directly cause axonal damage, changes in membrane permeability and ion concentrations.[7] Alternatively, microglia primed to a prior trauma may undergo full activation following repeated exposure to head injuries and secrete excitotoxins which may ultimately result in CTE neuropathology.[8] Unquestionably, these hypotheses may clarify some of the pathologic features of CTE, yet the primary causative mechanism leading later on to neurodegeneration remains missing. In addition, it is not entirely clear how a single exposure to an mTBI may lead to CTE pathology even without recurrent concussions later in life.[5] Indeed, understanding the mechanisms underlying the neuropathological changes in CTE is fundamental in order to uncover and then develop potential therapeutic approaches and for the detection of molecules to be used as potential biomarkers for this condition.

The blood−brain barrier (BBB) plays a pivotal role in creating a highly restricted environment in the brain, to maintain its homeostasis and protect it from systemic fluctuations, by preventing the contact of blood-borne factors with the brain parenchyma.[9] Following a blast injury, due to either the direct impact or to the acceleration-deceleration forces applied to the head, a breakdown of tight vascular junctions may occur resulting in increased permeability of the BBB to blood-borne factors.[10,11] Furthermore, the damage of microvessels activates the coagulation cascade leading to intracerebral generation of thrombin.[9,12] Thrombin is a key serine protease involved in the coagulation cascade and it is generated following the cleavage of prothrombin by activated Factor X and many studies have implicated prothrombin activation mechanisms in neurodegeneration. Blood is the major source of prothrombin; yet, it has been demonstrated that the transcripts for both prothrombin and Factor X are present in the CNS.[13,14] In the brain, thrombin mediates multiple actions through the activation of the protease-activated receptors (PARs). PARs belong to the superfamily of G-protein−coupled receptors and are activated by a unique mechanism requiring a proteolytic cleavage.[15] Through PAR-1 activation, thrombin induces astrogliosis, microglia activation, local reactive oxygen and nitrogen species (ROS and RNS) and proinflammatory factors production, to ultimately induce neuronal dysfunction and neurodegeneration.[9,16] High concentrations of thrombin are found in some neurodegenerative diseases leading to dementia[17−19] and are associated with tau pathology.[19] Thrombin, administered intracerebrally, was shown to be neurotoxic and reduce memory performance. Thrombin is degraded by protease nexin-1 (PN-1), a 44 kDa protease belonging to the serpins family, which is known to be expressed in the brain[20,21]; however, its role in physiology and pathophysiology has not been fully elucidated. Levels of both PN-1 and thrombin are elevated in brain in response to insults such as ischemia, suggesting roles in neural injury and reparative processes. We and others have further demonstrated that high concentrations of thrombin impair normal synaptic transmission, LTP and hippocampal learning and memory.[22−24] Recently, using a mouse model of concussion injury,[25] we have observed that thrombin activity and PAR-1 levels rise in the brain following trauma.[26] These findings correlate well with behavioral memory deficits and decreased levels of LTP in the hippocampus of these animals. Interestingly, the use of PAR-1 antagonists seems to mitigate the behavioral deficits as well as restore the ability to evoke LTP in the injured animals.[26] These data may hint toward a fundamental role of thrombin in the pathophysiology of mTBI-induced cognitive disturbances and, quite possibly, in CTE.

An additional consequence of mTBI is the onset of seizures and epilepsy,[4] as a result of a localized and transient BBB breakdown,[27,28] which leads to changes in the brain extracellular ionic environment and in albumin and TGF-beta mediated astrocytic transformation and inflammatory processes.[29,30] On the other hand, the loss of BBB integrity may directly cause epilepsy. In this respect, serine proteases normally found in the brain at a very low level[31] may have an abnormal increase in their cerebral expression following BBB breakdown. In particular, although there remains a paucity of information concerning the absolute amount of thrombin that crosses the BBB in specific neurological disorders, it has been demonstrated that thrombin levels increase more than 200-fold (from 100 pM to 25 nM) in the cerebrospinal fluid of patients with subarachnoid cerebral hemorrhage.[32] Undeniably, should bleeding occur directly within brain tissue, active thrombin and other proteases would freely diffuse into the brain parenchyma, and seizures are a direct consequence of the contact of thrombin with the brain. Indeed, intracerebral injections of thrombin result in focal motor seizures[33] whereas application of thrombin together with its inhibitor alpha-(2-naphthylsulfonyl-glycyl)-4 amidinophenylalanine piperidide (alpha-NAPAP) does not cause any sign of either clinical or electrographic seizures.[33] Knockout mice for PN-1, the endogenous thrombin inhibitor, have an increased susceptibility to kainic acid-induced seizures.[34] We[23] and others[35] have provided evidence that thrombin modulates synaptic transmission[36] and induces seizures[23,24] through the activation of PAR-1; this receptor is G-protein coupled and activated by cleavage of part of its N-terminal extracellular domain that then acts as a tethered ligand. Specifically, in hippocampal slices, thrombin at a concentration of 5 nM (1 U/mL) has been shown to increase spontaneous firing of CA3 pyramidal cells[24] and induce epileptic discharges under conditions mimicking BBB breakdown in the slice after such exposure to elevated [K +] or low levels of glutamate.[37,38] The facilitatory action of thrombin on the production of seizure-like activity is independent on N-methyl-D-aspartate receptors (NMDA-Rs), and it is most likely due to the effects on synaptic transmission in hippocampal CA3 neurons. Here, thrombin has been shown to enhance both frequency and amplitude of miniature Excitatory Postsynaptic Currents while reducing frequency and amplitude of miniature Inhibitory Postsynaptic Currents.[23] An additional mechanism by which BBB breakdown could promote epileptogenesis, apart from extravasation/brain accumulation of serum proteins and edema formation, is by triggering specific signaling pathways in glial and neuronal cells. In this respect, serum albumin may potently induce calcium signaling and DNA synthesis in astrocytes both in culture[39] and in brain slices.[40] Furthermore, upon local BBB disruption, albumin has been reported to be selectively transported into astrocytes via TGF-beta receptors, where it triggers transcriptional and functional changes, resulting in neuronal hyperexcitability.[29] Finally, in the presence of BBB dysfunction, astrocytic signaling can mediate transcriptional changes that include down-regulation of potassium inward rectifying channels (Kir4.1), water channels (AQP4), gap junction proteins and glutamate transporters,[41] as well as proinflammatory molecules such as cyclooxygenase-2 and interleukin-1β.[42] Seizures drastically affect the neurovascular unit, resulting in: (1) dramatic increases in brain metabolism and cerebral blood flow during the ictus period; (2) disruption of the BBB; (3) an acute loss of cerebral pressure autoregulation; and (4) a delayed impairment of cerebrovascular reactivity to various stimuli.[43] Regional patterns of BBB breakdown have been reported during epileptiform seizures induced in animal models by the use of various convulsive agents.[44,45] This may be due to the direct consequence of an increase in cerebral blood flow occurring during a seizure.[46] In this setting, besides the direct neuronal effect on vasculature exerted by catecholamines, acetylcholine, neuropeptides, or NO, astrocytes are critically involved in regulation of hemodynamic responses.[47] Indeed, astrocytic processes form close contacts to interact with both the synapses and the abluminal surface of vessels.[48] Astrocytes equipped with neurotransmitter receptors and transporters may release vasoactive substances such as

NO, arachidonic acid derivatives, adenosine, ATP, and influence vascular permeability.[48] This seems to be a peculiar property of activated astrocytes at the epileptic focus whose altered intracellular calcium release may ultimately lead to BBB breakdown.[49] Indeed, astrocyte—pericyte interactions have been identified as determinants of functional hyperemia at the microcirculation level.[50] They may induce vascular remodeling as well, by inducing alteration of thrombospondin signaling and regulation of the activity of matrix metalloproteases.[51] It is therefore interesting to speculate as to what the contribution of BBB breakdown in mTBI and CTE might be. Indeed, in these conditions an enduring BBB breakdown due to uncontrolled seizures may lead to a continuous leak of thrombin into the brain that, in turn, may sustain the epileptic process. If thrombin is then the major reason for seizures in this condition, it is tempting to speculate that PAR-1 antagonists and/or thrombin inhibitors may possibly act as potential antiepileptic drugs.[28,42]

MTBI: NOVEL THERAPEUTICAL IMPLICATIONS

Given the myriad of factors that, together, underpin mTBI neuropathology [brain edema, neuroinflammation, free radical generation (ROS, RNS), DNA damage, glutamate-induced excitoxicity, and others], a successful treatment should potentially target any number or combination of factors (as the relevance and amount of each may be different following distinct insults and across diverse individuals). An efficacious treatment would also need to produce its therapeutic effects when administered at a delayed time from the injury that is feasible for medical intervention. Hence when targeting a biological cascade triggered by TBI as a therapeutic approach, it is both essential to engage the target while it is mechanistically relevant to the ensuing damage, as well as to select a target and intervention time that is translatable to the human condition. Using the nonsurgical weight-drop model of mTBI and evaluating deficits in Novel Object Recognition (NOR) performance as an indication of cognitive impairment, our collaborative group has found a number of promising therapeutic agents targeting different secondary injury features.

Neuroinflammation and Apoptosis

A key target following any form of TBI is the rapidly ensuing neuroinflammation, which is a key component of secondary injury. In this regard, there are numerous antiinflammatory approaches and, as recently reviewed by,[52] although many have been evaluated in animal models, few have translated to effective clinical development. An interesting agent under recent evaluation by our collaborative group is the small synthetic candidate drug 3,6'-dithiothalamide that inhibits the synthesis of tumor necrosis factor-alpha (TNF-α).[53] TNF-α is an early proinflammatory cytokine identified as initiating and regulating molecular cascades contributing to inflammation, and has been suggested as a primary mediator of neurotoxicity following closed head injury. Whereas initiation of an inflammatory response can be essential to promote neuroreparative mechanisms in response to a physiological insult (whether TBI, stroke or a bacterial infection), if this is excessive or unregulated, it can augment neuronal dysfunction and degeneration by inducing a self-propagating pathological cascade of neuroinflammation that can ultimately drive pathological processes.[54,55] Shortly following TBI, substantial synthesis and release of proinflammatory cytokines occur from microglia and astrocytes, in particular TNF-α, with its mRNA and protein levels become acutely elevated within as little as 17 minutes after injury, as evaluated in post-mortem brains from patients expiring shortly after a TBI.[56] An analogous rapid sequence has been reported in rodent TBI animal models in which an elevation in brain TNF-α precedes the appearance of subsequent cytokines.[57] Contingent on signaling pathways activated, TNF-α can exacerbate trauma and oxidative stress within the brain and contribute to glutamate release and BBB disruption, which can then instigate further influx of inflammatory factors from blood to brain to drive pathological processes.[58] In this regard, increased mRNA expression of TNF-α by up to 30-fold as well as upregulation of the protein itself has been shown in rodent models as the result of closed head injury.[57] Such a rise in brain TNF-α is often transient and, in the case of weight-drop mTBI, becomes rapidly elevated immediately following injury, peaks at 12 hours and declines by 18 hours.[59] When the TNF-α synthesis inhibitor 3,6′-dithiothalamide was administered, even at a low, single dose of 28 mg/kg up to 12 hour post-weight drop injury, the drug fully mitigated the rise in brain TNF-α, ameliorated the diffuse neuronal cell loss that occurred consequent to mTBI, and protected against mTBI-induced NOR impairment evaluated 7 and 30 days later. In contrast, when treatment was delayed beyond 12 hours (initiated at 18 hour post-mTBI, i.e., 6 hours beyond the mTBI-induced spike in brain TNF-α levels), no mitigation of neuronal loss or cognitive impairment was evident.[59] These results are clearly promising for translation to clinical studies in light of elevated levels of TNF-α post-TBI in human studies, the wide therapeutic window of 12 hours to initiate treatment,[59] and the effectiveness of this agent and treatment strategy across other neurodegenerative disorders such as Alzheimer's disease and stroke in which there, likewise, is a neuroinflammatory component centered on TNF-α.[60,61] Notably, a close clinical analog of 3,6′-dithiothalamide, specifically pomalidomide, demonstrated similarly impressive activity in ameliorating neuroinflammation, neuronal cell loss and impairments in functional behavioral outcomes in a moderate to severe model of controlled cortical impact (CCI) TBI,[62] and yet more potent TNF-α lowering analogs are already in evaluation. In light of the fact that lowering TNF-α is a validated approach in the effective treatment of rheumatoid arthritis (with protein-based biologicals that bind and clear TNF-α before it activates its target receptors), despite the prior failure of more classical antiinflammatory approaches to treat this same disorder, the investigation of small brain permeant drugs to lower TNF-α represents a promising approach for mTBI and may, likewise, prove effective despite the failure of more classical nonsteroidal antiinflammatory drugs in TBI clinical trials.

The therapeutic window for target engagement after TBI is clearly critical for responsivity and efficacy. To mechanistically evaluate this window and to separate cells undergoing immediate necrotic cell death from potentially reversible apoptotic cell death, one can utilize small molecular weight p53 inactivators (tetrahydrobenzo thiazoles and oxazoles)[63] that have become widely used as pharmacological tools in the neurosciences to both inhibit and characterize apoptosis.[64,65] In animal models of stroke (transient middle cerebral artery occlusion), for example, studies have demonstrated that infarct volume can be reduced by >50% by p53 inhibition, resulting in improved neurological outcome with a window of opportunity of 3 hours.[66] A newly developed neuronal specific conditional p53 KO (CamcreTRP53$^{loxP/loxP}$) mouse in which neuron p53 ablation reduces stroke volume by 50%,[67] recently confirms these studies. Our studies across mild and moderate (CCI) TBI rodent models with p53 inhibitors,[68,69] likewise, demonstrate that a substantial portion of dying neurons undergo apoptotic cell death and, importantly, are amenable to rescue. Critically, such rescue mitigates TBI-induced cognitive impairment, as evaluated by NOR and other quantitative cognitive measures, with a window of 5–7 hours in moderate CCI and up to 12 hours in mTBI—thereby, defining the time-dependent opportunity for clinical intervention and human translational studies. How this specific window (5–12 hours) determined in rodents translates into humans remains to be determined—is there a 1:1 time-dependent translation across species or, quite possibly, is the window longer in the larger human brain?

Neurotrophic and Neuroprotective Agents

Balancing pro-apoptotic pathways leading to cell dysfunction and death following a brain insult are multiple biochemical cascades that promote cell survival. In this regard, increasingly well-characterized neurotrophic/protective actions have been achieved by glucagon-like peptide-1 receptor (GLP-1R) activation in cellular and animal models of acute and long-term neurological injuries.[70] This drug target, the GLP-1R, has clinical relevance for type 2 diabetes mellitus and is gaining increasing interest in neurological disorders.[70] GLP-1 is an endogenous 30 amino acid insulinotropic peptide that, with glucose-dependent insulinotropic polypeptide (GIP) of 42 amino acids, regulates blood glucose levels through activation of their respective receptors on pancreatic β-cells.[71] These insulinotropic actions are glucose-dependent and, hence, incretin-based therapies are not associated with the development of hypoglycemia, in contrast to most other antidiabetic drug classes.[71] Notably, GLP-1 not only provides insulinotropic actions at pancreatic β cells but, importantly, acts as a trophic agent, stimulating pancreatic β-cell proliferation and neogenesis, and inhibiting β-cell apoptosis.[71] These findings hastened the development of long-acting GLP-1R agonists for treatment of type 2 diabetes mellitus, and such agents [Exendin-4 (Ex-4), also known as exenatide, and liraglutide] are both well tolerated and broadly used.[71] Of note, the GLP-1R is expressed on numerous nonislet cells throughout the body and, in particular, on neurons throughout the central and peripheral nervous system. GLP-1 is also produced within brain, chiefly in the nucleus of the solitary tract in brainstem,[72] as well as within M2 phenotype (antiinflammatory) microglia, and systemic GLP-1 and associated longer-acting peptide analogs readily enter the brain.[70]

The GLP-1R is a G-protein–coupled receptor that is coupled to the cAMP second messenger pathway, increases in which are associated with neuroprotection[73]—a function very different from its prior known role in brain in the regulation of food intake and satiety.[71] Numerous recent cellular and animal studies of GLP-1 and analogs have demonstrated promising actions across a number of neurodegenerative disease models,[73,74] suggestive of the efficacy of this potential treatment approach in TBI.

We hypothesized that GLP-1R agonists would be useful to mitigate TBI on two complementary levels: (1) as neuroprotective/neurotrophic agents to ameliorate neuronal cell death and cognitive impairment and (2) as antihyperglycemic agents[70]—since TBI-induced hyperglycemia is associated with increased mortality and morbidity in humans.[75] To vigorously test this hypothesis and provide a translational basis for clinical TBI studies, three complimentary models of TBI (weight-drop mTBI in mice),[68,76] CCI moderate TBI in rats,[77] and blast-induced mTBI in mice[78] were evaluated utilizing clinically translatable doses and routes of administration of the long-acting GLP-1R agonist, Ex-4. The dose appraised in rodents was selected as equivalent to 30%—50% of the FDA approved human dose in a 60—85 kg subject for diabetes treatment, following appropriate normalization of body surface area between species, in accord with FDA guidelines. Across all of these models, whether administration was initiated prior to or following TBI, Ex-4 significantly mitigated TBI-induced deficits in cognition.[76–78] It also reduced neuronal cell death in hippocampus and, notably, largely reversed many gene pathway expressions up- and down-regulated following TBI (including those associated with oxidative stress, neuroinflammation, ribosomal and electron transport chain, neurogenesis, and, remarkably, AD), returning them back to control levels.[76,78] Notably, this occurred at both the pathway analysis and individual gene level.[76,78] Although treatment was limited to a 7 day regimen, mitigation of cognitive impairments was evident at both day 7 onward as well as when evaluated on day 30 onward in a parallel series of animals, indicating protection from TBI-induced pathology rather than mere symptomatic effects.[79] This was supported by mitigation of TBI-induced losses in synaptic markers evaluated in both cerebral cortex and hippocampus. Taken together these data suggest a strong beneficial action of Ex-4 in managing TBI secondary damage across animal models. To cross-validate this, a clinically translatable dose of liraglutide was evaluated in mice subjected to weight-drop mTBI, and cognitive impairments were, likewise mitigated,[80] as well as by a synthetic dual incretin receptor agonsist that activates both the GLP-1R and the GIP receptor.[81]

Oxidative Stress and Antioxidant Approaches

A further key target to potentially mitigate TBI-induced neuronal damage and impairment is to ameliorate the oxidative stress that ensues. In this regard, N-acetyl-L-cycteine (NAC), the active agent in the FDA approved medication Mucomyst, has been found to have neuroprotective effects when tested in multiple TBI models.[82,83] The therapeutic mechanisms that underpins this appears to be twofold, combating both oxidative stress and inflammation. Not only is NAC an antioxidant itself, but also it is a precursor of the important endogenous antioxidant glutathione, which prevents damage from ROS and RNS, particularly at the level of mitochondria. A 100 mg/kg dose of NAC combined with a 30 mg/kg dose of topiramate (an antiepileptic medication), administered 1 hour following a mild weight-drop injury was shown to ameliorate cognitive deficits.[82] In this representative study, whereas the mTBI mouse group had a markedly reduced performance from the sham vehicle (control) group at 7 and 30 days in both a NOR and Y-maze paradigm, the mTBI-drug treatment group was not found to significantly differ from the sham vehicle group at either time. In the same study, rats challenged with FPI and treated with NAC, likewise, demonstrated mitigation of cognitive impairment when evaluated in the Morris water maze; demonstrating activity across TBI models, species, and behavioral paradigms.[82] Notably, a parallel dose given to active duty military personnel in the first human study of its kind was found to improve auditory, vestibular, and cognitive function sequelae following an mTBI blast injury,[84] providing an excellent example of successful translation, as well as a preclinical methodological strategy to approach human studies.

An alternative approach to administering an exogenous antioxidant is to up regulate endogenous antioxidant levels. Tert-butylhydroxiquinone (tBHQ) is a chemical activator of nuclear factor erythroid-2 related factor 2(Nrf2), a basic leucine zipper protein that functions as a transcription factor which, in turn, is known to activate antioxidant and oxidative stress genes that protect against oxidative damage triggered by injury and inflammation. Under normal physiological, unstressed conditions, Nrf2 primarily exists within the cytoplasm where it interacts with Kelch like-ECH-associated protein 1 (Keap1) and Cullin 3 that rapidly degrade Nrf2 by ubiquitination[85] (half-life 20 minutes).[86] During conditions of oxidative stress, Nrf2 is not degraded but, instead, translocates to the nucleus where it binds to a DNA promoter and initiates transcription of antioxidative genes and their proteins. tBHQ is able to cross the BBB and disassociate Nrf2 from its cytoplasmic protein interactions to thereby elevate Nrf2 levels and nuclear translocation. Mice that are deficient in Nrf2 have been demonstrated to exhibit increased apoptosis and inflammatory signaling following a moderate TBI. A 2012 study determined a tBHQ dose of 33.4 mg/kg, to be effective in rescuing a NOR deficit 7 days post-injury and showed a positive trend but not significant difference in a parallel series of TBI challenged mice at day 30.[87] tBHQ and other drugs that stimulate the Nrf2 pathway are being evaluated across a number of neurological and systemic disorders involving oxidative stress.[88]

An additional potential therapeutic target for TBI is the unfolded protein response (UPI or ER stress). Possible prevention of cell death could be either blocking the pro-apoptotic arm or activating the translational/adaptive one. Thus, we used the phosphatase inhibitor Salubrinal that by inhibiting de-phosphorylation of the translation initiation factor over stressed cells induced sparing from apoptotic cell death. To test this hypothesis, a dose of 1 mg/kg Salubrinal was administered 24 hour post-injury and was found to be effective at preventing neuronal degeneration 72 hour post-injury and reversing NOR deficits at both 7 and 30 days later.

A further approach, still, to optimize and augment endogenous compensatory mechanisms that are naturally instigated following a physiological challenge, such as occurs from a TBI, is the pharmacological use of the experimental drug (−)-phenserine tartrate (often known as Phenserine). (−)-Phenserine was originally developed as an anticholinesterase with a high selectivity for the acetyl (AChE) form of the enzyme and with a high brain uptake following parental administration (brain plasma ratio (−)-phenserine 8:1).[89] Past and recent research has demonstrated that (−)-phenserine has a broad range of noncholinergic actions of potential value for TBI as well as chronic neurodegenerative conditions, such as Alzheimer's disease and mild cognitive impairment. These involve the mitigation of preprogrammed neuronal cell death, as induced by glutamate excitotoxicity, oxidative stress or poisons like soman[90]; the upregulation of endogenous antioxidant mechanisms that include superoxide dismutase 1 and 2, and glutathione peroxidase [GPx],[91] the amelioration of neuroinflammation,[92] and lowering the levels of select proteins that comprise amyloid precursor protein as well as cleavage products like amyloid-β peptide,[93,94] and of α-synuclein at the level of their mRNA translation in neuronal cells. As a consequence of these actions, many of which appear to be involved in the secondary phase of TBI, clinically translatable doses of (−)-phenserine were found to significantly inhibit cognitive impairments-induced by weight-drop mTBI in mice evaluated at 7 days,[91] and to dramatically reduce markers of neuroinflammation and cell loss at 72-hour post-injury. Such agents that provide therapeutic benefit via multiple pathways have the potential to advantageously translate across not only different forms of TBI but also across diverse neurodegenerative disorders in which these multiple mechanisms differentially contribute.

Protease-Activated Receptors and Antagonists

Our collaborative group recently demonstrated that SCH79797, a PAR-1 antagonist, is able to alleviate trauma-induced amnesia in mice that have undergone mTBI. Thrombin is a serine protease that plays an essential role in the blood coagulation cascade.[95] Subsequent to its formation, following the enzymatic cleavage of prothrombin by activated Factor X, thrombin regulates a cascade of proteolytic events that ultimately lead to the formation of blood clots. Recently, however, novel signaling cascades mediated by thrombin have been discovered.[95] Specifically, through the activation of the PARs, thrombin appears to directly affect the activity of multiple cell types and regulate a variety of biological functions that include inflammation, leukocyte migration, cellular proliferation, vascular permeability and tone, edema formation, and other processes related to tissue repair.[15,96] PARs belong to a unique family of G-protein−coupled receptors.[31] Their activation is instigated by an irreversible site-specific proteolytic cleavage within the N-terminal extracellular region of the protein. The uncovered N-terminal region then acts as a tethered ligand that activates the receptor.[97] As recently reviewed by Refs.[28,98] PARs are present within the nervous system and whereas PAR-2 acts as a class of trypsin/tryptase-activated receptors, PAR-1, PAR-3, and PAR-4 are most efficiently triggered by thrombin.[97] Within brain, PAR-1 is expressed on neurons and astrocytes, with stronger immunoreactivity evident on astrocytces in human brain—particularly in the hippocampus, cortex, and striatum.[99] Although the molecular cascades triggered by PAR-1 within astrocytes and neurons have yet to be fully characterized as are its various roles and modes of regulation, PAR-1 activation is reported to modulate synaptic transmission and plasticity by augmenting NMDA-R currents,[24,33,97] and impacting LTP. Notably, PAR-1 knockout animals present with substantial impairments in hippocampus-dependent learning and memory processes.[100,101] In synopsis, PAR-1 may have a key role in memory formation and synaptic plasticity,[28,36] which can be regulated in a concentration-dependent manner by thrombin under physiological and pathological conditions. Interestingly, thrombin concentrations rise in the brain just a few minutes following a mTBI,[26] with such an increase in concentrations related to poor NOR performance in animals challenged by brain trauma. Notably, injection of the PAR-1 antagonist SCH79797 prevents memory deficits and rescues LTP in injured mice. These results may therefore indicate a potential new therapeutic strategy aimed at PAR-1 inhibition for alleviating amnesia and possibly other cognitive and behavioral deficits following mTBI in humans. Modulating this pathway may also have a beneficial effect on the long-term consequences of mTBI, and provide an interesting avenue for further research. It is important to note, however, that this potential therapeutic strategy possesses potential risks that warrant further preclinical investigation, as thrombin and/or PAR-1 inhibition may complicate trauma in the event that excessive bleeding occurs within the brain. Like other strategies involving potential therapeutic targets that have concentration-dependent and time-dependent roles in both physiological and pathological processes, a fine balance needs to be maintained in relation to both time and concentration dependence in an attempt to optimize beneficial actions and minimize potentially adverse ones, as well as channeling the approach toward a patient population/disease state that may better respond.

CONCLUSIONS

TBI research is a major area of investigation in the search and preclinical/clinical development of novel therapeutic tools to alleviate brain damage of the exposed population. With our ever-increasing knowledge of the pathophysiological mechanisms that appear to underpin the secondary injury phase of mTBI are still under, several promising therapeutic targets have been revealed in recent years. The time-dependent window within which these targets are available to engage across animal models and humans requires to be understood, as do both on and off target actions of experimental drugs. Hence, additional studies are needed to validate these approaches as having restorative brain function under pathological conditions in translational studies where drugs are administered as both treatments and tests to evaluate mechanism-based hypotheses.

References

1. Schreiber S, Barkai G, et al. Long-lasting sleep patterns of adult patients with minor traumatic brain injury (mTBI) and non-mTBI subjects. *Sleep Med* 2008;**9**(5):481−7.
2. Daneshvar DH, Riley DO, et al. Long-term consequences: effects on normal development profile after concussion. *Phys Med Rehabil Clin N Am* 2011;**22**(4):683−700.
3. Kondo A, Shahpasand K, et al. Antibody against early driver of neurodegeneration cis P-tau blocks brain injury and tauopathy. *Nature* 2015;**523**(7561):431−6.
4. Werner C, Engelhard K. Pathophysiology of traumatic brain injury. *Br J Anaesth* 2007;**99**(1):4−9.
5. Goldstein LE, Fisher AM, et al. Chronic traumatic encephalopathy in blast-exposed military veterans and a blast neurotrauma mouse model. *Sci Transl Med* 2012;**4**(134). 134ra160.
6. Saulle M, Greenwald BD. Chronic traumatic encephalopathy: a review. *Rehabil Res Pract* 2012;**2012**:816069.
7. McKee AC, Cantu RC, et al. Chronic traumatic encephalopathy in athletes: progressive tauopathy after repetitive head injury. *J Neuropathol Exp Neurol* 2009;**68**(7):709−35.
8. Blaylock RL, Maroon J. Immunoexcitotoxicity as a central mechanism in chronic traumatic encephalopathy—a unifying hypothesis. *Surg Neurol Int* 2011;**2**:107.
9. Chodobski A, Zink BJ, et al. Blood-brain barrier pathophysiology in traumatic brain injury. *Transl Stroke Res* 2011;**2**(4):492−516.
10. Ghabriel MN, Zdziarski IM, et al. Changes in the blood-CSF barrier in experimental traumatic brain injury. *Acta Neurochir Suppl* 2010;**106**:239−45.
11. Readnower RD, Chavko M, et al. Increase in blood-brain barrier permeability, oxidative stress, and activated microglia in a rat model of blast-induced traumatic brain injury. *J Neurosci Res* 2010;**88**(16):3530−9.
12. Stein SC, Chen XH, et al. Intravascular coagulation: a major secondary insult in nonfatal traumatic brain injury. *J Neurosurg* 2002;**97**(6):1373−7.

13. Dihanich M, Kaser M, et al. Prothrombin mRNA is expressed by cells of the nervous system. *Neuron* 1991;**6**(4):575–81.
14. Shikamoto Y, Morita T. Expression of factor X in both the rat brain and cells of the central nervous system. *FEBS Lett* 1999;**463**(3):387–9.
15. Coughlin SR. Thrombin signalling and protease-activated receptors. *Nature* 2000;**407**(6801):258–64.
16. Suo Z, Wu M, et al. Participation of protease-activated receptor-1 in thrombin-induced microglial activation. *J Neurochem* 2002;**80**(4):655–66.
17. Akiyama H, Ikeda K, et al. Thrombin accumulation in brains of patients with Alzheimer's disease. *Neurosci Lett* 1992;**146**(2):152–4.
18. Ishida Y, Nagai A, et al. Upregulation of protease-activated receptor-1 in astrocytes in Parkinson disease: astrocyte-mediated neuroprotection through increased levels of glutathione peroxidase. *J Neuropathol Exp Neurol* 2006;**65**(1):66–77.
19. Arai T, Miklossy J, et al. Thrombin and prothrombin are expressed by neurons and glial cells and accumulate in neurofibrillary tangles in Alzheimer disease brain. *J Neuropathol Exp Neurol* 2006;**65**(1):19–25.
20. Citron BA, Ratzlaff KT, et al. Protease nexin I (PNI) in mouse brain is expressed from the same gene as in seminal vesicle. *J Mol Neurosci* 1996;**7**(3):183–91.
21. Festoff BW, Smirnova IV, et al. Thrombin, its receptor and protease nexin I, its potent serpin, in the nervous system. *Semin Thromb Hemost* 1996;**22**(3):267–71.
22. Han KS, Mannaioni G, et al. Activation of protease activated receptor 1 increases the excitability of the dentate granule neurons of hippocampus. *Mol Brain* 2011;**4**:32.
23. Maggio N, Cavaliere C, et al. Thrombin regulation of synaptic transmission: implications for seizure onset. *Neurobiol Dis* 2012;**50**:171–8.
24. Maggio N, Shavit E, et al. Thrombin induces long-term potentiation of reactivity to afferent stimulation and facilitates epileptic seizures in rat hippocampal slices: toward understanding the functional consequences of cerebrovascular insults. *J Neurosci* 2008;**28**(3):732–6.
25. Zohar O, Rubovitch V, et al. Behavioral consequences of minimal traumatic brain injury in mice. *Acta Neurobiol Exp (Wars)* 2011;**71**(1):36–45.
26. Itzekson Z, Maggio N, et al. Reversal of trauma-induced amnesia in mice by a thrombin receptor antagonist. *J Mol Neurosci* 2014;**53**(1):87–95.
27. Friedman A. Blood-brain barrier dysfunction, status epilepticus, seizures, and epilepsy: a puzzle of a chicken and egg? *Epilepsia* 2011;**52**(Suppl 8):19–20.
28. Maggio N, Blatt I, et al. Treating seizures and epilepsy with anticoagulants? *Front Cell Neurosci* 2013;**7**:19.
29. Ivens S, Kaufer D, et al. TGF-beta receptor-mediated albumin uptake into astrocytes is involved in neocortical epileptogenesis. *Brain* 2007;**130**(Pt 2):535–47.
30. Marchi N, Angelov L, et al. Seizure-promoting effect of blood-brain barrier disruption. *Epilepsia* 2007;**48**(4):732–42.
31. Luo W, Wang Y, et al. Protease-activated receptors in the brain: receptor expression, activation, and functions in neurodegeneration and neuroprotection. *Brain Res Rev* 2007;**56**(2):331–45.
32. Suzuki M, Ogawa A, et al. Thrombin activity in cerebrospinal fluid after subarachnoid hemorrhage. *Stroke* 1992;**23**(8):1181–2.
33. Lee KR, Drury I, et al. Seizures induced by intracerebral injection of thrombin: a model of intracerebral hemorrhage. *J Neurosurg* 1997;**87**(1):73–8.
34. Luthi A, Van der Putten H, et al. Endogenous serine protease inhibitor modulates epileptic activity and hippocampal long-term potentiation. *J Neurosci* 1997;**17**(12):4688–99.
35. Isaeva E, Hernan A, et al. Thrombin facilitates seizures through activation of persistent sodium current. *Ann Neurol* 2012;**72**(2):192–8.
36. Maggio N, Itsekson Z, et al. Thrombin regulation of synaptic plasticity: implications for physiology and pathology. *Exp Neurol* 2013;**247**:595–604.
37. Chen Y, Swanson RA. Astrocytes and brain injury. *J Cereb Blood Flow Metab* 2003;**23**(2):137–49.
38. Beart PM, O'Shea RD. Transporters for L-glutamate: an update on their molecular pharmacology and pathological involvement. *Br J Pharmacol* 2007;**150**(1):5–17.
39. Nadal A, Fuentes E, et al. Plasma albumin is a potent trigger of calcium signals and DNA synthesis in astrocytes. *Proc Natl Acad Sci USA* 1995;**92**(5):1426–30.

40. Nadal A, Sul JY, et al. Albumin elicits calcium signals from astrocytes in brain slices from neonatal rat cortex. *J Physiol* 1998;**509**(Pt 3):711—16.

41. David Y, Cacheaux LP, et al. Astrocytic dysfunction in epileptogenesis: consequence of altered potassium and glutamate homeostasis? *J Neurosci* 2009;**29**(34):10588—99.

42. Marchi N, Granata T, et al. Inflammatory pathways of seizure disorders. *Trends Neurosci* 2013;**37**(2):55—65.

43. Zimmermann A, Domoki F, et al. Seizure-induced alterations in cerebrovascular function in the neonate. *Dev Neurosci* 2008;**30**(5):293—305.

44. Danjo S, Ishihara Y, et al. Pentylentetrazole-induced loss of blood-brain barrier integrity involves excess nitric oxide generation by neuronal nitric oxide synthase. *Brain Res* 2013;**1530**:44—53.

45. Nitsch C, Klatzo I. Regional patterns of blood-brain barrier breakdown during epileptiform seizures induced by various convulsive agents. *J Neurol Sci* 1983;**59**(3):305—22.

46. Kovacs R, Heinemann U, et al. Mechanisms underlying blood-brain barrier dysfunction in brain pathology and epileptogenesis: role of astroglia. *Epilepsia* 2012;**53**(Suppl 6):53—9.

47. Filosa JA. Vascular tone and neurovascular coupling: considerations toward an improved in vitro model. *Front Neuroenergetics* 2010;**2**.

48. Haydon PG, Carmignoto G. Astrocyte control of synaptic transmission and neurovascular coupling. *Physiol Rev* 2006;**86**(3):1009—31.

49. Carmignoto G, Haydon PG. Astrocyte calcium signaling and epilepsy. *Glia* 2012;**60**(8):1227—33.

50. Peppiatt CM, Howarth C, et al. Bidirectional control of CNS capillary diameter by pericytes. *Nature* 2006;**443**(7112):700—4.

51. Risher WC, Eroglu C. Thrombospondins as key regulators of synaptogenesis in the central nervous system. *Matrix Biol* 2012;**31**(3):170—7.

52. Bergold PJ. Treatment of traumatic brain injury with anti-inflammatory drugs. *Exp Neurol* 2015;**275**(Pt 3):367—80.

53. Greig NH, Mattson MP, et al. New therapeutic strategies and drug candidates for neurodegenerative diseases: p53 and TNF-alpha inhibitors, and GLP-1 receptor agonists. *Ann NY Acad Sci* 2004;**1035**:290—315.

54. McCoy MK, Ruhn KA, et al. TNF: a key neuroinflammatory mediator of neurotoxicity and neurodegeneration in models of Parkinson's disease. *Adv Exp Med Biol* 2011;**691**:539—40.

55. Tweedie D, Sambamurti K, et al. TNF-alpha inhibition as a treatment strategy for neurodegenerative disorders: new drug candidates and targets. *Curr Alzheimer Res* 2007;**4**(4):378—85.

56. Frugier T, Morganti-Kossmann MC, et al. In situ detection of inflammatory mediators in post mortem human brain tissue after traumatic injury. *J Neurotrauma* 2010;**27**(3):497—507.

57. Shohami E, Gallily R, et al. Cytokine production in the brain following closed head injury: dexanabinol (HU-211) is a novel TNF-alpha inhibitor and an effective neuroprotectant. *J Neuroimmunol* 1997;**72**(2):169—77.

58. Tuttolomondo A, Pecoraro R, et al. Studies of selective TNF inhibitors in the treatment of brain injury from stroke and trauma: a review of the evidence to date. *Drug Des Devel Ther* 2014;**8**:2221—38.

59. Baratz R, Tweedie D, et al. Transiently lowering tumor necrosis factor-alpha synthesis ameliorates neuronal cell loss and cognitive impairments induced by minimal traumatic brain injury in mice. *J Neuroinflam* 2015;**12**:45.

60. Tweedie D, Ferguson RA, et al. Tumor necrosis factor-alpha synthesis inhibitor 3,6'-dithiothalidomide attenuates markers of inflammation, Alzheimer pathology and behavioral deficits in animal models of neuroinflammation and Alzheimer's disease. *J Neuroinflam* 2012;**9**:106.

61. Yoon JS, Lee JH, et al. 3,6'-Dithiothalidomide improves experimental stroke outcome by suppressing neuroinflammation. *J Neurosci Res* 2013;**91**(5):671—80.

62. Wang JY, Huang YN, et al. Pomalidomide mitigates neuronal loss, neuroinflammation, and behavioral impairments induced by traumatic brain injury in rat. *J Neuroinflam* 2016;**13**(1):168.

63. Zhu X, Yu QS, et al. Novel p53 inactivators with neuroprotective action: syntheses and pharmacological evaluation of 2-imino-2,3,4,5,6,7-hexahydrobenzothiazole and 2-imino-2,3,4,5,6,7-hexahydrobenzoxazole derivatives. *J Med Chem* 2002;**45**(23):5090—7.

64. Culmsee C, Zhu X, et al. A synthetic inhibitor of p53 protects neurons against death induced by ischemic and excitotoxic insults, and amyloid beta-peptide. *J Neurochem* 2001;**77**(1):220—8.

65. Plesnila N, von Baumgarten L, et al. Delayed neuronal death after brain trauma involves p53-dependent inhibition of NF-kappaB transcriptional activity. *Cell Death Differ* 2007;**14**(8):1529—41.

66. Leker RR, Aharonowiz M, et al. The role of p53-induced apoptosis in cerebral ischemia: effects of the p53 inhibitor pifithrin alpha. *Exp Neurol* 2004;**187**(2):478–86.
67. Filichia E, Shen H, et al. Forebrain neuronal specific ablation of p53 gene provides protection in a cortical ischemic stroke model. *Neuroscience* 2015;**295**(1-10).
68. Rachmany L, Tweedie D, et al. Cognitive impairments accompanying rodent mild traumatic brain injury involve p53-dependent neuronal cell death and are ameliorated by the tetrahydrobenzothiazole PFT-alpha. *PLoS One* 2013;**8**(11):e79837.
69. Yang LY, Chu YH, et al. Post-trauma administration of the pifithrin-alpha oxygen analog improves histological and functional outcomes after experimental traumatic brain injury. *Exp Neurol* 2015;**269**:56–66.
70. Greig NH, Tweedie D, et al. Incretin mimetics as pharmacologic tools to elucidate and as a new drug strategy to treat traumatic brain injury. *Alzheimers Dement* 2014;**10**(1 Suppl):S62–75.
71. Campbell JE, Drucker DJ. Pharmacology, physiology, and mechanisms of incretin hormone action. *Cell Metab* 2013;**17**(6):819–37.
72. Alvarez E, Martinez MD, et al. The expression of GLP-1 receptor mRNA and protein allows the effect of GLP-1 on glucose metabolism in the human hypothalamus and brainstem. *J Neurochem* 2005;**92**(4):798–806.
73. Perry T, Greig NH. The glucagon-like peptides: a double-edged therapeutic sword? *Trends Pharmacol Sci* 2003;**24**(7):377–83.
74. Holscher C. Central effects of GLP-1: new opportunities for treatments of neurodegenerative diseases. *J Endocrinol* 2014;**221**(1):T31–41.
75. Moppett IK. Traumatic brain injury: assessment, resuscitation and early management. *Br J Anaesth* 2007;**99**(1):18–31.
76. Tweedie D, Rachmany L, et al. Exendin-4, a glucagon-like peptide-1 receptor agonist prevents mTBI-induced changes in hippocampus gene expression and memory deficits in mice. *Exp Neurol* 2013;**239**:170–82.
77. Eakin K, Li Y, et al. Exendin-4 ameliorates traumatic brain injury-induced cognitive impairment in rats. *PLoS One* 2013;**8**(12):e82016.
78. Tweedie D, Rachmany L, et al. Blast traumatic brain injury-induced cognitive deficits are attenuated by preinjury or postinjury treatment with the glucagon-like peptide-1 receptor agonist, exendin-4. *Alzheimers Dement* 2015;**12**(1):34–48.
79. Rachmany L, Tweedie D, et al. Exendin-4 attenuates blast traumatic brain injury induced cognitive impairments, losses of synaptophysin and in vitro TBI induced in vitro hippocampal cellular degeneration. *Sci Rep* 2017;**7**(1):3735. Available from: https://doi.org/10.1038/s41598-017-03792-9.
80. Li Y, Bader M, et al. Liraglutide is neurotrophic and neuroprotective in neuronal cultures and mitigates mild traumatic brain injury in mice. *J Neurochem* 2015;**135**(6):1203–17.
81. Tamargo IA, Bader M, et al. Novel GLP-1R/GIPR co-agonist "twincretin" is neuroprotective in cell and rodent models of mild traumatic brain injury. *Exp Neurol* 2017;**288**:176–86.
82. Eakin K, Baratz-Goldstein R, et al. Efficacy of N-acetyl cysteine in traumatic brain injury. *PLoS One* 2014;**9**(4):e90617.
83. Hicdonmez T, Kanter M, et al. Neuroprotective effects of N-acetylcysteine on experimental closed head trauma in rats. *Neurochem Res* 2006;**31**(4):473–81.
84. Hoffer ME, Balaban C, et al. Amelioration of acute sequelae of blast induced mild traumatic brain injury by N-acetyl cysteine: a double-blind, placebo controlled study. *PLoS One* 2013;**8**(1):e54163.
85. Itoh K, Ishii T, et al. Regulatory mechanisms of cellular response to oxidative stress. *Free Radic Res* 1999;**31**(4):319–24.
86. Kobayashi A, Ohta T, et al. Unique function of the Nrf2-Keap1 pathway in the inducible expression of antioxidant and detoxifying enzymes. *Methods Enzymol* 2004;**378**:273–86.
87. Saykally JN, Rachmany L, et al. The nuclear factor erythroid 2-like 2 activator, tert-butylhydroquinone, improves cognitive performance in mice after mild traumatic brain injury. *Neuroscience* 2012;**223**:305–14.
88. Saso L, Firuzi O. Pharmacological applications of antioxidants: lights and shadows. *Curr Drug Targets* 2014;**15**(13):1177–99.
89. Greig NH, De Micheli E, et al. The experimental Alzheimer drug phenserine: preclinical pharmacokinetics and pharmacodynamics. *Acta Neurol Scand Suppl* 2000;**176**:74–84.
90. Lilja AM, Luo Y, et al. Neurotrophic and neuroprotective actions of (-)- and (+)-phenserine, candidate drugs for Alzheimer's disease. *PLoS One* 2013;**8**(1):e54887.

91. Tweedie D, Fukui K, et al. Cognitive impairments induced by concussive mild traumatic brain injury in mouse are ameliorated by treatment with phenserine via multiple non-cholinergic and cholinergic mechanisms. *PLoS One* 2016;**11**(6):e0156493.

92. Reale M, Di Nicola M, et al. Selective acetyl- and butyrylcholinesterase inhibitors reduce amyloid-beta ex vivo activation of peripheral chemo-cytokines from Alzheimer's disease subjects: exploring the cholinergic anti-inflammatory pathway. *Curr Alzheimer Res* 2014;**11**(6):608−22.

93. Lahiri DK, Chen D, et al. The experimental Alzheimer's disease drug posiphen [(+)-phenserine] lowers amyloid-beta peptide levels in cell culture and mice. *J Pharmacol Exp Ther* 2007;**320**(1):386−96.

94. Shaw KT, Utsuki T, et al. Phenserine regulates translation of beta-amyloid precursor protein mRNA by a putative interleukin-1 responsive element, a target for drug development. *Proc Natl Acad Sci USA* 2001;**98**(13):7605−10.

95. Siller-Matula JM, Schwameis M, et al. Thrombin as a multi-functional enzyme. Focus on in vitro and in vivo effects. *Thromb Haemost* 2011;**106**(6):1020−33.

96. Sambrano GR, Weiss EJ, et al. Role of thrombin signalling in platelets in haemostasis and thrombosis. *Nature* 2001;**413**(6851):74−8.

97. Gingrich MB, Traynelis SF. Serine proteases and brain damage—is there a link? *Trends Neurosci* 2000;**23**(9):399−407.

98. Ben Shimon M, Lenz M, et al. Thrombin regulation of synaptic transmission and plasticity: implications for health and disease. *Front Cell Neurosci* 2015;**9**:151.

99. Junge CE, Lee CJ, et al. Protease-activated receptor-1 in human brain: localization and functional expression in astrocytes. *Exp Neurol* 2004;**188**(1):94−103.

100. Almonte AG, Hamill CE, et al. Learning and memory deficits in mice lacking protease activated receptor-1. *Neurobiol Learn Mem* 2007;**88**(3):295−304.

101. Almonte AG, Qadri LH, et al. Protease-activated receptor-1 modulates hippocampal memory formation and synaptic plasticity. *J Neurochem* 2013;**124**(1):109−22.

The Application of Story Structural Concepts and Elements to Clarify Interpretation of Reported mild TBI Symptoms

Kendall Haven[1] and Carey D. Balaban, PhD[2]

[1]Story Consultant, Fulton, CA, United States [2]Departments of Otolaryngology, Neurobiology, Communication Sciences & Disorders, and Bioengineering, University of Pittsburgh, Pittsburgh, PA, United States

INTRODUCTION

Symptoms and symptom clusters are often characterized as medically explained or medically unexplained.[1−8] Medically explained symptoms fit a medical diagnostic story line that is linked to biological or psychological processes with a history and prognostic trajectory. Patients with medically unexplained symptoms may be designated as fitting empirically defined diagnostic story lines, such as somatoform disorders, chronic fatigue syndrome, irritable bowel syndrome or fibromyalgia. If we consider definitions of mild traumatic brain injury (mTBI) or concussion (see Chapter 1), the symptoms are medically unexplained but are attributed to a concussion story line based purely history of a traumatic incident. The challenge to clinicians is identifying symptom clusters that map onto neurologic and psychological processes related to pathophysiology and recovery.

The symptoms associated with current mTBI or concussion questionnaires include features associated with medically unexplained symptoms, such as dizziness, balance problems/unsteadiness, headache, difficulty remembering, fogginess, fatigue, contusion and drowsiness (e.g., SCAT5 symptom questionnaire). As discussed in a recent publication,[9] analyses based upon standard questionnaires show gender differences that are consistent with differences in reporting headaches and dizziness in other contexts. This begs the issue of whether the test instruments are providing an accurate narrative of patient perceptions, both within the context of a medical story ("I have a concussion") and independent of contamination by that extrinsic story line.

Narrative theory has developed over many centuries of story analysis. However, prior to advances in neural imaging over the past two decades, all of that analytical effort was constrained to treat the brains of the audience (the actual target of all narratives) as a classic black box. It is obvious that the effects and influence sought by every narrative communicator happen in the brain/mind of audience members. However, the design and structure of those communications have had to rely not on direct (or objective) assessment of the mental impact of a narrative, but on inferences gleaned from analysis of surrogate indirect indicators (physical, facial, and vocal response).

Much work in recent years has been focused at the intersection between the established narrative theory and emerging neural science of story. This work has attempted to confirm narrative theory by directly observing and measuring the neural effects of story and of individual story elements, and by identifying the story informational pathway between sensory organs and conscious mind and memory.[10,11]

The resulting neural story science, based on story science research, has the potential to explain major portions of the gender discrepancies found in rates, patterns, and vocabulary used by patients to report patterns of nonspecific symptoms in conditions such as mTBI.

In this chapter we will present the applicable elements of current story science findings and demonstrate their potential benefit for improving the elicitation and interpretation of reported TBI symptoms. We develop basic concepts for using story structural elements as the foundation for clarifying symptom descriptions in terms of the story lines for diagnostic entities.

THE NEURAL STORY NET

It is well-recognized that storytelling is a fundamental and characteristically human activity. Human minds automatically seek specific story information in order to understand and create meaning from the world around us. We think in story form. We make sense in story form. We create meaning in story form. We remember and recall in stories. This drive to focus on story information can be seen in babies only a few months old.[10] Gottschall[12] (p. 8) introduces his book, *The Story Telling Animal: How Stories Make Us Human*, with the statement: "Story's role in human life extends far beyond conventional novels or films. Story…dominates human life." This statement echoes the recognition of the centrality of story in human perception and thinking[10] from a list that includes important contributors to the fields of developmental psychology, evolutionary biology, neural biology, and cognitive sciences such as Pinker,[13,14] Bransford,[15,16] Bruner,[17–20] Schank,[21,22] Turner,[23] Egan,[24] Applebee,[25] Anderson,[26] Kotulak,[27] Crossley,[28] Lakoff and Johnson,[29,30] and Fisher.[31]

The ubiquity of storytelling as a fundamental human activity leads to the obvious hypothesis that storytelling is the product of neural networks characteristic to the human brain. In the words of Damasio[32] (p. 293), "Storytelling is something brains automatically do, naturally and implicitly… It should be no surprise that stories pervade the entire fabric of human societies and cultures." As argued by McAdams,[33] life stories define personal identity and interact with story lines defining peoplehood, cultures, nationhood and potential individual roles. As pointed out by Hacker[34] in the book, *Crusaders, Criminals, Crazies: Terror and Terrorism in Our Time*, different story lines and narratives provide motivational scripts for mass murders in our time.

There is also wide recognition that the ability to formulate, tell, and understand stories is a key tool for advantageous, adaptive sense-making and situation assessment. Story structure *is* how we learn, how we perceive, and how we communicate. Gottschall[12] (p. XIV) summarized this point in the phrase: "Humans: the great ape with the storytelling mind." Story structure can, thus, be regarded as the *lingua franca* of neural sense-making structure. In this vein, Cron[35] (p. 9) observed that: "Neuroscientists believe the reason our already overloaded brain devotes so much precious time, energy, and space to allowing us to get lost in a story is that without stories, we'd be toast. Stories allow us to simulate intense experience without having to actually live through them. Stories allow us to experience the world before we have to actually experience it." This comment amplifies a similar perspective from cognitive scientist Pinker[13] (p. 543) who wrote that: "Stories supply us with a mental catalog of the fatal conundrums we might face someday and the outcomes of strategies we could deploy in them. Because we need that vicarious experience, our brains are wired to think in stories. We are truly *homo narratus*, story animals." Although the final comment may confute cause and effect, a point seems clear. Stated epigrammatically, our conscious story lines represent the updated output of our current neural models of ourselves.

Recent research has been directed at identification of the literal and physical neural networks engaged in story generation, communication, and understanding.[11] Experimental studies have ensconced story structural and architectural elements more firmly in the center of the neuroscience of human perception, thinking, and memory. A first step has been definition of terms. The linked neural network of brain regions that perform the story development and processing has been termed as the *Neural Story Net*—the regions you use to create the specific elements of your stories. Haven[10,11] has previously described the development of the conceptual basis for this neural circuit. The identification of connectivity networks and patterns of dynamic network activity subserving the Neural Story Net, though, remains elusive. Neuroimaging methods have been applied to localizing neural correlates of activation of connected networks for processes such as narrative production and comprehensions.[36] However, the challenge has been identifying the dimensions of story structure for visualizing differential network activation with imaging (fMRI and PET) and recording (EEG and MEG) methods.

HEURISTIC FRAMEWORK FOR THE NEURAL STORY NET IN SYMPTOM INTERPRETATION AND REPORTING

As reviewed by Haven,[10,11] story-based research has shown that the human brain fulfills this compelling mandate to make sense of information and experience (the *Make Sense Mandate*) in story form. That is, Neural Story Nets form incoming information and experience into specific story form in order to make it make sense to the individual. The Neural Story Net distorts, augments, interprets, and assumes as needed to create a storied version of the actual incoming sensations and information that makes sense, is understandable, and is consistent with the individual's world- and personal-view. It is, therefore, reasonable to propose that the effects of TBI are interpreted and given meaning within the individual in story form, and are then expressed based on these same story elements and constructs. These story-based symptom reports should also vary from patient to patient (even for identical physical traumas) as a function of other elements in the self-created story and as a function of the individual's life experience.

A schematic view of the role of the Neural Story Net in symptom reporting is shown in Fig. 7.1, modified from a schema describing the perception of nausea.[37] Symptom attribution is represented heuristically as the result an interactive process that involves sensorimotor, interoceptive, and cognitive mechanisms. The prodromal signs and symptoms are vague and neither specific nor localizing, and the certainty of an attribution increases with time. Symptom identification, reporting, and attribution are nothing more than a hypothesis-driven search to resolve ambiguity and construct a consistent story to explain sensations, perceptions, and physical features. Assumption of a story-based sick role is one potential outcome.

This schema also encompasses the following key heuristic concepts for the application of story theory[11] to TBI symptom analysis:

1. The Neural Story Net lies *between* human sensory organs (eyes and ears) and the conscious mind. Nothing reaches the conscious mind (and, thus, memory) without first being massaged into story form and structure.
2. Subconscious elements in the brain turn incoming narrative and experiential information into story form *before* it reaches the conscious mind.

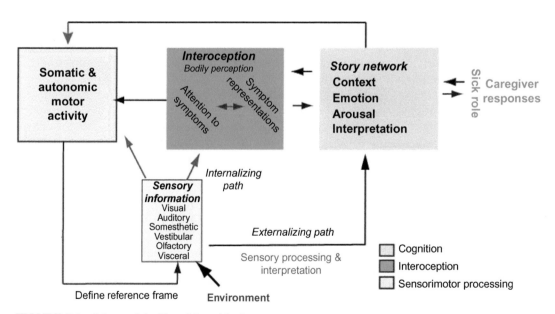

FIGURE 7.1   Schema of the Neural Story Net for symptoms.

3. What reaches the conscious mind is a self-created, story-based interpretation of what was recorded by sensory organs, distorted from the original in order to make it make sense to that specific individual.

THE INFORMATIONAL ELEMENTS OF NEURAL STORY STRUCTURE

The Neural Story Net converts incoming experiential and narrative information into story form before it reaches the conscious mind. The key question is: "What are the informational story elements that form these stories and how are they selected and updated?"

The story structure that an individual creates determines the *relevance* of the new information. Relevance, in this sense, is an internal metric to describe the closeness of the relationship or importance of the information to the story. Relevance answers the question: what does this mean to me (and to my goals, issues, and concerns). Information deemed relevant may be incorporated to strengthen, augment or modify the story. On the other hand, information deemed to be irrelevant is ignored to preserve a story line.

Experiments conducted by Haven,[11] supported by extensive observation testing and audience trials by others,[10,11] have identified the core narrative informational elements used by the human mental Neural Story Net to construct story architectures in its effort to initially make sense of, and to understand, incoming experiential and narrative information.

Those eight essential elements are listed on Table 7.1 (from Haven[11]).

In summary form, the core structure of a story may be stated as follows:

> A *character* has a tangible stated *goal* that is explained by a set of *motives* that explain why that specific goal is important to the individual. However, immediate attainment of that goal is blocked by some combination of *problems* (that could include *conflicts*) that each creates both *risk* and *danger* for the character. The character must then *struggle* to overcome those obstacles, facing the risk & danger in order to attain the goal. The story is made vivid, real, and compelling by the sensory **details** included in its presentation.

Stories may also be embedded (or nested) within stories, such that each core informational element may itself be a story and/or an element of other linked stories.

Five of these core informational elements that build the framework of the story structural model are most important for improved interpretation of reported TBI symptoms.

TABLE 7.1   The *Eight Essential Elements* of Story Structure

1. *Characters*: The characters that populate essential character positions in the story.
2. *Traits*: Selected elements of character description used to control receiver attitude toward story characters.
3. *Goal*: What a character needs/wants to do/get in a story.
4. *Motives*: The drivers that make a goal important to a character.
5. *Conflicts and Problems*: The sets of obstacles that stand between a character and an established goal.
6. *Risk and Danger*: The likelihood of failure (risk) and the consequences of failure (danger).
7. *Struggles*: The sequence of events a character undertakes to reach a goal highlighted by the climax scene (confrontation with the last and greatest obstacle) and the resolution scene.
8. *Details*: The character, sensory, scenic, and event specific descriptors used to create, direct, and control receivers' story imagery.

Character

We find experimentally that human brains are preprogrammed to structure incoming experiential and narrative information into story form following a specific structural template. Three central story character positions dominate that structural template. The human brain always attempts to fill those character positions with available story characters.

The structurally most important of these is the main character of the story—defined as that character whose primary goal is resolved at the end of the story. The main character is the character the story is "about." For self-created personal stories—and especially for personal life stories—the main character is the individual, himself or herself, in virtually all cases.

The second of these central character roles is that of antagonist. By definition, the antagonist is the physical embodiment of the greatest single obstacle (problem) blocking the main character from achieving their primary goal. This is the "bad guy," the villain, the story role that everyone loves to hate. It is not essential that the antagonist be a sentient being. While the story is made stronger by having a character in the antagonist role, any problem (e.g., perceived disabilities since a blow to the head or blast exposure) can fulfill the mandates of that role.

The final of this triumvirate of central character roles is that of the climax character. This is the story power position, often dubbed the "hero" position. By definition, the climax character is that one story character who possesses the power to make the climax play out as that character wants it to. It is not essential that the climax character exercises that power. Stories with a negative ending often play out that way specifically because the climax character failed to act at the critical moment.

Goal

A story goal is the specific thing that a character has decided that they need to do or get in this story. An effective (meaningful) goal must be a physical, tangible thing. Patient short-term and long-term goals that are impeded by the perceived injury are not solicited routinely. However, without this knowledge, the significance and meaning of specific vocabulary and reporting patterns by the patient may go unrecognized.

Given only character and goal, the human mind will always construct the architectural framework of a story. An example:

> Once there was a girl named Mary who wanted an ice cream cone.

There, in one sentence, is a character and a goal. Given only those two pieces of information, a variety of audiences and individuals were asked to state how the story would end. Every tested subject stated that the story would end when Mary either got her ice cream or when she realized that she would not get it.[11]

Given a character and a goal, the human mind automatically constructs a story framework that requires that the story ends when the primary goal of the main character is resolved—one way or the other. It is not that life, nature, or the world around us automatically follows that pattern. It is that the human Neural Story Net *mandates* that structure in its attempt to make sense of the incoming information. Without knowledge of character and goal, story events and other elements (such as story problems and obstacles) cannot assume meaning or relevance.

Motive(s)

Motives are the driving forces that lie behind any goal. Motives spring from personal beliefs, values, and attitudes. These are where tribal, cultural, religious, family, community, regional, team, and/or group values, attitudes, and beliefs manifest in individual life stories. The key question is not *what* a person is after (their goal), but rather *why* they believe that is an important goal.

All experiences and learning are filtered through this story-based lens of motives in order to be assigned meaning and value. In a very real sense, who I believe I am (or am supposed to be) is defined by the motives of the group(s) I adopt and ascribe to. In this way, motives serve as a key to accurate interpretation of symptoms related to mild head trauma and of the vocabulary chosen for that reporting. For example, motives to get back to a combat unit can underlie a symptom report of "Never felt better, Sir" from a person who has signs of injury.

Problem

Stories require the existence of problems in order to explain why a stated goal has not already been achieved. A story problem is defined as that which blocks a character from reaching a goal. Within the context of a story, "problems" only assume relevance if they can be demonstrated to block (even temporarily) a character from achieving a goal. A problem that does not impede goal attainment has no role or significance is a story (other than serving as an interesting character trait). We believe that both the physical brain injury, and its reported symptoms, are perceived, and given significance, by patients in story terms as *problems attributed to the traumatic event*.

Hence, TBI symptoms should be described by patients in language that reflects strongly the *effect* (or incongruous denial of the effect) of the physical injury on their major or minor goal attainment. Change the perceived patient goal, and you will also change the language used to describe the symptoms of the injury. This means that "symptoms" can have no definitive context until a goal is identified and stated.

An example: *George wanted to walk next door to visit a friend. However, his car was out of gas.*

Given those two sentences, tested individuals consistently respond (in general) with: "Who cares if the car is out of gas? He plans to walk next door." That is, the problem (car out of gas) is not relevant and has no story significance because it does not impede attainment of the stated goal.

When presented with these sentences, a significant minority of respondents tried to change (or augment) the story so as to force the problem statement to be relevant. This supports another observed pattern of the Neural Story Net reported by Haven[11]: If information is included in a story, the Neural Story Net assumes that it must be relevant and will distort the story as needed to make it appear to be relevant.

Risk and Danger

Risk is the mathematical probability of failure—the chances that something will go wrong. Danger is a measure of the magnitude of what bad things will happen if things go wrong—the magnitude of the consequences of failure. The mathematical product of normalized risk and normalized danger serves as an accurate metric for instantaneous story excitement and is a prime determinant of story tension. (As goes tension, so goes attention.) The greater the tension, the greater the internal focus on that portion or aspect of a story. Increase risk and/or danger and you increase the internal mental attention dedicated to that aspect or moment in a story. This increases the relative attention paid to that same aspect or moment of a story when it is later recalled and retold.

A significance point is that perceived risk and danger are metrics of how likely it is that a stated problem will prevent or significantly retard goal attainment, and the magnitude of the catastrophic impact if that particular goal is not attained. One would expect that the perceived risk and danger of any permanent, career threatening physical injury for a high-performance athlete would be far greater than would the perception of the same physical injury for a noncompetitive person. This shift in perceived risk and danger should significantly alter the intensity and severity of the descriptive language used to report the injury's symptoms. Certainly, this symptom reporting principle should impact significantly on subjective reports after mild head trauma.

From this research work, we can draw several key conclusions worth pursuing within the current context of TBI assessment and treatment.

Firstly, TBI symptoms will be described in language that is substantially dependent on the perceived story-based *effect* of the physical injury that will adhere to the elements and concepts of story structure. Patients perceive and evaluate that effect by estimating the degree to which the injury will impede their efforts to attain various short-term and long-term goals, combined with their estimation of the severity of the consequences of failure to attain that goal. For example, balance dysfunction and migraine-like symptoms are frequently comorbid with anxiety, linked to the risk and danger associated with a sense of postural threat or a scenario of a serious underlying medial problem.[38–41]

Secondly, reporting attitude and language will be controlled by a life view that is a product of the dominant motives adopted by that individual.

Thirdly, interpretation of these patient-reported TBI symptoms requires the researcher (or clinician) to obtain some sense of patient goals, motives, and resulting life story.

Fourthly, gender differences in reporting patterns and in reporting language will reflect, in large part, gender differences in the perceived role of the physical injury. That role will be internally determined by the various goals that the injury—even temporarily—impedes. If the sets of significant short-term goals are different for the two genders, then gender TBI symptom reporting must, in kind, be different.

THE IMPLICIT STORY STRUCTURE OF MEDICAL DIAGNOSIS

By their very nature, medical diagnoses can be considered as stories that describe predisposing factors, etiologies, symptoms, signs and prognoses. These stories may rely heavily on physical findings and laboratory tests, such as a sprained ankle or a fractured tibia. Other stories may rely more heavily on symptom reports, subjective observations relative to contextually rich narrative scenarios or archetype descriptions, such as the entry for narcissistic personality disorder in the Diagnostic and Statistical Manual (DSM-5). Differential diagnostic clinical tools are designed to differentiate between these clinical story lines. As a result, "good" questionnaires about symptoms are designed explicitly within the constraints imposed by these story lines. The goal becomes fitting the patient within a diagnostic category, not illuminating the relationship between symptoms and underlying etiologies.

The 2016 ICD-10-CM definition of concussion[42] incorporates story lines that share the common element of "sequelae of a head injury." (Concussion represents a subheading of the nonspecific code S06.0X; concussions are stratified into subcodes based upon the duration of loss of consciousness.) The definition, then, is simply an organization of a patient's otherwise nonspecific symptoms into a story line of "having a concussion":

- A concussion is a type of brain injury. It is a short loss of normal brain function in response to a head injury. Concussions are a common type of sports injury. You can also suffer from one if you suffer a blow to the head or hit your head after a fall. After a concussion, you may have a headache or neck pain. You may also experience nausea, ringing in your ears, dizziness, or tiredness. You may feel dazed or not your normal self for several days or weeks after the injury. Consult your health professional if you notice any of your symptoms getting worse, or if you have more serious symptoms such as seizures or trouble walking or sleeping.
- A nonspecific term used to describe transient alterations or loss of consciousness following closed head injuries. The duration of unconsciousness generally lasts a few seconds, but may persist for several hours. Concussions may be classified as mild, intermediate, and severe. Prolonged periods of unconsciousness (often defined as greater than 6 hours in duration) may be referred to as post-traumatic coma (coma, post-head injury).
- A violent jar or shock, or the condition which results from such an injury.

Symptom reporting has a dominant role in the diagnosis of mTBI. For example, the American Academy of Neurological Surgeons provides the following narrative for a diagnosis of mTBI[43]:

> Like concussions, mild injuries to the brain may not be observable in routine neurological examinations. Diagnostic tests typically will not show any changes. Therefore, diagnosis is based on the nature of the incident and the presence of specific symptoms, confusion being a primary one.

The three principal features of confusion are:

- Inability to maintain a coherent stream of thought.
- A disturbance of awareness with heightened distractibility.
- Inability to carry out a sequence of goal-directed movements.

The following are concussion symptoms:

- prolonged headache,
- vision disturbances,

- dizziness,
- nausea or vomiting,
- impaired balance,
- confusion,
- memory loss,
- ringing ears,
- difficulty concentrating,
- sensitivity to light,
- loss of smell or taste, etc.

The signs of a concussion, according to the NCAA,[44] are as follows:

- amnesia,
- confusion,
- headache,
- loss of consciousness,
- balance problems,
- double or fuzzy vision,
- sensitivity to light or noise,
- nausea,
- feeling sluggish,
- concentration or memory problems,
- slowed reaction time, and
- feeling unusually irritable.

Hence, it is not surprising that the standard symptom questionnaire used for sports concussion in the SCAT5 requests a ranking of 22 symptom descriptors on a seven-point labeled adjective scale (none to severe). They include headache, "pressure in the head," neck pain, nausea or vomiting, dizziness, blurred vision, balance problems, sensitivity to light, sensitivity to noise, feeling slowed down, feeling like "in a fog," "don't feel right," difficulty concentrating, difficulty remembering, fatigue or low energy, confusion, drowsiness, trouble falling asleep, more emotional than usual, irritability, sadness, and nervousness or anxiousness. The reported intensities on these descriptors generate both symptom scores and severity scores that can be related to the narrative schema for mTBI. In this sense, they are regarded as elements in a diagnostic narrative of mTBI.

The list of symptoms of mTBI, reflected in Fig. 7.1, includes terms that have multiple implicit, underlying story lines, which one may call a personal psychophysical filter.

THE APPLICATION OF STORY STRUCTURAL SCIENCE TO TRAUMATIC BRAIN INJURY PATIENT-REPORTED SYMPTOM INTERPRETATION

A story-based model approach posits that the way that an injury and its concurrent symptoms are experienced, internalized, and later reported are as much (if not more) a function of that individual's current and projected life *story* as of the injury, itself (see Fig. 7.1)—even though the reporting of the symptoms is completely conscious and the structure and nature of that life story is primarily subconscious. This line of reasoning implies that revisions to existing symptom inventories and symptom collection protocols need to be developed to solicit relevant story information in addition to patient symptom description and symptom impact assessment.

Research suggests that both the experience of, and the reporting of, injury symptoms are dependent on the internal story. Each individual subconsciously creates that creates personal context within which the symptoms are given relevance, importance, and meaning. During World War II, Dr. Henry Beecher compared the self-reported level of pain and need for morphine by soldiers receiving bullet wounds (during the Anzio landing) to civilian patients receiving identical bullet wounds being treated at his Boston emergency clinic (before he entered the war). While 100% of the civilian patients reported severe pain and regular need for morphine, only 25% of the soldiers did. Beecher concluded that the level of pain experienced by each individual varied dramatically depending on the context created by the story that came with the bullet.[45,46]

This concept applies equally well to other sources of injury and negative symptoms, certainly including mTBI and concussion. There are two general ways in which the elements of an individual's life story may be impacted by (1) physical consequences of a TBI and (2) acceptance of the story line of "being brain damaged."

1. The TBI symptoms will be perceived as a problem, as an obstacle impeding goal attainment. We believe that this is the dominant and most common TBI perception. Typical groups viewing TBI in this way will include athletes and military. One common response is denial or reverse malingering, the "Never felt better, Sir" or "Good to go, Coach" response. On the other end of the spectrum, others may be sensitized to report normally subclinical sensations as symptoms.
2. Other individuals (including, for example, most of Beecher's soldiers) view their own symptoms in a radically different way: as a goal enabler, as a necessary step in achieving some other important, positive goal. Examples of this group will include post-brain surgery patients (where the brain injury caused by the cranial surgery is a necessary side effect of movement toward another, greater goal) and patients for whom the diagnosis of TBI explains a set of vague, diffused symptoms that created anxiety in excess of the physical discomfort of the TBI symptoms, themselves. For many of these patients, the diagnosis creates a renewed confidence (assurance) in their overall health and also places this patient into a community (TBI patients) from whom this patient can receive reassurance.

In either case, the injury merges into, and alters, the patient's current and projected life story. The magnitude of that alteration is a measure of the significance, relevance, and personal importance of the injury and its resultant symptoms.

In this way, the various essential elements of a person's life story act as a set of distortion lenses distorting the experience of a TBI-related perceptions away from objective reality and toward cohesive integration into an existing life story. Experiences pass through and are distorted into relevant story form by the Neural Story Net upon entering the brain and before conscious consideration and memory. These same elements, then, can then be used as corrective filters to remove those story-based distortions from the reported symptoms to produce a much more objective symptoms report.

The construction of these "corrective story lenses," will require the conversion of story influences into a discrete number of quantified variables. We believe that two or three of these scaling lenses can be developed relatively easily and that these two can correct for much of the variability in symptom reporting. Questionnaires and interviews constrain symptom descriptions to story contexts; a "corrective story filter" may simply be the engagement of the patient as a character in carefully structured stories to elicit their personal story in other contexts.

This approach will require the development of new interview questions to obtain data on five story-based elements. We believe that these elements exert the greatest influence over the language, rate, and nature of reported symptoms. This same list of story variables can serve as the basis for development of a specific protocol for patient interrogation that should measurable improve the interpretation of reported symptoms and that should also explain much of the gender-related and same-sex patient-to-patient variation) in the language and reporting patterns.

The five story variables most critically important to include are:

- Goals: Short-term (immediate) and mid-term goals and life goals.
- Motives: The driving beliefs and values that underpin each goal.
- Problem perspective: How patient perceives that this injury impedes goal attainment.
- Risk and Danger: Personal significance of those goals (a measure of perceived risk and danger).
- Personality traits: Beliefs and attitudes about the desirability, benefits (or lack there or), and social acceptability of reporting injury symptoms.

From this new interview data, we envision creating two vocabulary scales

a. *The Goal Intensity Scale*: Technically, this scale must be a mathematical function of goal, motive, and the relative perceived magnitude of the associated risk and danger. We believe that we can numerically scale a relative value for the criticality of stated motives with a numerical representation of risk and danger onto a 10-point scale that will then be applied to each significant goal.

This effort will include the development of specific goal/motive language to reflect each numerical step on the scale. We currently envision that this scale will range, as an example, from 10 = "life critical; no alternate path" down to 1 = "I occasionally enjoy playing the sport."

b. *The Propensity to Report Scale*: This scale will be based on a consolidation of personality-based character traits and related group/cultural norms. Some people report every nuance of every injury in shrill and excruciating detail. Some "John Wayne" their injuries. ("Shucks, ma'm. 'Taint nothin'. It is only my left arm that's been ripped off and is squirtin' blood. It's not worth mentionin.") This stoic end of the spectrum tends to excessively minimize their verbal reporting as much as the other extreme tends to over dramatize and over verbalize it. Someone who craves to be the center of attention and will milk any malady for all of the attention they can get would describe identical TBI symptoms quite differently than would someone who shuns attention and would prefer to grit their teeth and quietly take care of it themselves.

Understanding the vocabulary used to self-report an injury must use this scale to normalize the medical significance of the injury. Thus, we can devise and test specific language to reflect each step on this 1–10 scale.

To the extent that we can quantify and scale these variables, they will serve as corrective lenses (or filters) to screen and normalize symptom reporting. In effect, the combine scales will act as a translation matrix to convert individual symptom reporting vocabulary and detain into a standardized reporting style and language. We posit that this should remove much of the reporting biases and variability from patient self-reported symptoms.

THE INCLUSION OF STORY ANALYSIS INTO SYMPTOM INVENTORIES: AN EXAMPLE

The language used by patients to self-report symptoms of TBI is dependent on both the injury itself and also on the automatic, self-created story of the experience and effect of the injury. The story-dependency of this reporting language significantly reduces the accuracy of those patient reports for medical diagnostic and treatment purposes.

As a quick conceptual example, consider the Dizziness Handicap Inventory (DHI) a list of 25 questions designed to assess the extent of a person's disability due to dizziness.[47] In story terms, virtually every question in the inventory asks a patient to assess various aspects of the risk (the probability that this negative outcome will occur) and the danger (the magnitude of the negative consequences) created by the problem of dizziness.

However, each patient's assessment of these risks and dangers that have been created by a problem (in this case: dizziness) only have personal relevance to the extent that they block a character from achieving a stated goal. Dizziness would be perceived as a vastly different problem for someone who aspired to be a racecar driver than for someone who worked as a home-based telemarketer. Without knowing the person's goals, motives, and current life story that create context and meaning for TBI symptoms, one cannot make a meaningful assessment of answers that qualitatively rank risk and danger.

Similarly, a person motivated by a core belief that any admission of injury, illness, or physical problem is an unacceptable admission of weakness and failure would answer the DHI questions quite differently than someone who was motivated to build a compelling worker comp claim—even though they experienced exactly the same degree of dizziness.

In order to apply the DHI as it currently exists, a medical professional must assume that *all* patients have virtually identical life goals and that they *all* are driven by virtually identical sets of motives. This certainly is not the case. Yet those assumptions are implicit in the DHI.

The additions of the key questions we advocate to assess goal and motive, and the use of the associated corrective scales, would provide a much more consistently objective Inventory picture to the medical professional. An identical argument can be developed for the HIT-6 Headache Impact Test or any item-based symptom or quality of life questionnaire.

The two initial steps required to launch this process will be:

1. The development of both story-based vocabulary/language for the key story elements and development of the Goal Intensity Scale and the Personality Profile Scale.
2. Creation and refinement of prototypical life story templates to represent major target populations.

Once these concepts and approaches have been validated, we can develop appropriate protocols and quantitative analytical tools to make the translation matrix readily and easily applied.

CONCLUSION

This chapter offers a story approach, based on emerging story science, that provides a rational mechanism to explain noted variances in reported TBI and mTBI symptoms. The authors have presented recent key findings from neural story research and have shown how they can be applied to benefit patient symptom inventories with a specific emphasis on TBI and mTBI symptom reporting.

Human brains are hardwired to automatically perceive, experience, make sense of, remember, and report TBI and mTBI (and related) symptoms in story terms and within the context of their ongoing life story which, itself, is automatically perceived according to a specific story model and structural template. The injury and its related symptoms will be internalized and remembered as part of that ongoing and revised life story and will be assigned relevance and meaning based on the story role the injury is given by that individual. In this paper, we have presented recent experimental developments that identify the informational narrative terms and organizational structure of those stories as well as their functional relationships.

We envision only two plausible roles that a TBI can play in terms of the patient's ongoing story: most commonly as a "problem"—as something that blocks the individual from achieving some stated goal. Alternately, in a relatively few situations, TBI and its associated symptoms could be perceived in the story role of Climax Character: part of the force that enables a stated goal. (e.g., the symptoms following brain surgery that removed a life-threatening brain tumor.) The assigned structural role defines the individual's attitude toward, experience of, and reporting of the resulting symptoms. Thus, an individual's goals and motives greatly influence the language and emotional charge used to report symptoms and should be inventoried along with the extent of the symptoms' intrusion into normal life functions.

Substantial individual variation has been noted in symptom reports for TBI athletes and military personnel. The key question is whether or not that language variation represents a corresponding variation in the nature and severity of the original injury. We believe that a large portion of this variation is the result of the human brain's automatic reliance on the core elements of effective story structure to create meaning, relevance, and understanding from the injury event. The event, the injury, and its effect will, therefore, be remembered, recalled, and reported in story form. In this sense, the stories can be designed to be therapeutic, incorporating a theme of growth through adversity.[48,49] Accurate decoding of reported TBI symptoms then requires initial story interpretation.

Two immediate efforts are required to successfully integrate essential story questions into existing symptom inventories. The first, as described, involves the development of two story-based scaling factors that we have titled the Goal Intensity Scale and the Personality Profile Scale. These scaling factors will then direct the interpretation of key story questions to be used as part of patient symptom inventories.

References

1. Brown RJ. Psychological mechanisms of medically unexplained symptoms: an integrative conceptual approach. *Psychol Bull* 2004;**130**:793–812.
2. Engel CC, Adkins JA, Cowan DN. Caring for medically unexplained physical symptoms after toxic environmental exposures: effects of contested causation. *Environ Health Perspect* 2002;**110**:641–7.
3. Ferguson E, Cassaday H, Erskind J, Delahaye G. Individual differences in the temporal variability of medically unexplained symptom reporting. *Br J Health Psychol* 2004;**9**:219–40.
4. Reuber M, MItchell AJ, Howlett SJ, Crimlisk HL, Grünewald RA. Functional symptoms in neurology: questions and answers. *J Neurol Neurosurg Psychiatry* 2005;**76**:307–14.
5. Rief W, Broadbent E. Explaining medically unexplained symptoms—models and mechanisms. *Clin Psychol Rev* 2007;**27**:821–41.
6. Smith RC, Dwamena FC. Classification and diagnosis of patients with medically unexplained symptoms. *J Gen Internal Med* 2007;**22**:685–91.
7. Barsky AJ, Boras JF. Functional somatic syndromes. *Ann Internal Med* 1999;**130**:910–21.
8. Barsky AJ, Saintfort R, Rogers MP. Nonspecific medication side effects and the nocebo phenomenon. *JAMA* 2002;**287**:622–7.
9. Hoffer ME, Szczupak M, Kiderman A, Crawford J, Murphy S, Marshall K, et al. Neurosensory symptom complexes after acute mild traumatic brain injury. *PLoS One* 2016;**11**:e0146039.
10. Haven K. *Story proof: the science behind the startling power of story.* Westprot, CT: Libraires Unlimited; 2009.
11. Haven K. *Story smart: using the science of story to persuade, influence, inspire, and teach.* Santa Barbara, CA: Libraries Unlimited; 2014.
12. Gottschall J. *The storytelling animal: how stories make us human.* Boston, NY: Houghton Mifflin Harcourt; 2012.
13. Pinker S. *How the mind works.* New York: W.W. Norton & Company; 1997.
14. Pinker S. *The language instinct.* New York: Perenial Classic; 2000.
15. Bransford J, Brown A. *How people learn.* Washington, DC: National Academy Press; 2000.
16. Bransford J, Stein B. *The ideal problem solver.* 2nd ed. New York: Freeman; 1993.
17. Bruner J. Life as narrative. *Soc Res* 1987;**54**:11–32.
18. Bruner J. *Acts of meaning.* Cambridge, MA: Harvard University Press; 1990.
19. Bruner J. The narrative construction of reality. In: Beilin H, Pufall P, editors. *Piaget's theory: prospects and possibilities.* Hillsdale, NJ: Lawrence Erlbaum; 1992. p. 229–48.
20. Bruner J. *Making stories: law, literature, life.* Cambridge, MA: Harvard University Press; 2003.
21. Schank R. *Tell me a story.* New York: Charles Scribner's Sons; 1990.
22. Schank R. Every curriculum tells a story. *Tech Direct* 2000;**62**:25–9.
23. Turner M. *The literary mind: the origins of thought and language.* New York: Oxford University Press; 1996.
24. Egan K. *The educated mind: how cognitive tools shape our understanding.* Chicago, IL: University of Chicago Press; 1997.
25. Applebee A. *The child's concept of story.* Chicago, IL: University of Chicago Press; 1998.
26. Anderson J, Martin P. Narratives and healing: exploring one family's stories of cancer survivorship. *Health Commun* 2003;**15**:133–43.
27. Kotulak R. *Inside the brain: revolutionary discoveries of how the mind works.* Kansas City, MO: Andrews McNeal Publishing; 1999.
28. Crossley M. *Introducing narrative psychology.* London: Open University Press; 2000.
29. Lakoff G, Johnson M. *Philosophy in the flesh: the embodied mind and its challenge to western thought.* New York: Basic Books; 1999.
30. Lakoff G, Johnson M. *Metaphors we live by.* Chicago, IL: University of Chicago Press; 2003.

31. Fisher W. The narrative paradigm: in the beginning. *J Commun* 1985;**35**:74−89.
32. Damasio AR. *Self comes to mind: constructing the conscious brain*. New York: Pantheon; 2010.
33. McAdams DP. The psychology of life stories. *Rev Gen Psychol* 2001;**5**:100−22.
34. Hacker FJ. *Crusaders, criminals, crazies: terror and terrorism in our time*. New York: W.W. Norton; 1976.
35. Cron L. *Wired for story: the Writer's guide*. New York: Ten Speed Press (Random House); 2012.
36. AbdulSabur NY, Xu Y, Liu S, Chow HM, Baxter M, Carson J, et al. Neural correlates and network connectivity underlying narrative production and comprehension: a combined fMRI and PET study. *Cortex* 2014;**57**:107−27.
37. Balaban CD, Yates BJ. What is nausea? A historical analysis of changing views. *Autonom Neurosci: Basic Clin* 2017;**202**:5−17.
38. Coelho CM, Balaban CD. Visuo-vestibular contributions to anxiety and fear. *Neurosci Biobehav Rev* 2015;**48**:148−59.
39. Staab JP, Balaban CD, Furman JM. Threat assessment and locomotion: clinical applications of an integrated model of anxiety and postural control. *Semin Neurol* 2013;**33**:297−306.
40. Balaban CD, Jacob RG. Background and history of the interface between anxiety and vertigo. *J Anxiety Disorders* 2001;**15**:27−51.
41. Balaban CD, Jacob RG, Furman JM. Neurologic bases for comorbidity of balance disorders, anxiety disorders and migraine: neurotherapeutic implications. *Expert Rev Neurother* 2011;**11**:379−94.
42. Codes, I.C.D., 2016. ICD-10-CM Diagnosis Codes: concussion.
43. AANS, 2016. Patient information: concussion.
44. NCAA, 2016. Concussion.
45. Beecher HK. Experimental pharmacology and measurement of the subjective response. *Science* 1952;**116**:157−62.
46. Beecher HK. The powerful placebo. *JAMA* 1955;**159**:1602−6.
47. Jacobson GP, Newman CW. The development of the dizziness handicap index. *Arch Otolayngol Head Neck Surg* 1990;**116**:424−7.
48. Joseph S, Linley PA. Positive adjustment to threatening events: an organismal valuing theory of growth through adversity. *Rev Gen Psychol* 2005;**9**:262−80.
49. Linley PA. Positive adaptation to trauma:wisdom as both process and outcome. *J Traumat Stress* 2003;**16**:601−10.

Neuropsychological and Psychiatric Comorbidities of Mild Traumatic Brain Injury

Jeffrey P. Staab, MD, MS and Matthew R. Powell, PhD, LP

Department of Psychiatry and Psychology, Mayo Clinic, Rochester, MN, United States

INTRODUCTION

In this chapter, we will review the neuropsychological and psychiatric sequelae of mild traumatic brain injury (mTBI). We will confine our discussion to mTBI because it is by far the most common severity of brain injury, constituting at least 80% of identifiable cases,[1] and because the association of neuropsychological and psychiatric problems with mTBI is far more controversial than similar sequelae of more severe brain injuries. One area of controversy is the definition and extent of mTBI. In this chapter, we will use the definition of mTBI promulgated by the US Department of Veterans Affairs and Department of Defense (VA/DoD) in a comprehensive guideline for diagnosis and management of military service members and veterans with histories of brain injury.[2] The events that may cause mTBIs include blunt force blows to the head (i.e., head striking an object or an object striking the head), whiplash type of injuries (i.e., abrupt acceleration/deceleration movement without a direct blow to the head), and direct exposure to other external forces that do not cause objects to penetrate the skull (e.g., blasts or explosions). Penetrating brain injuries are by definition moderate or severe because they cause gross structural damage to the brain. Following any of these events, mTBI is defined by any alteration in mental state or focal neurological deficits with loss of consciousness of 30 minutes or less, altered consciousness of 24 hours or less, posttraumatic amnesia of 24 hours or less, Glasgow Coma Scale score of 13–15 within the first 24 hours, and absence of structural lesions on clinical neuroimaging.[2] The VA/DoD definition is the most common one in current use in clinical and research settings. The Mayo Classification System for TBI Severity subdivides the VA/DoD mTBI group into two classes: Mild (probable) TBI which includes individuals with loss of consciousness lasting less than 30 minutes, posttraumatic amnesia lasting less than 24 hours, or nonpenetrating injury to the skull with intact dura, and Symptomatic (possible) TBI which includes those with no loss or consciousness, posttraumatic amnesia, or injury to the skull, but at least one symptom of feeling dazed or confused, headache, nausea, dizziness, blurred vision, or transient focal neurologic symptoms after exposure to a brain injury event.[3] This subdivision is meant to separate patients who have symptoms and signs thought to be more specific for injuries to the brain, itself, from patients with symptoms and signs that might arise from other causes following one of the brain injury events listed earlier.[4]

A second area of controversy and a much more difficult problem is the diagnostic classification of patients with persistent post-mTBI symptoms. There are no established biomarkers for mTBI. As a result, patients, family members, and friends; healthcare professionals of many specialties and disciplines; lawyers, judges, and juries; and representatives of healthcare and disability systems often battle across the divide between neurological (real brain injury) and psychological (not real brain injury) causes of symptoms. This struggle is rooted in mind-body dualism and is tainted by the dichotomous hierarchy of the 20th century that reified "objective" diagnostic tests despite the fact that they have limited power to predict the daily level of functioning or quality of life of individual patients with any chronic medical condition. In all major clinical specialties, long-term outcomes have a very human variability that is not captured well by blood work, imaging, or standardized diagnostic tests. These statements are not meant to denigrate the ever-expanding range of biomarkers of human physiology in health and disease that have been developed over the last several decades, but rather to put them in proper perspective. They each measure one aspect of human disease. Emerging biomarkers of mTBI will do the same. They will not rid us of the difficult problem of trying to understand why one person fares well after the same type of brain injury event that fells another quite badly. At the same time, it is just as important to realize that the answer to this dilemma does not lie exclusively within the psychological realm, though the logic of the dichotomous hierarchy would place it there. Psychological assessments, like their structural counterparts, have limitations that fall well short of predicting individual outcomes. Thus, the care of patients who have sustained TBIs will continue to be a combination of structural, functional, and psychological assessments and treatment interventions tailored as best possible to the needs of individuals who are living in their own personal contexts with the consequences of their injuries.

ACUTE NEUROCOGNITIVE EFFECTS OF MILD TRAUMATIC BRAIN INJURY

For an excellent discussion of the complex pathophysiological changes that occur within the brain at the time of injury and during the early postacute (subacute) recovery period, please see the review by Giza and Hovda.[5] For 80%–90% patients with histories of mTBI, acute mental status changes and focal neurological symptoms resolve relatively quickly.[6] Cognitive symptoms recover gradually over a period of 1–2 weeks on average, with minor residua lasting no more than 3 months for most individuals.[7,8] During recovery, patients often experience slowed cognition, attention problems, and memory difficulties.

Functional neuroimaging research in humans and physiologic studies in animals suggest that brain recovery follows a similar time course,[5] but there is some suggestion that full brain recovery may lag behind symptom resolution. If healing of the brain lags symptom recovery, then there would be obvious but currently unknowable implications for clinical management, particularly for return to activities with the potential for reinjury (e.g., athletics, military service, physically demanding occupations). Investigations into the timeframe of brain recovery are ongoing.[9,10]

POSTACUTE NEUROCOGNITIVE RECOVERY OF MILD TRAUMATIC BRAIN INJURY

The sport concussion research paradigm that sprang forth in the mid-1980s was a turning point in understanding subacute and later postacute neuropsychological recovery following mTBI.[11] Investigators were able to test athletes involved in contact sports at predetermined baselines (e.g., the start of a season) and then compare those players who suffered mTBIs against matched controls on variables of interest. Although there are some limitations to the generalizability of this research (i.e., most athletes are younger and healthier than the general population), this methodology permitted prospective and well controlled investigations of mTBI from the moment of injury until maximal recovery while tracking symptomatic, cognitive, and neurophysiological measures.[12] These methods were applied more recently to United States and allied miltary service members deployed to the combat zones of Iraq and Afghanistan.[13,14] Studies of military cohorts also offered well matched comparisons between individuals who suffered mTBIs and those who did not, but these investigations also have limitations in applying their results to the general populace. Combat veterans, like athletes, are younger and healthier than the civilian population at large, men still outnumber women in military units, and high force explosives may produce different injuries than lower impact blunt force trauma (although combat veterans also are at increased risk for accidents, assaults, and falls that mimic the most common brain injuries suffered by civilians[1,2]).

There have been a number of meta-analyses of neuropsychological data obtained from these lines of inquiry. In most prospective, well controlled group studies, postacute neuropsychological effects of mTBI appear to resolve by 3 months,[12,15−17] though some experts have argued that over-reliance on group data in meta-analyses obscures persisting effects for individuals or subgroups of patients.[18] For example, patients recruited from clinic-based samples or from medicolegal cohorts may have longer recovery periods.[19] It is possible that medical comorbidities (e.g., coexisting orthopedic injuries), more severe post-mTBI symptoms that prompt patients to seek medical care, and social factors such as involvement in litigation or applications for disability may prolong their cognitive recovery.[20] A small number of patients report new or worsening cognitive symptoms that develop weeks, months or even years post-mTBI. This subset of patients often has preexisting physical or psychiatric illnesses or problems such as depression, anxiety, or chronic pain after injury. They also tend to have complicated psychosocial circumstances such as limited support or involvement in legal or disability proceedings.[19,21−23] McCrea[8] conceptualized the postacute recovery period following mTBI within a neurobiopsychsocial framework. He emphasized that interactions among neurobiological, emotional, cognitive, occupational, and legal factors (i.e., structural, functional, and psychological variables and patients' context) all affect recovery and outcome.

PERSISTING NEUROCOGNITIVE AND PSYCHIATRIC EFFECTS OF MILD TRAUMATIC BRAIN INJURY

Approximately 10%–20% of individuals experience post-mTBI symptoms that persist beyond the expected window of recovery of 3 months, even if they have had an opportunity for appropriate treatment and rehabilitative interventions.[1,2,6–8] This condition is called postconcussion syndrome (PCS) (aka postconcussive or postconcussional syndrome). A validated set of diagnostic criteria for PCS does not yet exist, but it is commonly characterized as in the *International Classification of Diseases*, 10th edition[24] or the *Diagnostic and Statistical Manual of Mental Disorders*, 4th edition (DSM-IV)[25] by a constellation of cognitive, somatic, vegetative, behavioral, and emotional symptoms that develop following a mTBI. The most common symptoms of PCS are listed in the first column of Table 8.1.

TABLE 8.1   Symptoms of PCS and Common Post-mTBI Psychiatric Disorders

PCS	PTSD	Major Depressive Episode	Generalized Anxiety Disorder/ Panic Disorder
EMOTIONAL AND BEHAVIORAL SYMPTOMS			
Depressed mood	X	X	
Irritability	X	X	X
Apathy	X	X	
Anxiety	X	X	X
Reduced tolerance for stress or emotional excitement	X	X	x
VEGETATIVE PROBLEMS			
Fatigue		X	X
Insomnia	X	X	X
COGNITIVE COMPLAINTS			
Memory problems	X	X	
Loss of concentration	X	X	X
SOMATIC SYMPTOMS			
Dizziness			X
Headache			x

X, Symptom is explicitly listed in the DSM-5 diagnostic criteria for these conditions[26]; x, symptom is described as commonly occurring with these conditions.[26]

Of note, the DSM-5 does not define PCS. It only contains diagnostic criteria for major and minor cognitive disorders following TBI.[26] PCS should not be diagnosed until an individual experiences symptoms for 3 months or more.[25] Patients with residual deficits following moderate to severe brain injury should not be diagnosed with PCS. PCS appears to be a heterogenous condition; some individuals report very circumscribed clinical symptoms (i.e., only headache), whereas others report symptoms that span the full range listed in Table 8.1 and more (e.g., chronic tinnitus, photophobia, or hyperacusis).

Despite controversies about the nature and extent of PCS, there is evidence from animal studies that mild brain injury can cause cognitive deficits and pathological changes in the brain.[27] For example, rats with mild brain injury were found to have decreased synaptic density in specific hippocampal regions relative to controls. These changes were subtler than the lesions found on gross inspection in mice with severe brain injuries, yet the mice with mild injuries performed just as poorly as their more severely injured counterparts on certain experimental memory tasks.[27]

In humans, there is not a distinct neuropsychological profile that is universally associated with PCS, highlighting the fact that cognitive tests cannot be used as a diagnostic standard for PCS. Coexisting problems such as depression, medication side-effects, and other confounds, explain an equal amount (or more) of the variance in cognitive performance in patients during the postconcussive period when compared against acute concussion, making it difficult to interpret the cause of abnormal test results in those who present for examination temporally remote from their brain injury events.[7] Nevertheless, neuropsychometric tests can be useful to quantify the state of an individual's neurocognitive functioning at a given point during recovery, as long as appropriate confounds are carefully considered during the interpretation of the results.

The most common cognitive symptoms reported by patients beyond 3 months after mTBI are attention problems, slowed information processing speed,[28] and reduced memory functioning.[28,29] It has been hypothesized that mTBI may be associated with persisting cognitive symptoms because of underlying microscopic neuropathologic abnormalities, particularly diffuse axonal injury.[30] Mild brain injury stresses frontal-subcortical networks and decreases axonal integrity in the acute phase of injury, which is thought to correlate with persisting cognitive symptoms.[5] Research using functional magnetic resonance imaging demonstrated that disruption of right hemisphere attentional networks correlated with cognitive symptom reported by athletes in the acute period following mTBI, but not the postacute period.[31] Axonal injury assessed via serum biomarkers drawn at time of injury was associated with subjective cognitive complaints at 6 months postinjury.[32] Initial and subsequent analysis of biomarkers of axonal injury in boxers failed to correlate with cognitive function, but was associated with slowed reaction time at 2 weeks after concussion.[33] This mix of structural and biochemical results presents an intriguing but quite incomplete picture of the neurobiology of PCS. Questions about how long postconcussive cognitive (and other) symptoms may persist due to the direct effects of neurobiological factors and what roles cognitive reserve[34] and psychosocial stressors play in the clinical manifestations of PCS remain unanswered. Despite all the technology available today, including advanced neuroimaging, serum markers, and genetic studies, there is still not a compelling, comprehensive neurobiological explanation for PCS. In planning future research, it has been recommended that multiple neuroimaging technologies be combined with biomarkers in prospective investigations to better characterize any biological underpinnings to PCS and then examine subgroups of the syndrome.[35] To that, we would suggest equal attention to psychosocial variables.

Factors other than strutural brain deficits can explain persisting symptoms following mTBI.[20] The symptoms of PCS are nonspecific. They may occur in healthy individuals, though usually transiently and not in aggregate. More importantly, they may occur in patients experiencing other sequelae of brain injury events including posttraumatic stress disorder (PTSD), major depressive disorder, anxiety disorders, substance use disorders, and chronic pain.[36−39] Persisting complaints have been correlated with female gender, positive premorbid psychiatric history, comorbid depressive symptoms, and posttraumatic anxiety.[40] Table 8.1 gives a side by side comparison of the symptoms of PCS, PTSD, major depressive episodes, and anxiety disorders, which illustrates their overlapping nature. This may create difficult diagnostic dilemmas. For example, in a study of 4462 Vietnam veterans, more patients with PTSD, anxiety, or depressive disorders (50%−57%) met DSM-IV criteria for PCS than patients with mTBI (32%).[41] In disability and forensic settings, data like these have been used to discount diagnoses of PCS for given patients, and sometimes to argue against the construct of PCS, in general. The problem with this line of reasoning is that it uses commonalities to blur distinctions. Even measurable signs such as body temperature are nonspecific as evidenced by the wide differential diagnosis of fever. In situations like the evaluation of fever of unknown origin,[42] the diagnostic dilemma cannot be solved by focusing on common elements in an attempt to rule out illnesses, but by identifying distinctive features that allow active conditions to be ruled in. This approach has been applied to PCS. In a study of 213 veterans from Iraq and Afghanistan, Morrisette et al.[43] used structural equation modeling to show that nonoverlapping features of PCS mediated the effects of TBI on coexisting PTSD and depression. Table 8.2 lists clinical features that overlap least among PCS and common post-mTBI psychiatric disorders. It is important to interpret Table 8.2 properly. The presence of the listed features suggests the existence of the associated diagnoses (possible rule in), but their absence does not exclude the diagnosis (cannot rule out). For example, a patient with multiple PCS symptoms and recurrent suicidal thoughts after a mTBI does not have PCS alone, but also a coexisting depressive or related disorder that explains his suicidal ideation. In contrast, the absence of suicidal ideation does not preclude a diagnosis of a depressive disorder if all other features are present, even if some overlap with PCS symptoms. Similarly, a patient with all of the major symptoms of PTSD and chronic daily headache and dizziness after a mTBI does not have PTSD alone, but likely a component of PCS, posttraumatic headache, or chronic vestibular syndrome to explain her daily headache and dizziness.

Psychological adjustment to injury can influence speed of recovery following mTBI.[3,37] Depression affects the experience and reporting of PCS symptoms. Outpatients with a history of mTBI plus depression reported more PCS symptoms than patients without depression or patients with depression but no history of mTBI.[44] Coexisting clinical diagnoses of depression, anxiety, and pain disorders as well as self-perceived cognitive disturbances affected disability and work status.[45] Psychiatric comorbidity, especially PTSD, increased utilization of psychotherapy services among military veterans with histories of mTBI.[46] Misattributing all post-mTBI symptoms to a diagnosis of structural brain injury rather than apportioning them to PTSD, depression, anxiety, or pain when these problem coexist

TABLE 8.2   Features That May Distinguish PCS From Common Post-mTBI Psychiatric Disorders

PCS	PTSD	Major Depressive Episode	Generalized Anxiety Disorder/Panic Disorder
Headache (chronic daily headache or frequent migraine headache)			
Dizziness (often a chronic symptom exacerbated by exercise)			
	Intrusion symptoms related to mTBI (flashbacks, nightmares)		
	Excessive avoidance of reminders of the mTBI		
		Suicidal ideations, plans, or behaviors	
		Excessive feelings of worthlessness	
			Chronic worry about multiple topics (often predates mTBI)
			Frequent, unexpected panic attacks (unrelated to mTBI)

may lead patients to the erroneous conclusion that their problems are permanent.[2] How can one recover from a damaged brain? The resulting decrease in self-efficacy can serve to maintain PCS symptoms.[2,37] Patients, like their clinicians, may fall into the trap of the dichotomous hierarchy, spending inordinate time and effort searching for the person or test that will reveal their suspected brain damage, while giving short shrift to properly addressing psychological morbidity. The resultant frustration may exacerbate their symptoms and alienate them from needed medical, and especially psychological care, potentially increasing their disability.

PSYCHIATRIC DISORDERS FOLLOWING MILD TRAUMATIC BRAIN INJURY

Epidemiological and clinical studies have used various methods to investigate the psychiatric sequelae of TBI over many years. Unfortunately, most older reports have been small and of modest quality. In 2009, Carlson et al.[47] performed a comprehensive review of 1107 references for the VA. The largest and most detailed study that they identified was conducted by the RAND Corporation on approximately 2000 US service members and veterans of deployments to Iraq and Afghanistan. That investigation reported a point prevalence of 19.5% for probable TBI, 13.8% for PTSD, and 6.6% for coexisting probable TBI and PTSD. The rate of coexisting probable TBI and PTSD was 2.4 times the rate of a chance cooccurrence indicating that a probable TBI more than doubled the risk of developing PTSD above and beyond other exposures associated with deployment. In a more recent study, Lagarde et al.[48] compared the development of PTSD and PCS in 534 civilian accident victims who sustained mTBIs compared to 827 patients with nonhead injuries who were followed prospectively after emergency department evaluations. At 3 months after injury, 8.8% of patients with mTBIs and 2.2% of patients without brain injuries met diagnostic criteria for PTSD, again suggesting that mTBI carries an increased risk of PTSD compared to other exposures (odds ratio, 4.47; 95% CI: 2.38−8.40). In additional findings that stirred doubts about the validity of PCS as a unique construct, Lagarde et al.[48] reported that 21.2% of patients with mTBI and 16.3% of the comparison group without head injuries met the DSM-IV diagnosis of PCS with exposure to mTBI carrying no added risk for PCS (odds ratio, 1.13; 95% CI: 0.82−1.55). They further concluded from a correspondence analysis that PCS symptoms acted like PTSD hyperarousal symptoms, which is where the two syndromes have the greatest overlap (i.e., shared symptoms of irritability, concentration problems, and insomnia). However, they found no clustering of other PCS symptoms or unique relationships to mTBI.

The incidence and prevalence of major depression also are increased among individuals who have sustained mTBIs. Hoge et al.[14] investigated 2525 US Army infantry soldiers 3−4 months after their return from a 1-year deployment to Iraq. In that cohort, 124 soldiers (4.9%) reported injuries with loss of consciousness—that is, mild (probable) TBI in the Mayo classification.[3] An additional 260 soldiers (10.3%) reported injuries with altered mental status—that is, Symptomatic (possible) TBI in the Mayo classification.[3] Rates of major depression were significantly increased in the former group at 22.9%, but not in the latter group at only 8.4%, which was comparable to the remainder of the study cohort. Studies of civilians have reported a wide range for the prevalence of major depression after TBI, but best estimates suggest an incidence of 18%[49] and prevalence of 33%−42% within 1 year after injury.[50] A 5-year prospective study of patients with moderate to severe (not mild) TBI illustrated the time course of post-TBI psychiatric morbidity.[51] In 161 civilians, three-quarters of those who developed depressive, anxiety, or substance use disorders did so within the first year after injury. This was followed by a natural decline in psychiatric morbidity of about one-quarter per year from the second through fifth years. Depressive and substance use disorders were more likely to persist than anxiety disorders. Other psychiatric consequences of brain injury events are more circumscribed but potentially disruptive problems such as specific phobias. An example is a specific phobia of driving or riding in an automobile after a motor vehicle accident that severely limits a person's mobility.[52]

The VA/DoD clinical practice guidelines strongly recommends screening patients with post-mTBI symptoms for psychiatric morbidity including PTSD, depression, substance use disorders, and suicidality.[2] That recommendation is well-suited to civilian populations as well and could be extended to include anxiety disorders. To aid in the identification of psychiatric morbidity in patients with histories of mTBI, widely available self-report questionnaires and clinician-rated instruments for PTSD, depression, anxiety disorders, and substance use disorders may be used—for example, the 9-item Patient Health Questionnaire (PHQ-9) for depression. Two caveats must be kept in mind. First, there have been no studies that fully tested the validity of these measures in patients with mTBI.[47] Second, positive self-report scores or clinician-rated findings do not necessarily mean that the identified traumatic stress, depressive, or anxiety symptoms are secondary to the mTBI. Proper diagnosis would depend on full consideration of premorbid medical and psychiatric history and other potential sequelae of brain injury events—for example, other physical injuries, persistent pain, and family, occupational, financial, and legal consequences.[53]

LATE NEUROCOGNITIVE OF MILD TRAUMATIC BRAIN INJURY

A third major area of controversy is the potential for brain injury to be a risk factor for later development of neurodegenerative disorders. Here we will not cover pugilistic parkinsonism or chronic traumatic encephalopathy (CTE) in detail. For those interested in more information, please see the review of CTE by Iverson et al.[54] and refer to the article by Giza and Hovda[5] for an evidence-based discussion of potential pathophysiological mechanisms that may link repetitive mTBI to an increased risk of neurodegeneration. Apart from the cases of Muhammed Ali and former National Football League players that have captured headlines,[55] the existing body of epidemiological evidence is mixed regarding a potential association between the duration of exposure to subconcussive blows (e.g., years of participation in contact sports) and later life neurodegenerative disorders.[56,57] While there is some evidence that a history of mTBI, cumulative effects of repetitive mTBI,[5] and more serious levels of brain injury[18] may be risk factors for development of neurodegeneration, it is not yet known if exposure to a single mTBI with loss of consciousness or a limited number of incidental mTBIs leads to an acceleration of amyloid deposition and increased risk of Alzheimer's disease. In one study,[58] a self-reported history of brain injury with loss of consciousness was linked to amyloid deposition, but variability in the results suggested that some individuals may have inherent vulnerabilities, whereas others may possess intrinsic protective factors, none of which is well understood. Taken together, these incomplete and inconsistent results illustrate the urgent need for more definitive research and serve as a reminder that caution is still warranted before drawing any firm conclusions for individual patients between their histories of mTBI and risk of neurodegenerative disorders.[54]

TREATMENT OF NEUROPSYCHOLOGICAL AND PSYCHIATRIC SYMPTOMS FOLLOWING MILD TRAUMATIC BRAIN INJURY

Treatment of patients with histories of mTBI depends on the length of time it has been since the brain injury event that prompted their symptoms. Within the first few weeks after injury, it is best to separate incident symptoms (i.e., those that developed de novo after the brain injury event) from preexisting problems that may have been exacerbated by injury. For incident symptoms, the first step is to set reasonable expectations for recovery.

Most patients will improve substantially within the first 2 weeks and at least 80% will recover within the first 3 months after their brain injury events. During this time, the recovery environment is important.[59] Patients should be encouraged to set regular schedules to ensure adequate sleep and nutrition. They also should be supported in maintaining activities of daily living, work, and recreation, though these activities may have to be paced with breaks during the recovery period. Activities inside and outside the home that risk reinjury are best avoided until symptoms and signs of injury have resolved. There is a great deal of research underway on test procedures to guide return to play, work, and duty for individuals involved in high risk activities (e.g., athletics, physical labor, military service), but these investigations have not yet coalesced around specific metrics. For more information on these topics, please see the review by Cancelliere et al.,[60] guidelines from the US Centers for Disease Control and Prevention (https://www.cdc.gov/headsup/providers/return_to_activities.html), and patient education information from the Brain Injury Association of America (https://www.biausa.org/brain-injury/about-brain-injury/concussion/return-to-play).

For patients who have preexisting illnesses (e.g., mood, anxiety, traumatic stress, substance use, or cogntive disorders) that were exacerbated by the brain injury event, the first step is to reassess the efficacy of the preexisting treatment plan. If the increase in symptoms is mild, then the conservative measures just described may be enough to restore adequate control. If the exacerbation of preexisting problems is more than mild, then the brain injury event may have exposed vulnerabilites in treatment. In the latter situation, it may be necessary to reexam the efficacy of pharmacotherapy or provide added sessions of psychotherapy.

For post-mTBI cognitive, emotional, or behavioral symptoms that remain problematic after a few weeks ($\sim$30 days), further evaluation is indicated.[2] There is no global intervention for emerging PCS symptoms or developing psychiatric comorbidity. Rather, treatment is directed at specific symptom clusters (e.g., cognitive complaints) or identifiable disorders (e.g., PTSD, major depressive, anxiety, or substance use disorders). For cognitive symptoms, formal neuropsychological assessment may be useful to ascertain functional limitations and identify targets for treatment.[2] A course of therapist-directed cognitive rehabilitation may be indicated and is the treatment option with the best supporting evidence.[61,62] A variety of medications have been used off-label over the years in an effort to promote recovery from neurocognitive symptoms following brain injury. Examples include psychostimulants (methylphenidate and amphetamines) and nonamphetamine stimulants (modafinil) for attention and concentration problems and fatigue, memory preserving medications (primarily donepezil and memantine) and dietary supplements (gingko biloba) for memory complaints, and antidepressants (selective serotonin reuptake inhibitors and serotonin-norepinephrine reuptake inhibitors) to promote brain recovery across multiple domains. There are no data from large scale randomized controlled trials to support the efficacy of these pharmaceuticals. Available evidence has been obtained from small samples of patients with TBI severity ranging from mild to severe who were treated during acute, postacute, and chronic periods after injury. As a result, the VA/DoD practice guidelines,[2] reinforced at a consensus conference in 2017,[63] recommend against offering medications or supplements to treat neurocognitive symptoms in patients with histories of mTBI. In contrast, Talsky et al.[64] prepared a succinct summary of medication options and Wortzel and Arciniegas[65] offered an overly optimistic review of pharmacologic treatment choices.

For post-mTBI psychiatric morbidity (i.e., major mood, anxiety, traumatic stress, and substance use disorders) the VA/DoD guideline[2] recommends following standards of care for those disorders as established for patients without brain injuries. The VA consensus conference in 2017[63] updated this recommendation and cited emerging evidence that cognitive behavioral therapy is just as effective for PTSD in patients with TBI as it is in patients without TBI and that it also improves depressive symptoms, insomnia, general PCS symptom burden, and psychosocial functioning.[63,66,67] In contrast, there have not been adequate clinical trials that compared the relative efficacy of medications indicated for major mood, anxiety, traumatic stress, and substance use disorders in patients with histories of TBI versus uninjured cohorts. Therefore, current practice is to purse medication management based on general treatment guidelines for psychiatric disorders identified in patients with histories of mTBI, whether they emerged de novo or existed prior to brain injury events. Hammer and Sauvé[68] wrote a concise review of this topic.

Research has begun on other treatments for the sequelae of TBI, including neuropsychological and psychiatric symptoms. The first reports on transcranial magnetic stimulation and transcranial direct current stimulation,[69] and hyperbaric oxygen therapy[70] indicate potential benefit, but await confirmation in more definitive trails.

References

1. Centers for Disease Control and Prevention (CDC), National Center for Injury Prevention and Control. *Report to Congress on mild traumatic brain injury in the United States: steps to prevent a serious public health problem.* Atlanta, GA: Centers for Disease Control and Prevention; 2003.
2. *VA/DoD clinical practice guideline for the Management of Concussion-Mild Traumatic Brain Injury.* <https://www.healthquality.va.gov/guidelines/Rehab/mtbi/mTBICPGFullCPG50821816.pdf>; 2017 [accessed 10.12.17].
3. Malec JF, Brown AW, Leibson CL, Flaada JT, Mandrekar JN, Diehl NN, et al. The Mayo classification system for traumatic brain injury severity. *J Neurotrauma* 2007;24(9):1417–24.
4. Friedland DP. Improving the classification of traumatic brain injury: the Mayo classification system for traumatic brain injury severity. *J Spine* 2003;S4:0051.
5. Giza CC, Hovda DA. The new neurometabolic cascade of concussion. *Neurosurgery* 2014;75(suppl 4):S24–33.
6. Katz DI, Cohen SI, Alexander MP. Mild traumatic brain injury. *Handb Clin Neurol* 2015;127:131–56. Available from: https://doi.org/10.1016/B978-0-444-52892-6.00009-X.
7. Iverson GL. Outcome from mild traumatic brain injury. *Curr Opin Psychiatry* 2005;18(3):301–17.
8. McCrea M. *Mild traumatic brain injury and post-concussion syndrome: the new evidence base for diagnosis and treatment.* New York: Oxford Press; 2008.
9. Barr WB, Prichep LS, Chabot R, Powell MR, McCrea M. Measuring brain electrical activity to track recovery from sport-related concussion. *Brain Inj* 2012;26(1):58–66.
10. Kamins J, Bigler E, Covassin T, Henry L, Kemp S, Leddy JJ, et al. What is the physiological time to recovery after concussion? A systematic review. *Br J Sports Med* 2017;51(12):935–40.
11. Barth JT, Alves W, Ryan T, Macciocchi S, Rimel R, Jane JJ. Mild head injury in sports: neuropsychological sequelae and recovery of function. In: Levin H, Eisenberg J, Benton A, editors. *Mild head injury.* Oxford: New York; 1989. p. 257–75.
12. Belanger HG, Vanderploeg RD. The neuropsychological impact of sports-related concussion: a meta-analysis. *J Int Neuropsychol Soc* 2005;11(4):345–57.
13. Morissette SB, Woodward M, Kimbrel NA, Meyer EC, Kruse MI, Dolan S, et al. Deployment-related TBI, persistent postconcussive symptoms, PTSD, and depression in OEF/OIF veterans. *Rehabil Psychol* 2011;56:340–50.

14. Hoge CW, McGurk D, Thomas JL, Cox AL, Engel CC, Castro CA. Mild traumatic brain injury in U.S. soldiers returning from Iraq. *N Engl J Med* 2008;**358**:453−63.
15. Schretlen DJ, Shapiro AM. A quantitative review of the effects of traumatic brain injury on cognitive functioning. *Int Rev Psychiatry* 2003;**15**(4):341−9.
16. McCrea M, Iverson GL, McAllister TW, Hammeke TA, Powell MR, Barr WB, et al. An integrated review of recovery after mild traumatic brain injury (MTBI): implications for clinical management. *Clin Neuropsychol*. In press.
17. Frencham KA, Fox AM, Maybery MT. Neuropsychological studies of mild traumatic brain injury: a meta-analytic review of research since 1995. *J Clin Exp Neuropsychol* 2005;**27**(3):334−51.
18. Bigler ED. Traumatic brain injury, neuroimaging, and neurodegeneration. *Front Hum Neurosci*. 2013;**7**:395.
19. Belanger HG, Curtiss G, Demery JA, Lebowitz BK, Vanderploeg RD. Factors moderating neuropsychological outcomes following mild traumatic brain injury: a meta-analysis. *J Int Neuropsychol Soc* 2005;**11**(3):215−27.
20. Tarsh MJ, Royston C. A follow-up study of accident neurosis. *Br J Psychiatry* 1985;**146**:18−25.
21. Vanderploeg RD, Curtiss G, Belanger HG. Long-term neuropsychological outcomes following mild traumatic brain injury. *J Int Neuropsychol Soc* 2005;**11**(3):228−36.
22. Lange RT, Brickell TA, Ivins B, Vanderploeg RD, French LM. Variable, not always persistent, postconcussion symptoms after mild TBI in U.S. Military service members: a five-year cross-sectional outcome study. *J Neurotrauma* 2013;**30**(11):958−69.
23. Binder LM, Rohling ML, Larrabee GJ. A review of mild head trauma. Part i: meta-analytic review of neuropsychological studies. *J Clin Exp Neuropsychol* 1997;**19**(3):421−31.
24. World Health Organization. *International classification of diseases, 10th edition, postconcussional syndrome (F07.81)*. <http://www.icd10data.com/ICD10CM/Codes/F01-F99/F01-F09/F07-/F07.81>; 2018 [accessed 20.03.18].
25. American Psychiatric Association. *Diagnostic and statistical manual of mental disorders*. 4th ed. Washington, DC: American Psychiatric Association; 1994.
26. American Psychiatric Association. *Diagnostic and statistical manual of mental disorders (DSM-5)*. 5th ed. Washington, DC: American Psychiatric Association; 2013.
27. Darwish H, Mahmood A, Schallert T, Chopp M, Therrien B. Mild traumatic brain injury (MTBI) leads to spatial learning deficits. *Brain Inj* 2012;**26**(2):151−65.
28. Bigler ED. Neuropsychological results and neuropathological findings at autopsy in a case of mild traumatic brain injury. *J Int Neuropsychol Soc* 2004;**10**(5):794−806.
29. Anderson SD. Mild traumatic brain injury and memory impairment. *Arch Phys Med Rehabil* 2004;**85**(5):862.
30. Bigler ED. Neurobiology and neuropathology underlie the neuropsychological deficits associated with traumatic brain injury. *Arch Clin Neuropsychol* 2003;**18**(6):595−621 discussion 3-7.
31. Hammeke TA, McCrea M, Coats SM, Verber MD, Durgerian S, Flora K, et al. Acute and subacute changes in neural activation during the recovery from sport-related concussion. *J Int Neuropsychol Soc* 2013;**19**(8):863−72.
32. De Kruijk JR, Leffers P, Menheere PP, Meerhoff S, Rutten J, Twijnstra A. Prediction of post-traumatic complaints after mild traumatic brain injury: early symptoms and biochemical markers. *J Neurol Neurosurg Psychiatry* 2002;**73**(6):727−32.
33. Neselius S, Brisby H, Marcusson J, Zetterberg H, Blennow K, Karlsson T. Neurological assessment and its relationship to CSF biomarkers in amateur boxers. *PLoS One* 2014;**9**(6):e99870.
34. Oldenburg C, Lundin A, Edman G, Nygren-de Boussard C, Bartfai A. Cognitive reserve and persistent postconcussion symptoms—a prospective mild traumatic brain injury (mTBI) cohort study. *Brain Inj* 2016;**30**(2):146−55.
35. Shenton ME, Hamoda HM, Schneiderman JS, Bouix S, Pasternak O, Rathi Y, et al. A review of magnetic resonance imaging and diffusion tensor imaging findings in mild traumatic brain injury. *Brain Imaging Behav* 2012;**6**(2):137−92.
36. Iverson GL, Lange RT, Gaetz M, Zasler ND, Mild TBI. In: Zasler ND, Katz D, Zafonte RD, editors. *Brain injury medicine*. New York: Demos Medical Publishing; 2007. p. 333−71.
37. Iverson GL, Zasler ND, Lange RT. Post-concussive disorder. In: Zasler ND, Katz DI, Zafonte RD, editors. *Brain injury medicine: principles and practice*. New York: Demos Medical Publishing; 2007. p. 373−405.
38. Iverson GL, Lange RT, Franzen MD. Effects of mild traumatic brain injury cannot be differentiated from substance abuse. *Brain Inj* 2005;**19**(1):11−18.
39. Iverson GL, McCracken LM. 'Postconcussive' symptoms in persons with chronic pain. *Brain Inj* 1997;**11**(11):783−90.

40. Scheenen ME, Spikman JM, de Koning ME, van der Horn HJ, Roks G, Hageman G, et al. Patients "at risk" of suffering from persistent complaints after mild traumatic brain injury: the role of coping, mood disorders, and post-traumatic stress. *J Neurotrauma* 2017;**34**(1):31–7.

41. Donnell AJ, Kim MS, Silva MA, Vanderploeg RD. Incidence of postconcussion symptoms in psychiatric diagnostic groups, mild traumatic brain injury, and comorbid conditions. *Clin Neuropsychol* 2012;**26**:1092–101.

42. FUO.

43. Morissette SB, Woodward M, Kimbrel NA, Meyer EC, Kruse MI, Dolan S, et al. Deployment-related TBI, persistent postconcussive symptoms, PTSD, and depression in OEF/OIF veterans. *Rehabil Psychol* 2011;**56**:340–50.

44. Lange RT, Iverson GL, Rose A. Depression strongly influences postconcussion symptom reporting following mild traumatic brain injury. *J Head Trauma Rehabil* 2011;**26**:127–37.

45. Xiong C, Martin T, Sravanapudi A, Colantonio A, Mollayeva T. Factors associated with return to work in men and women with work-related traumatic brain injury. *Disabil Health J* 2016;**9**:439–48.

46. Miles SR, Harik JM, Hundt NE, Mignogna J, Pastorek NJ, Thompson KE, et al. Delivery of mental health treatment to combat veterans with psychiatric diagnoses and TBI histories. *PLoS One* 2017;**12**:e0184265.

47. Carlson K, Kehle S, Meis L, Greer N, MacDonald R, Rutks I, et al. *The assessment and treatment of individuals with history of traumatic brain injury and post-traumatic stress disorder: a systematic review of the evidence.* Washington, DC: U.S. Department of Veterans Affairs, Evidence-based Synthesis Program; 2009.

48. Lagarde E, Salmi L-R, Holm LW, Contrand B, Masson F, Ribéreau-Gayon R, et al. Association of symptoms following mild traumatic brain injury with posttraumatic stress disorder vs postconcussion syndrome. *JAMA Psychiatry* 2014;**71**(9):1032–40.

49. Rao V, Bertrand M, Rosenberg P, Makley M, Schretlen DJ, Brandt J, et al. Predictors of new-onset depression after mild traumatic brain injury. *J Neuropsychiatry Clin Neurosci* 2010;**22**:100–4.

50. Jorge RE, Robinson RG, Moser D, Tateno A, Crespo-Facorro B, Arndt S. Major depression following traumatic brain injury. *Arch Gen Psychiatry* 2004;**61**:42–50.

51. Alway Y, Gould KR, Johnston L, McKenzie D, Ponsford J. A prospective examination of Axis I psychiatric disorders in the first 5 years following moderate to severe traumatic brain injury. *Psychol Med* 2016;**46**.1331–41.

52. Sutherland J, Middleton J, Ornstein TJ, Lawson K, Vickers K. Assessing accident phobia in mild traumatic brain injury: the accident fear questionnaire. *Rehabil Psychol* 2016;**61**:317–27.

53. Donders J, Pendery A. Clinical utility of the patient health questionnaire-9 in the assessment of major depression after broad-spectrum traumatic brain injury. *Arch Phys Med Rehabil* 2017;**98**:2514–19.

54. Iverson GL, Gardner AJ, McCrory P, Zafonte R, Castellani RJ. A critical review of chronic traumatic encephalopathy. *Neurosci Biobehav Rev* 2015;**56**:276–93.

55. Lehman EJ, Hein MJ, Baron SL, Gersic CM. Neurodegenerative causes of death among retired National Football League players. *Neurology* 2012;**79**(19):1970–4.

56. Janssen PH, Mandrekar J, Mielke MM, Ahlskog JE, Boeve BF, Josephs K, et al. High school football and late-life risk of neurodegenerative syndromes, 1956–1970. *Mayo Clin Proc* 2017;**92**(1):66–71.

57. Savica R, Parisi JE, Wold LE, Josephs KA, Ahlskog JE. High school football and risk of neurodegeneration: a community-based study. *Mayo Clin Proc* 2012;**87**(4):335–40.

58. Mielke MM, Savica R, Wiste HJ, Weigand SD, Vemuri P, Knopman DS, et al. Head trauma and in vivo measures of amyloid and neurodegeneration in a population-based study. *Neurology* 2014;**82**(1):70–6.

59. Mittenberg W, DiGiulio DV, Perrin S, Bass AE. Symptoms following mild head injury: expectation as aetiology. *J Neurol Neurosurg Psychiatry* 1992;**55**(3):200–4.

60. Cancelliere C, Hincapié CA, Keightley M, Godbolt AK, Côté P, Kristman VL, et al. Systematic review of prognosis and return to play after sport concussion: results of the international collaboration on mild traumatic brain injury prognosis. *Arch Phys Med Rehabil* 2014;**95**(3 Suppl):S210–29.

61. Cooper DB, Bowles AO, Kennedy JE, Curtiss G, French LM, Tate DF, et al. Cognitive rehabilitation for military service members with mild traumatic brain injury: a randomized clinical trial. *J Head Trauma Rehabil* 2017;**32**(3):E1–15.

62. Mittenberg W, Tremont G, Zielinski RE, Fichera S, Rayls KR. Cognitive-behavioral prevention of postconcussion syndrome. *Arch Clin Neuropsychol* 1996;**11**(2):139–45.

63. Scholten J, Vasterling JJ, Grimes JB. Traumatic brain injury clinical practice guidelines and best practices from the VA state of the art conference. *Brain Injury* 2017;**31**(9):1246–51.

II. OVERVIEW OF NEUROSENSORY CONSEQUENCES

64. Talsky A, Pacione LR, Shaw T, Wasserman L, Lenny A, Verma A, et al. Pharmacological interventions for traumatic brain injury. *Br Columb Med J* 2010;**53**(1):26–31.
65. Wortzel HS, Arciniegas DB. Treatment of post-traumatic cognitive impairments. *Curr Treat Options Neurol* 2012;**14**(5):493–508.
66. Ponsford J, Lee NK, Wong D, McKay A, Haines K, Alway Y, et al. Efficacy of motivational interviewing and cognitive behavioral therapy for anxiety and depression symptoms following traumatic brain injury. *Psychol Med* 2016;**46**:1079–90.
67. Bryant R. Post-traumatic stress disorder vs traumatic brain injury. *Dialog Clin Neurosci* 2011;**13**(3):251–62.
68. Hammer PS, Sauvé WM. Psychopharmacology in treating posttraumatic stress disorder with co-occuring mild traumatic brain injury. *Primary Psychiatry*, July 8, 2014.
69. Dhaliwal SK, Meek BP, Modirrousta MM. Non-invasive brain stimulation for the treatment of symptoms following traumatic brain injury. *Front Psychiatry* 2015;**6**:119.
70. Harch PG, Andrews SR, Fogarty EF, Amen D, Pezzullo JC, Lucarini J, et al. A phase I study of low-pressure hyperbaric oxygen therapy for blast-induced post-concussion syndrome and post-traumatic stress disorder. *J Neurotrauma* 2012;**29**:168–85.

Tauopathies in Traumatic Brain Injury

Jonathan Pace, MD, Berje Shammassian, MD
and S. Alan Hoffer, MD

Department of Neurological Surgery, The Neurological Institute, University Hospitals
Cleveland Medical Center, Cleveland, OH, United States

INTRODUCTION

Repetitive mild traumatic brain injury (mTBI) is a defined risk factor for developing two entities associated with tauopathy. Although the increased incidence of both Alzheimer's disease (AD) and chronic traumatic encephalopathy (CTE) is well-defined in this population, the progression of pathology prior to clinically evident disease is less established. There have been great strides in the field from understanding the molecular basis of the disease process with different isomers of tau posing greater threat, to noninvasive methods of diagnosis such as magnetic resonance imaging (MRI) and positron emission tomography (PET) scanning, and retrospective and prospective studies that aid in identifying populations of people at greatest risk for developing CTE and early onset AD. There has been some recent data[1a-d] suggesting that there is an overlap between TBI and the development of CTE, AD, mild cognitive delay with posttraumatic stress disorder (PTSD), and anxiety.

In pursuit of increased understanding of the pathophysiology and clinical response to head trauma, animal models of TBI have undergone development as early as the 1940s. These animal models continue to be refined to reflect the improved technology available for animal testing as well as through the development of new injury models to study new classification of TBI as it is encountered clinically, namely blast injury. Despite the advances and discoveries made, the early identification and subsequent treatment of patients remains elusive at this time as the only definitive diagnosis is made post-mortem.

HISTORY

Although CTE has only recently received robust attention, the clinical and pathologic entity has been studied since the early to mid-20th century. Punch-drunk syndrome seen in boxers was initially described in 1928 by Martland and eventually began to be referred to as "Dementia Pugilistica".[1e] The first pathological correlate to the syndrome was described as a case report in 1954 by Brandenburg and Hallervorden.[1f] Not until 20 years later did the first definitive series emerge. In early 1973, Corsellis and colleagues described a number of post-mortem pathological findings among a series of 15 boxers.[2–4] These changes included septal abnormalities, supratentorial ventriculomegaly, and cerebral atrophy. In addition to these gross findings, there was concomitant microscopic presence of neurofibrillary tangles (NFTs), neuropil threads, and beta amyloid plaques, the latter of which was identified upon further studies to be present in the overwhelming majority of these patients. These findings were initially suspicious because, pathologically, they appeared identical to specimens obtained from AD patients many years older.

Tau originally functions to stabilize and elongate microtubules under low phosphorylation conditions. However, when tau becomes phosphorylated, it then has a low affinity for microtubules.[5,6] Thus, the phosphorylation and stability of the microtubules is directly related to the phosphorylated state of tau and the kinases that breakdown this protein.[7]

Simon and colleagues recently described a way that muscarinic receptors M1/3 on cholinergic neurons interact with tau, thereby disrupting the function of the neuron and leading to its loss—a mechanism by which tau becomes disseminated throughout the brain in AD.[8] This also may be the basis behind detection of tau and its breakdown products in cerebrospinal fluid.

EPIDEMIOLOGY

TBI is a significant disease entity associated with a large socioeconomic burden secondary to the amount of people affected by this process. mTBI, which occurs in approximately 3 million people annually, is often as a result of concussion sustained in sports such as football, soccer, rugby, and boxing.[9] It may also be associated with other disease states, such as physical abuse.[10] Most commonly, there is complete recovery from mTBI, but a subset of individuals may be subject to long-term sequelae of the mTBI, such as mild cognitive impairment, behavioral changes, CTE, and early onset dementia.[11] Moreover, there is some evidence that, even after "recovery," there may be late life cognitive sequelae and mTBI may influence subsequent development of dementia. While the link between mTBI and subsequent neurodegeneration is still controversial, a number of epidemiological studies have documented a strong association between TBI and the development of dementia syndromes in later life.[12–21] In addition, data from gene array studies performed in rodents support a link between concussive and blast TBI and dementia, illustrated by the identification of gene sets and pathways associated with AD and Parkinson disease observed by Days 3 and 14 after injury (e.g., genes such as Blalock a1 AD incipient, AD down and up, and the Parkin pathway).[22–24] It is, therefore, possible that mTBI predisposes individuals to future development of neuropathology and cognitive impairment.

The likelihood of developing long-term impairment from TBI relates to both the severity and frequency of exposure. Often, patients with diagnosed late-stage CTE also clinically meet the diagnostic criteria for AD[25] and, as such, effort is made to differentiate these two similar disease entities.

"Second impact syndrome" occurs when an individual sustains a second head injury while still symptomatic from an initial injury, which may produce rapid cerebral swelling and neurologic decline.[9,26−28] Frequently, the second insult is milder compared to the initial injury, but rapidly there is the development of severe cerebral edema and vascular engorgement. Mori and colleagues report that most individuals sustaining this event are young males, most commonly football players, but also hockey, boxing, and martial arts.[27] The pathophysiology of this syndrome is thought to be the result of lost autoregulation and marked catecholamine release, which results in the clinically evident diffuse, severe cerebral edema.[29]

Patients sustaining moderate TBI, as defined by the Glascow Coma Scale score of 9−13, and severe TBI, as defined by the Glascow Coma Scale score of 3−8, are at high risk of secondary injury following the direct insult due to excitotoxicity, hypotension, hypoxia, and cerebral edema to name a few.[30] In addition, there is significant neuroinflammation and apoptosis, probably secondary to activation of genes such as TNFα and p53. These topics, which are complex and have a host of issues related to them, will not be discussed here as it is outside the aim and scope of this text.

Blast injury, when inflicted, may range from a mTBI to severe TBI, depending on the size of the explosion and proximity to the origin of the blast. Initially described as "shell shock" during World War I,[9] where patients described symptoms of headache, memory loss, and neurocognitive changes, blast injury has come to the forefront following the increased frequency service members and civilians are exposed to explosions. Pertinently, according to a recent study by Frieden and Collins, up to 1/5 of the US military troops deployed the warzone in the Middle East are affected by some degree of TBI, and most of these injuries are due to blast injury.[31] In addition to the neurologic effects described earlier, there are reports of soldier with history of TBI developing neuropathologic changes consistent with CTE.[32]

mTBI, a term that is often used interchangeably with concussion, is a mild brain injury that may or may not result in a brief unconscious episode. The forces acting upon the head are often acceleration/deceleration as well as linear or rotational. Rotational injuries are the most common type to involve a loss of consciousness.[33] Several investigators have demonstrated that the accelerating and rotating injuries tend to cause a deformation of the brain, resulting in stretching of neuroglia, with axons being the most susceptible to this phenomenon. When stretched, the cell membranes have altered permeability, resulting in cross-membrane transit of ions and neurotransmitters, and causing resultant neurotoxicity in mTBI.[34,35]

mTBI often affects axons and cell compartment such as the corpus callosum, cerebellum, and mesial temporal lobes; the perivascular space as well as the vasculature itself is often where tau deposits are found in both TBI subjects as well as those with CTE and early onset AD secondary to the aggregation and misfolding of several proteins, including tau, beta-amyloid, and alpha-synuclein, that are associated with neurodegenerative disorders.[9,36,37] Indeed, a meta-analysis performed by Fleminger and colleagues reports that males suffering a single episode of TBI with associated loss of consciousness was associated with a 50% increased risk of developing AD; this risk further increased with increasingly severe head injuries.[38] This increased risk of developing AD has been similarly demonstrated in a population of war veterans.[39,40]

Individuals who sustain TBI are at risk for other disorders as well as from the direct injury and the development of CTE and AD. There is also an association with mood disorders, such as PTSD, anxiety, and depression, as well as addictive syndromes and sleep disorders.[9,41,42] As with the development of CTE, the risk of developing a mood disorder is also related to the severity and quantity of exposure to TBI. Clinically, both conditions demonstrate alterations in executive functioning, working memory, complex decision making, empathy, and emotional lability, along with behavioral changes.[32]

Aside from the association of CTE with disorders such as PTSD, anxiety, and depression, as noted earlier, there are also associations with other neurologic conditions. Lehman and colleagues identified an increased risk of amyotrophic lateral sclerosis (ALS) and motor neuron disease in patients with prolonged exposure to TBI.[42a] ALS is also predominant among other populations who suffer frequent concussions, such as soccer players as outlined earlier.[43] Mckee and colleagues took this finding one step further and identified that 11% of patients with diagnosed CTE developed ALS.[9]

Clinically, as noted earlier, one of the subtle early findings of CTE is mild cognitive impairment, which is nonspecific and may be seen with dementia and depression and following concussion. There is also a progressive decline in memory and executive functioning as well as other mood disturbances related to the gross regions of the brain affected.[9,25] The mood and behavioral disturbances may go beyond anxiety and depression and include apathy, anger, irritability, suicidality, and aggressiveness.

CTE disease progression is thought to occur slowly and progressively over the course of decades, with early findings again being subtle and nonspecific, including mild cognitive impairment as well as other signs of postconcussive syndrome, namely, difficulty with concentration, memory lapses, irritability, and headache.[44] This slow progression makes diagnosis difficult as CTE must be distinguished from age-related changes in brain.

As patients progress into stage II, paranoia and suicidality may become prominent. In the latter stages of CTE, prominent memory loss is often identified as well as progressive signs of executive dysfunction. Aggression and suicidality are seen in stage III, with executive dysfunction and dementia predominating in stage IV—the terminal aspect of this disease.

NEUROPATHOLOGY

Tau is expressed in normal as well as pathological brain samples. There are several ways to identify and study tau in the brain, which include ELISA, immunohistochemistry, and western blot techniques to identify the different isoforms and cleaved proteins derived from tau (Table 9.1).

Tau exists in an expected isoform ratio in AD. In the normal adult brain, Goedert and colleagues describe the ratio of 3-repeat tau as being equal to that of 4-repeat tau, 1:1.[45] Tau tangles in patients with AD are represented in a similar ratio of 3-repeat to 4-repeat isomers,[46] yet there is a shift of the ratio of mRNA expression in varying areas of the brain, such as CA1 of the hippocampus.[47]

Tau is clearly linked to both AD and CTE, although the direct relationship is not clearly defined. Tau deposition was the reason for the CTE diagnosis in the majority of cases, and

TABLE 9.1 Criteria for Pathological Diagnosis of CTE as Developed by the National Institute of Neurological Disorder and Stroke (NINDS) TBI/CTE Consensus Group

Required	Deep sulcal microperivascular neurons, astrocytes, and cell processes containing p-tau aggregates
Supportive	p-Tau-related

1. p-Tau aggregates and NFTs predominantly within cortical layers II–III
2. Hippocampal CA2 p-tau aggregates, NFTs, or extracellular tangles
3. Hippocampal CA4 prominent proximal dendritic swelling
4. Neuronal and astrocytic p-Tau aggregates in subcortical nuclei
5. Periventricular p-Tau thorny astrocytes
6. p-Tau positive large "grain-like" and "dot-like" structures

Gross anatomic findings
1. Parenchymal signs of prior trauma
2. Abnormalities of the septum pellucidum
3. Atrophy of the mamillary bodies
4. Ventricular dilatation (disproportionately the third ventricle)

Other histologic findings
1. TDP-43 cytoplastmic inclusions within the hippocampus, anteromedial temporal cortex, and amygdala

Adapted from McKee AC, Cairns NJ, Dickson DW, et al. The first NINDS/NIBIB consensus meeting to define neuropathological criteria for the diagnosis of chronic traumatic encephalopathy. Acta Neuropathol 2016;131(1):75–86. doi:10.1007/s00401-015-1515-z.

yet biochemical markers were only collected from two boxers, which demonstrated the expected presence of tau deposition in the brain.[48] However, when evaluated more fully, these NFTs differed significantly from those seen in AD in both form and tau isomer ratio.

CTE can only be diagnosed on autopsy, and, until recently, there was no consensus regarding criteria for diagnosis or biomarkers of the disease to aid in the diagnosis. Criteria for diagnosis included cerebral atrophy with concomitant "hydrocephalus ex vacuo" in which the ventricles enlarge secondary to the brain atrophy experienced as well as scarring and neuronal loss. NFTs are common, with immunohistochemistry staining positive for hyperphosphorylated tau. In 2016, a joint NINDS/NIBIB meeting released consensus criteria for the pathological diagnosis of CTE.[49]

As outlined earlier, the most recognizable features of CTE involve marked atrophy of the cerebrum, including the frontotemporal lobes and mesial temporal lobes, as well as diminished size of the thalamus and hypothalamus, and mammillary bodies. There has been a recent attempt to assign stages of progressive pathology based on the distribution and volume of tauopathy present. The current system in use was initially described in 2013 after analysis of 68 brains with CTE among 85 individuals with clinical histories of repetitive mTBI.[50] Researchers have identified tau pathology clustering in perivascular neurons following TBI, suggesting a link between TBI, neurons, and the adjacent vasculature, termed the neurovascular unit.[32] This may indicate a principal concept termed "trophic uncoupling," in which the proximity of the several types of cells are dependent upon the others for survival. When this aspect of the microenvironment is destabilized, such as secondary to injury, it will lead to malfunction of the other elements and possible cellular death. Further, perivascular accumulations of hyperphosphorylated tau, which comprise NFTs, and TDP-43 positive neurites in the white matter have been found after concussion, further reinforcing the axonal injury theory as directly related to the perivascular deposits of tau observed in mTBI[37]—often accompanied by microhemorrhage, which may also be related to tau deposition.

While the detection of tau with basic laboratory testing is important for the research and discovery aspects of TBI research in relation to tauopathy, it will be important to have this type of work translatable to the bedside. As such, the pathologic tau forms need to be able to be identified in a clinically meaningful way. Following TBI, tau may be identified in cerebrospinal fluid in its full length, cleaved, and PHF1-positive forms with full length tau being elevated in the majority of TBI patients.[51–54] This process is reproduced in both the cortical contusion injury animal model and fluid percussion animal model outlined below. Importantly, a caveat for the detection of tau within CSF is the source of the fluid itself. There have been reports of a higher concentration of tau within the ventricular system as opposed to the lumbar cistern.[55]

Indeed, oligomeric forms of tau may be a potentially pathologic form of tau, which may be a target for diagnosis and therapy. Hawkins and colleagues recently demonstrated in a fluid percussion injury rat model that following parasagittal injury, the rat model developed significant accumulation of tau oligomers as identified with ELISA,[56] thought to relate directly to the development of trauma-induced dementia and tauopathies, such as early-onset AD or CTE. The mechanism is unique for CTE, which is theorized to be related to direct, pathological accumulation along perivascular neurons and glia, and to be irregularly distributed in the cortical sulci.[57–59]

These findings are mirrored histologically as Albrayram and colleagues have recently demonstrated. Developing a polyclonal antibody that is able to distinguish between different isoforms of hyperphosphorylated tau (*cis* and *trans*) may play different roles in patients suffering from TBI.[60] Phosphorylated tau serves to disrupt microtubule binding and structure, with subsequent impaired axonal transport and neuronal function.[61] It has been found that the *cis* isomer is a precursor of neurodegeneration and cognitive impairment, both following sport-related and military-related TBI, and plays a role in the early cognitive changes associated with chronic TBI sequelae.[60,62] This discovery may pave the way for future diagnostic and therapeutic interventions for patients with TBI and associated AD and CTE. Targeted therapies to bind and facilitate removal of this tau isomer may be in the future of treatment, with trials currently underway.

Aside from tau being detected directly within CSF obtained from patients with TBI, there is evidence that tau may also be detected in serum, with higher elevations corresponding with more severe TBI in rat models. These findings are identified early following TBI—peaks within 24–48 hours, with a normalization following this spike.[63]

Analysis of neural-derived and astrocyte-derived exosomes (ADEs) can provide direct information about neuroinflammatory and neurodegenerative pathophysiology in brain. Exosomes, 50–200 nm-sized membranous vesicles, are generated and released by most viable cells and accumulate in biological fluids, including the blood, where they can be sampled in a time-dependent manner. The careful selection of the cell type from which exosomes derive by use of defined markers expressed on their surface, such as L1CAM, allows the immunoprecipitation of exosomes that are enriched for neural origin. Analysis of the contents of such exosomes provides a window to neural cells within the brain in relation to their response to physiological challenges, disease, and its progression and responses to drugs. Hence, plasma exosomes have recently been used as circulating biomarkers preclinically and clinically for the definitive diagnosis and monitoring of therapeutic responses. Exosomes derived from astrocytes allow evaluation of a variety of neural processes because astrocytes maintain ion, metabolic, and neurochemical homeostasis in the brain and respond to numerous physiological and pathological brain challenges to initiate homeostatic and reparative processes. Astrocytes accumulate at sites of injury within the brain and overexpress astrocyte-specific genes/proteins, such as the glial fibrillary acid and inflammatory proteins. Astrocytes also accumulate in regions of Aβ-peptide deposition in the brain, where they internalize and degrade aggregated peptides in an apparently protective process. A subset of astrocytes expresses amyloid precursor protein (APP) and associated β- and γ-secretases required for generation of Aβ, whose production is increased in the presence of oligomeric Aβ42 and pro-inflammatory cytokines. Immunochemical techniques have recently been developed to permit the isolation of plasma ADEs to allow characterization of their cargo,[64] for example, enriching for ADEs by using a mouse antihuman glutamine aspartate transporter (GLAST) (ACSA-1) biotinylated antibody (Miltenyi Biotec, Inc., Auburn, CA, United States). Studies of human ADEs and rodent cell cultures have indicated that levels of APP species as well as secretase levels are greater in ADEs than in neural-derived exosomes.[64] ADEs also allow evaluation of levels of pro- and antiinflammatory cytokines, such as TNF-α, IL-1, IL-6, IL-10, and TGFβ.

CTE encompasses four separate stages that occur along a spectrum of increasing tauopathy while considering the presence of findings about TDP-43 inclusions found within neurons and glia[9]; A beta amyloid inclusions, which are found in roughly half of cases; and axonal damage. Inflammation is also a driver with CTE as elevated numbers of reactive microglia are seen in the white matter of these subjects. The initial study also provided descriptions of clinical symptoms of individuals within the stages, attempting to demonstrate a relationship between severity of clinical perturbations and pathological severity of CTE seen in specimens. It is important to acknowledge that the studies on which the staging system is based are post-mortem in nature and lend to particular biases especially when formulating a chronological progression of pathological disease. In addition, there are expected limitations of these studies when attempting to ascribe clinical manifestations to pathological findings.

The majority of pathological findings in stage I occur microscopically. NFTs are mostly confined to the sulcal perivascular spaces of the frontal lobe cortices but can be visualized within the locus coeruleus. Although there is an absence of AB plaques in stage I, TDP-43 inclusions are found in roughly half of specimens.[9]

Stage II retains the location of the pathology mostly within the frontal lobes, but roughly half of brains show the gross changes characteristically associated with the disease, such as ventriculomegaly and septal abnormalities. Clusters of perivascular hyperphosphorylated tau are found, primarily in the regions of expected future atrophy, the frontal and temporal lobes, and insula. NFTs may also be found in the thalamus and brainstem.[9]

Stage III shows a progression of gross anatomic pathology seen in stage II, including further frontotemporal atrophy. The mesial temporal lobes and entorhinal cortex degenerate, with microscopically more diffuse and densely packed NFTs within the cortex in addition to the presence within the limbic system and cerebellum. Within this stage, A beta plaques begin to be seen.[9]

Gross frontotemporal atrophy is significant in stage IV CTE with noticeable progressive degeneration. Principal findings include dense packing of NFTs throughout the brain, with associated neuronal loss and scarring. Interestingly, the occipital lobes responsible for vision are usually spared.[9]

IMAGING BIOMARKERS

To aid in the diagnosis of tauopathies and their relation to TBI, the delivery of timely diagnostic imaging modalities to guide treatment will be important. Among the newly devised imaging modalities are PET, MRI, and electroencephalography (EEG).

Positron Emission Tomography

PET may be employed for the imaging of tau. There are many tracers that may be tailored to label the various isoforms and cleaved products of the tau protein, allowing for visualization of tau. Tracers have been developed to specifically bind various isomers or cleavage products, which include primarily naphthols and arylquinolone derivatives.[65]

Magnetic Resonance Imaging and Functional Magnetic Resonance Imaging

Other imaging biomarkers that have been developed include magnetic resonance imaging for structural and quantitative imaging. Functional MRI (fMRI) may demonstrate early changes usually found in prefrontal activation and working-memory—related changes in the context of prior history of concussion as well as changes seen in mild cognitive impairment or dementia, while key structures may remain intact.[66]

fMRI shows promise in the evaluation of TBI, both in the acute setting as well as long-term, as it may be utilized to test for changes in cognitive function and recruitment of different regions of the brain compared to controls. Further, fMRI may be useful in the evaluation of dementia and tauopathies such as AD and CTE. The prefrontal cortex is used for several executive functions, such as cognitive control, organization, and efficient use of resources, among others.[66] In TBI, compensatory changes in the cognitive control and activation of the prefrontal cortex is observed; when TBI is coupled with dementia, this compensation diminishes.[67–71]

fMRI can also be used to evaluate interconnected regions prior to the application of a cognitive stimulus. This may play a role in the evaluation of the brain network as a whole, in which the analysis of the intrinsic brain function, on a quantitative level, may serve as a means for evaluating pathologic changes following TBI, with or without neurodegenerative disease.[72] Moreover, this may allow for evaluation of changes over time and for recognition of advanced aging signs as might be seen from early-onset AD or CTE.

Resting state fMRI is likely the most useful in patients following TBI as this modality does not require the subject's cooperation or participation. It is easy to test and interpret because the default resting network will show abnormalities. Patients who have suffered TBI may demonstrate changes, which are stimulus independent, to show less connectivity between other areas of the network, increased activation during tasks while also demonstrating increased deactivation during rest.[73] The regions of this network include the mesial temporal lobes, lateral temporal region, anterior and posterior midlines, and temporo-parietal junction.

Aberrations have also been identified in the connections between the default network and networks controlling goal-oriented behavior and drives.[74] Bonnelle and colleagues have demonstrated that alterations in these networks may be seen in TBI patients, when less deactivation of the default network described earlier is coupled with impaired control mechanisms; in other words, these patients may demonstrate disinhibition and emotional lability.[75,76]

Electroencephalography

EEG has advantages over MRI and PET imaging given lower cost, ease of acquisition, and lack of exclusion criteria. Further, EEG is a real-time test, which allows for detection of abnormalities as they occur, and it can track these changes over time.[66] However, the current use of EEG while evaluating those people who have suffered TBI is limited.

ANIMAL MODELS

To better investigate the effects of TBI on the brain, several preclinical models have been developed to evaluate this pathological process. Early animal models of TBI included the use of nonhuman primates, dogs, cats, guinea pigs, and rabbits, whereas the majority of the current models involve rodents as the study vehicle. However, as was importantly outlined by Abisambra and colleagues, it is necessary to highlight the differences between murine and human tau sequences, which are 88% similar.[77,78] As delineated earlier by Goedert and colleagues, humans express roughly equal numbers of the 3-repeat and 4-repeat isomers, whereas mice express solely 4-repeat isomers and do not form tau tangles.[45,79] Tau NFTs can be formed in transgenic knockout mice when endogenous tau is no longer expressed, and instead is replaced with disease-associated mutant tau or wild-type human tau.[80,81] The most common animal models utilized for TBI include the weight drop model, the fluid percussion model, cortical contusion model, and the blast injury model.

Weight Drop Model

The weight drop model is a model in which an object is guided to drop onto the animal's head, and was first described by Pilcher et al in 1937 in a dog animal model.[82] There have been other, more sophisticated weight drop models developed, including a model in which cats underwent TBI by a weight falling onto a column of water that was in contact with the dura of the cat brain.[83] Subsequently Feeney and colleagues developed a weight drop model where a craniotomy was performed on rats, with subsequent TBI inflicted by a footplate at the end of a guide tube coming into contact with dura.[84]

More current models have been developed which allow for injury without the exposure of the skull or brain of the rodent. The advantages of these systems revolve around the simplicity with animal preparation, and the minimal sedation requirements for the animals. Blaha and colleagues describe a rat model for inflicting TBI for the study of diffuse brain injury.[85] The Marmarou model, one of the best characterized weight drop models, involves a metal disc being fixated to the exposed skull of the rat. The rat is positioned on a foam pad to absorb energy and produce an acceleration/deceleration type of injury when the weight is dropped onto the animal's head.[86,87] This allows the findings of TBI in this animal model to be more consistently applied as a translational model. However, this model is prone to variable degrees of injury severity, due to the method of injury induction.

A variety of techniques have been developed for inflicting injury in mouse models, which were designed to look at a variety of diffuse brain injuries, as well as mild, concussion-type injuries.[88–91] Importantly, the use of mice allows studies on transgenic animal models in which various molecules can be overexpressed or deleted to test mechanistic hypothesis.

Fluid Percussion Model

The fluid percussion model is one of the more common animal models used to study TBI. There have been several improvements in the fluid percussion model, primarily in cats and rabbits initially.[92–94] Over time, this approach has been adapted to several other animal models, such as in dogs, sheep, rats, and mice. This a useful tool in mice also for studying changes using transgenic animals.[95,96] Essentially, a fluid filled reservoir is fit to an animal's head following a craniotomy, with a pendulum striking the fluid reservoir from a set distance. This creates an impulse which is then transmitted to the brain. Currently, one of the most popular methods to employ the fluid percussion model involves making the craniotomy just lateral to midline.[97,98]

Cortical Contusion Injury Model

The cortical contusion injury model was initially developed in the ferret; this model allows for a craniotomy to be made over the area of brain to withstand the injury.[99] Since its development, the cortical contusion injury model has been modified for use in smaller mammals, such as the mouse and rat.[100] As earlier, its implementation in a mouse model allows for the study of brain injury in a transgenic model. This model is able to be modified easily to cause a range of injuries from mild to severe.[101]

The majority of the craniotomies performed were initially over the parietal regions, although a bifrontal injury model has also been developed.[102,103] These models, interestingly in mice, also demonstrate associated dysfunction including hippocampal injury and neuronal loss. Indeed, this model is associated with neuronal loss not only in the hippocampus, but also in the cortex and striatum and is associated with gliosis, inflammation, blood−brain barrier disruption, and behavioral dysfunction.[21,77]

As outlined earlier, these models have the ability to aid in the study of TBI across a wide range of severities. Further, they are both historic as well as modern in technique and inception. Below, we will also discuss blast injury models that have become popular to aid in studying the complex injuries that arise following warfare. This has gained importance over the past decade, following the conflicts in Iraq and Afghanistan and the injuries observed in civilians and soldiers suffering blast-induced TBI.

Blast Injury Model

To adequately study blast injury and subsequent TBI development, it is important to develop a model that replicated the forces delivered to the brain. Up to this point, the injury models outlined earlier did a good job of mimicking direct injury to the brain and head. However, the secondary injuries delivered to the brain during a blast injury were initially not modeled in a satisfactory way. There are more recent animal models for such blast injury, using the blast tube and open field blasts[104] which are much better approximations of the clinical situation, both in terms of behavior and pathophysiology.

In conclusion, the key role of phosphorylated tau offers not only a molecular mechanistic approach to TBI but also a potential therapeutic pathway. While normally tau is critical for microtubule function, drugs that interact with the cis hyperphosphorylated moieties may offer new and innovative treatments.

CONCLUSION AND FUTURE AIMS

The knowledge concerning the relationship between mTBI and tauopathies continues to be refined, from both an etiological as well as a therapeutic standpoint. There is data suggesting isolated minor TBI may lead to long-term sequelae, but there is clearly evidence relating both the number and severity of TBI incidents and the development of CTE. With the advances made at the benchtop identifying associated molecules, which may be causative in the clinical syndromes encountered, the future of diagnosis and treatment of TBI, CTE, and its associated neurocognitive dysfunction appears bright.

References

1a. Mufson EJ, Perez SE, Nadeem M, et al. Progression of tau pathology within cholinergic nucleus basalis neurons in chronic traumatic encephalopathy: A chronic effects of neurotrauma consortium study. *Brain Inj* 2016;**30**(12):1399−413. Available from: https://doi.org/10.1080/02699052.2016.1219058.

1b. Osborn AJ, Mathias JL, Fairweather-Schmidt AK. Prevalence of anxiety following adult traumatic brain injury: A meta-analysis comparing measures, samples and postinjury intervals. *Neuropsychology* 2016;**30**(2):247−61. Available from: https://doi.org/10.1037/neu0000221.

1c. Moretti L, Cristofori I, Weaver SM, Chau A, Portelli JN, Grafman J. Cognitive decline in older adults with a history of traumatic brain injury. *Lancet Neurol* 2012;**11**(12):1103−12. Available from: https://doi.org/10.1016/S1474-4422(12)70226-0.

1d. Klein M, Houx PJ, Jolles J. Long-term persisting cognitive sequelae of traumatic brain injury and the effect of age. *J Nerv Ment Dis* 1996;**184**(8):459–67. http://www.ncbi.nlm.nih.gov/pubmed/8752074. Accessed September 3, 2018.

1e. Martland HS. Punchdrunk. *J Am Med Assoc* 1928;**91**(15):1103. Available from: https://doi.org/10.1001/jama.1928.02700150029009.

1f. Bradenburg W, Hallervorden J. Dementia pugilistica with anatomical findings. *Virchows Arch Pathol Anat Physiol Klin Med [Internet]* 1954;**325**(6):680–709. [cited 2017 Oct 9] Available from: http://www.ncbi.nlm.nih.gov/pubmed/13226712.

2. Ling H, Neal JW, Revesz T. Evolving concepts of chronic traumatic encephalopathy as a neuropathological entity. *Neuropathol Appl Neurobiol* 2017;**46**(6):467–76. Available from: https://doi.org/10.1111/nan.12425.

3. Kiernan PT, Montenigro PH, Solomon TM, McKee AC. Chronic traumatic encephalopathy: a neurodegenerative consequence of repetitive traumatic brain injury. *Semin Neurol* 2015;**35**(1):20–80. Available from: https://doi.org/10.1055/s-0035-1545080.

4. Corsellis JA, Bruton CJ, Freeman-Browne D. The aftermath of boxing. *Psychol Med [Internet]* 1973;**3**(3):270–303. [cited 2017 Oct 20]. Available from: http://www.ncbi.nlm.nih.gov/pubmed/4729191.

5. Sengupta A, Kabat J, Novak M, Wu Q, Grundke-Iqbal I, Iqbal K. Phosphorylation of tau at both Thr231 and Ser 262 is required for maximal inhibition of its binding to microtubules. *Arch Biochem Biophys* 1998;**357**(2):299–309.

6. Illenberger S, Drewes G, Trinczek B, Biernat J, Meyer HE, Olmsted JB, et al. Phosphorylation of microtubule-associated proteins MAP2 and MAP4 by the protein kinase p110mark. Phosphorylation sites and regulation of microtubule dynamics. *J Biol Chem* 1996;**271**(18):10834–43.

7. Gong CX, Grundke-Iqbal I, Damuni Z, Iqbal K. Dephosphorylation of microtubule-associated protein tau by protein phosphatase-1 and -2C and its implication in Alzheimer disease. *FEBS Lett* 1994;**341**(1):94–8.

8. Simon D, Hernandez F, Avila J. The involvement of cholinergic neurons in the spreading of tau pathology. *Front Neurol* 2013;**4**:74.

9. McKee AC. DDH. *The neuropathology of Traumatic brain injury.* 2015;**15**:45–66.

10. Daneshvar DH, Nowinski CJ, McKee AC, Cantu RC. The epidemiology of sport-related concussion. *Clin Sports Med [Internet]* 2011;**30**(1):1–17. [cited 2017 Oct 20] Available from: http://www.ncbi.nlm.nih.gov/pubmed/21074078.

11. Langlois JA, Rutland-Brown W, Wald MM. The epidemiology and impact of traumatic brain injury: a brief overview. *J Head Trauma Rehabil [Internet]*;21(5):375–378. [cited 2017 Oct 20] Available from: http://www.ncbi.nlm.nih.gov/pubmed/16983222

12. Abner EL, Nelson PT, Schmitt FA, Browning SR, Fardo DW, Wan L, et al. Self-reported head injury and risk of late-life impairment and AD pathology in an AD center cohort. *Dement Geriatr Cogn Disord [Internet]* 2014;**37**(5–6):294–306. [cited 2017 Oct 20] Available from: http://www.ncbi.nlm.nih.gov/pubmed/24401791.

13. Barnes DE, Kaup A, Kirby KA, Byers AL, Diaz-Arrastia R, Yaffe K. Traumatic brain injury and risk of dementia in older veterans. *Neurology [Internet]* 2014;**83**(4):312–19 [cited 2017 Oct 20] Available from: http://www.ncbi.nlm.nih.gov/pubmed/24966406.

14. Gardner RC, Burke JF, Nettiksimmons J, Kaup A, Barnes DE, Yaffe K. Dementia risk after traumatic brain injury vs nonbrain trauma. *JAMA Neurol [Internet]* 2014;**71**(12):1490. [cited 2017 Oct 20] Available from: http://www.ncbi.nlm.nih.gov/pubmed/25347255.

15. Lee Y.-K., Hou S.-W., Lee C.-C., Hsu C.-Y., Huang Y.-S., Su Y.-C. Increased risk of dementia in patients with mild traumatic brain injury: a nationwide cohort study. Zhang XY, editor. *PLoS One [Internet]* 2013;8(5):e62422. [cited 2017 Oct 20] Available from: http://www.ncbi.nlm.nih.gov/pubmed/23658727.

16. Nordström P, Michaëlsson K, Gustafson Y, Nordström A. Traumatic brain injury and young onset dementia: a nationwide cohort study. *Ann Neurol [Internet]* 2014;**75**(3):374–81. [cited 2017 Oct 20] Available from: http://www.ncbi.nlm.nih.gov/pubmed/24812697.

17. Seichepine DR, Stamm JM, Daneshvar DH, Riley DO, Baugh CM, Gavett BE, et al. Profile of self-reported problems with executive functioning in college and professional football players. *J Neurotrauma [Internet]* 2013;**30**(14):1299–304. [cited 2017 Oct 20] Available from: http://online.liebertpub.com/doi/abs/10.1089/neu.2012.2690.

18. Stamm JM, Bourlas AP, Baugh CM, Fritts NG, Daneshvar DH, Martin BM, et al. Age of first exposure to football and later-life cognitive impairment in former NFL players. *Neurology [Internet]* 2015;**84**(11):1114–20. [cited2017 Oct 20] Available from: http://www.neurology.org/cgi/doi/10.1212/WNL.0000000000001358.

19. Sundström A, Nilsson L-G, Cruts M, Adolfsson R, Van Broeckhoven C, Nyberg L. Increased risk of dementia following mild head injury for carriers but not for non-carriers of the APOE epsilon4 allele. *Int Psychogeriatrics [Internet]* 2007;**19**(1):159−65. [cited 2017 Oct 20] Available from: http://www.journals.cambridge.org/abstract_S1041610206003498.

20. Wang H-K, Lin S-H, Sung P-S, Wu M-H, Hung K-W, Wang L-C, et al. Population based study on patients with traumatic brain injury suggests increased risk of dementia. *J Neurol Neurosurg Psychiatry [Internet]* 2012;**83**(11):1080−5. [cited 2017 Oct 20] Available from: http://www.ncbi.nlm.nih.gov/pubmed/22842203.

21. Wang T-Y, Wei H-T, Liou Y-J, Su T-P, Bai Y-M, Tsai S-J, et al. Risk for developing dementia among patients with posttraumatic stress disorder: a nationwide longitudinal study. *J Affect Disord [Internet]* 2016;**205**:306−10. [cited 2017 Oct 20] Available from: http://linkinghub.elsevier.com/retrieve/pii/S0165032716307686.

22. Tweedie D, Rachmany L, Kim DS, Rubovitch V, Lehrmann E, Zhang Y, et al. Mild traumatic brain injury-induced hippocampal gene expressions: the identification of target cellular processes for drug development. *J Neurosci Methods [Internet]* 2016;**272**:4−18. [cited 2017 Oct 20] Available from: http://www.ncbi.nlm.nih.gov/pubmed/26868732.

23. Tweedie D, Rachmany L, Rubovitch V, Zhang Y, Becker KG, Perez E, et al. Changes in mouse cognition and hippocampal gene expression observed in a mild physical- and blast-traumatic brain injury. *Neurobiol Dis [Internet]* 2013;**54**:1−11. [cited 2017 Oct 20] Available from: http://www.ncbi.nlm.nih.gov/pubmed/23454194.

24. Tweedie D, Rachmany L, Rubovitch V, Lehrmann E, Zhang Y, Becker KG, et al. Exendin-4, a glucagon-like peptide-1 receptor agonist prevents mTBI-induced changes in hippocampus gene expression and memory deficits in mice. *Exp Neurol [Internet]* 2013;**239**:170−82. [cited 2017 Oct 20] Available from: http://www.ncbi.nlm.nih.gov/pubmed/23059457.

25. Stern RA, Daneshvar DH, Baugh CM, Seichepine DR, Montenigro PH, Riley DO, et al. Clinical presentation of chronic traumatic encephalopathy. *Neurology [Internet]* 2013;**81**(13):1122−9. [cited 2017 Oct 9] Available from: http://www.ncbi.nlm.nih.gov/pubmed/23966253.

26. Saunders RL, Harbaugh RE. The second impact in catastrophic contact-sports head trauma. *JAMA [Internet]* 1984;**252**(4):538−9. [cited 2017 Oct 20] Available from: http://www.ncbi.nlm.nih.gov/pubmed/6737652.

27. Mori T, Katayama Y, Kawamata T. Acute hemispheric swelling associated with thin subdural hematomas: pathophysiology of repetitive head injury in sports. *Acta Neurochir Suppl [Internet]* 2006;**96**:40−3. [cited 2017 Oct 20] Available from: http://www.ncbi.nlm.nih.gov/pubmed/16671421.

28. Cantu RC, Gean AD. Second-impact syndrome and a small subdural hematoma: an uncommon catastrophic result of repetitive head injury with a characteristic imaging appearance. *J Neurotrauma [Internet]* 2010;**27**(9):1557−64. [cited 2017 Oct 20]Available from: http://www.liebertonline.com/doi/abs/10.1089/neu.2010.1334.

29. Strebel S, Lam AM, Matta BF, Newell DW. Impaired cerebral autoregulation after mild brain injury. *Surg Neurol [Internet]* 1997;**47**(2):128−31. [cited 2017 Oct 20] Available from: http://www.ncbi.nlm.nih.gov/pubmed/9040813.

30. Hukkelhoven CWPM, Rampen AJJ, Maas AIR, Farace E, Habbema JDF, Marmarou A, et al. Some prognostic models for traumatic brain injury were not valid. *J Clin Epidemiol [Internet]* 2006;59(2):132−43. [cited 2017 Oct 9] Available from: http://www.ncbi.nlm.nih.gov/pubmed/16426948

31. National Center for Injury Prevention C, Institutes of Health N. *Report to Congress on traumatic brain injury in the United States: understanding the public health problem among current and former military personnel.* 2013; [cited 2017 Oct 20] Available from: https://www.cdc.gov/traumaticbraininjury/pdf/report_to_congress_on_traumatic_brain_injury_2013-a.pdf

32. Goldstein LE, Fisher AM, Tagge CA, Zhang XL, Velisek L, Sullivan JA, et al. Chronic traumatic encephalopathy in blast-exposed military veterans and a blast neurotrauma mouse model. *Sci Transl Med* 2012;**4**(134):134ra60.

33. Meaney DF, Smith DH, Shreiber DI, Bain AC, Miller RT, Ross DT, et al. Biomechanical analysis of experimental diffuse axonal injury. *J Neurotrauma [Internet]* 1995;**12**(4):689−94. [cited 2017 Oct 9] Available from: http://www.ncbi.nlm.nih.gov/pubmed/8683620.

34. Povlishock JT, Erb DE, Astruc J. Axonal response to traumatic brain injury: reactive axonal change, deafferentation, and neuroplasticity. *J Neurotrauma [Internet]* 1992;**9**(Suppl 1). S189-200. [cited2017 Oct 9] Available from: http://www.ncbi.nlm.nih.gov/pubmed/1588608.

35. Prins ML, Hovda DA. Mapping cerebral glucose metabolism during spatial learning: interactions of development and traumatic brain injury. *J Neurotrauma [Internet]* 2001;**18**(1):31−46. [cited 2017 Oct 20] Available from: http://www.ncbi.nlm.nih.gov/pubmed/11200248.

36. Nemetz PN, Leibson C, Naessens JM, Beard M, Kokmen E, Annegers JF, et al. Traumatic brain injury and time to onset of Alzheimer's disease: a population-based study. *Am J Epidemiol [Internet]* 1999;**149**(1):32–40. [cited 2017 Oct 20] Available from: http://www.ncbi.nlm.nih.gov/pubmed/9883791.

37. McKee AC, Daneshvar DH, Alvarez VE, Stein TD. The neuropathology of sport. *Acta Neuropathol [Internet]* 2014;**127**(1):29–51. [cited 2017 Oct 9] Available from: http://www.ncbi.nlm.nih.gov/pubmed/24366527.

38. Fleminger S, Oliver DL, Lovestone S, Rabe-Hesketh S, Giora A. Head injury as a risk factor for Alzheimer's disease: the evidence 10 years on; a partial replication. *J Neurol Neurosurg Psychiatry [Internet]* 2003;**74**(7):857–62. [cited 2017 Oct 20] Available from: http://www.ncbi.nlm.nih.gov/pubmed/12810767.

39. Corkin S, Rosen TJ, Sullivan EV, Clegg RA. Penetrating head injury in young adulthood exacerbates cognitive decline in later years. *J Neurosci [Internet]* 1989;**9**(11):3876–83. [cited 2017 Oct 20] Available from: http://www.ncbi.nlm.nih.gov/pubmed/2585058.

40. Plassman BL, Havlik RJ, Steffens DC, Helms MJ, Newman TN, Drosdick D, et al. Documented head injury in early adulthood and risk of Alzheimer's disease and other dementias. *Neurology [Internet]* 2000;**55**(8):1158–66. [cited 2017 Oct 20] Available from: http://www.ncbi.nlm.nih.gov/pubmed/11071494.

41. Guskiewicz KM, Marshall SW, Bailes J, Mccrea M, Harding HP, Matthews A, et al. Recurrent concussion and risk of depression in retired professional football players. *Med Sci Sport Exerc [Internet]* 2007;**39**(6):903–9. [cited 2017 Oct 20] Available from: http://www.ncbi.nlm.nih.gov/pubmed/17545878.

42. Kerr ZY, Evenson KR, Rosamond WD, Mihalik JP, Guskiewicz KM, Marshall SW. Association between concussion and mental health in former collegiate athletes. *Inj Epidemiol [Internet]* 2014;**1**(1):28. [cited 2017 Oct 20] Available from: http://www.ncbi.nlm.nih.gov/pubmed/27747661.

42a. Lehman EJ, Hein MJ, Baron SL, Gersic CM. Neurodegenerative causes of death among retired National Football League players. *Neurology* 2012;**79**(19):1970–4. Available from: https://doi.org/10.1212/WNL.0b013e31826daf50.

43. Chiò A, Benzi G, Dossena M, Mutani R, Mora G. Severely increased risk of amyotrophic lateral sclerosis among Italian professional football players. *Brain [Internet]* 2005;**128**(Pt 3):472–6. [cited2017 Oct 20] Available from: https://academic.oup.com/brain/article-lookup/doi/10.1093/brain/awh373.

44. Daneshvar DH, Riley DO, Nowinski CJ, McKee AC, Stern RA, Cantu RC. Long-term consequences: effects on normal development profile after concussion. *Phys Med Rehabil Clin N Am [Internet]* 2011;**22**(4):683–700. [cited 2017 Oct 20] Available from: http://www.ncbi.nlm.nih.gov/pubmed/22050943.

45. Goedert M, Spillantini MG, Jakes R, Rutherford D, Crowther RA. Multiple isoforms of human microtubule-associated protein tau: sequences and localization in neurofibrillary tangles of Alzheimer's disease. *Neuron* 1989;**3**(4):519–26.

46. de Silva R, Lashley T, Gibb G, Hanger D, Hope A, Reid A, et al. Pathological inclusion bodies in tauopathies contain distinct complements of tau with three or four microtubule-binding repeat domains as demonstrated by new specific monoclonal antibodies. *Neuropathol Appl Neurobiol.* 2003;**29**(3):288–302.

47. Ginsberg SD, Che S, Counts SE, Mufson EJ. Shift in the ratio of three-repeat tau and four-repeat tau mRNAs in individual cholinergic basal forebrain neurons in mild cognitive impairment and Alzheimer's disease. *J Neurochem* 2006;**96**(5):1401–8.

48. Zetterberg H, Hietala MA, Jonsson M, Andreasen N, Styrud E, Karlsson I, et al. Neurochemical aftermath of amateur boxing. *Arch Neurol* 2006;**63**(9):1277–80.

49. McKee AC, Cairns NJ, Dickson DW, Folkerth RD, Dirk Keene C, Litvan I, et al. The first NINDS/NIBIB consensus meeting to define neuropathological criteria for the diagnosis of chronic traumatic encephalopathy. *Acta Neuropathol* 2016;**131**(1):75–86.

50. McKee AC, Stein TD, Nowinski CJ, Stern RA, Daneshvar DH, Alvarez VE, et al. The spectrum of disease in chronic traumatic encephalopathy. *Brain* 2013;**136**(1):43–64.

51. Kay AD, Petzold A, Kerr M, Keir G, Thompson E, Nicoll JA. Alterations in cerebrospinal fluid apolipoprotein E and amyloid beta-protein after traumatic brain injury. *J Neurotrauma* 2003;**20**(10):943–52.

52. Zemlan FP, Jauch EC, Mulchahey JJ, Gabbita SP, Rosenberg WS, Speciale SG, et al. C-tau biomarker of neuronal damage in severe brain injured patients: association with elevated intracranial pressure and clinical outcome. *Brain Res* 2002;**947**(1):131–9.

53. Franz G, Beer R, Kampfl A, Engelhardt K, Schmutzhard E, Ulmer H, et al. Amyloid beta 1-42 and tau in cerebrospinal fluid after severe traumatic brain injury. *Neurology* 2003;**60**(9):1457–61.

54. Zemlan FP, Rosenberg WS, Luebbe PA, Campbell TA, Dean GE, Weiner NE, et al. Quantification of axonal damage in traumatic brain injury: affinity purification and characterization of cerebrospinal fluid tau proteins. *J Neurochem* 1999;**72**(2):741−50.

55. Blennow K, Nellgard B. Amyloid beta 1-42 and tau in cerebrospinal fluid after severe traumatic brain injury. *Neurology* 2004;**62**(1):159. author reply 159-60.

56. Hawkins BE, Krishnamurthy S, Castillo-Carranza DL, Sengupta U, Prough DS, Jackson GR, et al. Rapid accumulation of endogenous Tau oligomers in a rat model of traumatic brain injury: possible link between traumatic brain injury and sporadic tauopathies. *J Biol Chem* 2013;**288**(23):17042−50.

57. Clavaguera F, Bolmont T, Crowther RA, Abramowski D, Frank S, Probst A, et al. Transmission and spreading of tauopathy in transgenic mouse brain. *Nat Cell Biol* 2009;**11**(7):909−13.

58. Frost B, Diamond MI. Prion-like mechanisms in neurodegenerative diseases. *Nat Rev Neurosci* 2010;**11**(3):155−9.

59. Le MN, Kim W, Lee S, McKee AC, Hall GF. Multiple mechanisms of extracellular tau spreading in a non-transgenic tauopathy model. *Am J Neurodegener Dis* 2012;**1**(3):316−33.

60. Albayram O, Herbert MK, Kondo A, Tsai C-Y, Baxley S, Lian X, et al. Function and regulation of tau conformations in the development and treatment of traumatic brain injury and neurodegeneration. *Cell Biosci* 2016;**6**(59):1−6. Available from: https://doi.org/10.1186/s13578-016-0124-4.

61. Mandelkow EM, Mandelkow E. Biochemistry and cell biology of tau protein in neurofibrillary degeneration. *Cold Spring Harb Perspect Med* 2012;**2**(7):a006247.

62. Kondo A, Shahpasand K, Mannix R, Qiu J, Moncaster J, Chen C-H, et al. Antibody against early driver of neurodegeneration cis P-tau blocks brain injury and tauopathy. *Nature [Internet]* 2015;**523**(7561):431−6. Available from: http://www.nature.com/doifinder/10.1038/nature14658.

63. Gabbita SP, Scheff SW, Menard RM, Roberts K, Fugaccia I, Zemlan FP. Cleaved-tau: a biomarker of neuronal damage after traumatic brain injury. *J Neurotrauma [Internet]* 2005;**22**(1):83−94. [cited 2017 Oct 20] Available from: http://www.liebertonline.com/doi/abs/10.1089/neu.2005.22.83.

64. Goetzl EJ, Kapogiannis D, Schwartz JB, Lobach IV, Goetzl L, Abner EL, et al. Decreased synaptic proteins in neuronal exosomes of frontotemporal dementia and Alzheimers disease. *FASEB J [Internet]* 2016;**30**(12):4141−8. [cited 2017 Oct 9] Available from: http://www.ncbi.nlm.nih.gov/pubmed/27601437.

65. Dani M, Edison P, Brooks DJ. Imaging biomarkers in tauopathies. *Park Relat Disord* 2016;**22**:S26−8. Available from: https://doi.org/10.1016/J.PARKRELDIS.2015.08.011.

66. Esopenko C., Levine B. Aging, Neurodegenerative disease, and traumatic brain injury: the role of neuroimaging. J Neurotrauma 2015;32(4):209-20. https://doi.org/10.1089/neu.2014.3506.

67. Hillary FG, Medaglia JD, Gates K, Molenaar PC, Slocomb J, Peechatka A, et al. Examining working memory task acquisition in a disrupted neural network. *Brain* 2011;**134**(Pt 5):1555−70.

68. Grady C. The cognitive neuroscience of ageing. *Nat Rev Neurosci* 2012;**13**(7):491−505.

69. Turner GR, McIntosh AR, Levine B. Prefrontal compensatory engagement in TBI is due to altered functional engagement of existing networks and not functional reorganization. *Front Syst Neurosci* 2011;**5**:9.

70. Turner GR, Levine B. Augmented neural activity during executive control processing following diffuse axonal injury. *Neurology* 2008;**71**(11):812−18.

71. McAllister TW, Flashman LA, McDonald BC, Saykin AJ. Mechanisms of working memory dysfunction after mild and moderate TBI: evidence from functional MRI and neurogenetics. *J Neurotrauma* 2006;**23**(10):1450−67.

72. Buckner RL, Andrews-Hanna JR, Schacter DL. The brain's default network: anatomy, function, and relevance to disease. *Ann N Y Acad Sci* 2008;**1124**:1−38.

73. Sharp DJ, Beckmann CF, Greenwood R, Kinnunen KM, Bonnelle V, De Boissezon X, et al. Default mode network functional and structural connectivity after traumatic brain injury. *Brain* 2011;**134**(Pt 8):2233−47.

74. Spreng RN, Sepulcre J, Turner GR, Stevens WD, Schacter DL. Intrinsic architecture underlying the relations among the default, dorsal attention, and frontoparietal control networks of the human brain. *J Cogn Neurosci* 2013;**25**(1):74−86.

75. Sharp DJ, Scott G, Leech R. Network dysfunction after traumatic brain injury. *Nat Rev Neurol* 2014;**10**(3):156−66.

76. Bonnelle V, Ham TE, Leech R, Kinnunen KM, Mehta MA, Greenwood RJ, et al. Salience network integrity predicts default mode network function after traumatic brain injury. *Proc Natl Acad Sci USA* 2012;**109**(12):4690−5.

II. OVERVIEW OF NEUROSENSORY CONSEQUENCES

77. Abisambra JF, Scheff S. Brain injury in the context of tauopathies. *J Alzheimer's Dis* 2014;**40**(3):495–518. Available from: https://doi.org/10.3233/jad-131019.

78. Poorkaj P, Kas A, D'Souza I, Zhou Y, Pham Q, Stone M, et al. A genomic sequence analysis of the mouse and human microtubule-associated protein tau. *Mamm Genome* 2001;**12**(9):700–12.

79. Goedert M, Spillantini MG, Potier MC, Ulrich J, Crowther RA. Cloning and sequencing of the cDNA encoding an isoform of microtubule-associated protein tau containing four tandem repeats: differential expression of tau protein mRNAs in human brain. *Embo J* 1989;**8**(2):393–9.

80. Lewis J, McGowan E, Rockwood J, Melrose H, Nacharaju P, Van Slegtenhorst M, et al. Neurofibrillary tangles, amyotrophy and progressive motor disturbance in mice expressing mutant (P301L) tau protein. *Nat Genet* 2000;**25**(4):402–5.

81. Santacruz K, Lewis J, Spires T, Paulson J, Kotilinek L, Ingelsson M, et al. Tau suppression in a neurodegenerative mouse model improves memory function. *Science (80-)* 2005;**309**(5733):476–81.

82. Pilcher C. Experimental cerebral trauma. *Arch Surg [Internet]* 1937;**35**(3):512. [cited2017 Oct 20]Available from: http://archsurg.jamanetwork.com/article.aspx?doi = 10.1001/archsurg.1937.01190150095009.

83. Walker AE, Kollros JJ, Case TJ. The physiological basis of concussion. *J Neurosurg [Internet]* 1944;**1**(2):103–16. [cited 2017 Oct 20] Available from: http://thejns.org/doi/10.3171/jns.1944.1.2.0103.

84. Feeney DM, Boyeson MG, Linn RT, Murray HM, Dail WG. Responses to cortical injury: I. Methodology and local effects of contusions in the rat. *Brain Res* 1981;**211**(1):67–77.

85. Blaha M, Schwab J, Vajnerova O, Bednar M, Vajner L, Michal T. Intracranial pressure and experimental model of diffuse brain injury in rats. *J Korean Neurosurg Soc* 2010;**47**(1):7–10.

86. Foda MA, Marmarou A. A new model of diffuse brain injury in rats. Part II: Morphological characterization. *J Neurosurg* 1994;**80**(2):301–13.

87. Marmarou A, Foda MA, van den Brink W, Campbell J, Kita H, Demetriadou K. A new model of diffuse brain injury in rats. Part I: Pathophysiology and biomechanics. *J Neurosurg* 1994;**80**(2):291–300.

88. Hall ED. High-dose glucocorticoid treatment improves neurological recovery in head-injured mice. *J Neurosurg* 1985;**62**(6):882–7.

89. Kupina NC, Nath R, Bernath EE, Inoue J, Mitsuyoshi A, Yuen PW, et al. The novel calpain inhibitor SJA6017 improves functional outcome after delayed administration in a mouse model of diffuse brain injury. *J Neurotrauma* 2001;**18**(11):1229–40.

90. Tang YP, Noda Y, Hasegawa T, Nabeshima T. A concussive-like brain injury model in mice (I): impairment in learning and memory. *J Neurotrauma* 1997;**14**(11):851–62.

91. Kane MJ, Angoa-Perez M, Briggs DI, Viano DC, Kreipke CW, Kuhn DM. A mouse model of human repetitive mild traumatic brain injury. *J Neurosci Methods* 2012;**203**(1):41–9.

92. Lindgren S, Rinder L. Experimental studies in head injury. I. Some factors influencing results of model experiments. *Biophysik* 1965;**2**(5):320–9.

93. Sullivan HG, Martinez J, Becker DP, Miller JD, Griffith R, Wist AO. Fluid-percussion model of mechanical brain injury in the cat. *J Neurosurg* 1976;**45**(5):521–34.

94. Groat RA, Windle WF, Magoun HW. Functional and structural changes in the monkey's brain during and after concussion. *J Neurosurg [Internet]* 1945;**2**(1):26–35. [cited 2017 Oct 20] Available from: http://thejns.org/doi/10.3171/jns.1945.2.1.0026.

95. Millen JE, Glauser FL, Fairman RP. A comparison of physiological responses to percussive brain trauma in dogs and sheep. *J Neurosurg* 1985;**62**(4):587–91.

96. Carbonell WS, Maris DO, McCall T, Grady MS. Adaptation of the fluid percussion injury model to the mouse. *J Neurotrauma* 1998;**15**(3):217–29.

97. McIntosh TK, Vink R, Noble L, Yamakami I, Fernyak S, Soares H, et al. Traumatic brain injury in the rat: characterization of a lateral fluid-percussion model. *Neuroscience* 1989;**28**(1):233–44.

98. Chen W, Guo Y, Yang W, Chen L, Ren D, Wu C, et al. Phosphorylation of connexin 43 induced by traumatic brain injury promotes exosome release. *J Neurophysiol [Internet]* 2017. jn.00654.2017. [cited 2017 Oct 20] Available from: http://www.ncbi.nlm.nih.gov/pubmed/29046426.

99. Lighthall JW. Controlled cortical impact: a new experimental brain injury model. *J Neurotrauma* 1988;**5**(1):1–15.

100. Dixon CE, Clifton GL, Lighthall JW, Yaghmai AA, Hayes RL. A controlled cortical impact model of traumatic brain injury in the rat. *J Neurosci Methods* 1991;**39**(3):253–62.

101. Cherian L, Robertson CS, Contant Jr. CF, Bryan Jr. RM. Lateral cortical impact injury in rats: cerebrovascular effects of varying depth of cortical deformation and impact velocity. *J Neurotrauma* 1994;**11**(5):573–85.

102. Smith DH, Soares HD, Pierce JS, Perlman KG, Saatman KE, Meaney DF, et al. A model of parasagittal controlled cortical impact in the mouse: cognitive and histopathologic effects. *J Neurotrauma* 1995;**12**(2):169–78.

103. Hoffman SW, Fulop Z, Stein DG. Bilateral frontal cortical contusion in rats: behavioral and anatomic consequences. *J Neurotrauma* 1994;**11**(4):417–31.

104. Rubovitch V, Ten-Bosch M, Zohar O, et al. A mouse model of blast-induced mild traumatic brain injury. *Exp Neurol* 2011;**232**(2):280–9. Available from: https://doi.org/10.1016/J.EXPNEUROL.2011.09.018.

NEUROSENSORY DISORDERS IN CLINICAL PRACTICE

Vestibular Dysfunction Associated With Mild Traumatic Brain Injury (mTBI)

Abdulaziz A. Alkathiry, PT, PhD[1], Patrick J. Sparto, PT, PhD[2], Anthony P. Kontos, PhD[3] and Joseph M. Furman, MD, PhD[4]

[1]Department of Physical Therapy, Majmaah University, Al Majmaah, Saudi Arabia
[2]Department of Physical Therapy, University of Pittsburgh, Pittsburgh, PA, United States
[3]Department of Orthopaedic Surgery, University of Pittsburgh, Pittsburgh, PA, United States
[4]Department of Otolaryngology, University of Pittsburgh, Pittsburgh, PA, United States

OVERVIEW OF THE VESTIBULAR SYSTEM

The primary purposes of the vestibular system are to maintain gaze stability, control balance, and provide spatial orientation. These functions are distributed and coordinated amongst many central and peripheral components. The peripheral vestibular system consists of the semicircular canals and the otolithic organs. The semicircular canals consist of three perpendicular canals: the horizontal, anterior, and posterior canals, which detect and respond to angular acceleration of the head. The otolithic organs consist of the saccule and the utricle, which detect linear acceleration. The ampullae, which are parts of the semicircular canals, house the hair cells that detect and transmit angular acceleration through the ampullary vestibular nerve. The maculae, which are the receptors of the otolithic organs, are composed of hair cells and calcium carbonate crystals (the otoconia). The maculae detect and transmit linear acceleration through the vestibular nerve.

Information transmitted by the peripheral vestibular system to the central vestibular system is used for two main purposes: to maintain eye position with head movement and to maintain balance. The central vestibular system encompasses the vestibular nuclei in the brainstem, cerebellum, thalamus, and several cortical regions. The central vestibular

133

system organizes and integrates information from the peripheral vestibular, visual, and somatosensory systems, and produces appropriate motor responses to the eyes and body to accomplish gaze stabilization and maintain upright posture. Eyes are maintained on target during head movement using the vestibulo-ocular reflex (VOR), which moves the eyes with equal magnitude and opposite direction to the head movement using sensory feedback from the semicircular canals and otolithic organs. Optimal balance maintenance requires the integration of information from the visual, somatosensory and vestibular systems. The vestibular system provides angular and linear acceleration feedback to the balance system via the vestibulospinal tract.[1]

PREVALENCE OF VESTIBULAR DISORDERS AFTER MILD TRAUMATIC BRAIN INJURY

Different parts of the vestibular system are susceptible to injury following mild traumatic brain injury (mTBI) (i.e., concussion).[2] For example, Ernst et al. conducted a retrospective study on 63 patients complaining of vertigo after TBI and/or neck injury to investigate vestibular deficits following TBI. Several combinations of vestibular disorders were reported in trauma patients including benign paroxysmal positional vertigo (BPPV) (57%), cervicogenic vertigo (27%), otolith disorder (25%), labyrinthine concussion (19%), secondary endolymphatic hydrops (EH) (19%), perilymphatic fistulae (5%), and central vestibular disorders (5%).[2] Each of these vestibular disorders involves specific symptoms and impaired function that require a comprehensive assessment and individualized treatment and rehabilitation plan. In our experience with mTBI resulting from sport-related impacts, the prevalence of peripheral disorders is less and prevalence of central disorders more compared with the Ernst study. The characteristics of these disorders will be discussed in the following paragraphs.

BPPV[3,4] is a common cause of dizziness after mTBI with an incidence rate ranging from 28% to 61% of individuals with dizziness after TBIs.[5,6] The head impact during mTBI causes the otoconia to dislodge from the macula and escape into the semicircular canals. Movement of the otoconia inside the affected canal moves the hair cells and stimulates the vestibular nerve of that canal causing the vertigo.[7]

Labyrinthine concussion is an injury to the membranous labyrinth.[8] Transmitted forces of the head trauma may cause shearing forces to rupture the membranous labyrinth. Labyrinthine concussion symptoms include hearing loss, tinnitus, and dizziness.[9]

EH is a pathologic process caused by presumed increased endolymphatic pressure, resulting in vertigo, hearing loss, and tinnitus in the affected ear. If it appears spontaneously, it is referred to as primary EH (i.e., Meniere's disease), but if there appears to be a precipitating factor such as trauma, it is called secondary EH. Reports of EH after mTBI are rare, but one retrospective study reported that 12 out of 63 patients who reported posttraumatic vertigo had secondary EH, as determined using electrocochleography.[2] Interestingly, these patients did not have hearing loss or tinnitus.

Perilymphatic fistulae result from an abnormal opening of the round window or the oval window.[10] Head trauma may lead to rupture of the round and/or oval window that connects the middle ear and the inner ear perilymphatic spaces, which cause the perilymphatic fluids to leak from the inner ear to the middle ear.[11] Perilymphatic fistulae symptoms include: vertigo, postural instability, sensorineural hearing loss, deafness, or tinnitus.[8]

In addition to the peripheral vestibular disorders mentioned above, central vestibular disorders including vestibular migraine, convergence insufficiency, convergence spasm, nonspecific central VOR imbalance, and central suppression are frequently encountered after mTBI. Of these disorders, vestibular migraine is the most common. The diagnostic criteria for vestibular migraine have been detailed by the Barany Society and International Headache Society.[12] The main features of vestibular migraine include at least five episodes of vestibular symptoms, a current or past history of migraine according to International Classification of Headache Disorders (ICHD) criteria, and at least one migraine feature during the vestibular episodes.[12] Posttraumatic migraine has been recognized for decades,[13,14] although there is not a separate distinct classification for it in the ICHD. It has not been reported how many individuals with posttraumatic headaches or migraine would satisfy the criteria for vestibular migraine.

Dizziness has also been attributed to cervical spine disorders that are frequently reported after mTBI and whiplash incidents. Cervicogenic dizziness is considered after diagnostic evidence of vestibular dysfunction is ruled out, and the dizziness has some relationship with cervical dysfunction, such as pain and stiffness.[15] Obviously, the co-occurrence of cervical spine impairments with direct mechanical trauma to the head would lead a possibility of cervicogenic origin for dizziness if neck complaints are significant. The retrospective review by Ernst et al.[2] identified cervicogenic dizziness in 27% of the sample.

VESTIBULAR-RELATED SYMPTOMS AND IMPAIRMENT AFTER MILD TRAUMATIC BRAIN INJURY

Definition

Physical symptoms of mTBI include headache, dizziness, nausea, balance problems, visual problems, vomiting, fatigue, sensitivity to light, and sensitivity to noise.[16] Dizziness is a hallmark symptom with vestibular disorders. When people report dizziness after mTBI, it can represent a diverse set of perceptions such as vertigo (spinning), lightheadedness, wooziness, imbalance and others, so it is critical to follow up with additional questions in order to understand the true sensation. These characteristics of dizziness are particularly important in determining if the injury involves peripheral (inner ear) or central (brain) components.

Vertigo is the illusory sensation of spinning or whirling movement of self or the surrounding. Vertigo typically suggests a peripheral vestibular disorder, but it can also occur in central vestibular disorders.[17] If vertigo is accompanied by nystagmus, or involuntary rapid eye movements, then an acute peripheral vestibular disorder should be investigated. The other dizziness perceptions are more common after concussion and likely represent a general central vestibular disorder.

Balance has been defined as "the dynamics of body posture to prevent falling."[18] The word "balance" is commonly used in rehabilitation settings and is often used with other terms such as stability and postural control; however these terms have no universally accepted definitions.[19] Imbalance and unsteadiness during standing and walking implicate the vestibular system through the actions of the vestibulospinal system. These symptom reports are nonspecific and nonlocalizing and could indicate peripheral vestibular injury to the otolith organs, or central vestibular injury to the sensory integration system that receives input from the visual, somatosensory, and vestibular systems, and coordinates the motor responses.

Nausea and vomiting also can be manifestations of a vestibular disorder, but they are also general indicators of head trauma. However, vestibular system problems should be explored if one presents with nausea and vomiting after mTBI.

Difficulties with reading and focusing on objects can represent problems with oculomotor functions such as accommodation and convergence.[20,21] In addition, because of the tight linkage of vestibular and oculomotor systems in maintaining gaze stability, these symptoms can represent an impairment to VOR function.

Prevalence

Several recent large sample studies have investigated symptom prevalence after mTBI (Table 10.1).[22-27] These studies primarily looked at symptom reporting after sports-related concussion. We extracted the prevalence of vestibular-related symptoms, in addition to headache. Headache is the most frequently-reported symptom after mTBI, ranging from 72% to 95%.

Of the vestibular-related symptoms, dizziness was most common, ranging from 59% to 98% of the populations. The consistency of the values across different samples is remarkable. The 59% prevalence in one military sample is probably affected by recall bias, because the soldiers were asked about their symptoms months after the mTBI. The 98% estimate from another military population may have been larger than the other studies because the symptoms were provoked. Also of note is the combined estimate with balance problems in the survey from Marshall et al.,[25] which likely would have overestimated the prevalence of dizziness alone. Unfortunately, recent estimates of the various dizziness descriptors, such as vertigo, are unavailable.

In surveys where imbalance was recorded independently from dizziness, in was endorsed in approximately one-third of the respondents (26%–37%). Symptom questionnaires have included imbalance or balance problems as a unitary construct; therefore, estimates of difficulty during standing balance or during gait are unavailable. The occurrence of nausea or nausea and vomiting, also affects about a third of the individuals with a sports-related concussion.

Other symptoms that may be attributed to vestibular system dysfunction have also been reported in the literature. For example, blurred vision (50%) and visual disturbances (22%–29%) have been reported in several studies, although these terms are relatively imprecise. Migraine-like sensitivity to light (47%–49%) and noise (31%–39%) have also been examined.

TABLE 10.1 Estimates of Vestibular-Related Symptom Prevalence Immediately After mTBI in Representative Studies

Study	Subjects and Source of Data	Headache (%)	Dizziness (%)	Imbalance	Nausea and Vomiting	Other
Hoffer et al.[26]	Military personnel deployed in Iraq within 3 days of blast exposure, $n = 81$	72	98	NR	NR	NR
Marar et al.[22]	High-school athletes, $n = 1936$National High School Sports-Related Injury Surveillance System	94	76	NR	N: 31%	NR
Marshall et al.[25]	High school and collegiate athletes, $n = 375$ Concussion Prevention Initiative	87	77 (combined dizziness and balance problems)		N: 35% V: 8%	Blurred vision: 50%
O'Connor et al.[23]	High-school athletes, $n = 2004$ National Athletic Treatment, Injury and Outcomes Network (NATION)	95	75	32%	29%	Light sens: 47% Noise sens: 39% Visual disturb: 22%
Terrio et al.[27]	US Army soldiers deployed to Iraq, $n = 907$	81	59	26%	NR	NR
Wasserman et al.[24]	Collegiate athletes, $n = 1670$ NCAA Injury Surveillance Program	92	69	37%	N/V: 31%	Light sens: 49% Noise sens: 31% Visual disturb: 29% Tinnitus: 9%

Light sens, light sensitivity; noise sens, noise sensitivity; NR, not reported; N, nausea; V, vomiting; visual disturb, visual disturbances.

Because of their relationship to gaze stabilization, it is useful to document the prevalence of oculomotor impairments after mTBI. Such impairments may include dysfunction associated with pursuit/tracking and saccadic eye movements, accommodative and convergence insufficiencies, and problems associated with reading. In military personnel after blast injury, accommodation and/or convergence insufficiencies were observed in 24% of the 21 subjects.[28] In an outpatient polytrauma rehabilitation setting that treated mTBI mostly from blast injuries, close to 50% of patients had accommodation and convergence insufficiencies.[29,30] In a larger retrospective study consisting of patients with TBI (mild or severe) treated at an outpatient vision rehabilitation clinic, 56% of the patients had vergence impairments, and 41% had accommodation impairments.[31] With regard to pursuit and saccadic eye movements, researchers report that approximately 33%−51% of individuals with mTBI are referred for treatment for these problems.[30,31] However, these estimates may not represent the overall population, as the patients in these studies were a select group that had been referred for vision problems, but are none-the-less illustrative of the oculomotor problems that can occur following mTBI.

In other research on oculomotor dysfunction, Pearce and colleagues examined convergence insufficiency in a prospective study of 78 adolescent athletes.[32] These researchers reported that 42% of athletes had a convergence insufficiency of ≥5 cm, and that patients with convergence insufficiency performed worse on memory, processing speed, and reaction time tests following concussion. These findings support that influence of oculomotor impairments on other systems following mTBI.

ASSESSMENT OF VESTIBULAR FUNCTION AFTER MILD TRAUMATIC BRAIN INJURY

Vestibular Ocular Reflex

Vestibular function testing in individuals after mTBI has been reported in several studies. In 1970, Toglia et al. completed vestibular function tests in 235 individuals who reported dizziness after a closed head or whiplash injury.[33] There was little difference in test results between the closed head injury and whiplash groups. Thirty-six percent of the patients had spontaneous nystagmus without fixation, 63% had an abnormal caloric exam, and 47% of the patients had abnormal rotational chair responses.[33] Davies and Luxon retrospectively investigated vestibular abnormalities after head injury in 100 subjects with vestibular symptoms that resulted from the head injury.[34] The severity of head injury was classified as minor in 72 subjects (i.e., mTBI), and moderate or severe in 28 subjects (characterized by presence of a skull fracture). Across all severity groups, they found that 74% of the subjects had positive vestibular abnormality findings, indicated by a positive caloric or electronystagmography exam. Of the subjects with an mTBI, 74% had an abnormal vestibular exam. Sixty-one patients had a history of BPPV, although only 15 patients had a positive Dix-Hallpike test.[34] More recently, Zhou and colleagues evaluated vestibular function in 42 children and adolescents who had prolonged dizziness and imbalance after a sports-related concussion.[35] Spontaneous nystagmus was observed in 24%, abnormal caloric responses in 21%, and abnormal rotational chair testing in approximately 25% of the patients. Dynamic visual acuity testing was performed and 57% of this sample had reduced performance. One important caveat of the estimated percentage of vestibular function test abnormalities, a large portion of which imply peripheral vestibular dysfunction, is that all of the patients presented to a tertiary center with dizziness or imbalance after mTBI, and thus the results are not representative of all individuals who have a mTBI.[35]

The head impulse test (HIT) is a clinical test of peripheral vestibular function that assesses VOR responses to high acceleration, high velocity, low amplitude head impulses.[36] The HIT is performed by rotating the head in the plane of one pair of the semi-circular canals, usually the horizontal semicircular canals. Recently, the HIT was combined with video-oculography to be able to objectively quantify eye movement during head impulses.[37] The video head impulse Test (vHIT) was found to be equivalent to the scleral search coil technique in recording eye movement in response to head movement.[37] Our group used the vHIT to examine vestibular function in 56 individuals (adults and children) post-mTBI.[38] No patients had an abnormal head impulse response using a gain threshold of 0.7 established from previous work.[39–41] Balaban et al. assessed the HIT using a computer controlled rotation chair rather than manual stimuli, and discovered that the gain was decreased in 62 out of 100 participants with a mTBI (mean time of test was 2.5 days after injury) compared with controls.[42] They used a threshold of 0.90 based on a 95% confidence interval of their large control sample. It is uncertain why there is such disparity in results between the recent vHIT studies, but possible reasons include the acuity of the injury, method of delivering the impulses, and threshold for abnormality.

Vestibular and Ocular-Motor Screening

The vestibular and ocular-motor screening (VOMS) is a tool designed to screen the vestibular-ocular and ocular-motor systems following concussion.[43] The VOMS consists of seven components including smooth pursuits, horizontal and vertical saccades, near point of convergence (NPC), horizontal and vertical VOR, and visual motion sensitivity test. Participants are asked to rate headache, dizziness, nausea, and fogginess symptoms following each component, using a scale of 0 (none) to 10 (severe). Symptoms are also assessed before VOMS testing (i.e., baseline) to help determine changes in symptoms following each VOMS component. In addition, NPC distance is measured three times to provide an average NPC distance across the three trials. In a study on 85 children and adolescents with a sport-related concussion (aged $M = 14$, SD = 2.75) and 85 controls (aged $M = 12.7$, SD = 1.8) researchers reported a significant difference between groups in all items of the VOMS. Using a cutoff point of ≥ 2 points in VOMS items or a NPC distance of ≥ 5 cm indicated an increased likelihood of having a concussion that ranged from 25% to 44%.[43] None of the VOMS items were correlated with the Balance Error Scoring System (BESS) which measures the vestibulospinal system, suggesting that the VOMS measures different components of the vestibular system than the BESS. As such, the use of both measures is warranted to provide a more complete assessment of vestibular system involvement following concussion.

In a study of 263 uninjured NCAA Division I collegiate student-athletes, VOMS was reported to be internally consistent (Cronbach $\alpha = 0.97$).[44] Using the cutoff scores of ≥ 2

for any item of the VOMS and NPC distance of ≥ 5 cm,[43] Kontos et al. found a false-positive rate of 11%.[44] The researchers also reported an increased likelihood of ≥ 1 VOMS score above cutoff associated with being female [*odds ratio (OR)* = 2.99, *95% confidence interval (CI)* = 1.34−6.70, *P* = .006] and history of motion sickness (*OR* = 7.7, *95% CI* = 1.94−30.75, P = . 009).[44] In fact, 72% of participants with false positives on the VOMS also had a personal or family history of motion sickness, suggesting that a majority of false positives on the VOMS are a result of preexisting vestibular system issues. Therefore, clinicians should consider premorbid factors such as history of motion sickness when interpreting postconcussion VOMS scores.

With regard to post-injury VOMS scores, researchers have reported gender differences specific to the VOR component.[45] In their study of 64 athletes (28 females), Sufrinko et al. reported that females had greater symptoms during the VOR item in the first 21 days following a concussion.[45] In fact, a regression revealed that gender represented 45% of the variance in postconcussion VOR scores. In the same study, females performed similar to males on the remaining VOMS components as well as the BESS. These findings highlight the importance of factors such as gender that may be associated with post-mTBI impairment on the VOMS and should, therefore, be considered by clinicians when interpreting clinical findings on the VOMS.

Balance

Balance deficits are commonly reported in individuals with mTBI.[46−49] Tests of static standing balance can be divided into two categories: instrumented tests and noninstrumented tests. In noninstrumented tests the assessor evaluates the performance; while in instrumented tests, tools are used to measure certain aspects of the task. Most clinical balance assessments incorporate noninstrumented methods to assess balance while lab-based balance assessments incorporate tools such as accelerometers and force plates.

Noninstrumented balance assessment involves a variety of tests, including the modified Clinical Test of Sensory Interaction in Balance (mCTSIB),[50] and BESS.[51] These tests primarily test one's ability to maintain balance with modification of sensory inputs and base of support. The mCTSIB assesses the ability to stand for up to 30 seconds in a minimum of four conditions, usually eyes open and eyes closed on a level surface, and eyes open and eyes closed on a foam surface. These conditions can be followed by using a visual conflict dome on level and foam surfaces. The BESS consists of six conditions performed for 20 seconds, all with eyes closed with hands placed on hips. There are three stance conditions: double leg standing (feet in contact side by side), single leg standing on the nondominant leg with the dominant leg flexed 20 degree at the hip and 45 degree at the knee, and tandem standing (dominant foot placed in front of the nondominant foot). All stance conditions are performed on firm and foam surfaces.

The modified BESS (mBESS), which eliminates the foam conditions, is used as a part of the Sport Concussion Assessment Tool 5 (SCAT5),[52] which was recommended as one tool to be used in the acute (<3 days) time period to assess athletes with concussion by the 2016 Berlin Consensus Statement on Concussion in Sport.[53] No cutoff score is available to distinguish balance abnormalities; interpretation of BESS scores depends on comparing pre-injury and post-injury scores of the individual tested. A number of reliability studies have been performed on the BESS, and have examined the effect of different factors on the reliability.[54] Most of the studies have demonstrated at least moderate reliability. Reference values have been established for children, adolescents, and adults, and a decrease in BESS score has been observed from young children to young adults, with a subsequent increase in older adults.[55-57] The practice effect of BESS has been considered an important factor to be acknowledged when administering BESS to track recovery in athletes. Valovich et al. tested 32 healthy adolescents (mean age 17 years, SD 2 years) using BESS over four visits (Day 1, 3, 5, 7, and 30) and found significant improvement on the total BESS on Day 5 and 7 compared with Day 1. They also found significant improvement of BESS foam scores on Day 7 compared with Day 1, while no significant effect of visit was seen during BESS on a firm surface.[58]

In a study comparing BESS scores between 94 collegiate athletes with sport-related concussion and 56 matched controls, statistically significant differences were reported between groups on the total BESS score at the time of concussion.[59] However, these reported differences resolved within 3–5 days postconcussion. Similarly, in another study involving the BESS in 375 high school and collegiate athletes, researchers reported that concussed athletes returned to baseline levels of balance within 3 days of injury.[59] Together, these findings suggest that either balance impairment is short-lived following concussion or that the BESS may not be sensitive enough to detect impairment beyond the acute post-injury time period.

With the relatively recent development of low-cost body sway accelerometers and inertial measurement units, instrumented assessment of standing balance after concussion has become of focus for several groups. A benefit of these sensors is their applicability to sideline and military environments. King et al.[60] assessed balance in 13 children with concussion and 13 matched controls using the instrumented BESS.[60] Instrumentation consisted of affixing an inertial measurement unit (IMU) at the participants lower back while performing the BESS. They found that the instrumented BESS was superior to the BESS in classifying children with concussion. Sensitivity and specificity were found to be (31%/85%) for the mBESS and (54%/100%) for the instrumented mBESS.[60] Using a larger sample of 52 collegiate athletes post-mTBI tested 2 days after injury on average, and 76 controls, the same group found that the RMS acceleration in the mediolateral direction obtained during the feet together condition provided the best measure for distinguishing between the two groups.

Force platforms use load cells to measure ground reaction forces and moments between the individuals and the ground. The forces and moments are used to calculate the center of pressure (COP), which is the primary driver of center of mass movement. Drawbacks of using force platforms include their cost and relative importability in field settings. However, force platform-based studies have demonstrated impairments in balance longer after mTBI, compared with BESS scores. For example, Powers et al. measured the using a force plate with nine athletes with concussion and nine healthy athletes to investigate the effect of concussion on sway. They found elevated COP velocity in the mTBI group that was significant even after return to play clearance (mean 26 days post-mTBI).[61] In a sample of 49 collegiate athletes who had a mTBI, increased COP sway during standing with eyes closed compared with eyes open was observed during tests that occurred 7 and 15 days after injury, but had returned to baseline values by Day 30.[62]

A common instrumented test that utilizes a force platform is the Sensory Organization Test (SOT). The SOT identifies abnormalities in the patient's use of the three sensory systems that contribute to postural control: somatosensory, visual, and vestibular.[63,64] Peterson et al. compared the composite SOT scores between 26 athletes with mTBI and 18 controls and found balance differences between the two groups 10 days postconcussion.[47] Consequently it appears that instrumented assessments of standing balance may provide more sensitive measures of recovery compared with noninstrumented testing.

Gait

Gait speed is the most simple measure of gait that can be assessed in the clinic, and is usually recorded over a distance of at least 4 m. Gait speed has been shown to be reduced in young adults with mTBI compared with age- and gender-matched controls.[65] Furthermore, gait speed was shown to improve at discharge from vestibular rehabilitation compared with at the initial evaluation in children and adults with mTBI.[66] The Dynamic Gait Index (DGI) assesses the ability to walk while performing head movements, obstacle avoidance, and stair climbing.[67] The DGI has eight items that are ordinally scaled from 0 to 3. The Functional Gait Assessment (FGA) evolved from the DGI in order to overcome some of the ceiling effects of the DGI, and have quantitative benchmarks for the criterion scores.[68] These outcome measures have been examined in just a few studies to date.[66,69] The DGI and FGA were both reduced in individuals with mTBI (adolescents and adults) at entry into vestibular rehabilitation, and both significantly improved at discharge from treatment.[66,70]

The High Level Mobility Assessment Tool (HiMAT) comprises 13 items ranging from timed walking to running, skipping, and walking up and down stairs.[71-73] Timed scores are transformed into ordinal scores from 0 to 4. The HiMAT was originally developed to assess mobility in individuals with moderate to severe TBI.[71-73] The tests has excellent interrater and test–retest reliability for individuals with mTBI (intraclass correlation coefficient = 0.95).[74]

Dual-Task Balance and Gait Performance

Sports activities require high performance on cognitive and balance function simultaneously. Cognitive function impairments and balance deficits are common postconcussion.[46-49,75] Assessing postural stability and cognitive function concurrently by using dual-task methodologies may provide another tool for managing concussions. In theory, performance of a dual task should stress the balance and cognitive systems of individuals with mTBI to a greater degree compared with controls, and thus may be a more robust indicator of recovery. When examining dual-task studies, it is important to understand which balance components are being assessed, as well as which cognitive functions, as there are myriad tasks, and one of the causes of conflicting results may be the task-dependent nature of the tests.[76]

A couple of studies have examined dual-task standing balance performance in individuals with mTBI. Dorman et al. compared static standing postural stability between 18 adolescents with concussion and 26 injury-free adolescents.[77] Four balance conditions were tested: single-task with eyes open and closed and dual-task with eyes open and closed. Participants with concussion were tested within 10 days from the injury and were retested again three times along the course of their recovery. Controls were tested twice with 1 week between tests. Both groups produced increased sway in dual-task balance tests compared to single-task balance tests. On the first visit, significant differences between groups were found in both single and dual-task conditions, while on second visit, significant differences between groups were found only in the dual-task conditions. Rochefort et al., discovered that 33 adolescents who had an mTBI ranging from 28 to 40 days prior to testing, had elevated body COP measures as they performed a secondary Stroop task while standing on a force platform, compared with controls. Furthermore, they found no difference in sway between subjects with mTBI who reported balance problems and those who did not, suggesting that self-report of balance symptoms may not be a strong indicator of recovery.[78]

Many more investigations of the effect of secondary cognitive task performance on gait measures have been performed in a series of studies by Chou et al. The general paradigm was to have subjects walk on a level surface (single task), or walk while performing a secondary cognitive task (dual-task). The dual-task conditions included verbal question and answer (such as serial subtraction, spelling words backwards), auditory reaction time, and auditory Stroop tasks. Video motion analysis was used to measure kinematics of the center of mass and joint excursions. Eight to 10 trials were performed for each condition. Initial assessments occurred within 3 days of the mTBI, and at up to four follow-up visits (1 week, 2 weeks, 1 month, and 2 months after mTBI). One group of studies compared responses of young adults with mTBI and age-matched controls and found that individuals with mTBI walked more slowly during all conditions, and had lesser anteroposterior and greater mediolateral center of mass motion during a question and answer dual task, but not the auditory reaction time dual task during the initial assessment.[65,79,80] While gait speed recovered to control values by Day 5, elevated values of center of mass velocity were observed up to 28 days after injury.[80]

In another series of experiments that investigated factors that affected gait performance, Howell et al. tested 20 adolescents (mean age 15 years SD 1 year) within 3 days of an mTBI during single-task and dual-task conditions. The dual-task was walking while performing an auditory Stroop task in which subjects verbally indicated a high or low pitch of the congruent and incongruent computer played words "high" or "low." This procedure was repeated on four follow-up visits (1 week, 2 weeks, 1 month, and 2 months after SRC). The concussion group had a greater reduction in anterior center of mass velocity in the dual task condition relative to the single task, compared with the controls. The concussion group also had greater center of mass displacement in the frontal plane compared with controls, more so in the dual task condition compared with single task. Most of the gait parameters of the concussion group normalized to control values within 2 weeks of the injury.[81] Next, they examined the effect of cognitive task difficulty and observed that performance was degraded more with the question and answer dual task compared with the auditory Stroop task, up to 2 weeks post-mTBI.[76] There may be an age effect in performance, such that adolescents (mean age 15 years) demonstrate a prolonged return to control values compared with young adults (mean age 20 years).[82] In addition, it appears that there can be a worsening of gait performance after individuals return to full activity.[83] Altogether, these studies point to a valuable role for dual task gait assessment in individuals after mTBI.

SUMMARY

Vestibular dysfunction is common after mTBI and can result from both peripheral and central vestibular impairments. The manifestations of vestibular dysfunction include dizziness, vertigo, imbalance, nausea, and oculomotor insufficiency. Assessments of these problems have indicated differences between individuals with mTBI and healthy controls. A comprehensive assessment of vestibular-related problems can assist in the management of mTBI.

References

1. Guskiewicz KM. Balance assessment in the management of sport-related concussion. *Clin Sports Med* 2011;**30**(1):89–102.
2. Ernst A, Basta D, Seidl RO, Todt I, Scherer H, Clarke A. Management of posttraumatic vertigo. *Otolaryngol Head Neck Surg* 2005;**132**(4):554–8.
3. Bárány R. Diagnose von Krankheitserscheinungen im Bereiche des Otolithenapparatus. *Acta Otolaryngol Stock* 1921;2434–7.
4. Dix MR, Hallpike CS. The pathology symptomatology and diagnosis of certain common disorders of the vestibular system. *Proc R Soc Med* 1952;**45**(6):341–54.
5. Hoffer ME, Gottshall KR, Moore R, Balough BJ, Wester D. Characterizing and treating dizziness after mild head trauma. *Otol Neurotol* 2004;**25**(2):135–8.
6. Davies RA, Luxon LM. Dizziness following head injury: a neuro-otological study. *J Neurol* 1995;**242**(4):222–30.
7. Fife TD. Benign paroxysmal positional vertigo. *Semin Neurol* 2009;**29**(5):500–8.
8. Fife TD, Giza C. Posttraumatic vertigo and dizziness. *Semin Neurol* 2013;**33**(3):238–43.
9. Choi MS, Shin SO, Yeon JY, Choi YS, Kim J, Park SK. Clinical characteristics of labyrinthine concussion. *Korean J Audiol* 2013;**17**(1):13–17.
10. Hornibrook J. Perilymph fistula: fifty years of controversy. *ISRN Otolaryngol* 2012;**2012**:1–9.
11. Glasscock III ME, Hart MJ, Rosdeutscher JD, Bhansali SA. Traumatic perilymphatic fistula: how long can symptoms persist? A follow-up report. *Am J Otol* 1992;**13**(4):333–8.
12. Lempert T, Olesen J, Furman J, Waterston J, Seemungal B, Carey J, et al. Vestibular migraine: diagnostic criteria. *J Vestib Res Equilib Orientat* 2012;**22**(4):167–72.
13. Weiss HD, Stern BJ, Goldberg J. Post-traumatic migraine: chronic migraine precipitated by minor head or neck trauma. *Headache*. 1991;**31**(7):451–6. Available from: http://www.ncbi.nlm.nih.gov/pubmed/1774160.
14. Behrman S. Migraine as a sequela of blunt head injury. *Injury* 1977;**9**(1):74–6. Available from: http://www.ncbi.nlm.nih.gov/pubmed/338481.
15. Wrisley DM, Sparto PJ, Whitney SL, Furman JM. Cervicogenic dizziness: a review of diagnosis and treatment. *J Orthop Sports Phys Ther* 2000;**30**(12):755–66. Available from: http://www.jospt.org/doi/10.2519/jospt.2000.30.12.755.
16. Harmon KG, Drezner JA, Gammons M, Guskiewicz KM, Halstead M, Herring SA, et al. American Medical Society for Sports Medicine position statement: concussion in sport. *Br J Sport Med* 2013;**47**(1):15–26.
17. Furman JM, Cass SP, Whitney SL. *Vestibular disorders: a case study approach to diagnosis and treatment. 3rd ed.* New York: Oxford University Press; 2010.
18. Winter DA. Human balance and posture control during standing and walking. *Gait Posture*. 1995;193–214.
19. Pollock a S, Durward BR, Rowe PJ, Paul JP. What is balance? *Clin Rehabil* 2000;**14**(4):402–6.

20. Capó-Aponte JE, Urosevich TG, Temme LA, Tarbett AK, Sanghera NK. Visual dysfunctions and symptoms during the subacute stage of blast-induced mild traumatic brain injury. *Mil Med* 2012;**177**(7):804–13. Available from: http://www.ncbi.nlm.nih.gov/pubmed/22808887.

21. Goodrich GL, Kirby J, Cockerham G. Visual function in patients of a polytrauma rehabilitation center: a descriptive study. 2007. Available from: http://www.brainline.org/downloads/PDFs/VisualFunctionin Patients.pdf%5Cnpapers://2d58f8da-a316-4ec8-b1ac-62e5ed9dca49/Paper/p1824.

22. Marar M, McIlvain NM, Fields SK, Comstock RD. Epidemiology of concussions among United States high school athletes in 20 sports. *Am J Sports Med* 2012;**40**(4):747–55.

23. O'Connor KL, Baker MM, Dalton SL, Dompier TP, Broglio SP, Kerr ZY. Epidemiology of sport-related concussions in high school athletes: National Athletic Treatment, Injury and Outcomes Network (NATION), 2011–2012 through 2013–2014. *J Athl Train* 2017;**52**(3):175–85.

24. Wasserman EB, Kerr ZY, Zuckerman SL, Covassin T. Epidemiology of sports-related concussions in National Collegiate Athletic Association Athletes from 2009-2010 to 2013-2014. *Am J Sports Med* 2016;**44**(1):226–33.

25. Marshall SW, Guskiewicz KM, Shankar V, McCrea M, Cantu RC. Epidemiology of sports-related concussion in seven US high school and collegiate sports. *Inj Epidemiol* 2015;**2**(1):13.

26. Hoffer ME, Balaban C, Gottshall K, Balough BJ, Maddox MR, Penta JR. Blast exposure. *Otol Neurotol* 2010;**31**(2):232–6. Available from: http://www.ncbi.nlm.nih.gov/pubmed/20009782.

27. Terrio H, Brenner LA, Ivins BJ, Cho JM, Helmick K, Schwab K, et al. Traumatic brain injury screening. *J Head Trauma Rehabil* 2009;**24**(1):14–23. Available from: http://www.ncbi.nlm.nih.gov/pubmed/19158592.

28. Goodrich GL, Kirby J, Cockerham G, Ingalla SP, Lew HL. Visual function in patients of a polytrauma rehabilitation center: a descriptive study. *J Rehabil Res Dev* 2007;**44**(7):929–36. Available from: http://www.ncbi.nlm.nih.gov/pubmed/18075950.

29. Cockerham GC, Goodrich GL, Weichel ED, Orcutt JC, Rizzo JF, Bower KS, et al. Eye and visual function in traumatic brain injury. *J Rehabil Res Dev* 2009;**46**(6):811–18. Available from: http://www.ncbi.nlm.nih.gov/pubmed/20104404.

30. Brahm KD, Wilgenburg HM, Kirby J, Ingalla S, Chang C-Y, Goodrich GL. Visual impairment and dysfunction in combat-injured servicemembers with traumatic brain injury. *Optom Vis Sci* 2009;**86**(7):817–25. Available from: http://www.ncbi.nlm.nih.gov/pubmed/19521270.

31. Ciuffreda KJ, Wang B, Vasudevan B. Conceptual model of human blur perception. *Vision Res* 2007;**47**(9):1245–52. Available from: http://www.ncbi.nlm.nih.gov/pubmed/17223154.

32. Pearce KL, Sufrinko A, Lau BC, Henry L, Collins MW, Kontos AP. Near point of convergence after a sport-related concussion: measurement reliability and relationship to neurocognitive impairment and symptoms. *Am J Sport Med* 2015;**43**(12):3055–61. Available from: https://www.scopus.com/inward/record.uri?eid = 2-s2.0-84949009968&partnerID = 40&md5 = 9cbcad598ae071a09a6f77c3a757ebd9%5Cnhttp://www.ncbi.nlm.nih.gov/pubmed/26453625.

33. Toglia JU, Rosenberg PE, Ronis ML. Posttraumatic dizziness; vestibular, audiologic, and medicolegal aspects. *Arch Otolaryngol (Chicago, Ill 1960)* 1970;**92**(5):485–92. Available from: http://www.ncbi.nlm.nih.gov/pubmed/5506059.

34. Davies RA, Luxon LM. Dizziness following head injury: a neuro-otological study. *J Neurol* 1995;**242**(4):222–30. Available from: http://www.ncbi.nlm.nih.gov/pubmed/7798121.

35. Zhou G, Brodsky JR. Objective vestibular testing of children with dizziness and balance complaints following sports-related concussions. *Otolaryngol—Head Neck Surg* 2015;**152**(6):1133–9. Available from: http://www.ncbi.nlm.nih.gov/pubmed/25820582.

36. Halmagyi GM, Curthoys IS. A clinical sign of canal paresis. *Arch Neurol* 1988;**45**(7):737–9.

37. MacDougall HG, Weber KP, McGarvie LA, Halmagyi GM, Curthoys IS. The video head impulse test: diagnostic accuracy in peripheral vestibulopathy. *Neurology* 2009;**73**(14):1134–41.

38. Alshehri MM, Sparto PJ, Furman JM, Fedor S, Mucha A, Henry LC, et al. The usefulness of the video head impulse test in children and adults post-concussion. *J Vestib Res* 2017;**26**(5–6):439–46. Available from: http://www.ncbi.nlm.nih.gov/pubmed/28262647.

39. Hamilton SS, Zhou G, Brodsky JR. Video head impulse testing (VHIT) in the pediatric population. *Int J Pediatr Otorhinolaryngol* 2015;**79**(8):1283–7.

40. Mahringer A, Rambold HA. Caloric test and video-head-impulse: a study of vertigo/dizziness patients in a community hospital. *Eur Arch Oto-Rhino-Laryngol* 2014;**271**(3):463–72. Available from: http://www.ncbi.nlm.nih.gov/pubmed/23494283.

41. Migliaccio AA, Cremer PD. The 2D modified head impulse test: a 2D technique for measuring function in all six semi-circular canals. *J Vestib Res Equilib Orientat* 2011;**21**(4):227–34.
42. Balaban C, Hoffer ME, Szczupak M, Snapp H, Crawford J, Murphy S, et al. Oculomotor, vestibular, and reaction time tests in mild traumatic brain injury. *PLoS One* 2016;**11**(9):e0162168. Available from: http://www.pubmedcentral.nih.gov/articlerender.fcgi?artid = 5031310&tool = pmcentrez&rendertype = abstract.
43. Mucha A, Collins MW, Elbin RJ, Furman JM, Troutman-Enseki C, DeWolf RM, et al. A brief vestibular/ocular motor screening (VOMS) assessment to evaluate concussions: preliminary findings. *Am J Sports Med* 2014;**42**(10):2479–86.
44. Kontos AP, Sufrinko A, Elbin RJ, Puskar A, Collins MW. Reliability and associated risk factors for performance on the vestibular/ocular motor screening (VOMS) tool in healthy collegiate athletes. *Am J Sports Med* 2016;**44**(6). 0363546516632754-.
45. Sufrinko AM, Mucha A, Covassin T, Marchetti G, Elbin RJ, Collins MW, et al. Sex differences in vestibular/ocular and neurocognitive outcomes after sport-related concussion. *Clin J Sport Med* 2017;**27**(2):133–8. Available from: http://www.ncbi.nlm.nih.gov/pubmed/27379660.
46. Guskiewicz KM. Postural stability assessment following concussion: one piece of the puzzle. *Clin J Sport Med* 2001;**11**(3):182–9.
47. Peterson CL, Ferrara MS, Mrazik M, Piland S, Elliott R. Evaluation of neuropsychological domain scores and postural stability following cerebral concussion in sports. *Clin J Sport Med* 2003;**13**(4):230–7.
48. McCrea M, Barr WB, Guskiewicz KM, Randolph C, Marshall SW, Cantu RC, et al. Standard regression-based methods for measuring recovery after sport-related concussion. *J Int Neuropsychol Soc* 2005;**11**(1):58–69.
49. Furman GR, Lin CC, Bellanca JL, Marchetti GF, Collins MW, Whitney SL. Comparison of the balance accelerometer measure and balance error scoring system in adolescent concussions in sports. *Am J Sports Med* 2013;**41**(6):1404–10.
50. Shumway-Cook A, Horak F. Assessing the influence of sensory interaction of balance. Suggestion from the field. *Phys Ther* 1986;**66**(10):1548–50. Available from: http://www.ncbi.nlm.nih.gov/pubmed/3763708.
51. Riemann BL, Guskiewicz KM. Effects of mild head injury on postural balance testing. *J Athl Train* 2000;**35**(1):19–25. Available from: http://www.ncbi.nlm.nih.gov/pubmed/16558603.
52. Davis GA, Purcell L, Schneider KJ, Yeates KO, Gioia GA, Anderson V, et al. The child sport concussion assessment tool 5th edition (Child SCAT5). *Br J Sports Med* 2017. bjsports-2017-097492. Available from: http://bjsm.bmj.com/lookup/doi/10.1136/bjsports-2017-097492.
53. McCrory P, Meeuwisse W, Dvorak J, Aubry M, Bailes J, Broglio S, et al. Consensus statement on concussion in sport—the 5th international conference on concussion in sport held in Berlin, October 2016. *Br J Sports Med* 2017;**51**(11):838–47.
54. Bell DR, Guskiewicz KM, Clark MA, Padua DA. Systematic review of the balance error scoring system. *Sports Health* 2011;**3**(3):287–95. Available from: http://journals.sagepub.com/doi/10.1177/1941738111403122.
55. Hansen C, Cushman D, Anderson N, Chen W, Cheng C, Hon SD, et al. A normative dataset of the balance error scoring system in children aged between 5 and 14. *Clin J Sport Med* 2016;**26**(6):497–501. Available from: http://www.ncbi.nlm.nih.gov/pubmed/27783573.
56. Alsalaheen B, McClafferty A, Haines J, Smith L, Yorke A. Reference values for the balance error scoring system in adolescents. *Brain Inj* 2016;**30**(7):914–18. Available from: http://www.tandfonline.com/doi/full/10.3109/02699052.2016.1146965.
57. Iverson GL, Koehle MS. Normative data for the balance error scoring system in adults. *Rehabil Res Pract* 2013;**2013**:1–5. Available from: http://www.ncbi.nlm.nih.gov/pubmed/23577257.
58. Valovich TC, Perrin DH, Gansneder BM. Repeat administration elicits a practice effect with the Balance Error Scoring System but not with the Standardized Assessment of Concussion in high school athletes. *J Athl Train* 2003;**38**(1):51–6.
59. McCrea M, Guskiewicz KM, Marshall SW, Barr W, Randolph C, Cantu RC, et al. Acute effects and recovery time following. *J Am Med Assoc* 2003;**290**(19):2556–63.
60. King LA, Horak FB, Mancini M, Pierce D, Priest KC, Chesnutt J, et al. Instrumenting the balance error scoring system for use with patients reporting persistent balance problems after mild traumatic brain injury. *Arch Phys Med Rehabil* 2014;**95**(2):353–9.
61. Powers KC, Kalmar JM, Cinelli ME. Recovery of static stability following a concussion. *Gait Posture* 2014;**39**(1):611–14.

62. Slobounov S, Sebastianelli W, Hallett M. Residual brain dysfunction observed one year post-mild traumatic brain injury: combined EEG and balance study. *Clin Neurophysiol* 2012;**123**(9):1755–61. Available from: http://linkinghub.elsevier.com/retrieve/pii/S1388245712000661.

63. Nashner LM, Peters JF. Dynamic posturography in the diagnosis and management of dizziness and balance disorders. *Neurol Clin* 1990;**8**(2):331–49. Available from: http://www.ncbi.nlm.nih.gov/pubmed/2193215.

64. Nashner LM, Shupert CL, Horak FB, Black FO. Organization of posture controls: an analysis of sensory and mechanical constraints*Prog Brain Res* 1989;**80** 411-8-7. Available from . Available from: http://www.ncbi.nlm.nih.gov/pubmed/2699375.

65. Catena RD, Van Donkelaar P, Chou LS. Cognitive task effects on gait stability following concussion. *Exp Brain Res* 2007;**176**(1):23–31. Available from: http://www.ncbi.nlm.nih.gov/pubmed/16826411.

66. Alsalaheen BA, Mucha A, Morris LO, Whitney SL, Furman JM, Camiolo-Reddy CE, et al. Vestibular rehabilitation for dizziness and balance disorders after concussion. *J Neurol Phys Ther* 2010;**34**(2):87–93. Available from: http://content.wkhealth.com/linkback/openurl?sid = WKPTLP:landingpage&an = 01253086-201006000-00007.

67. Shumway-Cook A, Woollacott MH. Motor control: theory and practical applications [Internet]. Williams & Wilkins; 1995 [cited June 22, 2017]. 475 p. Available from: https://locatorplus.gov/cgi-bin/Pwebrecon.cgi?DB = local&v1 = 1&ti = 1,1&Search_Arg = 9507252&Search_Code = 0359&CNT = 20&SID = 1

68. Wrisley DM, Marchetti GF, Kuharsky DK, Whitney SL. Reliability, internal consistency, and validity of data obtained with the functional gait assessment. *Phys Ther* 2004;**84**(10):906–18. Available from: http://www.ncbi.nlm.nih.gov/pubmed/15449976.

69. Kleffelgaard I, Roe C, Soberg HL, Bergland A. Associations among self-reported balance problems, post-concussion symptoms and performance-based tests: a longitudinal follow-up study. *Disabil Rehabil* 2012;**34**(9):788–94. Available from: http://www.ncbi.nlm.nih.gov/pubmed/22149161.

70. Moore BM, Adams JT, Barakatt E. Outcomes following a vestibular rehabilitation and aerobic training program to address persistent post-concussion symptoms. *J Allied Health* 2016;**45**(4). e59–68. Available from: http://www.ncbi.nlm.nih.gov/pubmed/27915363.

71. Williams GP, Greenwood KM, Robertson VJ, Goldie PA, Morris ME. High-Level Mobility Assessment Tool (HiMAT): interrater reliability, retest reliability, and internal consistency. *Phys Ther* 2006;**86**(3):395–400. Available from: http://www.ncbi.nlm.nih.gov/pubmed/16506875.

72. Williams GP, Robertson V, Greenwood KM, Goldie PA, Morris ME. The high-level mobility assessment tool (HiMAT) for traumatic brain injury. Part 1: Item generation. *Brain Inj* 2005;**19**(11):925–32. Available from: http://www.ncbi.nlm.nih.gov/pubmed/16243748.

73. Williams GP, Robertson V, Greenwood KM, Goldie PA, Morris ME. The high-level mobility assessment tool (HiMAT) for traumatic brain injury. Part 2: Content validity and discriminability. *Brain Inj* 2005;**19**(10):833–43. Available from: http://www.ncbi.nlm.nih.gov/pubmed/16175843.

74. Kleffelgaard I, Roe C, Sandvik L, Hellstrom T, Soberg HL. Measurement properties of the high-level mobility assessment tool for mild traumatic brain injury. *Phys Ther* 2013;**93**(7). Available from: https://doi.org/10.2522/ptj.20120381. 900–10. Available from: https://academic.oup.com/ptj/article-lookup.

75. Broglio SP, Macciocchi SN, Ferrara MS. Neurocognitive performance of concussed athletes when symptom free. *J Athl Train* 2007;**42**(4):504–8.

76. Howell DR, Osternig LR, Koester MC, Chou LS. The effect of cognitive task complexity on gait stability in adolescents following concussion. *Exp Brain Res* 2014;**232**(6):1773–82. Available from: http://www.ncbi.nlm.nih.gov/pubmed/24531643.

77. Dorman JC, Valentine VD, Munce TA, Tjarks BJ, Thompson PA, Bergeron MF. Tracking postural stability of young concussion patients using dual-task interference. *J Sci Med Sport* 2015;**18**(1):2–7. Available from: http://www.ncbi.nlm.nih.gov/pubmed/24380848.

78. Rochefort C, Walters-Stewart C, Aglipay M, Barrowman N, Zemek R, Sveistrup H. Balance markers in adolescents at 1 month postconcussion. *Orthop J Sport Med* 2017;**5**(3). 232596711769550. Available from: http://www.ncbi.nlm.nih.gov/pubmed/28451603.

79. Catena RD, van Donkelaar P, Chou LS. Altered balance control following concussion is better detected with an attention test during gait. *Gait Posture* 2007;**25**(3):406–11. Available from: http://www.ncbi.nlm.nih.gov/pubmed/16787746.

80. Parker TM, Osternig LR, Van Donkelaar P, Chou LS. Gait stability following concussion. *Med Sci Sports Exerc* 2006;**38**(6):1032–40. Available from: http://www.ncbi.nlm.nih.gov/pubmed/16775541.

81. Howell DR, Osternig LR, Chou LS. Dual-task effect on gait balance control in adolescents with concussion. *Arch Phys Med Rehabil* 2013;**94**(8):1513–20. Available from: http://www.ncbi.nlm.nih.gov/pubmed/23643687.

82. Howell DR, Osternig LR, Chou L-S. Adolescents demonstrate greater gait balance control deficits after concussion than young adults. *Am J Sports Med* 2015;**43**(3):625–32. Available from: http://ajs.sagepub.com/lookup/doi/10.1177/0363546514560994.

83. Howell DR, Osternig LR, Chou L-S. Return to activity after concussion affects dual-task gait balance control recovery. *Med Sci Sports Exerc* 2015;**47**(4):673–80. Available from: http://content.wkhealth.com/linkback/openurl?sid = WKPTLP:landingpage&an = 00005768-201504000-00001.

Hearing Disorders Associated With Mild Traumatic Brain Injury (mTBI)

Tanya Singh, MS[1] and Michael D. Seidman, MD, FACS[2,3,4]

[1]Department of Medical Education, University of Central Florida College of Medicine, Orlando, FL, United States [2]Director Otologic/Neurotologic/Skull Base Surgery, Medical Director Wellness and Integrative Medicine, Advent Health (Celebration and South Campuses), Roslyn, NY, United States [3]Professor Otolaryngology Head and Neck Surgery, University of Central Florida College of Medicine, Orlando, FL, United States [4]Adjunct Professor Otolaryngology Head & Neck Surgery, University of South Florida College of Medicine, Tampa, FL, United States

INTRODUCTION

Due to increased rates of motor vehicle accidents, falls, concussive sports injuries, and military service related injuries, mild traumatic brain injury (mTBI) is becoming a topic of heightened regard in the medical community, as are the long term audiological sequalae. It has been estimated that 1.7 million people suffer a TBI annually in the United States, the leading causes of which were fall and motor vehicle accidents.[1] The prevalence of peripheral hearing loss following TBI is as high as 33% during the initial recovery period. Military conflicts in the Middle East, including Operation Enduring Freedom and Operation Iraqi Freedom (OIF), generated an increase in combat injuries and death related to the detonation of improvised explosive devices. Therefore, much of the recent epidemiological data regarding hearing disorders following TBI describes blast related injuries in the US military population.[2–5] The auditory system is the second most commonly affected body system among US veterans with service related disabilities. Together, tinnitus and hearing loss comprise greater than 90% of all auditory disabilities in veterans and are the two most prevalent service related disabilities overall at 7.4% and 5.4%, respectively.[6] In addition to the impaired quality of life and distress caused by these conditions, the economic burden is immense. Tinnitus and hearing loss accounted for an estimated 2 million

149

disabilities reported in 2015 among US veterans and more than 2 billion dollars went toward care and aural rehabilitation services.[6] Due to the complex nature of TBI and its overlapping functional sequelae, many hearing disorders are not diagnosed or treated until later in the recovery process. Damage to either the peripheral or central auditory system can lead to debilitating auditory problems. Here we review the most common hearing disorders associated with mTBI: tinnitus, hearing loss (sensorineural vs conductive), hyperacusis, and central auditory dysfunction (CAD).

TINNITUS

Tinnitus is a common phenomenon following mTBI, described as a high-pitched buzzing, hissing, or ringing sound in the ears which occurs in the absence of an external source of sound. In 2010, approximately 50 million US adults experienced some kind of tinnitus.[7] Although not a disease by itself, the impact of this symptom can range from minimally bothersome to effectively disabling, with 10% of chronic tinnitus sufferers eventually requiring intervention.[7] Tinnitus is the most common service related disability among US military veterans, affecting 7.4%, or more than 1.4 million service men and women, in 2015.[6] In a study of veterans who suffered specifically from blast injury during OIF, 38% experienced tinnitus.[8] In the overall US population, the prevalence of tinnitus has been shown to increase with age[7] and is associated with several mental health disorders including generalized anxiety disorder, depression, and insomnia.[7,9]

Clinical Characterization

The description of tinnitus is widely variable from patient to patient and can aid in distinguishing the underlying cause. Tinnitus can be described as objective or subjective, where objective tinnitus can be heard by an outside observer and subjective tinnitus can only be heard by the patient. Objective tinnitus occurs in less than 10% of all patients who present with tinnitus, and is typically described as pulsatile in nature, paralleling the patient's heartbeat.[7] Pulsatile tinnitus is usually associated with turbulent flow in the nearby vasculature and on rare occasion may be heard using a Toynbee stethoscope.[10] Rather than a result of damage, pulsatile tinnitus suggests the presence of an anomaly or impingement of the nearby vasculature and is therefore typically sensed unilaterally.[11] Additionally, tumors such as glomus tympanicum or even fluid in the middle ear can produce pulsatile tinnitus. Conversely, subjective tinnitus is more common, occurs in the absence of an auditory stimulus, and is generally related to hearing loss or damage along the auditory pathway. Tinnitus can be chronic or intermittent, can affect one or both ears, and can vary in loudness and pitch. Subjective tinnitus occurs in one out of every 10 adults, and is more common in older individuals.

Etiopathogenesis

Tinnitus can be a symptom of a broad variety of underlying conditions. Unilateral pulsatile tinnitus is typically suggestive of vascular pathology including dural arteriovenous

TABLE 11.1   Tinnitus Common Etiologies

Otologic	Presbycusis, sensorineural or CHL, Meniere's disease, trauma, idiopathic
Neurologic	Chiari malformation, multiple sclerosis, vestibular schwannoma, paraganglioma, trauma
Vascular	Benign intracranial hypertension, vascular malformations and tumors, stroke, pseudotumor cerebri, stenosis or dissection of internal carotid artery, small vessel disease, hypercholesterolemia, anemia
Infectious	Rubella, syphilis, lyme disease, meningitis, otitis media, measles, cytomegalovirus
Systemic	Autoimmune inner ear disease, rheumatoid arthritis, systemic lupus erythematosus, thyroid disease, diabetes mellitus, chronic renal failure, hyperparathyroidism
Medications	Salicylates, nonsteroidal antiinflammatory drugs, aminoglycoside antibiotics, loop diuretics, platins, vincristine

fistulas, arteriovenous malformations, aneurysm, congenital variants, stenosis, or dissection of nearby vasculature.[12,13] Systemic vascular disease can also cause pulsatile tinnitus, although this would present bilaterally.[12]

Subjective tinnitus, on the other hand, most commonly occurs in the setting of sensorineural hearing loss (SNHL).[14] High frequency hearing loss is a common risk factor for tinnitus and the majority of tinnitus cases are associated with SNHL.[11,15] Along the auditory axis, nontraumatic causes of subjective tinnitus include cerumen impaction, otosclerosis, Eustachian tube dysfunction, Meniere's disease, and vestibular schwannoma.[12] Other common etiologies of tinnitus (Table 11.1) include medications,[16] infectious diseases,[16] systemic conditions such as anemia,[17] and metabolic disorders such as thyroid disease and diabetes mellitus.[18,19] Tinnitus following mTBI can be due to direct trauma or completely unrelated to trauma such as medications used in mTBI for headache, emotional lability, depression, and anxiety.

Air filled organs such as the ear are particularly vulnerable to barotrauma from explosions. Tympanic membrane rupture is one of the most common blast-related ear injuries and can result in permanent conductive hearing loss (CHL) as well as tinnitus.[5,20] In a sample of veterans injured during OIF, 38% of those with blast related injury complained of tinnitus, compared with 18% in those injured through nonblast mechanisms.[8] In addition to trauma affecting the inner ear and middle ear, diffuse axonal damage can result from coup−contrecoup type injuries and blunt mechanical injury to the head, especially involving the temporal bone.[21]

Although the exact mechanism underlying tinnitus in the setting of mTBI remains elusive, possible explanations are grounded in the concept of neuroplasticity. Proposed mechanisms include reorganization of tonotopic maps, increased temporal synchrony, and reduced inhibition leading to hyperexcitability of the auditory cortex.[11,15] These theories are supported by positron emission tomography and functional magnetic resonance imaging (MRI) studies linking abnormal activity in the auditory cortex to the perception of tinnitus, although an exact neural correlate remains to be demonstrated.[11,22] Studies carried out in rat models of blast-induced tinnitus support the role of increased excitation in the auditory cortex as a mechanism underlying chronic tinnitus.[23]

Of note, tinnitus related to mTBI is particularly troublesome as it can exacerbate sleeplessness, restlessness and irritability compounding the impact of mTBI.[9] Coexisting conditions such as depression and hearing loss have been shown to worsen the perception of tinnitus.[7]

Diagnosis

The diagnosis of tinnitus largely depends upon clinical history, character of tinnitus (pulsatile vs rhythmic), and associated symptoms such as hearing loss and hyperacusis. Because pulsatile tinnitus is usually due to treatable underlying structural abnormalities, computed tomography angiogram (CTA) imaging is the recommended initial test in most cases.[24] Magnetic resonance angiogram is also widely used, although the resolution for osseous pathology is limited compared to CTA.[24] MRI should be used if idiopathic intracranial hemorrhage is suspected. In the case of subjective unilateral pulsatile tinnitus, it is important to first distinguish between venous and arterial causes.

Patients with asymmetric hearing loss or other associated neurological deficits should also undergo neuroimaging to rule out structural lesions. Neuroimaging studies including computed tomography (CT) and MRI of the brain are typically normal in mTBI. Although there are other imaging techniques such as magnetic resonance spectroscopy and diffusion tensor imaging that have the potential to increase sensitivity of MRI in mTBI, most symptoms in these patients are considered neuropsychiatric due to lack of objective diagnostic modalities.[25] Additionally, magnetoencephalography can noninvasively measure magnetic "images" of the brain and has been successfully used to map tinnitus to the brain.[26–28]

Pure tone audiometry is recommended in these patients and since most complain of blocked sensation in the ears, tympanometry can be useful. Audiologists can also measure the tone of the tinnitus (pitch match) and minimal masking level necessary to mask the patient's tinnitus.

Several validated surveys are available to measure the impact of tinnitus on quality of life and guide psychological management of tinnitus. The Tinnitus Functional Index (TFI)[29] and Tinnitus Handicap Inventory (THI)[30] are patient reported symptoms in various domains to capture the impact of tinnitus on daily living such as sleep pattern and ability to concentrate. The Tinnitus Reaction Questionnaire (TRQ) measures the associated psychological distress.[31] Cognitive speed may be helpful in determining the functional impact of tinnitus.[32] In addition to assessing the severity of tinnitus from the patient's perspective, these methods can be used to quantify the effects of treatment. For example, the THI has been shown to be useful in demonstrating effects of embolization therapy for pulsatile tinnitus.[33]

Treatment/Prognosis

Since there is no definitive cure or FDA approved treatment of tinnitus to date, current treatment regimens are aimed at improving symptoms and quality of life.[11] Most patients with tinnitus report significant comorbidities. Depression, anxiety, and insomnia are commonly associated with and can exacerbate tinnitus symptoms. These comorbidities should be addressed to the extent possible before considering more invasive approaches.[9,34] In addition, any medications which could potentially be triggering the tinnitus should be discontinued.

Other noninvasive treatment options include behavioral approaches to reduce the patient's perception of the tinnitus. Tinnitus retraining therapy (TRT) aims to habituate the patient to tinnitus symptoms through directive counseling and the use of low level noise generators to mask the tinnitus. Though up to 80% of patients experience improvement in symptoms, the long term effects are unknown and TRT may require 1–2 years to take effect.[35] Similarly, cognitive behavioral therapy (CBT) is the use of guided therapy to change the patient's attitudes and behaviors toward their tinnitus to reduce symptom severity. TRT and CBT have both been shown to improve quality of life for tinnitus patients with equal efficacy.[36,37]

Hearing aids or cochlear implants (CIs) can be considered for patients with tinnitus related to profound hearing loss.[38] In the case of SNHL, 75% of patients experience improved symptoms with CI.[39] Though the exact mechanism behind CI is unclear, it is thought that within the framework of reduced inhibition leading to hyperexcitability of the auditory cortex, CI may improve symptoms by providing consistent afferent stimulation. Similarly, hearing aids or general sound therapy can be used to amplify speech and environmental noise and mask the tinnitus, respectively.[15] However, limited data exist to support the efficacy of sound therapy.[40]

Patients with severe refractory tinnitus may require more invasive procedural interventions. Direct electrical stimulation of the auditory cortex may work to modify cortical hyperactivity linked with tinnitus and "sharpen" the tonotopic organization.[41] In the senior author's experience using implantable electrodes for electrical stimulation of the auditory cortex, some patients experienced sustained and significant reduction of symptoms while other patients did not.[41,42] Repeated transcranial magnetic stimulation has also been shown to alleviate symptoms in 40%–50% of patients with debilitating tinnitus at up to 26 weeks following treatment, although the long-term effects are still unclear.[43] Electrical stimulation to disrupt aberrant cortical activity is a promising strategy in the treatment of tinnitus and warrants further investigation.

Based on systematic reviews of randomized clinical trials as outlined in the American Academy of Otolaryngology Head and Neck Surgery Guidelines, antidepressants, anticonvulsants, anxiolytics, and intratympanic medications were found to be of limited benefit as compared to placebo for the treatment of tinnitus and are therefore not typically recommended by the guidelines.[14] Additionally, the use of alternative therapies such as Ginkgo biloba, melatonin, zinc, B vitamins, and other dietary supplements were not recommended for use.[14] However, many patients respond to herbal strategies, guided imagery, and certain medications such as alprazolam and amitriptyline, and the lead author often times recommends these strategies for his patients and there is compelling data for their use.[10,44–46]

HEARING LOSS

Hearing loss is common following TBI and has been reported in up to 56% of patients in the immediate aftermath of injury.[21] The temporal bone is particularly susceptible to

TABLE 11.2   Degrees of Decibel Loss

26−40 dB	Mild hearing loss
41−55 dB	Moderate hearing loss
56−70 dB	Moderately severe hearing loss
71−90 dB	Severe hearing loss
>90 dB	Profound hearing loss

fractures in head injury and can cause both SNHL and CHL, depending on the location of the fracture. Damage to the outer or middle ear typically results in CHL, while involvement of the inner ear causes SNHL, also known as nerve-related hearing loss. The Weber and Rinne bedside hearing tests can be used to differentiate SNHL from CHL and severity of hearing loss can range from mild to profound (Table 11.2).[47] Patients with hearing loss may also present with tinnitus, otalgia, vertigo, hemotympanum, tympanic membrane perforation, and difficulty with speech.[48]

SENSORINEURAL HEARING LOSS

SNHL, also known as nerve-related hearing loss, is frequently associated with blast-related mTBI. In a sample of 252 veterans injured during OIF, 62% with blast-related injury complained of hearing loss, compared with 44% in nonblast related injuries. Of note, SNHL was the most common type of hearing loss in this study.[8] SNHL is also associated with speech perception difficulties. Loss of high frequencies is more typical in traumatic injury than loss of low frequencies.[49]

Diagnosis

SNHL due to inner ear injury is difficult to examine directly, but damage in the case of asymmetric SNHL may be detected by the Weber tuning fork test or spontaneous horizontal nystagmus.[50-52] Perilymph fistula can cause SNHL and in addition to fluctuating or sudden SNHL, symptoms include Valsalva induced vertigo. Temporal bone CT may be used to demonstrate ossicular chain damage or labyrinthine concussion.[50-52] Temporal bone fractures should be evaluated early with bedside Weber and Rinne 512 Hz tuning fork test as well as an audiogram.[50-52] A threshold shift in pure tone noise indicates noise induced hearing loss and should be used in case of acute or new hearing loss with recent history of acoustic trauma.[50]

Mechanisms of Injury

The inner ear contains the cochlea, also known as the end organ of hearing, and the vestibular system. The vestibular system consists of the vestibule, utricle, saccule, and semicircular canals which function to maintain balance. These structures are encased in the most dense portion of the temporal bone, the otic capsule.[48,50]

SNHL results from inner ear lesions such as labyrinthine hemorrhage, labyrinthine concussion, perilymph fistula, or damage to the vestibulocochlear nerve, commonly seen in many sports related injuries.[48,50] Injury to the membranous labyrinth can result in inner ear hemorrhage seen as high intensity signal on T-1 weighted MRI sequences. Hearing loss due to labyrinthine concussion is often accompanied by complaints of vertigo and the presence of nystagmus.[50–52] Perilymph fistula is an abnormal channel between the middle and inner ear which allows for leakage of perilymph in to the middle ear.[53]

These injuries are associated with temporal bone fractures although notably, SNHL can also occur without any evidence of temporal bone fracture.[53,54] Temporal bone fractures are often described as longitudinal and transverse. Both can affect the otic capsule, but transverse fractures are more common and more likely to result in SNHL.[55]

Finally, SNHL can result from disruption in the central auditory pathway anywhere between the cochlea to the brainstem to the thalamus or projections to the auditory cortex. Depending on the level of lesion accounting for brainstem decussation, there may be contralateral hearing loss. Loud or repeated noise exposure is also known to result in SNHL.[50]

Treatment/Prognosis

Perilymph fistulas are treated by patching the oval or round window membrane, oral glucocorticoids, diuretics, bedrest, and stool softeners to minimize effects of the Valsalva maneuver.[50–52] Treatment for recent noise induced hearing loss is a steroid burst and taper and if that fails, consideration for intratympanic steroids is reasonable.[50] The prognosis for SNHL is worse than CHL in middle ear injuries.[48] Outcomes are improved with early steroid treatment following injury, so early evaluation is critical.[50–52] Middle ear damage may be corrected surgically.[48] For permanent hearing loss, hearing aids, contralateral routing of signal aids, bone conduction hearing aids, CIs can be considered.[50,56] Treatment for labyrinthine concussion is oral glucocorticoid therapy.[50–52]

CONDUCTIVE HEARING LOSS

Diagnosis

Common causes of CHL in the setting of TBI include laceration of external auditory canal, tympanic membrane perforation, middle ear fluid, or ossicular disruption.[50–52] CHL can also be caused by other disruptions in the transduction of sound to the inner ear such as otosclerosis, cerumen impaction, cholesteatoma, and otitis media.[57] The Rinne and Weber tests are inexpensive bedside hearing test which can be used as a preliminary screening tool for CHL, but formal audiogram should be used for definitive diagnosis.[58,59] A 512 Hz tuning fork is recommended and bone conduction greater than air conduction is suggestive of CHL.[58] Tympanometry can also be useful to guide diagnosis.[59] An audiogram can distinguish between conductive and SNHL as well as determine the degree of hearing loss.[59]

Mechanisms of Injury

The ossicular chain is comprised of the malleus, incus, and stapes. Together, these bones function to transduce acoustic vibrations from the tympanic membrane to the inner ear. Injury to the temporal bone or ossicular chain is common in traumatic head injuries.[60] Longitudinal rather than transverse temporal bone fractures are associated with conductive and mixed hearing loss.[55] Temporal bone fractures involving the ear canal often also involve TM perforation, suggesting inner or middle ear injury. Hemotympanum is a sign of temporal bone fracture.[50–52]

Blast injuries in particular are associated with a higher incidence of hearing loss due to TM injury.[20,21,61,62] TM perforation can be a result of acoustic or barotrauma and typically presents as sudden CHL with dizziness, ear pain, tinnitus, and nausea.[48,55] Roughly one third of severe head trauma cases present with a TM perforation and these patients should be evaluated for related injuries such as ossicular damage, undergo otoscopic evaluation, and Rinne and Weber hearing tests or audiometric testing.[48,55] More severe findings such as ossicular disruption, perilymph fistula, and greater than 40 dB hearing loss warrant referral to an otolaryngologist or hospitalization.[48,55] Basilar skull and temporal bone fractures are associated with severe head trauma and may result in hearing loss via blood accumulation in the middle ear, ossicular chain disruption, or cochlear damage.

Indirect forces to the ossicular chain such as traffic accidents, falls, or blow to the head and direct forces as seen in blast injury can cause CHL, as can trauma involving solely the middle ear.[60] Damage to the ossicular chain most commonly involves incudostapedial joint subluxation, incus dislocation, or fracture of the stapes crura.[54,60] CHL that lasts several weeks after a traumatic injury and is greater than 30 dB indicates ossicular injury.

Treatment/Prognosis

Early surgical intervention leads to favorable outcomes, which underscores the need for prompt diagnosis of ossicular injury following a traumatic injury to the head.[48,60] Unfortunately due to the severity and urgency of traumatic brain injuries, ossicular injuries are typically not diagnosed until weeks to years after the initial incident.[60]

HYPERACUSIS

Hyperacusis is a condition defined as diminished tolerance to ordinary environmental sounds and speech.[63] It is distinguished from phonophobia associated with migraines because where phonophobia typically refers to sensitivity to loud sounds, patients who suffer from hyperacusis find sounds of low intensity to be uncomfortably loud and even painful.[63,64] The comorbidity of hyperacusis and tinnitus is high. Up to 86% of patients with a primary complaint of hyperacusis also complain of tinnitus, suggesting a common underlying mechanism.[63,65] However, only about 30%−40% of patients with tinnitus complain of hyperacusis.[64]

Hyperacusis is associated with a wide variety of conditions outlined in Table 11.3.[63,64,66] The stapedial reflex, also called the attenuation reflex, is innervated by the facial nerve

TABLE 11.3   Causes of Hyperacusis

Infectious	Lyme disease, neurosyphilis, typhoid fever
Vascular	Vascular aneurysm, chiari malformation, vascular malformation, carotid aneurysm, middle cerebral aneurysm
Central nervous system disorders	Migraine, depression, PTSD, head injury, William's syndrome, autism
Disrupted attenuation reflex	Bell's Palsy, multiple sclerosis, Ramsey-Hunt syndrome, stapedectomy, perilymph fistula, Meniere's disease
Endocrine	Addison's disease, panhypopituitarism, hyperthyroidism
Medication-induced	Benzodiazepine withdrawal, phenytoin,
deficiencies	magnesium, pyridoxine

and functions to dampen the perceived intensity of incoming sound.[63] Disruption of this reflex in TBI may lead to hyperacusis.

Diagnosis of hyperacusis often involves measuring the uncomfortable loudness level (ULL) or loudness discomfort level (LDL), used interchangeably, across a range of frequencies.[63,66] A study of 381 hyperacusis patients demonstrated that LDLs decrease across the full range of frequencies independent of pattern of hearing loss, unlike tinnitus.[64] It has been proposed that a ULL of 70 dB hearing loss or less be used to diagnose hyperacusis.[66] Questionnaires available to objectively quantify a patient's experience of hyperacusis include the hyperacusis questionnaire,[67] the German Questionnaire on Hypersensitivity to Sound,[68] and the Multiple Activity Scale for Hyperacusis.[69]

Hyperacusis can be quite distressing for patients and a logical first instinct may be to protect the ears by wearing earplugs or ear muffs. Unfortunately, continuous protection from ordinary sounds is not recommended as treatment because it can worsen the severity of hyperacusis by increasing central auditory gain.[66] Treatment of hyperacusis involves many of the same strategies as used for tinnitus. In addition to counseling and education, CBT can help patients change their behavior in response to sounds by gradually exposing them to bothersome stimuli in a controlled environment and helping them to relax.[66] Although a gradual process, the benefits of CBT in one study were shown to persist at 1 year follow-up.[70] Exposure to continuous low level broadband noise may help to reduce symptoms in some, but not all hyperacusis patients.[66]

CENTRAL AUDITORY DYSFUNCTION

In CAD, patients complain of difficulty hearing despite a normal audiogram or normal peripheral auditory function. Symptoms of CAD can range from difficulty hearing in the presence of background noise, difficulty remembering and following verbal instructions, difficulty following verbal instructions, to difficulty understanding rapid speech.[8,71,72]

Subcortical differences appear to relate to performance on tests of auditory processing and perception, even in the absence of significant hearing loss on the audiogram. mTBI can result in neuronal changes within the subcortical auditory pathway that appear to relate to functional auditory outcomes.[73]

There may be disruption of the central auditory pathway in mTBI, but processing of auditory information can be impaired as a result of overall cognitive dysfunction such as delayed attention span, slow response time, executive dysfunction, and language. All these domains are involved in processing of auditory information. Among these, delayed attention span and reduced speed of information processing (slow mentation) are most consistently deficient and can linger for over 1 year after the injury.[74,75]

ELECTROPHYSIOLOGICAL STUDIES IN MILD TRAUMATIC BRAIN INJURY

In mTBI, electrophysiological assessments using scalp electrodes can help localize the neural impairment along the auditory processing pathway, which can be at the cortical, subcortical or cognitive levels.

Cortical

At the cortical level, the identification and perception of sound in the auditory cortex recorded as P1-N1-P2 is a long latency cortical auditory evoked potential (CAEP). It is a sensory potential that can be recorded in response to an auditory potential without the active participation of the patient. The CAEP has been studied in severe TBI patients; however, it has not been assessed frequently enough in mTBI patients to draw any meaningful conclusion. Of note, CAEP can be affected in individuals with auditory-based learning disorders and in aging related hearing disorders.

Subcortical

Auditory brainstem response (ABR) is a measure of sensory detection and encoding of acoustic elements of sound at subcortical level. It represents activity initiated at the base of the cochlea and moving toward the apex over a 4-ms time period. There is no evidence that an abnormal latency correlates with lingering postconcussion symptoms or low neuropsychological scores. The speech-evoked ABR does hold some promise to improve our understanding of subcortical auditory processing in mTBI, and is an area of active research.

Cognitive

The auditory P3 or P300 is the most commonly studied electrophysiological in TBI. The P3 response to both auditory and visual stimuli is used to test attention, memory, and processing speed by using an oddball task asking the patient to differentiate between a frequent and infrequent stimulus. There is data showing that auditory P3 which corresponds to large frequency changes in tones is sensitive in moderate to severe TBI.[76–78] Similar studies in the mTBI population have produced mixed results, showing either no difference or significant changes in P3 latency and/or amplitude using tonal stimuli in an oddball paradigm.

In recent years, there has been an emphasis on the use of evoked potentials, especially cortical potentials and auditory P3, to assess and monitor the effects of rehabilitation and auditory training.

MENTAL HEALTH ISSUES

Both hearing loss and tinnitus can cause depression, and can also be the cause of subjective tinnitus and hearing loss. Frequent tinnitus has been shown to be associated with generalized anxiety disorder, current depression, and insomnia [7,9,79] In Iraq and Afghanistan war veterans, hearing loss and tinnitus are associated with posttraumatic stress.[80] Behavioral problems after mTBI can range from fatigue and depression to irritability, anxiety, agitation, impulsivity, and aggression.[79] As many as 10%–70% patients with mTBI have depressive symptoms.[81]

FUTURE DIRECTIONS

Hearing disorders in mTBI are self-limiting and transient but can also last beyond the 3-month period along with other postconcussive symptoms. Currently there are no predictive models to know which patients will go on to have long-term symptoms following mTBI. While there is emerging literature to support the presence of dysfunction in auditory processing after mTBI, the lack of a standardized battery to assess auditory dysfunction, confounding due to the presence of lingering cognitive and psychological symptoms, and the heterogeneity in injury and population makes it difficult for providers to pinpoint the nature of the problem. Audiologists involved in the care of mTBI patients should conduct both tests for peripheral as well as CAD as per American Speech-Language-Hearing Association (2005).[82] The impact of cognitive postconcussive symptoms while interpreting the results of auditory processing should also be considered. Along with comprehensive early treatment of mTBI patients, otolaryngology-head and neck surgeons, neurosurgeons, neurologists, neuropsychologists, and proper acute rehabilitative services.

Baseline assessment of hearing in individuals at high risk of concussion, such as military personnel and athletes, early detection and preventative strategy is high priority and an active area of research.

CONCLUSION

Tinnitus, hearing loss, and hyperacusis are common and oftentimes cooccurring consequences of mTBI. These conditions tend to be diagnosed late due to the severe nature of head injuries and each is associated with several possible underlying etiologies, many of which can be ruled out with appropriate imaging and thorough clinical workup. Potential mechanisms linking tinnitus and hyperacusis with hearing loss may be related to hyperactivity and reorganization of tonotopic mapping in the auditory cortex as well as decreased inhibitory feedback from the peripheral auditory system. Insomnia, anxiety, and depression are common in patients who suffer from tinnitus, and may exacerbate symptoms. Though there is no cure for tinnitus, a variety of noninvasive behavioral and alternative treatment options as well as emerging surgical options are available. The treatment of tinnitus and hyperacusis are still very active areas of research, and further inquiry regarding the use of alternative therapies is warranted.

References

1. Faul M, Xu L, Wald MM, Coronado V, Dellinger AM. Traumatic brain injury in the United States: national estimates of prevalence and incidence, 2002–2006. *Inj Prev* 2010;**16**(Suppl. 1). A268-A.
2. Shah A, Ayala M, Capra G, Fox D, Hoffer M. Otologic assessment of blast and nonblast injury in returning Middle East-deployed service members. *Laryngoscope* 2014;**124**(1):272–7.
3. Helfer TM, Jordan NN, Lee RB, Pietrusiak P, Cave K, Schairer K. Noise-induced hearing injury and comorbidities among postdeployment U.S. Army soldiers: April 2003-June 2009. *Am J Audiol* 2011;**20**(1):33–41.
4. Yurgil KA, Clifford RE, Risbrough VB, Geyer MA, Huang M, Barkauskas DA, et al. Prospective associations between traumatic brain injury and postdeployment tinnitus in active-duty marines. *J Head Trauma Rehabil* 2016;**31**(1):30–9.
5. Dougherty AL, MacGregor AJ, Han PP, Viirre E, Heltemes KJ, Galarneau MR. Blast-related ear injuries among U.S. military personnel. *J Rehabil Res Dev* 2013;**50**(6):893–904.
6. Affairs UDoV. *Annual Benefits Report: Fiscal Year 2015*. Washington, DC: Department of Veterans Affairs; 2016.
7. Shargorodsky J, Curhan GC, Farwell WR. Prevalence and characteristics of tinnitus among US adults. *Am J Med* 2010;**123**(8):711–18.
8. Lew HL, Jerger JF, Guillory SB, Henry JA. Auditory dysfunction in traumatic brain injury. *J Rehabil Res Dev* 2007;**44**(7):921–8.
9. Folmer RL, Griest SE. Tinnitus and insomnia. *Am J Otolaryngol* 2000;**21**(5):287–93.
10. Ahmad N, Seidman M. Tinnitus in the older adult: epidemiology, pathophysiology and treatment options. *Drugs Aging* 2004;**21**(5):297–305.
11. Atik A. Pathophysiology and treatment of tinnitus: an elusive disease. *Indian J Otolaryngol Head Neck Surg* 2014;**66**(Suppl. 1):1–5.
12. Pegge SA, Steens SC, Kunst HP, Meijer FJ. Pulsatile tinnitus: differential diagnosis and radiological work-up. *Curr Radiol Rep* 2017;**5**(1):5.
13. Sismanis A. Pulsatile tinnitus. A 15-year experience. *Am J Otol* 1998;**19**(4):472–7.
14. Tunkel DE, Bauer CA, Sun GH, Rosenfeld RM, Chandrasekhar SS, Cunningham ER, et al. Clinical practice guideline: tinnitus. *Otolaryngol Head Neck Surg: Offic J Am Acad Otolaryngol-Head Neck Surg* 2014;**151**(2 Suppl): S1–s40.
15. Baguley D, McFerran D, Hall D. Tinnitus. *Lancet* 2013;**382**(9904):1600–7.
16. Han BI, Lee HW, Kim TY, Lim JS, Shin KS. Tinnitus: characteristics, causes, mechanisms, and treatments. *J Clin Neurol* 2009;**5**(1):11–19.
17. Patel R, Sabat S, Kanekar S. Imaging manifestations of neurologic complications in anemia. *Hematol Oncol Clin North Am* 2016;**30**(4):733–56.
18. Bhatia P, Gupta O, Agrawal M, Mishr S. Audiological and vestibular function tests in hypothyroidism. *The Laryngoscope* 1977;**87**(12):2082–9.
19. Kaźmierczak H, Doroszewska G. Metabolic disorders in vertigo, tinnitus, and hearing loss. *Int Tinnitus J* 2000;**7**(1):54–8.
20. DePalma RG, Burris DG, Champion HR, Hodgson MJ. Blast injuries. *N Engl J Med* 2005;**352**(13):1335–42.

21. Vander Werff KR. Auditory dysfunction among long-term consequences of mild traumatic brain injury (mTBI). *SIG 6 Perspect Hear Hear Disorders: Res Diagnost* 2012;**16**(1):3–17.

22. Lanting CP, de Kleine E, van Dijk P. Neural activity underlying tinnitus generation: results from PET and fMRI. *Hear Res* 2009;**255**(1–2):1–13.

23. Luo H, Pace E, Zhang J. Blast-induced tinnitus and hyperactivity in the auditory cortex of rats. *Neuroscience* 2017;**340**:515–20.

24. Ahsan SF, Seidman M, Yaremchuk K. What is the best imaging modality in evaluating patients with unilateral pulsatile tinnitus? *Laryngoscope* 2015;**125**(2):284–5.

25. Hofman PA, Stapert SZ, van Kroonenburgh MJ, Jolles J, de Kruijk J, Wilmink JT. MR imaging, single-photon emission CT, and neurocognitive performance after mild traumatic brain injury. *Am J Neuroradiol* 2001;**22**(3):441–9.

26. Bowyer SM, Seidman M, Elisevich K, De Ridder D, Mason KM, Dria J, et al. MEG localization of the putative cortical generators of tinnitus. *Int Congress Ser* 2007;**1300**:33–6.

27. Zhang JSGA, Zhang XG, Beydoun H, Seidman M, Elisevich K, Bowyer S, et al. Cortical electrical suppression of tinnitus and modulation of its related neural activity. *N Z Med J* 2010;**123**(1311):77–167.

28. Bowyer S, Seidman M, Moran J, Mason K, Jiang Q, Elisevich K, et al., editors. Coherence analysis of brain activity associated with tinnitus. In: *Biomagnetism—Transdisciplinary research and exploration: proceedings of the 16th international conference on biomagnetism*, Sapporo, Japan, August; 2008.

29. Meikle MB, Henry JA, Griest SE, Stewart BJ, Abrams HB, McArdle R, et al. The tinnitus functional index: development of a new clinical measure for chronic, intrusive tinnitus. *Ear Hear.* 2012;**33**(2):153–76.

30. Newman CW, Jacobson GP, Spitzer JB. Development of the tinnitus handicap inventory. *Arch Otolaryngol Head Neck Surg* 1996;**122**(2):143–8.

31. Wilson PH, Henry J, Bowen M, Haralambous G. Tinnitus reaction questionnaire: psychometric properties of a measure of distress associated with tinnitus. *J Speech Hear Res* 1991;**34**(1):197–201.

32. Das SK, Wineland A, Kallogjeri D, Piccirillo JF. Cognitive speed as an objective measure of tinnitus. *The Laryngoscope* 2012;**122**(11):2533–8.

33. Shiraishi K, Akioka N, Kashiwazaki D, Kuwayama N, Kuroda S. Semi-quantitative assessment of tinnitus before and after endovascular treatment for intracranial dural arteriovenous fistula: usefulness of the tinnitus handicap inventory (THI) score. *No Shinkei Geka Neurol Surg* 2017;**45**(1):21–6.

34. Crocetti A, Forti S, Ambrosetti U, Bo LD. Questionnaires to evaluate anxiety and depressive levels in tinnitus patients. *Otolaryngol Head Neck Surg: Offic J Am Acad Otolaryngol Head Neck Surg* 2009;**140**(3):403–5.

35. Andersson G, Lyttkens L. A meta-analytic review of psychological treatments for tinnitus. *Br J Audiol* 1999;**33**(4):201–10.

36. Grewal R, Spielmann PM, Jones SE, Hussain SS. Clinical efficacy of tinnitus retraining therapy and cognitive behavioural therapy in the treatment of subjective tinnitus: a systematic review. *J Laryngol Otol* 2014;**128**(12):1028–33.

37. Cima RF, Maes IH, Joore MA, Scheyen DJ, El Refaie A, Baguley DM, et al. Specialised treatment based on cognitive behaviour therapy versus usual care for tinnitus: a randomised controlled trial. *Lancet* 2012;**379**(9830):1951–9.

38. Fuller TE, Haider HF, Kikidis D, Lapira A, Mazurek B, Norena A, et al. Different teams, same conclusions? A systematic review of existing clinical guidelines for the assessment and treatment of tinnitus in adults. *Front Psychol* 2017;**8**:206.

39. Holder JT, O'Connell B, Hedley-Williams A, Wanna G. Cochlear implantation for single-sided deafness and tinnitus suppression. *Am J Otolaryngol* 2017;**38**(2):226–9.

40. Hobson J, Chisholm E, El Refaie A. Sound therapy (masking) in the management of tinnitus in adults. *Cochrane Database Syst Rev* 2010;(12)):Cd006371.

41. De Ridder D, De Mulder G, Verstraeten E, Seidman M, Elisevich K, Sunaert S, et al. Auditory cortex stimulation for tinnitus. *Acta Neurochir Suppl* 2007;**97**(Pt 2):451–62.

42. Seidman MD, Ridder DD, Elisevich K, Bowyer SM, Darrat I, Dria J, et al. Direct electrical stimulation of Heschl's gyrus for tinnitus treatment. *Laryngoscope* 2008;**118**(3):491–500.

43. Folmer RL, Theodoroff SM, Casiana L, Shi Y, Griest S, Vachhani J. Repetitive transcranial magnetic stimulation treatment for chronic tinnitus: a randomized clinical trial. *JAMA Otolaryngol Head Neck Surg* 2015;**141**(8):716–22.

III. NEUROSENSORY DISORDERS IN CLINICAL PRACTICE

44. Seidman MD, Moneysmith M. *Ch. 6: nutraceuticals and herbal supplements. Pharmacology and ototoxicity for audiologists.* Clifton Park, NY: Thomson Delmar Learning Publishers; 2005.

45. Seidman MD, Standring RT, Dornhoffer JL. Tinnitus: current understanding and contemporary management. *Curr Opin Otolaryngol Head Neck Surg* 2010;**18**(5):363–8.

46. Seidman MD, Babu S. Alternative medications and other treatments for tinnitus: facts from fiction. *Otolaryngol Clin North Am* 2003;**36**(2):359–81.

47. Clark JG. Uses and abuses of hearing loss classification. *ASHA* 1981;**23**(7):493–500.

48. Eagles K, Fralich L, Stevenson JH. Ear trauma. *Clin Sports Med* 2013;**32**(2):303–16.

49. Choi MS, Shin SO, Yeon JY, Choi YS, Kim J, Park SK. Clinical characteristics of labyrinthine concussion. *Korean J Audiol.* 2013;**17**(1):13–17.

50. Osetinsky LM, Hamilton 3rd GS, Carlson ML. Sport injuries of the ear and temporal bone. *Clin Sports Med* 2017;**36**(2):315–35.

51. Brodie H. Management of temporal bone trauma. *Bailey Byron J Johnson Jonas T Head Neck Surg–Otolaryngol* 2010;**2**:4.

52. Brodie HA, Thompson TC. Management of complications from 820 temporal bone fractures. *Am J Otol* 1997;**18**(2):188–97.

53. Grimm RJ, Hemenway WG, Lebray PR, Black FO. The perilymph fistula syndrome defined in mild head trauma. *Acta Otolaryngol Suppl* 1989;**464**:1–40.

54. Diaz RC, Cervenka B, Brodie HA. Treatment of temporal bone fractures. *J Neurol Surg Part B Skull Base.* 2016;**77**(5):419–29.

55. Nash JJ, Friedland DR, Boorsma KJ, Rhee JS. Management and outcomes of facial paralysis from intratemporal blunt trauma: a systematic review. *Laryngoscope* 2010;**120**(Suppl. 4). S214.

56. Lonsbury-Martin B, Martin G. Noise-induced hearing loss. In: Flint PWHB, Lund V, et al., editors. *Cummings otolaryngology: head & neck surgery.* 6th ed. Philadelphia, PA: Elsevier Saunders; 2015. p. 2345–68.

57. Uy J, Forciea MA. In the clinic. Hearing loss. *Ann Intern Med* 2013;**158**(7). ITC4-1; quiz ITC4-16.

58. Chole RA, Cook GB. The Rinne test for conductive deafness. A critical reappraisal. *Arch Otolaryngol Head Neck Surg* 1988;**114**(4):399–403.

59. Uy J, Forciea M. Hearing loss. *Ann Intern Med* 2013;**158**(7). ITC4-1.

60. Delrue S, Verhaert N, Dinther JV, Zarowski A, Somers T, Desloovere C, et al. Surgical management and hearing outcome of traumatic ossicular injuries. *J Int Adv Otol* 2016;**12**(3):231–6.

61. Belanger HG, Proctor-Weber Z, Kretzmer T, Kim M, French LM, Vanderploeg RD. Symptom complaints following reports of blast versus non-blast mild TBI: does mechanism of injury matter? *Clin Neuropsychol* 2011;**25**(5):702–15.

62. Johnson CM, Perez CF, Hoffer ME. The implications of physical injury on otovestibular and cognitive symptomatology following blast exposure. *Otolaryngol Head Neck Surg: Offic J Am Acad Otolaryngol Head Neck Surg* 2014;**150**(3):437–40.

63. Baguley DM. Hyperacusis. *J R Soc Med* 2003;**96**(12):582–5.

64. Sheldrake J, Diehl PU, Schaette R. Audiometric characteristics of hyperacusis patients. *Front Neurol* 2015;**6**(105):1–6

65. Anari M, Axelsson A, Eliasson A, Magnusson L. Hypersensitivity to sound—questionnaire data, audiometry and classification. *Scand Audiol* 1999;**28**(4):219–30.

66. Pienkowski M, Tyler RS, Roncancio ER, Jun HJ, Brozoski T, Dauman N, et al. A review of hyperacusis and future directions: part II. Measurement, mechanisms, and treatment. *Am J Audiol* 2014;**23**(4):420–36.

67. Khalfa S, Dubal S, Veuillet E, Perez-Diaz F, Jouvent R, Collet L. Psychometric normalization of a hyperacusis questionnaire. *ORL J Otorhinolaryngol Relat Spec* 2002;**64**(6):436–42.

68. Nelting M, Rienhoff NK, Hesse G, Lamparter U. The assessment of subjective distress related to hyperacusis with a self-rating questionnaire on hypersensitivity to sound. *Laryngorhinootologie* 2002;**81**(5):327–34.

69. Dauman R, Bouscau-Faure F. Assessment and amelioration of hyperacusis in tinnitus patients. *Acta Otolaryngol* 2005;**125**(5):503–9.

70. Juris L, Andersson G, Larsen HC, Ekselius L. Cognitive behaviour therapy for hyperacusis: a randomized controlled trial. *Behav Res Ther* 2014;**54**:30–7.

71. Lew HL, Thomander D, Chew KT, Bleiberg J. Review of sports-related concussion: potential for application in military settings. *J Rehabil Res Dev* 2007;**44**(7):963–74.

72. Jury MA, Flynn MC. Auditory and vestibular sequelae to traumatic brain injury: a pilot study. *N Z Med J* 2001;**114**(1134):286–8.

73. Vander Werff KR, Rieger B. Brainstem evoked potential indices of subcortical auditory processing after mild traumatic brain injury. *Ear Hear* 2017. 38(4):e200–e14.

74. Binder LM, Rohling ML, Larrabee GJ. A review of mild head trauma. Part I: Meta-analytic review of neuro-psychological studies. *J Clin Exp Neuropsychol* 1997;**19**(3):421–31.

75. Chan RC. Attentional deficits in patients with post-concussion symptoms: a componential perspective. *Brain Inj* 2001;**15**(1):71–94.

76. Lew HL, Thomander D, Gray M, Poole JH. The effects of increasing stimulus complexity in event-related potentials and reaction time testing: clinical applications in evaluating patients with traumatic brain injury. *J Clin Neurophysiol* 2007;**24**(5):398–404.

77. Duncan CC, Kosmidis MH, Mirsky AF. Closed head injury-related information processing deficits: an event-related potential analysis. *Int J Psychophysiol* 2005;**58**(2–3):133–57.

78. Duncan CC, Kosmidis MH, Mirsky AF. Event-related potential assessment of information processing after closed head injury. *Psychophysiology* 2003;**40**(1):45–59.

79. Vernon JA, Press LS. Characteristics of tinnitus induced by head injury. *Arch. Otolaryngol Head Neck Surg* 1994;**120**(5):547–51.

80. Swan AA, Nelson JT, Swiger B, Jaramillo CA, Eapen BC, Packer M, et al. Prevalence of hearing loss and tinni-tus in Iraq and Afghanistan veterans: a Chronic Effects of Neurotrauma Consortium study. *Hear Res* 2017;**349**:4–12.

81. Lew HL, Poole JH, Vanderploeg RD, Goodrich GL, Dekelboum S, Guillory SB, et al. Program development and defining characteristics of returning military in a VA Polytrauma Network Site. *J Rehabil Res Dev* 2007;**44**(7):1027–34.

82. Central auditory processing disorders American Speech-Language-Hearing Association, 2005. Available from: www.asha.org/policy.

Headache in Mild Traumatic Brain Injury

Teshamae S. Monteith, MD[1] and Tad Seifert, MD[2]

[1]Department of Neurology, Headache Division, University of Miami, Miller School of Medicine, Miami, FL, United States [2]Norton Sports Neurology, Norton Healthcare, University of Kentucky, Louisville, KY, United States

INTRODUCTION

Traumatic brain injury (TBI) is a common problem that occurs in the general population, but has gained increasing awareness especially due in military personnel and athletes including school aged children. In 2010, the Center for Disease Control and Prevention (CDC) estimated that TBI accounts for approximately 2.5 million emergency room visits, hospitalizations, and deaths in the United States.[1] Another estimate from the CDC noted that 75% of TBIs are mild or result in concussions.[2] Headache is one of the common symptoms following a head injury and can manifestation as a de novo secondary headache or worsening preexisting primary headache. The terms mild head injury, concussion, and posttraumatic headache (PTH) are sometimes used interchangeably; however, there are distinct differences (Fig. 12.1).[3] Mild TBI (mTBI) can present as PTH only or in association with other postconcussive sequela, adding to the clinical complexity. The understanding of PTH has grown over the past decade; however, skepticism remains in part due to the lack of biomarkers, the variability in clinical outcomes, litigation, cultural and psychological factors, and the lack of research progress. The focus of this chapter is headache associated with mild head injury. Other forms of headache due to moderate or severe TBI, whiplash, and craniotomy are also described in the International Classification of Headache Disorders 3rd edition (ICHD-3), but are beyond the scope of this chapter.[4]

EPIDEMIOLOGY

Headache is one of the most common symptoms experienced after a head injury.[5] It may occur variably in 30%–90% of individuals who are symptomatic after a mild head

Neurosensory Disorders in Mild Traumatic Brain Injury
DOI: https://doi.org/10.1016/B978-0-12-812344-7.00012-1

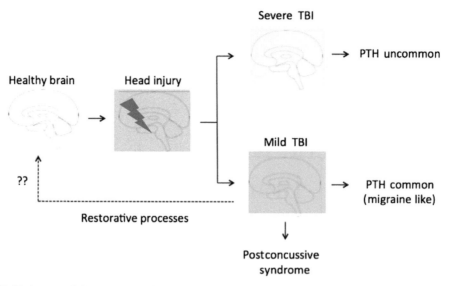

FIGURE 12.1   **PTH following TBI.** The majority of PTH occurs after mTBI with or without postconcussive syndrome. While most PTH resolves within weeks to months, brain changes in mTBI may persist along with comorbidities and is a risk factor for latent headache.

injury. Headache was the most common incident diagnosis following a TBI in service members, and was more commonly seen at 3 and 12 months after diagnosis as compared to control groups.[6] Up to 98% of Operation Enduring Freedom/Operation Iraqi Freedom (OEF/OIF) veterans reported headaches within 3 months of deployment-related concussion and 37% had headaches that lasted longer than 3 months. In same study, chronic daily headache was present in 27% of soldiers with posttraumatic headache compared with 14% of soldiers with primary headache.[7]

In the population based historical study, NordTrøndelag Health Study (HUNT), headache was investigated following head injury, with headache data from two large epidemiological surveys performed with an 11-year interval and hospital records on exposure to head injury occurring between the health surveys.[8] They found that individuals hospitalized due to mild head injury were more likely to report exacerbation of previously documented headache or develop new onset headache suffering as compared to the general population. The study provides case-control evidence to support the link between head injury and headache. In a US civilian inpatient sample, Lucas et al. conducted a longitudinal investigation of headaches in 212 mTBI subjects and followed the patients at 3, 6, and 12 months post-injury. After trauma, they found a cumulative incidence of 91% over 1 year.[9] About to half of headaches met the criteria for migraine and probable migraine; persistent headache occurred in greater than one third of subjects across all three follow-up time periods. In the first prospective cohort study in children following mTBI, migraine was also the most common headache type seen.[10]

There are a number of risk factors for persistent posttraumatic headache (PPTH) that have been identified in epidemiological and clinical based studies. A history of migraine is a risk factor for headache post-TBI.[11] Similar to population studies for migraine,[12] the female gender is also a risk factor for posttraumatic migraine.[13] Less recognized, individuals with migraine are at a greater risk for balance control impairments, increasing the risk for falls and mild head injuries.[14,15] Moreover, repetitive head and neck injuries are also risk factors of chronic headache.[16]

CLASSIFICATION

TBI is described as a multifaceted condition, as opposed to an event, that is broadly defined as an alteration in brain function or other evidence of brain pathology caused by an external, biomechanical force with or without loss of consciousness.[17] PTH is defined by the ICHD-3 as new or worsening headache developing within 7 days of the injury or after regaining consciousness from a TBI (Table 12.1).[4,18] In the case of headache associated with mTBI, there may be a loss of consciousness for 30 minutes or less, memory loss after the traumatic event for up to 24 hours, and a Glasgow Coma Scale (GCS) of 13–15. There are inherent controversies to the classification of PTH as the classification for TBI based on the GCS has some limitations.[20] The GCS has a high interobserver

TABLE 12.1   The ICHD-3 Diagnostic Criteria for Headache Attributed to Mild Head Injuries

Acute Headache Attributed to Mild Traumatic Injury to the Head	Persistent Headache Attributed to Mild Traumatic Injury to the Head

1. Headache fulfilling criteria for Acute headache attributed to traumatic injury to the head
2. Injury to the head fulfilling both of the following:
  a. Associated with none of the following:
    I. Loss of consciousness for >30 minutes
    II. Glasgow Coma Scale (GCS) score <13
    III. Posttraumatic amnesia lasting >24 hours
    IV. Altered level of awareness for >24 hours
    V. Imaging evidence of a traumatic head injury such as skull fracture, intracranial hemorrhage, and/or brain contusion
  b. Associated with one or more of the following symptoms and/or signs:
    I. Transient confusion, disorientation, or impaired consciousness
    II. Loss of memory for events immediately before or after the head injury
    III. Two or more of the following symptoms suggestive of mTBI:
      • Nausea
      • Vomiting
      • Visual disturbances
      • Dizziness and/or vertigo
      • Gait and/or postural imbalance
      • Impaired memory and/or concentration
	1. Any headache fulfilling criteria C and D
	2. Traumatic injury to the head[1] has occurred
	3. Headache is reported to have developed within 7 days after one of the following:
	  a. The injury to the head
	  b. Regaining of consciousness following the injury to the head
	  c. Discontinuation of medication(s) impairing ability to sense or report headache following the injury to the head
	4. Headache persists for >3 months after its onset
	5. Not better accounted for by another ICHD-3 diagnosis

variability among various providers, is inadequate to assess higher cortical functions, is influenced by drug and alcohol use, and is affected by language barriers.

According to ICHD-3, the acute phase of PTH begins within 7 days and may last up to 3 months before being considered PPTH. In recognition that headache may be latent, the term delayed-onset acute headache attributed to injury, ranging from mild to severe, has been placed in the Appendix of the ICHD-3 for further investigation. Longer cutoff durations have been proposed for the onset of PTH as opposed to the current 7-day cutoff. The requirement for headache onset within one week of a head injury has been argued to potentially miss 20–30% of PTH patients.[18–22] A longer latency for the onset of PTH is biologically plausible as brain plasticity may occur in later stages on the receptor level and therefore increase the risk of PTH.[23] However, the longer the latency, the greater likelihood of misattribution to TBI as primary headache disorders are common in the general population.

The definition does not account for the headache phenotype, which may resemble several kinds of primary headache such as tension type headache, migraine, as well as the trigeminal autonomic cephalalgias. It is unclear if further subtyping PTH by mechanism would be of any benefit. One study demonstrated a lack of association between mechanisms of injury and headache.[24] Moreover, the term persistent does not account for the frequency of headache nor does it differentiate continuous pain versus intermittent pain. Similar to proposed criteria for further classification of chronic migraine into intermittent and continuous forms under the appendix of the ICHD-3, the distinction between continuous and intermittent pain may be a useful according to one retrospective study at an army medical center.[25] In the study, PPTH was most likely be present with continuous pain and migraine was the most common diagnosis type. The investigators also found that the presence of continuous pain was associated with negative occupational outcomes while the diagnosis type was not.

PATHOPHYSIOLOGY

A broader view on the effects of brain injury on the generation of headache depends on a better understanding of the pathophysiology that occurs during TBI. Pain can be generated due to coup contrecoup and associated brain contusions and shearing or diffuse axonal injury even in relatively mild head injuries. The shearing forces disrupts axons and their connections. The vulnerability towards developing PTH may depend on epigenetic or genetic factors, gender, age related brain changes, neuroanatomical factors, physiological states, and biomechanics. A number of disturbances can lead to variety of pathology from cell injury to death, focal to widespread changes, and with effects on neurons, glia, other cellular types, and processes. There is a disruption of the blood brain barrier leading to the activation of cytokines and glia, proinflammatory mediators, the extravasation of cytotoxic peripheral blood components, dysregulation of molecules and ions, mitochondrial dysfunction, oxidative stress, and edema formation. Recently, immune biomarkers consisting of immune related genes for the diagnosis and prediction of mild brain injury has been demonstrated with higher sensitivity and specificity, but have not been specifically studied in PTH.[26] Despite these observations, the pathological processes that leads to PTH remains speculative.

Both the structural (i.e., axonal injury) and functional central nervous system network changes may result in the phenotypic expression of headache. Transient neurological disorders including headache following mild head injuries has also been theorized to occur secondary to cortical spreading depression, the underlying pathological substrate for the aura phase of migraine.[27]

Forces arising from acceleration/deceleration and energy dissipated through impact produce a cascade of acute events that disrupt the microarchitecture of the brain, including white matter damage evidenced as myelin disruption and axonal membrane injury. Evidence of dysfunctional pain modulation has also been observed in cases of PPTH, and it has been hypothesized that PTH may be a form of central pain.[28] During TBI, there is release of neurotransmitters, resulting in the loss of the imbalance between the excitatory and inhibitory neurotransmitters glutamate and GABA and alterations in cellular function.[23]

Disturbances in hormonal regulation has been shown in TBI,[29] and may be another potential contributor to PTH. Alterations in dopaminergic systems have been implicated with changes in working memory after mild headache injury; in addition, dopaminergic systems have also been linked to the premonitory phase of migraine and could therefore be linked to PTH. Trauma-induced hypothalamic dysfunction may also mediate headache through disturbances in sleep and/or circadian rhythms, endogenous rhythms with a periodicity of approximately 24 hours.

There have been a number of recent translations studies over the past few years designed to elucidate the mechanisms of PTH. Mild head injuries may produce pain generating from the calvarial periosteum, which has nociceptive sensory innervation and may produce headache of an extracranial origin.[30] Moreover, chronic sensitization may arise from both pericranial and intracranial tissue injury and lead to PPTH.[26] In a mouse model, persistent degranulation of dural mast cells has been demonstrated for at least 30 days after a concussive head injury, which was not responsive to sumatriptan, an anti-migraine drug, or cromolyn, a mast cell stabilizer.[31] Mast cell degranulation is thought to be an inflammatory response to head injury and can be induced by neuropeptides associated with neurogenic inflammation, including substance P and calcitonin gene-related peptide (CGRP).[32] Both substance P and CGRP are elevated in migraine, but only CGRP blocking agents show the potential for therapeutic translation in migraine and PTH.

Neuropeptide release and neuroinflammation appears to be important contributors to PTH. CGRP is a 37-amino acid peptide formed from the calcitonin family of peptides. It is widely distributed in the peripheral and central nervous system, and is well represented in the trigeminovascular system. CGRP also acts as a potent vasodilator, is involved in sensory nociception, and is a key player in the pathophysiology of migraine.[33] In one animal model, frequent mild head injuries was shown to promote reduced trigeminal allodynia thresholds, along with the greatest increases in CGRP levels.[34] Moreover, repetitive, mild, closed head injuries also resulted in astrogliosis in the central trigeminal system, increased astrocyte markers in the sensory cortex, and an increased number of microglia in the trigeminal nucleus caudalis.[34,35] Another study showed the development of CGRP-dependent pain and headache in a rat model of concussion.[34] Cephalic pain hypersensitivity was inhibited by sumatriptan, which lowers CGRP,[36] and an anti-CGRP antibody.

There are a number of other mechanisms that may theoretically explain headache as a defining feature of mTBI. Superficial branches of the trigeminal nerves and the occipital nerves are vulnerable to traumatic injuries, leading to neuralgic pain. Alternations in cerebral hemodynamics including autoregulation and cerebral vascular injury are associated with TBI and may result in alternations in the trigeminovascular system. The autonomic nervous system may become dysfunctional during after a mTBI, with may contribute to PTH similar to migraine. Altered hypothalamic functional connectivity with autonomic circuits and the locus coeruleus has been shown in migraine but has not been investigated in PTH.[37] In addition, parasympathetic outflow to the cranial cavity can enhance plasma protein extravasation and the release of proinflammatory mediators that activate perivascular nociceptors.[38] Activation of perivascular nociceptors may, therefore, lead to peripheral and central sensitization along the trigeminovascular pathway. Taken together, multiple structural and functional disturbances along the peripheral and central nervous system pain pathways could potentially account for PTH. Cervical injuries may also contribute to PTH, through the involvement of the trigeminocervicocomplex.

PTH often resembles migraine and is characterized similarly as moderate to severe throbbing pain. Individuals may have sensitivity to light, sound, smell, movements, and gastrointestinal symptoms. It is not clear if migraine-like headache after a TBI is the result of a de-novo mechanisms or lowers an individual's threshold to produce a migraine attack. Migraine is a heterogeneous disorder with genetic, epigenetic, and environmental factors. Migraine can be considered a sensory perceptual disorder given the prominence of multisensory disturbances. The broad sensory dysfunction suggests a problem with central modulation of afferent signals that may be disrupted during mTBI.[39] The exact pathological mechanisms are unknown although the pathophysiology is associated with neural mechanisms that mediate trigeminovascular activation or the perception of activation centrally.[39,40] The trigeminovascular system includes a pseudounipolar trigeminal ganglion that has sensory peripheral projections to the pain-producing dura mater, cranial blood vessels, and other structures as well as a central projection to the trigeminal nucleus caudalis and its cervical components, the trigeminocervical complex.[39] Trauma-induced activation of the trigeminovascular system, and/or the diencephalon and brainstem could conceivably contribute to PTH of the migraine type.[41] Patients with mTBI may have subtle injury in the thalamus, a region of the brain that receives convergent trigeminovascular projections and neurochemical pathways, important substrates for the modulation of sleep, stress, and anxiety.[42–44] Changes in cortical plasticity have also been described after TBI,[45] but studies are needed to better understand the potential relationship between cortical plasticity and PTH. Trauma-induced neurochemical derangements are associated with visual, auditory and vestibular processing abnormalities which may contribute to photophobia, phonophobia, and vestibular problems.[46]

Individuals with migraine may have particular intrinsic brain vulnerabilities that could lead to more symptomatology. For example, sensory processing in migraine patients is abnormal between attacks, as evidenced by increased amplitudes and decreased habituation of cortical evoked potentials. Furthermore, recent neurophysiological findings suggest that migraineurs experience high rates of cortical energy expenditure.[47] Less is known about the pathophysiology of tension type headache. However, trauma to soft tissues and the scalp may cause pericranial tenderness, activation of peripheral nociceptors, and the perception of head pain that resembles posttraumatic tension type headache.[48]

Imaging Studies

Routine structural imaging studies of headache associated with mild traumatic head injury including CT head and magnetic resonance imaging (MRI) are often normal. Widely used MRI machines with lower with lower magnetic field strengths cannot detect microscopic shearing and tearing. There are few studies yielding morphometric data specifically for PTH. In one study of cerebral blood flow which compared 35 patients with PPTH, 49 nonheadache controls and 92 patients with migraine, patients with PPTH had reduced cerebral blood flow and regional hemispheric asymmetries.[49] In another advanced imaging study, the investigators used magnetic resonance-based voxel-based morphometry and found that gray matter changes occur in relationship to PPTH.[50] Specifically, decreases in gray matter in the anterior cingulate gyrus and dorsolateral prefrontal cortex was found after 3 months and resolved after 1 year with resolution of headache. The same patients who developed chronic headache showed an increase of gray matter in antinociceptive brainstem centers, thalamus, and cerebellum 1 year after the accident.[50]

MR spectroscopy imaging has also been used to evaluate the metabolic changes that might occur after a mild head injury. In a cohort of patients experience PTH, the study illustrated reduced N-acetylaspartate (NAA), a marker of neuronal integrity, in the bilateral anterior regions of the frontal lobe white matter, anterior and posterior medial region of the frontal lobes and the medial region of parietal lobes. They also showed increased choline, a marker of cellular turnover, in the posterior region of the white matter of the right side frontal lobe, anterior medial region of the frontal lobe, and medial region of the parietal lobes.[51] In another study, proton MR spectroscopy correlated diffuse axonal abnormalities in participants with postconcussive symptoms after mTBI; headache occurred in 13 out of 15 patients along with other postconcussive symptoms including dizziness, sleep disturbances, memory deficits, and blurred vision.[52] Patients that had postconcussive symptoms were found to have lower white matter NAA than controls. Longitudinal studies are needed with specific headache characterization and comparisons with primary headache to determine if MR spectroscopy is useful to detect metabolic brain signatures in PTH.

In a study of adults with PPTH according to the ICHD-3 criteria, patients with PTH had less cortical thickness relative to healthy controls in the left and right superior frontal, caudal middle, frontal, and precentral cortex.[53] Patients also had significantly less cortical thickness in the right supramarginal, right superior and inferior parietal, and right precuneus region. A correlation analysis in regions where there was less cortical thickness demonstrated a negative correlation between headache frequency with the left and right superior frontal thickness. In terms of years lived with PTH, no association was found with regional cortical thickness. More frequent headaches were related to less thickness in the left and right superior frontal regions, potentially indicating that brain morphology changes in the superior frontal regions in patients with PPTH and are modified by headache frequency. Morphometric imaging was also used to compare brain structure in a cohort with PTH, as compared to migraine and controls. The investigators found differences in regional volumes, cortical thickness, surface area, and brain curvature.[54] Differences were also found in these regions in those with PPTH as compared to controls; however, there were no differences in migraine versus controls.

Resting state functional connectivity studies have also been investigated in TBI. Abnormal whole-brain functional network alterations have been shown early after a mTBI in a homogeneous mTBI population. The authors suggested that the cluster of increased functional connectivity in the right fronto-parietal network might underlie postconcussive symptoms including headache, sensitivity to light and sound. In sum, these studies support brain changes that occur in advanced imaging but are not routinely available on an individual case basis.

Imaging Guidelines

Neuroimaging aims after mTBI include detecting injuries that may benefit from early medical therapy, those requiring vigilant neurologic supervision, detecting injuries that may require immediate surgical intervention, or determining the prognosis of patients to establish the need for rehabilitative therapy.[55] Multiple neuroimaging techniques are available to assess patients presenting with TBI.

Generally, neuroimaging is not a standard element in the evaluation of PTH if the neurologic examination is normal; however, it should be considered when there is concern for skull fracture, intracranial hemorrhage, or associated spinal cord injury. Red flags that raise suspicion for intracranial lesions include abnormalities or asymmetries on physical examination, altered mental status, headache that is progressively worsening after an acute injury, acute onset of headache long after trauma, or other underlying risk factors such as hypercoagulable state. In the absence of red flags or if symptoms are improving, imaging generally not recommended.

Computerized tomography and MRI are the mainstay of neuroimaging options in the evaluation of PTH. In the future, studies such as functional MRI, magnetic resonance spectroscopy, and diffusion tensor imaging that reveal acute or chronic changes may aid in the management of PTH; however, standard neuroimaging paradigms do not currently utilize these advanced neuroimaging techniques after concussive injury.

Clinical Course and Comorbidities

Clinical considerations for PTH include its characterization, the relationship with other postconcussive symptoms and related comorbid conditions for optimal treatment and management. In terms of a clinical approach, it is important to try and localize the lesion with the understanding that mTBI may be multifocal. Cervical facet disease, tempomandibular joint dysfunction, and whiplash injury may occur concurrently. The history, examination, and further diagnostic tests are vital to ruling out potentially serious problems such as a subdural and epidural hematomas, arterial dissections, or insidious cerebrospinal fluid leaks. Medication overuse headache may occur with PPTH; and frequent use of acute analgesics may be motived by somatic pain and worsen headache outcomes.

The presence of migraine symptoms after a mild headache injury is associated with more cognitive impairment. In sport-related concussion (SRT), Kontos et al. found that posttraumatic migraine sufferers at 8–14 days were more likely to perform worse on verbal memory than those with headache without migraine symptoms.[56] The posttraumatic migraine group also did worse on visual memory, reaction time, and symptom severity than the no-headache group and also the headache group at 1−7 days and 8−14 days after injury. In posttraumatic migraine, a protracted recovery (>20 days) was more likely experienced as compared to both the no-headache and the headache groups. Mihalik et al. also found that individuals with posttraumatic migraines had delayed recovery and were more likely to be symptomatic.[13] Veterans with neurocognitive deficits following TBI were also more likely to have headaches with migraine features.[57] Overall, the posttraumatic migraine subtype appears to be an important phenotype with worse outcomes.

PTH is comorbid with psychiatric disorders, somatic pain and sleep disorders. Patients with PPTH were more likely to report anxiety and depression in comparison to the group without PTH.[58] PTH is also commonly associated with PTSD, and disability from PTH is compounded by PTSD.[59] The frequency of cognitive impairment, PTSD, sleep disorders, and headache are particularly common. However, more severe TBI is associated with a diminished risk of PTSD and headache.[24] More cognitive and somatic symptoms and work loss has been shown in a clinic-based study of 90 PPTH patients versus 45 chronic primary headache patients.[60] In addition, 31% in the chronic PTH group had scores meeting the Harvard Trauma Questionnaire criteria for PTSD. PTSD was also prevalent among US soldiers with chronic PTH. In this cohort, PTSD was not associated with more frequent headache and did not appear to affect short-term outcome.[61] In another study, TBI patients with insomnia were at a greater risk for headache and/or dizziness.[62] They also reported more symptoms of depression and anxiety.[61] Chronic traumatic encephalopathy, known as CTE, is condition due to repetitive head injuries and neuropsychiatric complications, including dementia and suicide. Headache has not been reported as a defining feature of the condition; however, specific studies are needed. Given the nature of postconcussive syndrome, a multidisciplinary approach for PTH is often advisable.

MEDICAL TREATMENT

Despite being the most common symptom after concussion, there are few high-quality studies investigating the diagnosis and treatment of PTH. The Consensus Statement on Concussion in Sport implored clinicians to pursue well designed studies to aid in providing further evidence-based studies from which treatment directive may be obtained.[63] As part of the Consensus Statement on Concussion in Sport, a systematic literature review of rest and treatment/rehabilitation following concussion was performed and identified only two studies that address medical treatment of PTH. The recommendation to rest and reduced activity might in part be driven by associated symptoms of PTH (light, sound, nausea, movement sensitivity, etc.) but has been challenged.[64] Although certain pharmacotherapeutics may be effective in treating PTH, recovery from SRT is not hastened.[65] Despite this current paucity of evidence, it is imperative that medical providers maintain a realistic approach of being "evidence- or consensus-guided," rather than "evidence hindered." Specifically, a lack of evidence is not a viable reason to approach challenging clinical scenarios through a nihilistic lens of treatment. Conversely, there are quite clear directives from the primary headache literature that have clearly highlighted the need for early, assertive, and consistent treatment approaches in those unique patient subsets presenting with underlying risk factors portending a potentially prolonged and refractory recovery course.[66,67]

A more recent study from the North Texas Concussion Registry examined changes in headache severity over a 3-month period in concussion patients with PTH.[68] The study compared treatment with triptans versus over-the-counter (NSAID/analgesic) or opioid medications. Patients treated with triptans were more likely to report severe headache 3 months after initial evaluation compared to those treated with NSAIDs or opioids. Specifically, individuals treated with triptans, compared to those treated with opioids or NSAIDs/analgesics, were 2.1 times as likely to report PPTH symptoms after 3 months of treatment. The explanation of the relative lack of triptan efficacy in this cohort is unclear; however, it is possible that underlying inflammatory processes contribute to PTH propagation and, thus, respond better to directed NSAID treatment. As this was a registry study, the results may also be explained by selection bias given patients with more severe migraine-like pain received prescriptions for triptans. Similar to acute migraine management, bultalbital-containing medications and opiates should not be the first line treatment for PTH.

While current migraine treatment guidelines include $5\text{-HT}_{1B/1D}$ agonists (i.e., triptans), in some patients, these agents do not provide sufficient pain relief.[69] The first emergency department prospective study of acute PTH investigated the use of metoclopramide 20 mg and diphenhydramine 25 mg in 21 patients enrolled. Sustained pain relief was the primary outcome measure and was achieved in 60% of patients with available data upon follow up by telephone Days 2 and 7.[70] Postconcussive symptoms measured by the Post-Concussion Symptom Scale (PCSS) at the time of discharge and 1 week after treatment.

Preventive treatment approaches consist of both pharmacological and nonpharmacological interventions with combination or monotherapy. Few studies have specifically investigated the benefits of pharmaceutical approaches. The current empiric approach to treating PTH is to treat based on the clinical phenotype. In a retrospective study of 100 patients using divalproex sodium for PPTH, the treatment appeared effective.[71] In small clinic based studies, there is a suggestion that propranolol and amitriptyline alone or in combination may be effective for chronic forms.[72] Bramley et al. reported improvement of acute PTH in a cohort of adolescent patients (age 13–18) treated with amitriptyline (median dose 25 mg, range 10–100 mg).[73] The medication was generally well tolerated, although 23% of patients reported mild side-effects such as over-sedation.

The blockade of CGRP has recently emerged as a viable therapeutic option in the treatment of episodic and chronic migraine.[74–76] There are currently two different classes of CGRP blockers in development: small molecule CGRP receptor antagonists and monoclonal antibodies. Three CGRP receptor antibodies have recently completed Phase III studies, (fremanazumab, galcanazumab, erenumab) with all three currently approved by the Food and Drug Administration (FDA).[77,78] The Vector study is a large, randomized, multicentered, placebo control trial investigating the use of fremanazumab, a CGRP monoclonal antibody, for prevention of PPTH (NCT03347188).[79] The treatment of migraine with anti-CGRP antibodies may also provide a viable approach in the setting of PTH.[34] There remains little evidence to support specific medical managements in SRC, including the treatment of associated PTH. Lastly, the role of endocannabinoid modulation and the potential for use of phytocannabinoids to treat posttraumatic headache is an area of needed research. It has been proposed that the endocannabinoid system may act as a modulator of the trigeminal pain response to concussion, regulate inflammation, and restore balance of the central nervous system.[80]

INTERVENTIONAL/PROCEDURAL TREATMENT

Peripheral nerve blocks are among the most common interventional procedures to treat PTH[81] Therapeutic sites include the greater occipital nerve (GON), lesser occipital nerve (LON), sphenopalatine ganglion (SPG), auriculotemporal nerve (ATN), supraorbital nerve (SON), and supratrochlear nerve (STN). By introducing local anesthesia to these nerves and/or ganglion, a reduction of afferent feedback is delivered to the trigeminal nucleus caudalis. Dubrovsky et al. used targeted peripheral nerve blocks of the scalp in a small cohort of adolescent patients.[82] The subjects each met the diagnostic criteria of acute or persistent headache attributed to mTBI according to the ICHD-3, beta version classification criteria.[83] Injection sites were determined by palpation of the points of maximal tenderness and generally targeted the GON and in some cases the LON or the SON. In the study, 93% of the cohort reported a "good" therapeutic effect (which was defined as benefit sustained >24 hours and/or the patient requested repeat nerve blocks).

Botulinum toxins are effective in trigeminal pain modulation via direct delivery into afferent terminals, as well as superficial extracranial dermatomes. In 2002, Loder and Biondi first reported improvement in PPTH following botulinum toxin injections.[84] More recently, Yerry et al. reported improved daily function in a retrospective cohort study of 64 active duty service members with chronic PTH of migrainous phenotype after OnabotulinumtoxinA treatment.[85] Randomized control trials are needed.

PROGNOSIS

Headache is typically the first symptom reported and is often the last to resolve after concussion. The majority of patients with PTH have complete resolution of symptoms within 3 months from the time of injury, although a small percentage of patients develop PPTH.[86] There is an inverse relationship between the development of PTH and the severity of injury. Faux and Sheedy found that 15% of those with minor head injury reported PPTH at 3 months, compared with 2% of controls [21].[87]

SPECIAL POPULATIONS

Sports Concussion Versus Migraine

Theoretically, migraine history could be an effect modifier for concussion. A personal history of migraine could represent inherent vulnerabilities that: (1) predispose an individual to sustaining the injury of concussion; (2) magnify both clinical (e.g., headache, nausea, and light sensitivity) and subclinical (e.g., intracellular and cerebrovascular) effects of concussion; and/or (3) increase the likelihood of a refractory recovery course post-injury.

Little is known about the spectrum of headache disorders in collegiate student-athletes, including primary headaches such as migraine; however in a 2017 study, Seifert et al. reported a prevalence of migraine of 23.7% ($n = 198$).[88] When compared to the general population this statistic seems elevated, although a previous study in university students observed similar migraine prevalence.[89] A similar retrospective study in professional American football players revealed the 1-year prevalence of migraine among retired players to be 92% (56% with episodic and 36% with chronic migraine), which is much more than the 6% with episodic and 0.5% with chronic migraine in the general adult male population.[90] Given that these studies were cross-sectional retrospective cohort survey designs, therefore, we cannot draw conclusions about causation, such as whether the association between migraine and concussion is unidirectional, bidirectional, effect modifying, or incidental. Future prospective studies that do not rely solely on self-reported diagnosis will help clarify uncertainties.

Individuals with preexisting headache conditions might be at increased risk for post-injury headaches. This was confirmed by one large-scale multisite study found that a personal history of migraine was associated with increased risk for having persistent symptoms, for more than 4 weeks, in children and adolescents following mild brain injury.[91] In 2017, Eckner and Seifert discovered a significant positive association between concussion and history of migraine in athletes.[92] As this study was also retrospective in nature, a cause—effect nature of this relationship could not be determined and it was unclear whether a predisposition to headaches existed before the documented concussion(s).

A 2018 study found that athletes with a pre-injury history of migraine may be at increased risk for a prolonged return to academics after concussion, particularly among females.[93] Additional prospective research is necessary to further establish the potential effects of a migraine diagnosis on concussion course. Until such data are available, migraine should be considered a modifying factor by clinicians caring for concussed athletes.

Children

Head injuries are common in pediatrics, and headaches are the most common complaint following mild head trauma. Although moderate and severe traumatic brain injuries occur less frequently, headaches can complicate recovery in such settings.[94] An emerging body of research suggests that repetitive, subconcussive head impacts play a larger role than concussive injury itself in risk of neurocognitive dysfunction later in life.[95] This increased awareness of repetitive head injuries and associated PTH has renewed interest in the study of those headaches occurring after concussion, particular those refractory cases influencing a return to sports, academics, and work. With that being said, there remains very little evidence in the treatment of pediatric PTH. A small number of case reports and cohort studies have previously been published; however, the level of evidence in such contexts is also lacking. There are no available data from randomized controlled trials evaluating specific medical interventions or their therapeutic efficacy in the treatment of PTH. While emerging therapies in migraine continue to show promise and will undoubtedly continue to translate to PTH clinical practice, objective data regarding within the space of PTH remain desperately needed.

Domestic Violence

It is estimated that as many as 23,000,000 women in the United States who have experienced domestic violence (DV) live with brain injury.[96] Experiencing DV also increases the risk for developing PTSD.[97] Specifically, women who experience DV are almost three times as likely to meet criteria for PTSD when compared to those who have not had such experiences.[98] PTSD is more common in women than in men, with the reporting of women's symptoms being higher than that of men's symptoms.[59] The symptomatology of TBI reflects that of PTSD, posing significant challenges in obtaining appropriate diagnosis and treatment. Increased severity of PTSD-type symptoms is significantly associated with increased headache disability in patients with PPTH.[99] This is consistent with studies suggesting that emotional health can impact headache disability PTH.[100]

Elderly

The prevalence of primary headache disorders decline after the age of 40, but secondary headache is more likely to be seen in the elderly.[101–103] Up to 15% of elderly patients presenting with headache ominous underlying etiologies, such as subarachnoid hemorrhage, temporal arteritis, trigeminal neuralgia, or intracranial hemorrhage, whereas only 1.6% of those under 65 have similar serious conditions.[102] Further analysis of PTH reporting in the elderly has found that patients older than 60 years report less severe headaches and are significantly less likely to report PTH overall.[99]

Additional analysis has highlighted the impact of age upon PTH. Lucas et al. found that patients older than 60 years were significantly less likely to report PTH.[18] Older age has also correlated significantly with decreased PTH severity.[18,99] Adherence to fall safety prevention and rigorous evaluations of driving capacity in the elderly may potentially lead to less occurrence of headache associated with mild head injuries.

CONCLUSION

Headache is a common outcome in mild traumatic brain injuries. Significant variabilities exist in the clinical trajectory with most outcomes being favorable. The greater societal attention and emerging science has led to greater awareness, management, and treatment. To date, there is no biomarker available to guide prognosis, return to play, treatment decisions, and disability assessments. In addition, translational studies are needed to better elucidate pathological mechanisms that may guide clinical trials.

References

1. Prevention CfDCa. Report to Congress on Traumatic Brain Injury in the United States: Epidemiology and Rehabilitation. National Center for Injury Prevention and Control; Division of Unintentional Injury Prevention; 2015.
2. Centers for Disease Control and Prevention (CDC). NCfIPaC. *Report to Congress on mild traumatic brain injury in the United States: steps to prevent a serious public health problem.* Altanta Centers for Disease Control and Prevention; 2003.
3. Monteith TS, Borsook D. Insights and advances in post-traumatic headache: research considerations. *Curr. Neurol Neurosci. Reports* 2014;**14**(2):428.
4. Headache Classification Committee of the International Headache Society (IHS). The International Classification of Headache Disorders, 3rd edition. *Cephalalgia* 2018;**38**(1):1–211.
5. Okie S. Traumatic brain injury in the war zone. *N Eng J Med* 2005;**352**(20):2043–7.
6. Armed Forces Health Surveillance Center (AFHSC). Incident diagnoses of common symptoms ("sequelae") following traumatic brain injury, active component, U.S. Armed Forces, 2000–2012. *Msmr* 2013;**20**(6):9–13.
7. Theeler BJ, Flynn FG, Erickson JC. Headaches after concussion in US soldiers returning from Iraq or Afghanistan. *Headache.* 2010;**50**(8):1262–72.
8. Nordhaug LH, Hagen K, Vik A, et al. Headache following head injury: a population-based longitudinal cohort study (HUNT). *J Headache Pain* 2018;**19**:8.
9. Lucas S, Hoffman JM, Bell KR, Dikmen S. A prospective study of prevalence and characterization of headache following mild traumatic brain injury. *Cephalalgia* 2014;**34**(2):93–102.
10. Kuczynski A, Crawford S, Bodell L, Dewey D, Barlow KM. Characteristics of post-traumatic headaches in children following mild traumatic brain injury and their response to treatment: a prospective cohort. *Dev Med Child Neurol* 2013;**55**(7):636–41.
11. Walker WC, Marwitz JH, Wilk AR, et al. Prediction of headache severity (density and functional impact) after traumatic brain injury: a longitudinal multicenter study. *Cephalalgia* 2013;**33**(12):998–1008.
12. Lipton RB, Stewart WF. Prevalence and impact of migraine. *Neurol Clin* 1997;**15**(1):1–13.
13. Mihalik JP, Register-Mihalik J, Kerr ZY, Marshall SW, McCrea MC, Guskiewicz KM. Recovery of posttraumatic migraine characteristics in patients after mild traumatic brain injury. *Am J Sports Med* 2013;**41**(7):1490–6.
14. Carvalho GF, Bonato P, Florencio LL, et al. Balance impairments in different subgroups of patients with migraine. *Headache* 2017;**57**(3):363–74.
15. Carvalho GF, Chaves TC, Dach F, et al. Influence of migraine and of migraine aura on balance and mobility—a controlled study. *Headache* 2013;**53**(7):1116–22.
16. Stovner LJ, Schrader H, Couch Jr JR, Lipton RB, Stewart WF, Scher AI. Head or neck injury increases the risk of chronic daily headache: a population-based study. *Neurology* 2008;**71**(5):383–5.
17. Manley GT, Maas AI. Traumatic brain injury: an international knowledge-based approach. *J Am Med Assoc* 2013;**310**(5):473–4.
18. Lucas S, Hoffman JM, Bell KR, Walker W, Dikmen S. Characterization of headache after traumatic brain injury. *Cephalalgia: Int J Headache* 2012;**32**(8):600–6.
19. Gill MR, Reiley DG, Green SM. Interrater reliability of Glasgow Coma Scale scores in the emergency department. *Annals of emergency medicine* 2004;**43**(2):215–23.
20. Hoffman JM, Lucas S, Dikmen S, et al. Natural history of headache after traumatic brain injury. *J Neurotrauma* 2011;**28**:1719–25.
21. Theeler BJ, Flynn FG, Erickson JC. Headaches after concussion in US soldiers returning from Iraq or Afghanistan. *Headache* 2010;**50**:1262–72.
22. Theeler BJ, Erickson JC. Post-traumatic headaches: time for a revised classification? *Cephalalgia* 2012;**32**:589–91.
23. Guerriero RM, Giza CC, Rotenberg A. Glutamate and GABA imbalance following traumatic brain injury. *Curr Neurol Neurosci Rep* 2015;**15**(5):27.
24. Mac Donald C, Johnson A. Prospectively assessed clinical outcomes in concussive blast vs nonblast traumatic brain injury among evacuated US military personnel. *JAMA Neurol* 2014;**71**(8):994–1002.

25. Finkel AG, Ivins BJ, Yerry JA, Klaric JS, Scher A, Sammy Choi Y. Which matters more? A retrospective cohort study of headache characteristics and diagnosis type in soldiers with mTBI/concussion. *Headache* 2017;**57**(5):719−28.

26. Petrone AB, Gionis V, et al. Immune biomarkers for the diagnosis of mild traumatic brain injury. *NeuroRehabilitation.* 2017;**40**(4):501−8. Available from: https://doi.org/10.3233/NRE-171437.

27. Oka H, Kako M, Matsushima M, Ando K. Traumatic spreading depression syndrome. Review of a particular type of head injury in 37 patients. *Brain: J Neurol* 1977;**100**(2):287−98.

28. Defrin R. Chronic post-traumatic headache: clinical finding and possible mechanisms. *J Manual Manipula Therapy* 2014;**22**(1):36−44.

29. Rosario ER, Aqeel R, Brown MA, Sanchez G, Moore C, Patterson D. Hypothalamic-pituitary dysfunction following traumatic brain injury affects functional improvement during acute inpatient rehabilitation. *J Head Trauma Rehabil* 2013;**28**(5):390−6.

30. Zhao J, Levy D. The sensory innervation of the calvarial periosteum is nociceptive and contributes to headache-like behavior. *Pain* 2014;**155**(7):1392−400.

31. Levy D, Edut S, Baraz-Goldstein R, et al. Responses of dural mast cells in concussive and blast models of mild traumatic brain injury in mice: potential implications for post-traumatic headache. *Cephalalgia* 2016;**36**(10):915−23.

32. Manning BM, Gruba SM, Meyer AF, et al. Neuropeptide-induced mast cell degranulation and characterization of signaling modulation in response to IgE conditioning. *ACS Chem. Biol.* 2016;**11**(11):3077−83.

33. Edvinsson L, Mulder H, Goadsby PJ, Uddman R. Calcitonin gene-related peptide and nitric oxide in the trigeminal ganglion: cerebral vasodilatation from trigeminal nerve stimulation involves mainly calcitonin gene-related peptide. *J Autonom Nervous Syst* 1998;**70**(1−2):15−22.

34. Bree D, Levy D. Development of CGRP-dependent pain and headache related behaviours in a rat model of concussion: implications for mechanisms of post-traumatic headache. *Cephalalgia* 2018;**38**(2):246−58.

35. Tyburski AL, Cheng L, Assari S, Darvish K, Elliott MB. Frequent mild head injury promotes trigeminal sensitivity concomitant with microglial proliferation, astrocytosis, and increased neuropeptide levels in the trigeminal pain system. *J Headache Pain.* 2017;**18**(1):16.

36. Buzzi MG, Carter WB, Shimizu T, Heath 3rd H, Moskowitz MA. Dihydroergotamine and sumatriptan attenuate levels of CGRP in plasma in rat superior sagittal sinus during electrical stimulation of the trigeminal ganglion. *Neuropharmacol* 1991;**30**(11):1193−200.

37. Moulton EA, Becerra L, Johnson A, Burstein R, Borsook D. Altered hypothalamic functional connectivity with autonomic circuits and the locus coeruleus in migraine. *PLoS One* 2014;**9**(4):e95508.

38. Yarnitsky D, Goor-Aryeh I, Bajwa ZH, et al. Wolff Award: Possible parasympathetic contributions to peripheral and central sensitization during migraine. *Headache* 2003;**43**(7):704−14.

39. Goadsby PJ. Pathophysiology of migraine. *Neurol Clin* 2009;**27**(2):335−60.

40. Goadsby PJ. Current concepts of the pathophysiology of migraine. *Neurol Clin* 1997;**15**(1):27−42.

41. Akerman S, Holland PR, Goadsby PJ. Diencephalic and brainstem mechanisms in migraine. *Nat Rev Neurosci* 2011;**12**(10):570−84.

42. Noseda R, Kainz V, Borsook D, Burstein R. Neurochemical pathways that converge on thalamic trigeminovascular neurons: potential substrate for modulation of migraine by sleep, food intake, stress and anxiety. *PLoS One* 2014;**9**(8):e103929.

43. Noseda R, Jakubowski M, Kainz V, Borsook D, Burstein R. Cortical projections of functionally identified thalamic trigeminovascular neurons: implications for migraine headache and its associated symptoms. *J Neurosci: Offic J Soc Neurosci* 2011;**31**(40):14204−17.

44. Tang L, Ge Y, Sodickson DK, et al. Thalamic resting-state functional networks: disruption in patients with mild traumatic brain injury. *Radiology* 2011;**260**(3):831−40.

45. De Beaumont L, Tremblay S, Poirier J, Lassonde M, Theoret H. Altered bidirectional plasticity and reduced implicit motor learning in concussed athletes. *Cereb Cortex* 2012;**22**(1):112−21.

46. Harris JL, Yeh HW, Choi IY, et al. Altered neurochemical profile after traumatic brain injury: (1)H-MRS biomarkers of pathological mechanisms. *J Cerebral Blood Flow Metab: Offic J Int Soc Cerebral Blood Flow Metab* 2012;**32**(12):2122−34.

47. Mayer CL, Huber BR, Peskind E. Traumatic brain injury, neuroinflammation, and post-traumatic headaches. *Headache* 2013;**53**(9):1523−30.

III. NEUROSENSORY DISORDERS IN CLINICAL PRACTICE

48. Drummond PD. Scalp tenderness and sensitivity to pain in migraine and tension headache. *Headache* 1987;**27**(1):45–50.

49. Gilkey SJ, Ramadan NM, Aurora TK, Welch KM. Cerebral blood flow in chronic posttraumatic headache. *Headache* 1997;**37**(9):583–7.

50. Obermann M, Nebel K, Schumann C, et al. Gray matter changes related to chronic posttraumatic headache. *Neurology* 2009;**73**(12):978–83.

51. Sarmento E, Moreira P, Brito C, Souza J, Jevoux C, Bigal M. Proton spectroscopy in patients with post-traumatic headache attributed to mild head injury. *Headache* 2009;**49**(9):1345–52.

52. Kirov II, Tal A, Babb JS, et al. Proton MR spectroscopy correlates diffuse axonal abnormalities with post-concussive symptoms in mild traumatic brain injury. *J Neurotrauma* 2013;**30**(13):1200–4.

53. Chong CD, Berisha V, Chiang CC, Ross K, Schwedt TJ. Less cortical thickness in patients with persistent post-traumatic headache compared with healthy controls: an MRI study. *Headache* 2018;**58**(1):53–61.

54. Schwedt TJ, Chong CD, Peplinski J, Ross K, Berisha V. Persistent post-traumatic headache vs. migraine: an MRI study demonstrating differences in brain structure. *J Headache Pain* 2017 Aug 22;**18**(1):87.

55. Wintermark M, Sanelli PC, Anzai Y, Tsiouris AJ, Whitlow CT. Imaging evidence and recommendations for traumatic brain injury: conventional neuroimaging techniques. *J Am College Radiol* 2015;**12**(2):e1–e14.

56. Kontos AP, Elbin RJ, Lau B, et al. Posttraumatic migraine as a predictor of recovery and cognitive impairment after sport-related concussion. *Am J Sports Med* 2013;**41**(7):1497–504.

57. Ruff RL, Ruff SS, Wang XF. Headaches among Operation Iraqi Freedom/Operation Enduring Freedom veterans with mild traumatic brain injury associated with exposures to explosions. *J Rehabil Res Develop* 2008;**45**(7):941–52.

58. Martins Hugo André de Lima, Martins Bianca Bastos Mazullo, et al. Life quality, depression and anxiety symptoms in chronic post-traumatic headache after mild brain injury. *Dement Neuropsychol* 2012;**6**(1):53–8.

59. Roper LS, Nightingale P, Su Z, Mitchell JL, Belli A, Sinclair AJ. Disability from posttraumatic headache is compounded by coexisting posttraumatic stress disorder. *J Pain Res* 2017;**10**:1991–6.

60. Kjeldgaard D, Forchhammer H, Teasdale T, Jensen RH. Chronic post-traumatic headache after mild head injury: a descriptive study. *Cephalalgia* 2014;**34**(3):191–200.

61. Rosenthal JF, Erickson JC. Post-traumatic stress disorder in U.S. soldiers with post-traumatic headache. *Headache* 2013;**53**(10):1564–72.

62. Hou L, Han X, Sheng P, et al. Risk factors associated with sleep disturbance following traumatic brain injury: clinical findings and questionnaire based study. *PLoS One* 2013;**8**(10):e76087.

63. McCrory P, Meeuwisse W, Dvorak J, et al. Consensus statement on concussion in sport-the 5(th) international conference on concussion in sport held in Berlin. October 2016 *Br J Sports Med* 2017;**51**(11):838–47.

64. Giza CC, Choe MC, Barlow KM. Determining if rest is best after concussion. *JAMA Neurol* 2018;**75**(4):399–400.

65. Schneider KJ, Leddy JJ, Guskiewicz KM, et al. Rest and treatment/rehabilitation following sport-related concussion: a systematic review. *Br J Sports Med* 2017;**51**(12):930–4.

66. Mathew NT. Pathophysiology of chronic migraine and mode of action of preventive medications. *Headache* 2011;**51**(Suppl 2):84–92.

67. Aurora SK, Nagesh V, Welch KMA. Functional imaging of subcortical nociceptive structures in response to treatment of chronic daily headache. *J Headache Pain* 2004;**5**(3):204–8.

68. Tejani ASME, Hynan L, et al. Treatment outcomes iwth triptans compared to NSAIDs/analgesics or opioid meidcations in post-concussive patients from North Texas Registry. *Headache* 2017;**57**(3). PS-84LB.

69. Thorlund K, Mills EJ, Wu P, et al. Comparative efficacy of triptans for the abortive treatment of migraine: a multiple treatment comparison meta-analysis. *Cephalalgia: Int J Headache* 2014;**34**(4):258–67.

70. Friedman BW, Babbush K, Irizarry E, White D, John Gallagher E. An exploratory study of IV metoclopramide + diphenhydramine for acute post-traumatic headache. *Am J Emerg Med* 2018;**36**(2):285–9.

71. Packard RC. Treatment of chronic daily posttraumatic headache with divalproex sodium. *Headache* 2000;**40**(9):736–9.

72. Weiss HD, Stern BJ, Goldberg J. Post-traumatic migraine: chronic migraine precipitated by minor head or neck trauma. *Headache* 1991;**31**(7):451–6.

73. Bramley H, Heverley S, Lewis MM, Kong L, Rivera R, Silvis M. Demographics and treatment of adolescent posttraumatic headache in a regional concussion clinic. *Pediatric Neurol* 2015;**52**(5):493–8.

74. Hershey AD. CGRP—the next frontier for migraine. *N Eng J Med* 2017;**377**(22):2190–1.
75. Tso AR, Goadsby PJ. Anti-CGRP monoclonal antibodies: the next era of migraine prevention? *Curr Treat Options Neurol* 2017;**19**(8):27.
76. Edvinsson L. The trigeminovascular pathway: role of CGRP and CGRP receptors in migraine. *Headache* 2017;**57**(Suppl 2):47–55.
77. Deen M, Correnti E, Kamm K, et al. Blocking CGRP in migraine patients—a review of pros and cons. *J Headache Pain* 2017;**18**(1):96.
78. https://www.clinicaltrials.gov/ct2/results?cond = migraine&term = CGRP&cntry = &state = &city = &dist = . USNLoMAf. Last accessed 17 February 2018.
79. https://clinicaltrials.gov/ct2/show/NCT03347188?term = fremanezumab&rank = 2.
80. Elliot MB, Ward SJ, Abood ME, et al. Understanding the endocannabinoid system as a modulator of the tri-geminal pain response to concussion. *Concussion* 2017;**2**(4). CNC49.
81. Pinchefsky E, Dubrovsky AS, Friedman D, Shevell M. Part II—Management of pediatric post-traumatic head-aches. *Pediatric Neurol* 2015;**52**(3):270–80.
82. Dubrovsky AS, Friedman D, Kocilowicz H. Pediatric post-traumatic headaches and peripheral nerve blocks of the scalp: a case series and patient satisfaction survey. *Headache* 2014;**54**(5):878–87.
83. Headache Classification Committee of the International Headache Society (IHS). The International Classification of Headache Disorders, 3rd edition (beta version). *Cephalalgia: Int J Headache* 2013;**33**(9):629–808.
84. Loder E, Biondi D. Use of botulinum toxins for chronic headaches: a focused review. *Clin J Pain* 2002;**18**(6 Suppl):S169–76.
85. Yerry JA, Kuehn D, Finkel AG. Onabotulinum toxin a for the treatment of headache in service members with a history of mild traumatic brain injury: a cohort study. *Headache* 2015;**55**(3):395–406.
86. Seifert TD, Evans RW. Posttraumatic headache: a review. *Curr Pain Headache Rep* 2010;**14**(4):292–8.
87. Faux S, Sheedy J. A prospective controlled study in the prevalence of posttraumatic headache following mild traumatic brain injury. *Pain Med* 2008;**9**(8):1001–11.
88. Seifert T, Sufrinko A, Cowan R, et al. Comprehensive headache experience in collegiate student-athletes: an initial report from the NCAA headache task force. *Headache* 2017;**57**(6):877–86.
89. Bigal ME, Bigal JM, Betti M, Bordini CA, Speciali JG. Evaluation of the impact of migraine and episodic tension-type headache on the quality of life and performance of a university student population. *Headache* 2001;**41**(7):710–19.
90. RW E. The prevalence of migraine and other neurological conditions among retired National Football League players: a pilot study. *Pract Neurol* 2017;21–5.
91. Zemek R, Barrowman N, Freedman SB, et al. Clinical risk score for persistent postconcussion symptoms among children with acute concussion in the ED. *J Am Med Assoc* 2016;**315**(10):1014–25.
92. Eckner JT, Seifert T, Pescovitz A, Zeiger M, Kutcher JS. Is Migraine Headache Associated With Concussion in Athletes? A Case-Control Study. *Clinical journal of sport medicine: official journal of the Canadian Academy of Sport Medicine* 2017;**27**(3):266–70.
93. Terry DP, Huebschmann N, Maxwell B, et al. Pre-injury migraine history as a risk factor for prolonged return to school and sports following concussion. *J Neurotrauma* 2018.
94. Choe MC, Blume HK. Pediatric posttraumatic headache: a review. *J Child Neurol* 2016;**31**(1):76–85.
95. Abbas K, Shenk TE, Poole VN, et al. Effects of repetitive sub-concussive brain injury on the functional connec-tivity of Default Mode Network in high school football athletes. *Develop Neuropsychol* 2015;**40**(1):51–6.
96. Smith TJHC. Assessment and treatment of brain injury in women impacted by intimate partner violence and post-traumatic stress disorder. *Prof Counselor* 2018;**8**(1):1–10.
97. National Center on Domestic Violence T, & Mental Health. Current evidence: intimate partner violence, trauma-related mental health conditions & chronic illness. <http://www.nationalcenterdvtraumamh.org/wp-content/uploads/2014/10/FactSheet_IPVTraumaMHChronicIllness_2014_Final.pdf> 2014.
98. Fedovskiy K, Higgins S, Paranjape A. Intimate partner violence: how does it impact major depressive disorder and post traumatic stress disorder among immigrant Latinas? *J Immigr Minor Health* 2008;**10**(1):45–51.
99. Ahman S, Saveman BI, Styrke J, Bjornstig U, Stalnacke BM. Long-term follow-up of patients with mild trau-matic brain injury: a mixed-method study. *J Rehabil Med* 2013;**45**(8):758–64.
100. Abu Bakar N, Tanprawate S, Lambru G, Torkamani M, Jahanshahi M, Matharu M. Quality of life in primary headache disorders: a review. *Cephalalgia: Int J Headache* 2016;**36**(1):67–91.

101. Prencipe M, Casini AR, Ferretti C, et al. Prevalence of headache in an elderly population: attack frequency, disability, and use of medication. *J Neurol Neurosurg Psychiatry* 2001;**70**(3):377–81.
102. Lipton RB, Stewart WF, Diamond S, Diamond ML, Reed M. Prevalence and burden of migraine in the United States: data from the American Migraine Study II. *Headache* 2001;**41**(7):646–57.
103. Pascual J, Berciano J. Experience in the diagnosis of headaches that start in elderly people. *J Neurol Neurosurg Psychiatry* 1994;**57**(10):1255–7.

Cognitive-Emotional-Vestibular Triad in Mild Traumatic Brain Injury

Nikhil Banerjee[1], Sarah J. Getz[2] and Bonnie E. Levin[1]

[1]Department of Neurology, University of Miami, Miller School of Medicine, Miami, FL, United States [2]Miller School of Medicine, Department of Neurology, Division of Neuropsychology, University of Miami, FL, United States

INTRODUCTION

Traumatic brain injury (TBI) is the most commonly acquired neurological insult, involving an estimated 2.4 million new cases each year in the United States.[1] Traumatic brain injuries pose a considerable public health burden, with some estimates reaching $60 billion in total lifetime costs.[2] Mild TBI (mTBI), otherwise known as concussion, accounts for upwards of 80% of all TBIs in the civilian population.[3] In this group, the leading causes of mTBI are falls, motor vehicle accidents, and being struck with an object.[4] Comparable rates have been reported in the military,[1] where blast-related injuries are predominant. Nearly 30% of servicemen and women returning from deployment screen positive for possible mTBI.[5] Among athletes, particularly in contact sports, mTBI may be twice as prevalent as in the general population.[1] Furthermore, it is widely believed that a substantial number of individuals do not report their mTBI or seek medical care, especially in sports. Thus, it is likely that the true incidence of mTBI in all the above-mentioned categories is underestimated.[6]

The neuropathology of mTBI involves a series of complex biomechanical processes. When mTBI occurs, there is deformation of neural tissue characterized by compression of cortical regions at the sight of impact with concurrent stretching of the parenchyma opposite to the site of impact. This mechanical strain triggers a cascade of biochemical alterations that typically persist for days to weeks. At the neuronal level, traumatic forces cause transient functional changes including abnormal neurochemical signaling via ion flux and glutamate release, as well as disturbed metabolic functioning by way of mitochondrial dysfunction.[7,8] Secondary inflammatory immune reactions can engender microglial activation and astrogliosis, which can result in eventual glial scarring.[9] In addition, axonal structure and function is particularly vulnerable to the biomechanical effects of mTBI, and as a result, diffuse axonal injury is a common pathological feature of mTBI.[10] At the structural level, there is evidence of reduced integrity of white-matter tracts and structures (e.g., corpus callosum, fornix, and anterior commissure) and displacement of brain regions known to be linked with cognitive and emotional processing as well as physiological regulation[11–13] (e.g., orbitofrontal cortex, medial temporal lobe, hippocampus, caudate, amygdala, and midbrain). It has been proposed that, collectively, the vulnerability of these regions and structures to the shearing forces associated with the injury may underlie some of the cognitive, emotional and physical symptoms associated with mTBI. This cascade of events is what underlies Bigler's[14] proposed model of postconcussion syndrome (PCS), which posits that "the biomechanics of brain injury simultaneously disrupt neurological function in the upper brainstem, pituitary-hypothalamic axis, medial temporal lobe, and basal forebrain concomitant with irritative injury to the vasculature and meninges, which gives rise to the symptoms observed in postconcussive state and the neuropsychological sequela associated with such an injury"[14] (p. 10).

There is a lack of consensus regarding the diagnostic taxonomy associated with mTBI sequelae. However, there is general agreement that mTBI patients experience a wide range of symptoms following their injury, which include physical and sensory complaints (e.g., nausea, dizziness, headache, blurred vision, fatigue, noise or light sensitivity, and sleep disturbance), cognitive changes (e.g., difficulty concentrating, forgetfulness, indecisiveness, and slowed thinking), and behavioral or psychiatric symptomatology (e.g., depression, anxiety, irritability, apathy, and emotional lability). Postconcussion syndrome (PCS) is a broad term used to describe this cluster of symptoms. Although this is not formally considered a clinical classification based on the DSM-5 or ICD-10, it is a widely used for research. The term persistent postconcussion syndrome (PPCS) is used when symptoms fail to resolve.[14] This constellation of symptoms should be solely attributable to the neurological sequelae of a remote head injury, rather than preexisting or comorbid conditions. However, PPCS remains a considerable diagnostic challenge because the symptoms are nonspecific and overlap with numerous psychiatric (e.g., anxiety, depression, and PTSD) and medical conditions.[15] This can lead both patients and clinicians to misattribute nonspecific symptoms to a head injury. In fact, some researchers have found evidence of a high likelihood of false-positive errors in assessing PPCS, as individuals without a history of TBI (e.g., healthy controls or non-TBI trauma controls) endorse comparably high rates of symptoms consistent with PPCS to mTBI patients.[16,17] Thus, it is difficult to accurately estimate the prevalence of PPCS. Some researchers argue that prevalence estimates of PPCS in the general population (i.e., 10%–20%) are inflated, with the true estimate lying closer to 5% or lower.[18]

Factors associated with persistent mTBI symptoms include female gender, older age, being a student, history of past brain injury, chronic pain, chronic medical complaints, life stress, having a preexisting neurological or psychiatric comorbidity (especially depression), and litigation seeking.[19,20] In addition, there is a growing literature indicating that psychological factors are robust predictors of poor mTBI outcome, even more so than traditional injury-related factors such as duration of loss of consciousness (LOC) or posttraumatic amnesia.[21,22] In a systematic review of multivariable models predicting mTBI prognosis,[22] early post-injury elevated anxiety, particularly in women, was among the strongest independent predictors for prolonged postconcussive symptoms. This finding corroborates previous reports.[23] Another recent prospective study found that elevated depressive symptoms during acute recovery predicted greater postconcussion symptoms 1-year later; interestingly, there was no significant relationship with intracranial white-matter abnormalities assessed with magnetic resonance imaging (MRI) or diffusion tensor imaging (DTI).[17] Finally, some researchers have proposed additional factors that may account for persistent reporting of mTBI symptoms. These include negative appraisals and reactions to the injury and its sequelae (e.g., negative injury perceptions and poor expectations for recovery), premorbid personality traits and disorders, iatrogenic effects, adoption of a sick-role, compensation seeking behavior, and the tendency to view oneself as healthier prior to the head injury and underestimate past problems (i.e., the "good old days" bias).[18,24] Altogether, these findings emphasize the importance of assessing psychological well-being when evaluating mTBI prognosis, and highlight a potential avenue for intervention by which early psychosocial treatments (e.g., CBT) may expedite the recovery trajectory.

COGNITIVE, EMOTIONAL, AND VESTIBULAR CHANGES IN TRAUMATIC BRAIN INJURY: A MULTISYSTEM MODEL

Mild TBI can have wide-ranging effects on cognitive, emotional, and neurosensory functioning.[25,26] While there is wide consensus that mTBI symptoms will fully resolve in most individuals, a significant minority will follow a different trajectory, exhibiting a more variable course, which can range from subclinical intermittent symptoms to frank cognitive and behavioral impairments. For this latter group of individuals, these symptoms can be debilitating, distressing, and persistent, and have a significant impact on quality of life.[27] This chapter will review the constellation of acute and postacute cognitive and emotional changes associated with mTBI, as well as effects on vestibular functioning. In particular, it will emphasize the unique relationships between cognition, emotion, and the vestibular system, an observation that was first reported nearly three decades ago,[28] and one that continues to be the subject of significant scientific interest.[29,30] While this area of research is largely unexplored in models of mTBI, emerging literature suggests that a greater understanding of the intersection between cognition and neurosensory function in mTBI will provide a valuable framework from which to study the complex array of cognitive, emotional, and behavioral changes following a mild traumatic head injury.

EFFECTS OF MILD TRAUMATIC BRAIN INJURY ON NEUROPSYCHOLOGICAL FUNCTION

Changes in neuropsychological functioning are among the most common but poorly defined sequelae of mTBI. This is largely because cognitive profiles of mTBI patients are notoriously heterogeneous, with a wide variety of premorbid risk factors, injury-related variables (e.g., injury severity), and psychological reactions that can shape the trajectory of cognitive recovery. In addition, research efforts to define the temporal course of cognitive outcomes in mTBI, particularly over the long-term, have been hampered by methodological issues, which has led to mixed findings.[24] The current review will consider several high quality reviews and meta-analyses[19,24] (see also Karr et al.)[31] that have helped shed light on some of mTBI's acute and postacute effects on neuropsychological functioning.

Acute Effects of Mild Traumatic Brain Injury

Neuropsychological deficits are a common feature of early recovery from mTBI, with the most pronounced cognitive deficits observed in the immediate 7–10 days following the injury.[24] During this period, the brain must recruit reserve networks and consume additional cognitive resources to function at a premorbid level, and is particularly vulnerable to cognitive load effects, over exertion, and reinjury.[6] For the majority, an estimated 80% or more of mTBI sufferers in the general population, cognitive function rebounds rapidly over the next 30 days,[32] followed by a period of more gradual recovery with eventual return to premorbid levels by 90 days post-injury.[19,24,33] Thus, 90 days post-injury has historically been cited as the demarcation between acute and postacute injury.[34] Although it has been suggested that cognitive recovery may be faster in sports-related mTBI, based on evidence showing negligible neuropsychological deficits as early as 1 week post-injury,[35] this observation may be confounded by the use of screening tools to assess return to play rather than more extensive cognitive batteries used in other TBI assessment settings.

There is an abundant literature examining domain-specific neuropsychological impairments during acute recovery. Yet, interstudy comparisons are difficult due to varying quality of research methodology, disparate assessment approaches, and diverse study samples. To address this issue, the International Collaboration on mTBI Prognosis (ICoMP) conducted a best evidence synthesis from 12 methodologically rigorous, exploratory longitudinal studies evaluating cognitive changes following nonsports mTBI in civilians.[24] They found that neuropsychological deficits are consistently observed within 2–14 days post-injury, with the most common and pronounced deficits involving attention, learning and memory, and information processing domains. Beyond the first 2 weeks of acute recovery, however, domain-specific findings were remarkably heterogeneous and difficult to interpret, largely due to methodological limitations. Specifically, important factors such as injury severity (e.g., LOC duration, posttraumatic amnesia duration), mechanism of injury, time since injury, cognitive-test selection, and clinical criteria used to evaluate outcome, were inadequately controlled.

Several meta-analyses have sought to examine the acute effects of mTBI on neuropsychological performance. Notably, in 2005, Belanger and colleagues analyzed data from 26 studies comparing controls with prospectively recruited nonsports mTBI patients who were either nonsymptomatic or not selected based on symptomology. Out of the nine cognitive domains examined, they found the largest effect sizes of mTBI to be on fluency (verbal, semantic, and visual; $d = 89$) and delayed memory recall (verbal and visual; $d = 1.03$). These neuropsychological deficits were no longer evident after 3 months. Other meta-analytic studies have also reported acute cognitive deficits in the verbal and visual memory domains.[33] Interestingly, the acute effects of mTBI on executive functions (based on the authors' classification of tests in this domain) appear to be marginal at best.[19,33] Overall, caution is warranted in drawing conclusions from meta-analyses in this literature due to their inclusion of studies with the same methodological shortcomings noted earlier.

Postacute (Chronic) Effects of Mild Traumatic Brain Injury

While there is general agreement that the acute effects of mTBI on neuropsychological functioning will resolve within 90 days for the majority of patients,[19,24] there is little consensus regarding a small proportion of individuals who will experience persistent cognitive deficits. According to the ICoMP best evidence synthesis, there is currently insufficient evidence from well-controlled longitudinal studies to indicate postacute effects of mTBI on cognition.[24] However, there is some preliminary evidence suggesting that these effects may exist. For example, the ICoMP report did recognize a phase II cohort study[36] showing that verbal learning deficits persisted at 6 months post-mTBI before resolving by 12 months. Likewise, a more recent population-based study in New Zealand found evidence of persistently depressed scores on a computer-based measure of complex attention in over 20% of participants at 6-month post-injury, which continued in over 16% at 12-month post-injury.[37]

There is, in fact, remarkable disagreement among researchers as to whether measurable long-term cognitive difficulties exist. Numerous meta-analyses report that neuropsychological deficits are no longer evident at 90 days post-mTBI[19,32,33,38]; others indicate evidence of persistent deficits in a select minority of patients.[14,39] For example, Pertab, James, and Bigler (2009)[39] reanalyzed a set of studies from two prior meta-analyses[34,38] that initially reported negligible postacute effects of mTBI, but in their reanalysis, found that deficits on select neuropsychological measures (i.e., verbal paired associates, coding tasks, and digit span tasks) persisted into the postacute recovery period. In turn, Rohling and colleagues (2011) responded with their own reanalysis of the same set of studies, and found nonsignificant domain-specific effects with the exception of subtle isolated deficit in working memory ($d = 19$). These authors argue that a long-term cognitively symptomatic subgroup is statistically improbable, and that meta-analytic evidence of postacute neuropsychological impairment is more likely a function of statistical error than a true effect.

Overall, research examining whether select patients continue to display true long-term objective neuropsychological deficits is inconsistent and remains the subject ongoing scientific debate. Carefully controlled longitudinal studies are needed to confirm previous reports of acute effects of mTBI on cognition, to clarify common patterns of domain-specific neuropsychological impairment, and to determine the existence of long-term effects of mTBI on neuropsychological outcomes.[24]

EFFECTS OF MILD TRAUMATIC BRAIN INJURY ON PSYCHIATRIC WELL-BEING

Difficulty regulating emotions is a prominent clinical feature following mTBI. In the early weeks to months after a mild head injury, patients often report elevated symptoms of depression, anxiety, irritability, angry outbursts, apathy, and emotional lability.[21,24] In addition, there is some research showing that mTBI may increase the risk of experiencing a clinical psychiatric disturbance. Fann et al. (2004)[40] looked at psychiatric illness in the year following mTBI and found higher prevalence rates than in a matched noninjured comparison group. The risk of a psychiatric diagnosis in the 6 months following mTBI was nearly threefold (relative risk = 2.8) among those without any prior diagnosis. This risk was sustained up to 18 months post-injury. Among those with a prior psychiatric diagnosis history in the year before the injury, the risk of post-injury psychiatric diagnosis was elevated (relative risk = 1.6). Another study found a small association in post-mTBI onset of schizophrenia in men, but not women.[41] In long-term post-mTBI, Konrad et al. (2011)[42] have shown that 6 years following a mild traumatic event, individuals who met criteria for mTBI showed significantly higher Beck Depression Inventory (BDI) scores as compared to controls indicating persisting emotional sequelae that may take longer to resolve than cognitive changes. One meta-analysis by Panayiotou, Jackson, and Crowe (2010)[43] reported that the effects of mTBI on self-reported emotional symptoms (i.e., depression, anxiety, coping, and psychosocial disability) were significant but small and arguably negligible. Collectively, these findings suggest that the risk for emotional changes and psychiatric diagnosis is raised following mTBI in select circumstances and may signal the need for careful and long-term monitoring of mental health changes in this population.

EFFECTS OF MILD TRAUMATIC BRAIN INJURY ON VESTIBULAR FUNCTION

The traumatic force associated with mTBI is sufficient to impact the vestibular system. It is well documented that mTBI can lead to otolith damage (e.g., utricular and saccular macula lesions), alterations to receptor functioning within the semicircular canals, semicircular canal dehiscence, vestibular nerve damage, or even damage to the brainstem or the visual and oculomotor pathways.[44] Accordingly, symptoms of vestibular dysfunction, including difficulties with balance and dizziness, are among the most commonly reported mTBI symptoms distinguishing mTBI patients from controls.[45] These changes typically emerge within 4–30 days post-injury.[46] In military populations, where blast exposure is particularly common, as many as 98% of service-members with mTBI experience dizziness in the early stage of recovery, and these difficulties persist in up to 84%.[46] In the civilian population, where blunt head trauma is more common, post-mTBI dizziness is among the most frequently observed symptoms[47] and is characterized by positional vertigo, dizziness upon exertion, migraine-associated dizziness, and spatial disorientation.[25] In fact, 21% of cases of benign paroxysmal positional vertigo are secondary to head trauma.[48] These highly prevalent vestibular disturbances can also be detected and quantified using objective techniques. Akin and Murnane (2011)[49] reported mTBI patients exhibit abnormal results on the rotational chair, caloric testing, optokinetic testing, and vestibular reflex testing under different degrees of challenge and exertion relative to control participants.

In light of growing evidence showing vestibular disturbance to be a reliable feature of mTBI, some researchers have begun to apply objective measurement of oculomotor and vestibular function to improve the diagnosis of mTBI. Balaban (2016)[50] utilized a novel goggle technology to assess objectively oculomotor (e.g., saccadic), vestibular, and reaction time differences between patients and controls. They found that the test battery yielded an 89% sensitivity and 95% specificity for confirming the presence of a mTBI. These research advancements support the view that the assessment of vestibular function may serve as a unique and powerful tool for diagnosing mTBI.

INTERRELATIONSHIPS BETWEEN VESTIBULAR, COGNITIVE, AND EMOTIONAL FUNCTION

Cognition

There is a growing literature describing relationships between vestibular and cognitive functioning.[29] In particular, vestibular dysfunction has been repeatedly linked to impaired visuospatial abilities (e.g., spatial memory, navigation, mental rotation, depth perception, and visuospatial construction). National data from the Baltimore Longitudinal Study of Aging examining elderly patients in the general population showed objective vestibular dysfunction is associated with impaired scores on an array of measures assessing visuo-spatial/visuomotor abilities and memory (e.g., Benton Visual Retention Test, Card Rotation Test, Purdue Pegboard, and Trail Making Test).[51] Evidence from experimental paradigms have shown that supra-threshold galvanic vestibular stimulation impairs short-term spatial memory and ego-centric mental rotation in healthy individuals.[52,53] Other experimental investigations have shown that caloric and galvanic vestibular stimulation can have the opposite effect and improve memory.[54,55]

Some of the most compelling evidence for the vestibular—cognitive link comes from studies showing impaired visuospatial and navigational cognitive abilities in patients with vestibulopathy. Brandt et al. (2005)[56] reported patients with a 5—10 year history of bilateral vestibular loss showed impaired performance on the virtual Morrison Water Maze, a test of navigation and spatial learning and memory skills, but not on measures of nonspatial memory. Furthermore, Brandt and colleagues found 16.9% smaller hippocampal volumes in the patient group relative to controls, which correlated with severity of spatial memory impairment. The mechanism by which vestibular failure might engender deleterious changes to the hippocampus remains poorly understood, although it appears that these changes develop with chronic vestibular dysfunction rather than acute.[57] Some researchers posit that vestibular input is fundamental for visuospatial processing and memory, and that long-term vestibular loss, especially when bilateral, can have a lasting impact on ana-tomical components of networks supporting both cognitive and vestibular processing (Smith, 2017). This notion is supported by zu Eulenburg, Stoeter, and Dieterich (2010),[58] who reported gray-matter atrophy not only in the posterior hippocampus of patients with vestibular loss, but also in higher-order processing regions such as the superior-temporal gyrus. They also found evidence of reorganized vestibular-cortical white-matter connec-tions, indicating that vestibular failure may have a downstream impact on the neurocogni-tive circuits involved in cognition.

There is also growing evidence linking the vestibular system with attention and infor-mation processing abilities. Studies in healthy individuals have shown that auditory atten-tion decreases when concurrent postural and balance demands are increased.[59] In these paradigms, performance on vestibular tasks was undisturbed, suggesting that limited cog-nitive resources may be recruited away from cognitive systems and preferentially diverted toward the vestibular system. Consistent with this notion is research showing that per-forming concomitant vestibular and cognitive processing tasks results in reduced cognitive efficiency that varies as a function of increasing attentional load demands.[60] In one study,[61] both controls and patients with unilateral vestibular dysfunction exhibited slower information processing during concurrent vestibular stimulation than without. This effect was pronounced in the patient group, suggesting that vestibular dysfunction may exacerbate the deleterious effects of vestibular challenge on cognitive efficiency by way of insufficient compensation.

Preliminary links between vestibular dysfunction and other areas of cognition have been proposed including executive functioning, memory, object recognition, and numerical cognition.[29] However, relative to research in visuo-spatial ability and attention/information processing, these areas of research remain largely unexplored.

EMOTION

There is a growing body of evidence showing that symptoms of vestibular dysfunction (e.g., balance difficulty, dizziness, and vertigo) frequently cooccur with symptoms of anxiety and depression.[62] One large cohort study found that nearly 60% of patients with chronic dizziness, of which TBI was a leading cause, had a comorbid anxiety disorder.[63] Other investigations have shown that patients with vestibular disorders (e.g., vestibular neuritis) endorse disproportionately high rates of depression and anxiety symptoms compared to healthy individuals, even among patients void of active dizziness symptoms.[64] This suggests that emotional reactions to symptom burden are unlikely to fully account for these high rates of comorbidity. Furthermore, decreases in vertigo symptoms are associated with decreases in anxiety symptoms,[65] and balance abnormalities and dizziness are common features among patients diagnosed with anxiety disorders such as panic disorder.[66,67] Although these findings do not suggest that vestibular disturbance alone is sufficient to cause anxiety, they provide preliminary evidence that vestibular alterations (e.g., dysregulation or stimulation) can impact the subjective sense of psychological well-being.[68]

NEUROANATOMICAL LINKS BETWEEN COGNITION, EMOTION AND VESTIBULAR FUNCTION

There are multiple potential neuroanatomical pathways within a broad vestibular-cortical network through which the vestibular system may be linked to cognition (reviewed by Hitier et al., 2014[69]). Broadly, afferents from the vestibular nuclei either directly or indirectly project to areas of the limbic system, neocortex, and other brain regions thought to be integral for spatial cognition as well as other cognitive abilities. Among the most commonly studied are the multiple pathways from vestibular apparatus to the hippocampus, an area known to play a critical role in navigation and spatial learning and memory.[57] One of these pathways is the *vestibulo-thalamo-cortical pathway*, comprised of vestibular afferents that synapse in the thalamus and terminate in the hippocampus via parietal and parahippocampal cortical intermediates.[70] It is believed that this pathway may be involved in processing spatial information in the environment as well as self versus nonself motion discrimination.[56] Like this pathway, the majority of pathways to the hippocampus are wired through the thalamus and ultimately the medial entorhinal cortex, which in concert with the hippocampus, plays a critical role in spatial cognition[70]. In addition to the hippocampus, other "cognitive" regions of the broad vestibulo-cortical network implicated in the group of skills involved in complex visual spatial learning and memory include the anterior cingulate, ventral tegmental nucleus, retrosplenial cortex, insula, superior temporal gyrus, inferior parietal lobule, basal ganglia, and cerebellum.[29,57] From a clinical perspective, it is interesting to note that the parieto-insular vestibular cortex, a region of the temporo-parietal junction that is regarded as the primary vestibular cortex, has been linked to hemispatial neglect.[71] Altogether, these data suggest a broad neural network underlying visuo-spatial and other cognitive abilities that is reliant on vestibular afferents.

Researchers have also identified the underpinnings of a complex link between vestibular and emotional processing systems, characterized by overlapping neuroanatomical and neurochemical features (see Ref.[72] for review). The vestibular nuclei are vastly connected to regions in the brainstem, limbic system, and neocortex, providing avenues by which somatic information about body position and movement can be integrated into autonomic and affective response networks. The vestibular nuclei have descending projections to the nucleus of the solitary tract and medullary reticular formation,[73] reflecting a direct connection to brainstem regions mediating autonomic control. In addition, the vestibular-parabrachial nucleus network (VPBN) provides the primary links between somatic-visceral information processing, autonomic control, the vestibular system, and higher limbic centers mediating anxiety, avoidance conditioning, and fear learning.[72] This is indicated by the organization of the VPBN which features dense reciprocal connections from the vestibular nuclei to the parabrachial nucleus, which in turn reciprocally projects to key regions involved in emotional processing and control, including the central amygdaloid nucleus, hippocampus, hypothalamus, insula, and prefrontal cortex.[74] In addition to being a critical relay center for processing information about body position and rotational velocity,[75] the parabrachial nucleus is frequently implicated in the etiology of panic and other anxiety disorders[76] as well as autonomic and emotional aspects of pain.[77] Neurons in caudal parabrachial nucleus show highly specialized vestibular responses to angular and linear acceleration[72] (Add McCandless CM Balaban CD Parabrachial nucleus neuronal responses to off-vertical axis rotation in macaques. Exp Brain Res. 2010 Apr;202(2):271−90. https://doi.org/10.1007/s00221-009-2130-9). In turn, this information is relayed and integrated into networks supporting autonomic regulation and affective responses to changes in interoceptive homeostasis.[77]

Vestibular and emotional processing systems also overlap at the cortical level. In particular, the vestibular nuclei project to cortical regions mutually supporting higher-level vestibular and affective processing via the vestibulo-thalamo-cortical pathway. The reciprocal nature of vestibular-cortical connections suggest that they may mediate regulatory feedback to the vestibular sensory system.[78] These regions include the anterior cingulate cortex, insula, temporo-parietal cortex, and prefrontal cortex. Interestingly, these cortical regions are implicated in numerous psychiatric conditions featuring vestibular dysfunction.[30]

The vestibular system may also interact with emotional processing by virtue of its connections with the raphe nuclei and locus coeruleus, two centers in the brainstem frequently implicated in anxiety, depression, and other psychiatric disorders.[30] The *raphe nuclear-vestibular network* features primarily serotonergic projections from the vestibular nuclei to the raphe nucleus, which in turn reciprocally connects with the central amygdaloid nucleus, infralimbic regions, and parabrachial nucleus,[79] suggesting a possible role for the vestibular system in the comodulation of autonomic components of emotion, the conscious perception of emotion, and fear conditioning.[80] Not only are vestibular nuclei particularly sensitive to serotonergic stimulation, treatment with SSRIs is associated with improvements in vertigo and anxiety, and conversely, discontinuation of SSRIs is associated with increased vestibular and anxiety symptoms.[72] In addition, the *coeruleo-vestibular network* consist of noradrenergic projections from the locus coeruleus to the vestibular nuclei, as well as collateral projections to cortical regions involved in emotion processing.[72] Accordingly, the locus coeruleus is implicated as a neural substrate of anxiety and panic.[76] The organization of this network suggests that the locus coeruleus mediates comodulation of vestibular responses (e.g., oculo-motor and postural) during changes in anxiety, vigilance, and arousal.[75] In summary, these two pathways suggest monoaminergic modulation of interactions among vestibular, autonomic, interoceptive, and affective processing networks mediating anxiety.

A novel principal component analysis of c-Fos protein (Fos)-like immunoreactivity, elicited in the cat brainstem by nausea-generating galvanic vestibular stimulation (GVS) provides insights into vestibular network links with nociceptive pathways and coping behaviors (Balaban CD, Ogburn SW, Warshafsky SG, Ahmed A, Yates BJ (2014) Identification of Neural Networks That Contribute to Motion Sickness through Principal Components Analysis of Fos Labeling Induced by Galvanic Vestibular Stimulation. PLoS ONE 9(1): e86730. https://doi. org/10.1371/journal.pone.0086730). One network included strong contributions from the inferior, lateral and medial vestibular nuclei, medial parabrachial nucleus and lateral division of the solitary nucleus with activation of locus coeruleus and the dorsal, ventral and ventro-lateral periaqueductal gray. The dorsal, ventral and ventrolateral periqueeductal gray and the medial parabrachial nucleus were also engaged with the superior vestibular nucleus, external cuneate nucleus and subtrigeminal nucleus in another independent component, while cFos labeling of the raphe nuclei (serotonergic and non-serotonergic neurons) was associated with a third statistically uncorrelated network. The importance of overlapping vestibular and emotional processing neural networks in mTBI cannot be understated. This is because elevated anxiety is both a common sequela of mTBI and a marker for increased risk of a prolonged recovery.[22] Likewise, vestibular dysfunction and associated complaints comprise a core feature of mTBI's clinical presentation. The summary above illustrates several examples of pathways supporting complex interactions between the vestibular system and autonomic and affective aspects of emotion, especially anxiety.

CHANGES IN NEUROLOGICAL NETWORK CONNECTIVITY AND FUNCTION IN MILD TRAUMATIC BRAIN INJURY

The neuroanatomical links described above are particularly relevant to understanding the cognitive, emotional, and neurosensory sequelae of mTBI in light of neuroimaging findings showing mTBI-related changes in neural connectivity and function. Specifically, more advanced neuroimaging techniques, such as functional magnetic resonance imaging (fMRI) and DTI, have allowed researchers to study subtle alterations of key neural networks that are undetectable with standard imaging techniques (e.g., CT or MRI).[81]

Several investigations have reported that mTBI-related white-matter abnormalities, detectable only by DTI, are associated with postconcussive symptomology. In one study,

Niogi et al.[82] found a link between microstructural white-matter lesions and impaired reaction time on an attention and reaction time test in mTBI patients with PCS. Bouix et al. (2013)[83] found that after several years post-mTBI (mean = 62.08 months), patients with persistent postconcussive symptoms exhibited significant increases in fractional anisotropy and gray-matter anisotropy compared with matched controls. In another study using both DTI and a visual tracking paradigm, Maruta et al.[84] showed that variability in tracking performance was correlated with reduced integrity of frontal white-matter tracts in mTBI patients. Additionally, tracking performance variability was associated with worse attentional and working memory performance. Given that the vestibular system is integral for oculomotor functioning, this research is consistent with the notion that microstructural changes in mTBI may impact both vestibulo-ocular function and cognitive processes.

Links between compromised functional connectivity and postconcussive symptomology have also been reported. A recent fMRI investigation by Palacios et al.[85] showed altered functional connectivity of resting state networks fundamental to cognitive processes at approximately two weeks post-mTBI. These include reduced connectivity within frontal areas of the default mode network (DMN), the orbitofrontal network, frontoparietal networks, and the dorsal attentional network. Changes in connectivity were positively associated with neuropsychological test performance at six months post-TBI, suggesting that disturbance of resting-state networks early on in mTBI may have enduring downstream consequences on cognitive recovery. Another investigation examined fMRI and DTI data from 75 mTBI patients and found that microstructural white-matter damage was related to abnormal functional connectivity.[86] These investigators also found that, compared with controls, patients exhibited decreased functional connectivity within the DMN as well as hyper-connectivity between the DMN and an executive control network involving the lateral prefrontal cortex, suggesting possible neural compensation for frontal dysfunction. Abnormal functional connectivity distinguished patients from control participants with 84% specificity, and predicted cognitive complaints up to three weeks post-injury. Building upon these findings, Stevens et al. (2012)[87] conducted a similar investigation and found altered functional connectivity not only in the DMN but also within each of the 12 separate resting state networks examined (e.g., visual processing, motor, limbic, and several implicated in higher-order executive control). These alterations were associated with severity of postconcussive symptomology, particularly in networks involving the anterior cingulate, a key neural region common to cognitive, emotional, and vestibular processing. Like Mayer et al. (2012),[86] these investigators also found evidence of neural compensation indicated by hyperconnectivity among select brain regions. A common finding across the studies noted above is that mTBI appears to not only disturb intranetwork functioning, but also the way in which different networks interact.

Changes in functional connectivity following mTBI have also been linked to emotional symptomology. Van der Horn, Liemburg, Aleman, Spikman, and van der Naalt[88]) drew on DTI and fMRI evidence and proposed that emotional postconcussive complaints following mTBI are associated with hyperactivity of the DMN and subsequent increases in activity of the executive and salience networks to overcome DMN interference, leading to mental fatigue. Elevated DMN activation has also been linked to increased rumination, which may impede top-down regulation by executive control circuitry. As noted previously, top-down regulation of circuits mediating affective and autonomic aspects of anxiety may also interact with the vestibular system.

Altogether, this field of research indicates that mTBI-related microsctructural changes may cause diffuse disturbances of neural networks implicated in an array of cognitive, emotional, and neurosensory processes. Detection of these network changes with DTI and fMRI technology shows promise for offering an objective marker for improving the assessment of mTBI.

VESTIBULAR–COGNITIVE–EMOTION RELATIONSHIPS IN MILD TRAUMATIC BRAIN INJURY

There is compelling evidence pointing to an interrelationship between cognitive, emotional, and neurovestibular function in mTBI. This association was first reported by Grimm et al. (1989)[28] who documented the cooccurrence of emotional difficulties and cognitive impairments (i.e., psychomotor speed, visuospatial construction, verbal learning, and visual sequencing) with vestibular dysfunction in patients with perilymph fistula syndrome secondary to mild head trauma. More recently, Hoffer et al. (2016)[26] used a principle component analysis to study neurosensory symptom complexes in acute mTBI, and showed that self-reported symptoms of vestibular dysfunction (i.e., dizziness, blurred vision, and balance difficulty) clustered with symptoms of cognitive dysfunction (i.e., difficulty concentrating, difficulty remembering, and confusion). In addition, there is growing field of research showing that increased attentional/cognitive demands disrupt gait stability in concussed patients but not controls, an effect that is potentially mediated by vestibular dysfunction.[89,90] These findings are consistent with other evidence showing that oculomotor abnormalities are uniquely correlated with poorer verbal memory performance (i.e., California Verbal Learning Test-II) in patients with mTBI but not controls.[91]

In conclusion, there is a growing body of evidence linking vestibular, cognitive and emotional symptoms in mTBI. This triad has been shown to interact in a complex and bidirectional fashion in non-mTBI populations, and these relationships are likely mediated by overlapping neural networks involving the parabrachial nucleus, hippocampus, monoaminergic pathways, and cortical processing centers. Thus, it is reasonable to suggest that the multisystem (i.e., vestibular, cognitive, and emotional) network described in this chapter may provide a framework for better understanding the diverse clinical presentation of mTBI. Further, it is also possible that mTBI-related cognitive and emotional difficulties, especially those persisting post-acutely, are rooted in vestibular dysfunction by way of deafferentation of higher brain centers involved in the integration of vestibular and cognitive-emotional information.[26] Overall, the study of mTBI is moving toward a multidimensional model that emphasizes vestibular dysfunction. Future studies are needed to determine whether technological advances using vestibular biomarkers to detect mTBI might offer novel insights into understanding the cognitive and emotional sequelae and improve rehabilitative efforts.[50]

References

1. Coronado VG, McGuire LC, Sarmiento K, Bell J, Lionbarger MR, Jones CD, et al. Trends in traumatic brain injury in the US and the public health response: 1995–2009. *J Safety Res* 2012;**43**(4):299–307.
2. Finkelstein E, Corso P, Miller T. *The Incidence and Economic Burden of Injuries in the United States*. New York: Oxford University Press; 2006.
3. Faul M, Xu L, Wald MM, Coronado VG. *Traumatic brain injury in the United States. Atlanta, GA: Centers for Disease Control and Prevention, National Center for Injury Prevention* and Control; 2010.
4. Langlois JA, Rutland-Brown W, Wald MM. The epidemiology and impact of traumatic brain injury: a brief overview. *J Head Trauma Rehabil* 2006;**21**(5):375–8.
5. Iverson GL, Langlois JA, McCrea MA, Kelly JP. Challenges associated with post-deployment screening for mild traumatic brain injury in military personnel. *Clin Neuropsychol* 2009;**23**(8):1299–314.
6. McCrea M. *Mild Traumatic Brain Injury and Post-Concussion Syndrome: The New Evidence Base for Diagnosis and Treatment*. New York: Oxford University Press; 2008.
7. Ramlackhansingh AF, Brooks DJ, Greenwood RJ, Bose SK, Turkheimer FE, Kinnunen KM, et al. Inflammation after trauma: microglial activation and traumatic brain injury. *Ann Neurol* 2011;**70**(3):374–83.
8. Signoretti S, Lazzarino G, Tavazzi B, Vagnozzi R. The pathophysiology of concussion. *Phys Med Rehab* 2011;**3**(10):S359–68.
9. Budde MD, Janes L, Gold E, Turtzo LC, Frank JA. The contribution of gliosis to diffusion tensor anisotropy and tractography following traumatic brain injury: validation in the rat using Fourier analysis of stained tissue sections. *Brain* 2011;**134**(8):2248–60.
10. Giza CC, Hovda DA. The new neurometabolic cascade of concussion. *Neurosurgery* 2014;**75**(suppl_4):S24–33.
11. Lipton ML, Gulko E, Zimmerman ME, Friedman BW, Kim M, Gellella E, et al. Diffusion-tensor imaging implicates prefrontal axonal injury in executive function impairment following very mild traumatic brain injury. *Radiology* 2009;**252**(3):816–24.
12. Mayer A, Ling J, Mannell M, Gasparovic C, Phillips J, Doezema D, et al. A prospective diffusion tensor imaging study in mild traumatic brain injury. *Neurology* 2010;**74**(8):643–50.
13. Viano DC, Casson IR, Pellman EJ, Zhang L, King AI, Yang KH. Concussion in professional football: brain responses by finite element analysis: part 9. *Neurosurgery* 2005;**57**(5):891–916.
14. Bigler ED. Neuropsychology and clinical neuroscience of persistent post-concussive syndrome. *J Int Neuropsychol Soc* 2008;**14**(1):1–22.
15. Iverson GL. Misdiagnosis of the persistent postconcussion syndrome in patients with depression. *Arch Clin Neuropsychol* 2006;**21**(4):303–10.
16. Meares S, Shores EA, Taylor AJ, Batchelor J, Bryant RA, Baguley IJ, et al. Mild traumatic brain injury does not predict acute postconcussion syndrome. *J Neurol Neurosurg Psychiatry* 2008;**79**(3):300–6.
17. Wäljas M, Iverson GL, Lange RT, Hakulinen U, Dastidar P, Huhtala H, et al. A prospective biopsychosocial study of the persistent post-concussion symptoms following mild traumatic brain injury. *J Neurotrauma* 2015;**32**(8):534–47.
18. Iverson GL, Zasler ND, Lange RT. Post-concussive disorder. *Brain Injury Med: Princ Pract* 2007;373–405.
19. Belanger HG, Curtiss G, Demery JA, Lebowitz BK, Vanderploeg RD. Factors moderating neuropsychological outcomes following mild traumatic brain injury: a meta-analysis. *J Int Neuropsychol Soc* 2005;**11**(3):215–27.
20. Ponsford J, Cameron P, Fitzgerald M, Grant M, Mikocka-Walus A, Schönberger M. Predictors of postconcussive symptoms 3 months after mild traumatic brain injury. *Neuropsychology* 2012;**26**(3):304.
21. Cassidy JD, Cancelliere C, Carroll LJ, Côté P, Hincapié CA, Holm LW, et al. Systematic review of self-reported prognosis in adults after mild traumatic brain injury: results of the International Collaboration on Mild Traumatic Brain Injury Prognosis. *Arch Phys Med Rehabil* 2014;**95**(3):S132–51.
22. Silverberg ND, Gardner AJ, Brubacher JR, Panenka WJ, Li JJ, Iverson GL. Systematic review of multivariable prognostic models for mild traumatic brain injury. *J Neurotrauma* 2015;**32**(8):517–26.
23. Dischinger PC, Ryb GE, Kufera JA, Auman KM. Early predictors of postconcussive syndrome in a population of trauma patients with mild traumatic brain injury. *J Trauma Acute Care Surg* 2009;**66**(2):289–97.
24. Carroll LJ, Cassidy JD, Cancelliere C, Côté P, Hincapié CA, Kristman VL, et al. Systematic review of the prognosis after mild traumatic brain injury in adults: cognitive, psychiatric, and mortality outcomes: results of the International Collaboration on Mild Traumatic Brain Injury Prognosis. *Arch Phys Med Rehabil* 2014;**95**(3):S152–73.

25. Hoffer ME, Balaban C, Nicholas R, Marcus D, Murphy S, Gottshall K. Neurosensory sequelae of mild traumatic brain injury. *Psychiatric Ann* 2013;**43**(7):318–23.
26. Hoffer ME, Szczupak M, Kiderman A, Crawford J, Murphy S, Marshall K, et al. Neurosensory symptom complexes after acute mild traumatic brain injury. *PLoS One* 2016;**11**(1):e0146039.
27. Levin HS, Diaz-Arrastia RR. Diagnosis, prognosis, and clinical management of mild traumatic brain injury. *Lancet Neurol* 2015;**14**(5):506–17.
28. Grimm R, Hemenway W, Lebray P, Black F. The perilymph fistula syndrome defined in mild head trauma. *Acta Oto-Laryngol* 1989;**108**(sup464):1–40.
29. Bigelow RT, Agrawal Y. Vestibular involvement in cognition: visuospatial ability, attention, executive function, and memory. *J Vestib Res* 2015;**25**(2):73–89.
30. Gurvich C, Maller JJ, Lithgow B, Haghgooie S, Kulkarni J. Vestibular insights into cognition and psychiatry. *Brain Res* 2013;**1537**:244–59.
31. Karr JE, Areshenkoff CN, Garcia-Barrera MA. The neuropsychological outcomes of concussion: A systematic review of meta-analyses on the cognitive sequelae of mild traumatic brain injury. *Neuropsychology* 2014;**28**(3):321–36.
32. Schretlen DJ, Shapiro AM. A quantitative review of the effects of traumatic brain injury on cognitive functioning. *Int Rev Psychiatry* 2003;**15**(4):341–9.
33. Rohling ML, Binder LM, Demakis GJ, Larrabee GJ, Ploetz DM, Langhinrichsen-Rohling J. A meta-analysis of neuropsychological outcome after mild traumatic brain injury: re-analyses and reconsiderations of Binder et al. (1997), Frencham et al. (2005), and Pertab et al. (2009). *Clin Neuropsychol* 2011;**25**(4):608–23.
34. Binder LM, Rohling ML, Larrabee GJ. A review of mild head trauma. Part I: Meta-analytic review of neuropsychological studies. *J Clin Exp Neuropsychol* 1997;**19**(3):421–31.
35. McCrea M, Guskiewicz KM, Marshall SW, Barr W, Randolph C, Cantu RC, et al. Acute effects and recovery time following concussion in collegiate football players: the NCAA Concussion Study. *J Am Med Assoc* 2003;**290**(19):2556–63.
36. Heitger MH, Jones RD, Dalrymple-Alford JC, Frampton CM, Ardagh MW, Anderson TJ. Motor deficits and recovery during the first year following mild closed head injury. *Brain Injury* 2006;**20**(8):807–24.
37. Barker-Collo S, Jones K, Theadom A, Starkey N, Dowell A, McPherson K, et al. Neuropsychological outcome and its correlates in the first year after adult mild traumatic brain injury: a population-based New Zealand study. *Brain Injury* 2015;**29**(13–14):1604–16.
38. Frencham KA, Fox AM, Maybery MT. Neuropsychological studies of mild traumatic brain injury: a meta-analytic review of research since 1995. *J Clin Exp Neuropsychol* 2005;**27**(3):334–51.
39. Pertab JL, James KM, Bigler ED. Limitations of mild traumatic brain injury meta-analyses. *Brain Injury* 2009;**23**(6):498–508.
40. Fann JR, Burington B, Leonetti A, Jaffe K, Katon WJ, Thompson RS. Psychiatric illness following traumatic brain injury in an adult healthMaintenance organization population. *Arch Gen Psychiatry* 2004;**61**(1):53–61.
41. Nielsen A, Mortensen P, O'Callaghan E, Mors O, Ewald H. Is head injury a risk factor for schizophrenia? *Schizophrenia Res* 2002;**55**(1):93–8.
42. Konrad C, Geburek A, Rist F, Blumenroth H, Fischer B, Husstedt I, et al. Long-term cognitive and emotional consequences of mild traumatic brain injury. *Psychol Med* 2011;**41**(6):1197–211.
43. Panayiotou A, Jackson M, Crowe SF. A meta-analytic review of the emotional symptoms associated with mild traumatic brain injury. *J Clin Exp Neuropsychol* 2010;**32**(5):463–73.
44. Akin FW, Murnane OD, Hall CD, Riska KM. Vestibular consequences of mild traumatic brain injury and blast exposure: a review. *Brain Injury* 2017;**31**(9):1188–94.
45. Paniak C, Reynolds S, Phillips K, Toller-Lobe G, Melnyk A, Nagy J. Patient complaints within 1 month of mild traumatic brain injury: a controlled study. *Arch Clin Neuropsychol* 2002;**17**(4):319–34.
46. Hoffer ME, Balaban C, Gottshall K, Balough BJ, Maddox MR, Penta JR. Blast exposure: vestibular consequences and associated characteristics. *Otol Neurotol* 2010;**31**(2):232–6.
47. Suarez H, Alonso R, Arocena M, Suarez A, Geisinger D. Clinical characteristics of positional vertigo after mild head trauma. *Acta Oto-Laryngol* 2011;**131**(4):377–81.
48. Boniver R. Benign paroxysmal positional vertigo: an overview. *Int Tinnitus J* 2008;**14**:159–67.

49. Akin FW, Murnane OD. Head injury and blast exposure: vestibular consequences. *Otolaryngol Clin N Am* 2011;**44**(2):323−34.
50. Balaban C, Hoffer ME, Szczupak M, Snapp H, Crawford J, Murphy S, et al. Oculomotor, vestibular, and reaction time tests in mild traumatic brain injury. *PLoS One* 2016;**11**(9):e0162168.
51. Bigelow RT, Semenov YR, Trevino C, Ferrucci L, Resnick SM, Simonsick EM, et al. Association between visuospatial ability and vestibular function in the Baltimore Longitudinal Study of Aging. *J Am Geriat Soc* 2015;**63**(9):1837−44.
52. Dilda V, MacDougall HG, Curthoys IS, Moore ST. Effects of galvanic vestibular stimulation on cognitive function. *Exp Brain Res* 2012;**216**(2):275−85.
53. Lenggenhager B, Lopez C, Blanke O. Influence of galvanic vestibular stimulation on egocentric and object-based mental transformations. *Exp Brain Res* 2008;**184**(2):211−21.
54. Bächtold D, Baumann T, Sandor P, Kritos M, Regard M, Brugger P. Spatial-and verbal-memory improvement by cold-water caloric stimulation in healthy subjects. *Exp Brain Res* 2001;**136**(1):128−32.
55. Wilkinson D, Nicholls S, Pattenden C, Kilduff P, Milberg W. Galvanic vestibular stimulation speeds visual memory recall. *Exp Brain Res* 2008;**189**(2):243−8.
56. Brandt T, Schautzer F, Hamilton DA, Brüning R, Markowitsch HJ, Kalla R, et al. Vestibular loss causes hippocampal atrophy and impaired spatial memory in humans. *Brain* 2005;**128**(11):2732−41.
57. Smith PF, Zheng Y, Horii A, Darlington CL. Does vestibular damage cause cognitive dysfunction in humans? *J Vestib Res* 2005;**15**(1):1−9.
58. zu Eulenburg P, Stoeter P, Dieterich M. Voxel-based morphometry depicts central compensation after vestibular neuritis. *Ann Neurol* 2010;**68**(2):241−9.
59. Furman JM, Müller ML, Redfern MS, Jennings JR. Visual−vestibular stimulation interferes with information processing in young and older humans. *Exp Brain Res* 2003;**152**(3):383−92.
60. Yardley L, Gardner M, Bronstein A, Davies R, Buckwell D, Luxon L. Interference between postural control and mental task performance in patients with vestibular disorder and healthy controls. *J Neurol Neurosurg Psychiatry* 2001;**71**(1):48−52.
61. Talkowski M, Redfern MS, Jennings J, Furman JM. Cognitive requirements for vestibular and ocular motor processing in healthy adults and patients with unilateral vestibular lesions. *J Cogn Neurosci* 2005;**17**(9):1432−41.
62. Balaban CD, Jacob RG. Background and history of the interface between anxiety and vertigo. *J Anx Disorders* 2001;**15**(1):27−51.
63. Staab JP, Ruckenstein MJ. Expanding the differential diagnosis of chronic dizziness. *Arch Otolaryngol−Head Neck Surg* 2007;**133**(2):170−6.
64. Guidetti G, Monzani D, Trebbi M, Rovatti V. Impaired navigation skills in patients with psychological distress and chronic peripheral vestibular hypofunction without vertigo. *Acta Otorhinolaryngol Italica* 2008;**28**(1):21.
65. Godemann F, Linden M, Neu P, Heipp E, Dörr P. A prospective study on the course of anxiety after vestibular neuronitis. *J Psychosomatic Res* 2004;**56**(3):351−4.
66. Furman JM, Jacob RG. A clinical taxonomy of dizziness and anxiety in the otoneurological setting. *J Anx Disorders* 2001;**15**(1):9−26.
67. Perna G, Dario A, Caldirola D, Stefania B, Cesarani A, Bellodi L. Panic disorder: the role of the balance system. *J Psych Res* 2001;**35**(5):279−86.
68. Winter L, Kruger TH, Laurens J, Engler H, Schedlowski M, Straumann D, et al. Vestibular stimulation on a motion-simulator impacts on mood states. *Front Psychol* 2012;**499**(3):1−7.
69. Hitier M, Besnard S, Smith PF. Vestibular pathways involved in cognition. *Front Integrat Neurosci* 2014;**8**(59):1−16.
70. Smith PF. The vestibular system and cognition. *Current opinion in neurology* 2017;**30**(1):84−9.
71. Karnath H-O, Dieterich M. Spatial neglect—a vestibular disorder? *Brain* 2005;**129**(2):293−305.
72. Balaban CD, Jacob RG, Furman JM. Neurologic bases for comorbidity of balance disorders, anxiety disorders and migraine: neurotherapeutic implications. *Expert Rev Neurotherap* 2011;**11**(3):379−94.
73. Balaban CD, Thayer JF. Neurological bases for balance−anxiety links. *J Anx Disorders* 2001;**15**(1):53−79.
74. Balaban CD, McGee DM, Zhou J, Scudder CA. Responses of primate caudal parabrachial nucleus and Kolliker-fuse nucleus neurons to whole body rotation. *J Neurophysiol* 2002;**88**(6):3175−93.

75. Balaban CD. Neural substrates linking balance control and anxiety. *Physiol Behav* 2002;**77**(4):469–75.
76. Gorman JM, Kent JM, Sullivan GM, Coplan JD. Neuroanatomical hypothesis of panic disorder, revised. *Focus* 2004;**157**:493–505.
77. Balaban CD. Projections from the parabrachial nucleus to the vestibular nuclei: potential substrates for autonomic and limbic influences on vestibular responses. *Brain Res* 2004;**996**(1):126–37.
78. Carmona JE, Holland AK, Harrison DW. Extending the functional cerebral systems theory of emotion to the vestibular modality: a systematic and integrative approach. *Psychol Bull* 2009;**135**(2):286.
79. Halberstadt A, Balaban C. Serotonergic and nonserotonergic neurons in the dorsal raphe nucleus send collateralized projections to both the vestibular nuclei and the central amygdaloid nucleus. *Neuroscience* 2006;**140**(3):1067–77.
80. Wilensky AE, Schafe GE, Kristensen MP, LeDoux JE. Rethinking the fear circuit: the central nucleus of the amygdala is required for the acquisition, consolidation, and expression of Pavlovian fear conditioning. *J Neurosci* 2006;**26**(48):12387–96.
81. Bigler ED, Maxwell WL. Neuropathology of mild traumatic brain injury: relationship to neuroimaging findings. *Brain Imaging Behav* 2012;**6**(2):108–36.
82. Niogi S, Mukherjee P, Ghajar J, Johnson C, Kolster R, Sarkar R, et al. Extent of microstructural white matter injury in postconcussive syndrome correlates with impaired cognitive reaction time: a 3T diffusion tensor imaging study of mild traumatic brain injury. *Am J Neuroradiol* 2008;**29**(5):967–73.
83. Bouix S, Pasternak O, Rathi Y, Pelavin PE, Zafonte R, Shenton ME. Increased gray matter diffusion anisotropy in patients with persistent post-concussive symptoms following mild traumatic brain injury. *PLoS One* 2013;**8**(6):e66205.
84. Maruta J, Suh M, Niogi SN, Mukherjee P, Ghajar J. Visual tracking synchronization as a metric for concussion screening. *J Head Trauma Rehabil* 2010;**25**(4):293–305.
85. Palacios EM, Yuh EL, Chang Y-S, Yue JK, Schnyer DM, Okonkwo DO, et al. Resting-state functional connectivity alterations associated with six-month outcomes in mild traumatic brain injury. *J Neurotrauma* 2017;**34**(8):1546–57.
86. Mayer AR, Mannell MV, Ling J, Gasparovic C, Yeo RA. Functional connectivity in mild traumatic brain injury. *Human Brain Map* 2011;**32**(11):1825–35.
87. Stevens MC, Lovejoy D, Kim J, Oakes H, Kureshi I, Witt ST. Multiple resting state network functional connectivity abnormalities in mild traumatic brain injury. *Brain Imaging Behav* 2012;**6**(2):293–318.
88. van der Horn HJ, Liemburg EJ, Aleman A, Spikman JM, van der Naalt J. Brain networks subserving emotion regulation and adaptation after mild traumatic brain injury. *Journal of Neurotrauma* 2016;**33**(1):1–9.
89. Catena RD, van Donkelaar P, Chou L-S. Cognitive task effects on gait stability following concussion. *Exp Brain Res* 2007;**176**(1):23.
90. Parker TM, Osternig LR, Lee H-J, van Donkelaar P, Chou L-S. The effect of divided attention on gait stability following concussion. *Clin Biomech* 2005;**20**(4):389–95.
91. Suh M, Basu S, Kolster R, Sarkar R, McCandliss B, Ghajar J, et al. Increased oculomotor deficits during target blanking as an indicator of mild traumatic brain injury. *Neurosci Lett* 2006;**410**(3):203–7.

14

Sleep Issues and Mild Traumatic Brain Injury

David Y. Goldrich[1], B. Tucker Woodson, MD, FACS[2],
Jasdeep S. Hundal, PsyD, ABPP-Cn[3,4] and
P. Ashley Wackym, MD, FACS, FAAP[5]

[1]Medical Student, Rutgers Robert Wood Johnson Medical School, New Brunswick, NJ,
United States [2]Division of Sleep Medicine and Upper Airway Reconstructive Surgery,
Department of Otolaryngology and Communication Sciences, Medical College Wisconsin,
Milwaukee, WI, United States [3]Departments of Medicine and Neurology, Rutgers Robert
Wood Johnson Medical School, New Brunswick, NJ, United States [4]Cancer Institute of New
Jersey, New Brunswick, NJ, United States [5]Department of Otolaryngology—Head and Neck
Surgery, Rutgers Robert Wood Johnson Medical School, New Brunswick, NJ, United States

INTRODUCTION

Sleep disorders are a common consequence of traumatic brain injury (TBI) with more than 50% of patients experiencing some form of sleep disturbance after TBI.[1] Of the 1.7 million TBIs sustained by Americans each year, roughly 70% (1.2 million) are considered mild traumatic brain injury (mTBI).[2,3] Disturbed sleep is among the most common complaints of patients with mTBI and contributes to increased morbidity and poor long-term outcomes.[1]

While TBI severity is generally associated with worse acute and chronic outcomes,[4–8] the link between TBI severity and sleep disorders is less clear due to limitations in existing literature. For example, Mathias and Alvaro observe that many TBI studies only focus on one particular severity of TBI, or include aggregate participants with mixed injury severity into one group.[1] Similarly, definitions of TBI, measurement methodologies (subjective versus objective) and criteria for identifying post-TBI sleep disorders can vary between studies. Therefore, types of sleep disturbances and disorders following mTBI and the extent to which they differ from those following other forms of TBI have not been clearly established.

199

Based on evaluation of current literature, we identified the following five questions as worthy of exploration:

1. Does mTBI contribute to the development of short-term and/or long-term sleep disorders?
2. Do preexisting sleep disorders increase/decrease mTBI risk?
3. Does the presence of sleep disorder symptoms (i.e., insomnia, hypersomnia, hyposomnia) identify those with mTBI who are at increased risk for severe/prolonged early impairments, neurologic catastrophe or chronic neurobehavioral impairment?
4. Do any sleep studies identify those at increased risk?
5. Do any sleep interventions enhance recovery, reduce recurrent concussion risk, or diminish long-term sequelae?

DOES MILD TRAUMATIC BRAIN INJURY CONTRIBUTE TO THE DEVELOPMENT OF SHORT-TERM AND/OR LONG-TERM SLEEP DISORDERS?

Sleep disturbance and sleep disorders are significant problems among patients who suffer mTBI, both in the short and long-term settings. The reported prevalence of sleep disturbance post-TBI ranges from 46% to 100%, with high variance based on measurement methodology, type of sleep disturbance studied, interval from injury to assessment, and patient's cognitive ability to report sleep symptoms.[9] For instance, patients with TBI report more sleep problems compared to controls or the general population,[1,10] with 30%−70% of patients (collapsed across all TBI severities) reporting subjective complaints of sleep-wake disturbance.[11−15] Sleep-wake complaints of any kind are reported by approximately one-third of mTBI patients within the first 10 days after injury and up to 50% report symptoms at 6 weeks post-injury.[16−18] These rates are lower than those seen among severe TBI patients, likely due to poor awareness, which decreases with TBI severity.[9] Surveys of US military service members with mTBI have found nearly all (92%−97%) of participants report problems with sleep.[19−21]

One meta-analysis of 21 studies found greater than 50% of patients experienced some chronic sleep dysfunction, the most common disturbances being insomnia (50%), difficulty maintaining sleep (50%), poor sleep efficiency on polysomnography (49%), early morning awakenings (38%), and nightmares (27%).[1] Other studies have shown 72% of patients reported sleep-wake disturbances 6 months post-TBI,[22] and 67% at 3 years.[13] One study reported patients with mTBI to have higher levels of sleep disturbance than those with severe TBI, potentially making them a more vulnerable TBI subpopulation.[23]

Some aspects of sleep disturbance can be attributed to postconcussion symptoms, a constellation of physical, behavioral, emotional, and cognitive symptoms that can include dizziness, headache, sleep disturbance, impaired concentration, forgetfulness, fatigue, apathy, irritability, anxiety, and depression. These symptoms are also associated with conditions such as chronic pain and mood disorders that can occur as complications of mTBI, complicating potential etiologies of sleep disorders in mTBI. While some have suggested sleep dysfunction following TBI can be accounted for by these comorbities,[21] studies have found significant relationship between TBI and sleep disturbance after controlling for factors such as depression and anxiety.[10,24,25] Because such sleep disturbances have been traditionally viewed purely as symptoms of mTBI rather than modifiable factors that can affect recovery, sleep disorders often go untreated in mTBI, causing a vicious cycle of exacerbating postconcussion symptoms which in turn worsen sleep disturbance.[2] Although problems with sleep are relatively common in the general population, general sleep disturbance, diagnosed sleep disorders, and sleep problems have all been shown to be significantly more prevalent following TBI.[1] Diagnosed sleep disorders seen include insomnia, hypersomnia, obstructive sleep apnea, periodic limb movement, and narcolepsy. Sleep problems include snoring, insomnia, poor sleep maintenance and sleep efficacy, delayed sleep initiation, nightmares, excessive daytime sleepiness, early awakenings, and sleepwalking.

Athletes are at particular risk of multiple TBIs, and sports-related mTBI and brain impact remain a major concern.[26] As identified by Gosselin et al.,[26] most sport-related concussions correspond to mTBI with Glasgow Coma Scale scores varying from 13 to 15, normal structural neuroimaging results and infrequent loss of consciousness or posttraumatic amnesia. History of concussion can increase risk of subsequent concussion sixfold.[27] Of note, 35%−70% of athletes suffering mTBI report sleep problems, fatigue, and vigilance disturbance postconcussion.[28-30] Gosselin found athletes with concussions to have more symptoms and worse sleep quality than control athletes.[26]

Hypersomnia

Hypersomnia, or excessive daytime sleepiness causing inability to maintain wakefulness/alertness and unintentional or inappropriate sleep, is a common symptom complaint following TBI of all severity including mTBI. Compared to the severe TBI population, daytime sleepiness was found to be less common among those with mTBI.[6,31] New onset daytime sleepiness was reported by 50%−85% of individuals after suffering TBI, and was present for months to years following injury.[11,12,32] In fact, hypersomnia prevalence in TBI may be underestimated as these patients tend to underestimate their levels of daytime sleepiness compared to non-TBI patients.[33] Severity of TBI as assessed with GCS was found to be significantly associated with presence of hypersomnia post-TBI.[34]

Similarly, 6 months following injury individuals with TBI were found to sleep 1−2 hours more per 24 hours than healthy controls, demonstrating pleiosomnia, or increased sleep need, to be an independent and potentially concomitant symptom of TBI.[33,35] Pleiosomnia was also seen at 18 months.[32] This excessive sleepiness differs from chronic fatigue, another commonly associated symptom of TBI, as it can be objectively assessed through physiologic signs of drowsiness,[36] whereas fatigue is a subjective state largely assessed via self-reported questionares.[14] While hypersomnia can cause or exacerbate post-TBI fatigue, fatigue can present independently as a symptom among TBI patients, and should be properly assessed for and treated.[37]

The pathophysiology of post-TBI hypersomnolence has been hypothesized to be due to hypothalamic injury during TBI. Posterolateral hypothalamic cells secrete hypocretin-1 (Orexin A), an important component to maintaining a state of wakefulness. Low cerebrospinal fluid levels of hypocretin-1 have been reported in 95% of moderate-severe TBI patients.

While this deficiency can improve months after injury, it may play a role in the 25% of hypersomnolent TBI patients whose symptoms fail to improve at 1-year post-injury.[12]

Hypersomnia can result from a number of different disorders following TBI. Narcolepsy, a chronic disorder characterized by a classic tetrad of excessive daytime sleepiness, cataplexy, hypnagogic or hypnopompic hallucinations, and sleep paralysis, is a potential cause of post-TBI excessive daytime sleepiness, although evidence of development of narcolepsy post-TBI is sparse.[12,38] One prospective study found that at 6 months post-TBI, 3% of patients met criteria for narcolepsy type 2 (narcolepsy without cataplexy),[22] and another found 6% at 64 months using multiple sleep latency testing,[15] both significantly greater than narcolepsy prevalence in the general population (<0.1%).[39] If sleep apnea and narcolepsy are ruled out, post-TBI excessive daytime sleepiness can be classified as posttraumatic hypersomnia, a diagnosis potentially applicable to 10%−30% of TBI patients.[15,22,40]

Obstructive Sleep Apnea

Hypersomnia is also commonly a core symptom of sleep-related breathing disorders. Obstructive sleep apnea occurs at higher rates among TBI patients than the general population, and has been reported in 35%−61% of TBI patients.[11,40] One military study found blunt trauma to be a predictor of obstructive sleep apnea development after TBI.[11] TBI patients with preexisting obstructive sleep apnea also experience greater neurocognitive impairment than TBI patients without obstructive sleep apnea. Obstructive sleep apnea can result in hypoxic brain injury, thus, increasing the likelihood of neurocognitive impairment.

Insomnia

Insomnia is another commonly presenting symptom following TBI. Diagnostic criteria for insomnia include the complaint of difficulty initiating or maintaining sleep despite adequate opportunity and circumstances for sleep, in addition to some form of daytime impairment. Symptoms can include difficulty initiating sleep, sleep fragmentation, early morning awakenings, and nonrestorative or poor-quality sleep, and are seen post-TBI. One study reported increased nighttime awakenings and longer sleep-onset latency following TBI, with increased frequency among mTBI patients unlike most post-TBI sleep disorders.[41] A retrospective study found 65% of mTBI patients complained of insomnia at 2 years post-injury, and 25% at 5 years.[42] A study of Iraqi military personnel found incidence of clinical insomnia increased in a dose-dependent manner with number of TBI episodes, and found increased severity across TBI groups after controlling for depression, posttraumatic stress disorder (PTSD), and concussion symptom severity.[43] A retrospective study found half of TBI patients to have symptoms of insomnia, and 29.4% met diagnostic criteria for insomnia syndrome.[44] Verma and colleagues found half of TBI patients with insomnia to have sleep-onset insomnia, and 76% to have sleep maintenance insomnia.[12] Another found 64% of mTBI patients reported waking up too early.

While mTBI patients appear to subjectively report insomnia more frequently than among severe TBI patients, when evaluated using objective measurements the subjective reports appear to overestimate the severity of insomnia.[45] This may be due to the state of increased arousal associated with mTBI insomnia affecting one's self-perception of symptoms.[46] The role of awareness has been posited to explain the apparent greater prevalence of insomnia among mTBI versus more severe TBI; patients with severe TBI may have decreased awareness of sleep difficulty, while those with mTBI may have increased awareness due to hyperarousal or postconcussive anxiety. Alternatively, Rao et al. posit that the diffuse axonal injury of mTBI can lead to impairment of higher function such as arousal more than severe or focal TBI.[47]

Like in hypersomnia, mTBI-induced insomnia can be confounded by comorbid factors such as pain and psychiatric disorders.[13]

Presence of insomnia correlated with decreased life satisfaction, as well as anxiety and depression.[48]

Circadian Rhythm Disturbance

Circadian rhythm disturbances appear to occur with increased frequency among TBI patients. These disorders consist of a recurrent pattern of sleep disturbance due to alteration of the circadian timing system or misalignment between endogenous circadian rhythm and exogenous factors that affects the timing or duration of sleep, leading to sleep complaints and impaired social or occupational function. These disorders can be misattributed to insomnia, and must be correctly identified as treatments can differ; one study found 36% of patients with complaint of insomnia post-mTBI to have circadian rhythm sleep disorders.[49] Most common is delayed sleep phase syndrome, a condition where one's sleep cycle is shifted to cause inability to fall asleep until late at night and resultant later waking times.

While further study is needed, circadian rhythm disturbance may be present in the acute phase post-TBI. One study of moderate to severe TBI patients within 10 days post-injury demonstrated severe sleep-wake fragmentation, possibly consistent with an irregular sleep-wake type circadian rhythm disorder.[50] TBI may cause decreased evening melatonin production, indicating circadian disruption.[25] Beyond circadian rhythm dysregulation and insomnia, this disruption may cause worse injury outcomes as melatonin has been shown to provide neuroprotection in animal models.[51,52] TBI with associated eye injuries has also been shown to correlate with a free running-type circadian rhythm disorder where sleep-wake times gradually shift over time due to loss of ability of light to entrain the circadian rhythm.[53]

Parasomnia

Parasomnias and sleep-related movement disorders may have increased incidence following TBI, both in the acute and chronic phases. Characteristics of these disorders include undesirable physical events occurring during entry to, duration of, or arousal from, sleep. These can include disorders of arousal, such as confusional arousals, somnambulism (sleepwalking), and sleep terrors, REM sleep disorders such as REM sleep behavior disorder, sleep paralysis, and nightmare disorders, and other disorders such as somniloquy (sleep talking), sleep-related bruxism (teeth grinding), and sleep-related enuresis. Verma et al. found 25% of patients had complaint of parasomnias 3 or more months post-TBI, with increased EMG tone and/or REM behavior disorder diagnosed in 13%.[12] A case-control study of mTBI patients 3 years post-injury found significant increase in somniloquy (42% versus 19%), bruxism (42 versus 6%), and enuresis (21% versus 0%), with no increase in rates of somnambulism.[54]

Sleep Disorders in Children With Posttraumatic Brain Injury

While the prevalence of sleep disorders among post-TBI children is difficult to estimate due to inadequate literature,[55] existing research appears to indicate consistency with the adult population. Significantly higher rates of sleep disturbances are seen among post-TBI children relative to healthy, siblings and orthopedic injury control groups.[56] In comparing moderate-severe pediatric TBI patients to siblings (controls for psychosocial, family and demographic factors), Sumter et al. found a significant association with actigraphy-measured sleep onset and sleep maintenance problems.[57] Another study comparing sleep disturbance in mTBI school-age children to a control group of orthopedic injury found that while parent-reported sleep difference was greater among mTBI group, no significant difference was seen in daytime sleepiness, child-reported sleep difficulties or actigraphy-measured sleep parameters.[58] Kaufman et al. found sleep disturbance persisted among mTBI adolescents 3 years post-injury, with findings confirmed by polysomnography and actigraphy.[54]

Balance, Hearing, and Cognitive Dysfunction

Additionally, mTBI-associated sleep disorders can worsen balance, hearing, and cognitive dysfunction. As shown by one study, chronic deprivation of proper sleep has been shown to cause dose-dependent deficits in cognitive performance, and "even relatively moderate sleep restrictions can seriously impair neurobehavioral functions in healthy adults."[59] Moreover, subjective sleepiness ratings suggested that patients were often unaware of these deficits. As sleep has been postulated to be essential for neural growth and plasticity as well as learning and memory consolidation, it follows that sleep disorders can be associated with deficits in cognitive function.[2] Cognitive symptoms seen in mTBI include attention difficulties, memory problems, and executive dysfunction.[60] Neuropsychological testing and evaluation should be considered in such patients if cognitive symptoms persist or prove disabling.

While balance and hearing disorders can be part of postconcussion symptoms in mTBI, these symptoms can be induced by sleep disorders as well. Undiagnosed sleep disorder can be a cause of unexplained auditory processing difficulty or dizziness,[61] and sleep disorders such as insomnia and obstructive sleep apnea have been reported to contribute to vestibular disorders and auditory dysfunction.[62] Abnormal vestibular function is common in patients with obstructive sleep apnea,[63] and obstructive sleep apnea has also been related to Menière disease.[61]

DO PREEXISTING SLEEP DISORDERS INCREASE/DECREASE CONCUSSION AND TRAUMATIC BRAIN INJURY RISK?

Preconcussion sleep deprivation is described as a risk factor for postconcussion symptoms.[64] Adolescents in the general population have high prevalence of disruption in sleep quantity, quality and circadian factors,[65] which may contribute to their likelihood of development of postconcussive symptoms. Among athletes, existing sleep disturbance may increase risk of athletic mTBI, particularly if performance is affected within contact sports.[46] Similarly, if athletic performance does not return to baseline due to sleep disturbance, an athlete may have increased risk of recurrent concussion.[46]

If a sleep disorder is identified through diagnostic testing, it can be difficult to determine if the disorder is pre-morbid or the result of TBI. Similarly, TBI and sleep disorders are each commonly complicated by comorbidities such as pain and mood disorders that can cause or result from their own sleep dysfunctions, making such cause and effect relationships difficult to tease apart. Patients with TBI with comorbid obstructive sleep apnea experience greater neurocognitive impairments in memory and attention than those without obstructive sleep apnea.[66]

DOES THE PRESENCE OF SLEEP DISORDER SYMPTOMS (I.E., INSOMNIA, HYPERSOMNIA, HYPOSOMNIA) IDENTIFY THOSE WITH CONCUSSIONS WHO ARE AT INCREASED RISK FOR SEVERE/ PROLONGED EARLY IMPAIRMENTS, NEUROLOGIC CATASTROPHE, OR CHRONIC NEUROBEHAVIORAL IMPAIRMENT?

One study of TBI patients in the acute rehabilitation setting demonstrated that those with sleep-wake cycle disturbance were functionally more impaired on admission and took longer to get to the same level of function on discharge when compared to non-sleep-wake cycle disturbance TBI patients.[67] Additionally, Makley et al. felt the longer length of stays in patients with sleep-wake cycle disturbance might be a marker for more severe injury.[67] Similarly, a study of primarily severe TBI patients in the acute rehabilitation setting found the presence of mild to severe sleep-wake cycle disturbance at one month helped significantly predict duration of posttraumatic amnesia and rehab length of stay.[9] While another study found no association between sleep-wake cycle disturbance and severity/localization of TBI, general clinical outcome, gender, pathological neurological findings and human leukocyte antigen typing, it did find correlation with impaired quality of life.[22]

A higher acute postconcussive symptom load tends to predict a higher risk for persistent insomnia complaints.[68]

DO ANY SLEEP STUDIES IDENTIFY THOSE AT INCREASED RISK?

Evaluation

Clinical guidelines recommend screening all mTBI patients with identified sleep problems for sleep/wake disturbances such as insomnia and excessive daytime sleepiness.[69]

Given the broad spectrum and prevalence of sleep disorders following TBI, patients presenting with sleep complaints should be evaluated with detailed history taking and subjective measures such as validated survey instruments, as well as objective testing such as actigraphy, polysomnography, or multiple sleep latency testing as appropriate. Screening for post-TBI sleep dysfunction can improve outcomes and reduce post-TBI adverse effects.[70] Objective sleep testing can play an important role in diagnosis, as TBI patients may be more inaccurate in subjective measurements; they tend to overestimate insomnia complaints and underestimate excessive daytime sleepiness and sleep need.[10,32,33,40,44,71]

In taking a history, questions should attempt to identify the nature of sleep complaint and identify potential etiologies. Interview questions should include multiple areas, including sleep quality, latency, duration, disturbances, medication use, and daytime sleepiness. The Pittsburgh Sleep Quality Index is a useful validated survey instrument for this task, and its use among TBI patients has been validated in several studies.[40,70,72] Patients' partners can also be questioned as they may be reliable sources of information concerning snoring or somnambulation, for example, that a patient may be unaware of. In addition, patients should be asked about medication and substance use, as many medications used in treatment of TBI, as well as alcohol and other substances, can cause daytime sleepiness or insomnia symptoms.

In patients predominantly complaining of daytime sleepiness, this complaint should be differentiated from other common complaints like fatigue or weakness. The Epworth Sleepiness Scale is used to quantify subjective sleepiness by assessing their likelihood of sleep during eight daytime situations, and its use among TBI patients has been validated in some studies.[40,70,72] The Stanford Sleepiness Scale can also be used, measuring one's present state of sleepiness using a 1–7 rating.[73] Habitual snoring can be a sign of obstructive sleep apnea and warrants polysomnography testing.

Patients predominantly complaining of insomnia should be asked questions to elicit description of sleep over a 24-hour period and patterns of sleep over time. A sleep diary can prove useful for this task, and can also play a role in identifying circadian rhythm disturbance, which can be objectively assessed with actigraphy. The Insomnia Severity Index is a useful questionnaire for assessing insomnia symptoms including sleep onset, sleep maintenance, early awakening, sleep satisfaction, the effect of sleep disturbance on daily functioning, and level of distress it causes (Table 14.1).[74] Scores range from 0 to 28, with ranges of 0–7 (no clinical insomnia), 8–14 (subthreshold insomnia), 15–21 (moderate severity clinical insomnia), 22–28 (severe clinical insomnia). For circadian rhythm disorders, the Morningness-Eveningness Questionnaire[75] (Table 14.2) or Sleep Timing Questionnaire[76] can be used to identify morning and evening sleep tendencies.

Given the frequency of psychiatric disorder comorbidities, history should also try to elicit symptoms of depression, anxiety or PTSD. A screening tool such as the Patient Health Questionnaire (PHQ-9) validated survey instrument is one reliable method for assessing depression (Table 14.3). Another is the Beck Depression Inventory, second edition (BDI-II). For anxiety, Beck Anxiety Inventory can be used. For PTSD, Checklist Civilian Version is a good resource. Spanish language versions are available for all three.

TABLE 14.1   Insomnia Severity Index

The Insomnia Severity Index has seven questions. The seven answers are added up to get a total score. When you have your total score, look at the Guidelines for Scoring/Interpretation below to see where your sleep difficulty fits.

For each question, please CIRCLE the number that best describes your answer.

Please rate the CURRENT (i.e., LAST 2 WEEKS) SEVERITY of your insomnia problem(s).

Insomnia Problem	None	Mild	Moderate	Severe	Very Severe
1. Difficulty falling asleep	0	1	2	3	4
2. Difficulty staying asleep	0	1	2	3	4
3. Problems waking up too early	0	1	2	3	4

4. How SATISFIED/DISSATISFIED are you with your CURRENT sleep pattern?

Very Satisfied	Satisfied	Moderately Satisfied	Dissatisfied	Very Dissatisfied
0	1	2	3	4

5. How NOTICEABLE to others do you think your sleep problem is in terms of impairing the quality of your life?

Not at all Noticeable	A Little	Somewhat	Much	Very Much Noticeable
0	1	2	3	4

6. How WORRIED/DISTRESSED are you about your current sleep problem?

Not at all Worried	A Little	Somewhat	Much	Very Much Worried
0	1	2	3	4

7. To what extent do you consider your sleep problem to INTERFERE with your daily functioning (e.g., daytime fatigue, mood, ability to function at work/daily chores, concentration, memory, mood, etc.) CURRENTLY?

Not at all Interfering	A Little	Somewhat	Much	Very Much Interfering
0	1	2	3	4

Guidelines for Scoring/Interpretation:

Add the scores for all seven items (questions 1 + 2 + 3 + 4 + 5 + 6 + 7) = _____ your total score

Total score categories:

0–7 = No clinically significant insomnia

8–14 = Subthreshold insomnia

15–21 = Clinical insomnia (moderate severity)

22–28 = Clinical insomnia (severe)

TABLE 14.2 Morningness-Eveningness Questionnaire

Name: _____ Date: _____

For each question, please select the answer that best describes you by checking the corresponding box. Make your judgments based on how you have felt in recent weeks.

1. *Approximately* what time would you get up if you were entirely free to plan your day?

☐ 5:00 a.m.–6:30 a.m.   5

☐ 6:30 a.m.–7:45 a.m.   4

☐ 7:45 a.m.–9:45 a.m.   3

☐ 9:45 a.m.–11:00 a.m.   2

☐ 11:00 a.m.–12 noon   1

2. *Approximately* what time would you go to bed if you were entirely free to plan your evening?

☐ 8:00 p.m.–9:00 p.m.   5

☐ 9:00 p.m.–10:15 p.m.   4

☐ 10:15 p.m.–12:30 a.m.   3

☐ 12:30 a.m.–1:45 a.m.   2

☐ 1:45 a.m.–3:00 a.m.   1

3. If you usually have to get up at a specific time in the morning, how much do you depend on an alarm clock?

☐ Not at all   4

☐ Slightly   3

☐ Somewhat   2

☐ Very much   1

4. How easy do you find it to get up in the morning (when you are not awakened unexpectedly)?

☐ Very difficult   1

☐ Somewhat difficult   2

☐ Fairly easy   3

☐ Very easy   4

5. How alert do you feel during the first half hour after you wake up in the morning?

☐ Not at all alert   1

☐ Slightly alert   2

☐ Fairly alert   3

☐ Very alert   4

(Continued)

TABLE 14.2 (Continued)

6. How hungry do you feel during the first half hour after you wake up?

    ☐ Not at all hungry   1

    ☐ Slightly hungry   2

    ☐ Fairly hungry   3

    ☐ Very hungry   4

7. During the first half hour after you wake up in the morning, how do you feel?

    ☐ Very tired   1

    ☐ Fairly tired   2

    ☐ Fairly refreshed   3

    ☐ Very refreshed   4

8. If you had no commitments the next day, what time would you go to bed compared to your usual bedtime?

    ☐ Seldom or never later   4

    ☐ Less than 1 hour later   3

    ☐ 1–2 hours later   2

    ☐ More than 2 hours later   1

9. You have decided to do physical exercise. A friend suggests that you do this for 1 hour twice a week, and the best time for him is between 7 and 8 a.m. Bearing in mind nothing but your own internal "clock," how do you think you would perform?

    ☐ Would be in good form   4

    ☐ Would be in reasonable form   3

    ☐ Would find it difficult   2

    ☐ Would find it very difficult   1

10. At *approximately* what time in the evening do you feel tired, and, as a result, in need of sleep?

    ☐ 8:00 p.m.–9:00 p.m.   5

    ☐ 9:00 p.m.–10:15 p.m.   4

    ☐ 10:15 p.m.–12:45 a.m.   3

    ☐ 12:45 a.m.–2:00 a.m.   2

    ☐ 2:00 a.m.–3:00 a.m.   1

11. You want to be at your peak performance for a test that you know is going to be mentally exhausting and will last 2 hours. You are entirely free to plan your day. Considering only your "internal clock," which one of the four testing times would you choose?

    ☐ 8 a.m.–10 a.m.   6

    ☐ 11 a.m.–1 p.m.   4

    ☐ 3 p.m.–5 p.m.   2

    ☐ 7p.m.–9 p.m.   0

(Continued)

TABLE 14.2 (Continued)

12. If you got into bed at 11 p.m., how tired would you be?

☐ Not at all tired	0
☐ A little tired	2
☐ Fairly tired	3
☐ Very tired	5

13. For some reason you have gone to bed several hours later than usual, but there is no need to get up at any particular time the next morning. Which one of the following are you most likely to do?

☐ Will wake up at usual time, but will not fall back asleep	4
☐ Will wake up at usual time and will doze thereafter	3
☐ Will wake up at usual time, but will fall asleep again	2
☐ Will not wake up until later than usual	1

14. One night you have to remain awake between 4 and 6 a.m. in order to carry out a night watch. You have no time commitments the next day. Which one of the alternatives would suit you best?

☐ Would not go to bed until the watch is over	1
☐ Would take a nap before and sleep after	2
☐ Would take a good sleep before and nap after	3
☐ Would sleep only before the watch	4

15. You have 2 hours of hard physical work. You are entirely free to plan your day. Considering only your internal "clock," which of the following times would you choose?

☐ 8 a.m.–10 a.m.	4
☐ 11 a.m.–1 p.m.	3
☐ 3 p.m.–5 p.m.	2
☐ 7 p.m.–9 p.m.	1

16. You have decided to do physical exercise. A friend suggests that you do this for 1 hour twice a week. The best time for her is between 10 and 11 p.m. Bearing in mind only your internal "clock," how well do you think you would perform?

☐ Would be in good form	1
☐ Would be in reasonable form	2
☐ Would find it difficult	3
☐ Would find it very difficult	4

17. Suppose you can choose your own work hours. Assume that you work a 5-hour day (including breaks), your job is interesting, and you are paid based on your performance. At *approximately* what time would you choose to begin?

☐ 5 hours starting between 4:00 and 8:00 a.m.	5
☐ 5 hours starting between 8:00 and 9:00 a.m.	4
☐ 5 hours starting between 9:00 a.m. and 2:00 p.m.	3
☐ 5 hours starting between 2:00 and 5:00 p.m.	2
☐ 5 hours starting between 5:00 p.m. and 4:00 a.m.	1

(Continued)

TABLE 14.2   (Continued)

18. At *approximately* what time of day do you usually feel your best?

☐ 5:00 a.m.−8:00 a.m.   5

☐ 8:00 a.m.−10:00 a.m.   4

☐ 10:00 a.m.−5:00 p.m.   3

☐ 5:00 p.m.−10:00 p.m.   2

☐ 10:00 p.m.−5:00 a.m.   1

19. One hears about "morning types" and "evening types." Which one of these types do you consider yourself to be?

☐ Definitely a morning type   6

☐ Rather more a morning type than an evening type   4

☐ Rather more an evening type than a morning type   2

☐ Definitely an evening type   0

Total _____

Add the numbers you circled for questions 1−19 here—you should only circle one per question. The total is your MEQ score.

Identifying Increased Risk

Important predictors of recovery and functional outcome of TBI in diffuse axonal injury include duration of posttraumatic amnesia, and age.[77] Another study by the same authors demonstrated improved sleep efficiency to correlate with resolution of posttraumatic amnesia, and identified actigraphy as suited to studying sleep patterns of these patients.[78]

Actigraphy is an objective measure of activity during sleep that uses an accelerometer combined with a light detector to detect patient motion during sleep, and can be correlated with a subjective counterpart such as a sleep diary.[79] Actigraphy can record activity over weeks to months and can be used in difficult populations such as pediatric or dementia patients, both advantages over polysomnography. It has been used in many studies of post-TBI patients.[22,50,78–81] One study offers guidelines for proper use of actigraphy in TBI, noting caution should be used when interpreting data from patients with comorbid motor impairment such as spasticity or paresis, or cognitive/behavioral impairments including agitation and impulsivity.[81]

Polysomnography is another important objective measure used for diagnosing sleep disorders in TBI. Polysomnography consists of monitoring a patient's sleep in a laboratory setting using a variety of physiologic monitoring devices, including EEG, EMG, EOG, and ECG and video and audio recording. Polysomnography is a diagnostic test for sleep-related breathing

TABLE 14.3   Patient Health Questionnaire (PHQ-9)

Name: _____ Date: _____

Over the past 2 weeks, how often have you been bothered by any of the following problems? (circle the number to indicate your answer)

	Not at all	Several days	More than half the days	Nearly every day
1. Little interest or pleasure in doing things	0	1	2	3
2. Feeling down, depressed or hopeless	0	1	2	3
3. Trouble falling or staying asleep, or sleeping too much	0	1	2	3
4. Feeling tired or having little energy	0	1	2	3
5. Poor appetite or overeating	0	1	2	3
6. Feeling bad about yourself—or that you are a failure or have let yourself or your family down	0	1	2	3
7. Trouble concentrating on things, such as reading the newspaper or watching television	0	1	2	3
8. Moving or speaking so slowly that other people could have noticed. Or the opposite—being so fidgety or restless that you have been moving around a lot more than usual	0	1	2	3
9. Thoughts that you would be better off dead, or of hurting yourself	0	1	2	3
Add columns		+	+	
TOTAL:				

10. If you checked off (circled) *any problems*, how *difficult* have these problems made it for you to do your work, take care of things at home, or get along with other people?	Not difficult at all	☐
	Somewhat difficult	☐
	Very difficult	☐
	Extremely difficult	☐

disorders such as sleep apnea, and be used together with other testing to diagnose narcolepsy, parasomnias, and other sleep disorders.[82] Polysomnography should be obtained for sleep complaints suspicious of sleep apnea such as excessive daytime sleepiness, snoring, or comorbid obesity, as it can confirm the diagnosis. Polysomnography has been shown to identify sleep changes in TBI. Studies involving polysomnography have found increased time spent awake, more frequent awakenings, and/or decreased sleep efficiency for a variety of TBI severities and post-injury time periods, validating the subjective complaint of poor sleep quality

TBI patients often report.[10,12,45,54,83–86] Survivors of severe TBI evaluated one to six months post-injury showed significantly decreased REM sleep percentage,[10,84] a finding reported among mTBI patients as well.[87] Decreased REM latency has also been identified among TBI patients using polysomnography (see Hypersomnia section).[15,45,86]

The EEG component of polysomnography has identified mTBI changes. One study monitored mTBI-affected adolescents at 72 hours, 6 and 12 weeks post-injury. It showed increased theta, delta and alpha waveforms within 72 hours of injury, with variable time to normalization for each waveform, particularly alpha waveforms returning last, and greatest changes recorded during non-REM sleep.[88] Another study examining mTBI patients on average 30 months post-injury found greater intrasubject variability in sigma, theta, and delta power during the sleep-onset period among mTBI patients relative to controls.[86] In study of mTBI-affected and unaffected athletes, Gosselin found no difference between groups on polysomnography sleep testing or REM or non-REM sleep quantitative EEG; however, mTBI athletes showed greater delta activity and less alpha activity during wakefulness than control athletes, correlating with reported poor sleep quality and daytime impairment.[26] As these groups reported clear differences on subjective questionnaire testing despite similar results on objective measures other than wakefulness, Gosselin highlighted the importance of incorporating objective measures in assessment of mTBI effects on sleep. Similarly, another study suggested mTBI disrupts sleep microarchitecture as evidenced on EEG power spectra during REM and non-REM sleep, and due to the difficulty of diagnosis of mTBI highlighted this method's potential use as an objective marker for brain injury.[47]

Multiple sleep latency testing is another objective test used in the TBI population that can be used to quantify patient's daytime sleepiness. Like polysomnography, it can consist of EEG, EMG, EOG, and ECG monitoring, but monitors a series of daytime naps rather than overnight sleep. It can be indicated for patients with chief complaint of excessive daytime sleepiness for whom polysomnography has ruled out sleep apnea and is useful for differentiating diagnosable sleep disorders from subjective sleepiness and post-TBI fatigue. By measuring an individual's mean sleep latency, or duration of time needed to fall asleep, multiple sleep latency testing can be used to diagnose certain TBI-related sleep disorders. Mean sleep-onset latency of less than 8 minutes is generally considered to be excessive daytime sleepiness. In the setting of excessive daytime sleepiness 3 or more months post-TBI, posttraumatic hypersomnia can be diagnosed with mean sleep latency of less than 8 minutes and less than two sleep-onset REM periods. Short mean sleep-onset latency in the presence of multiple sleep-onset REM periods can be diagnostic of posttraumatic narcolepsy versus insufficient sleep syndrome.[89]

While studies have shown reduced number of hypothalamic hypocretin (orexin) neurons in patients who died of severe TBI, low cerebrospinal fluid orexin in the acute period post-TBI, and an association between decreased orexin levels and post-TBI sleepiness[22,90,91]

DO ANY SLEEP INTERVENTIONS ENHANCE RECOVERY, REDUCE RECURRENT CONCUSSION RISK, OR DIMINISH LONG-TERM SEQUELAE?

Treatment of post-TBI sleep complaints can often follow an approach targeting symptoms much like in the non-TBI population. Comprehensive clinical practice guidelines for mTBI, including sleep symptom management, include the Veterans Authority/Department of Defense Clinical Practice Guidelines, the American Association of Neuroscience Nurses/ Association of Rehabilitation Nurses Clinical Practice Guidelines, and the Ontario Neurotrauma Foundation Guidelines.[92]

If medication is used in treatment of sleep disorders among mTBI patients, medications should be chosen to avoid producing dependency and minimal adverse effects, with the aim of producing a more regular sleep pattern.[69] These include trazodone, mirtazapine, and tricyclic antidepressants.[69] Benzodiazepines should be avoided, though newer non-benzodiazepines sedative-hypnotics can be considered for short-term use.[69]

Benzodiazepines are less useful in mTBI patients due to negative effects on sleep architecture, potential for abuse, and side effects such as dizziness, impaired memory, and altered psychomotor skills, as well as possibility of tolerance and rebound insomnia.[93] Animal studies have shown benzodiazepines can decrease neural recovery time in rats with TBI.[94,95] Use of hypnotics may also be associated with an increased risk of dementia among TBI patients with or without insomnia.[96] Similarly, anticholinergics are not ideal due to possible worsening effects on memory and attention among mTBI patients.

Nonbenzodiazepine sedative-hypnotics including zolpidem, zaleplon, zopiclone, and eszopiclone provide better alternatives due to less associated problems with tolerance, effect on sleep architecture, dependence, and other potential side effects of benzodiaze-penes.[93] Eszopiclon is the only sedative-hypnotic approved for long-term use, due to evidence of minimal residual daytime impairments and lack of development of tolerance.[97] However, little data exists specifically on the efficacy of these drugs in TBI or mTBI patients. One study comparing treatment of insomnia in TBI patients using a benzodiazepine versus nonbenzodiazepine found no difference in sleep duration, subjective sleep measures, or cognition between drugs when administered for 1 week, seemingly identifying the nonbenzodiazepine as an equally effective, but potentially less harmful alternative to benzodiazepenes.[98] Nonetheless, some caution against use of the nonbenzodiazepine drugs due to their potential effects on cognition, especially in populations with existing cognitive deficits.[99]

Trazodone, an antidepressant of the serotonin antagonist and reuptake inhibitor class, has been used off-label for treatment of insomnia, both in regular and frequently in TBI populations.[99]

Melatonin, used in treating sleep-wake cycle disorders by decreasing sleep latency,[100] has been shown to treat sleep disturbance post-TBI as well. Based on findings that TBI patients treated in the intense care unit have reduced melatonin levels, the study advocated for further investigation and use of melatonin in TBI treatment.[101] One randomized control study of chronic TBI patients compared melatonin versus amitriptyline found melatonin users reported improved daytime alertness compared to baseline, and amitriptyline users reported increased sleep duration compared to baseline.[102] While ramelteon, a synthetic melatonin agonist, has not been studied specifically in the TBI population, it should be considered for its superior side effect profile, as no significant side effects were observed in regard to nighttime balance and mobility in the elderly population or in regard to memory.[99]

Modafinil has been shown by Kaiser and coworkers to ameliorate excessive daytime sleepiness in TBI patients. Their randomized control trial compared 100—200 mg daily modafinil versus placebo in TBI patients over a 6-week period, and found significantly improved excessive daytime sleepiness among modafinil users relative to placebo without any clinically relevant side effects observed.[103] However, evidence remains mixed, with a 2008 study finding greater change with modafinil than placebo at week four but not 10 of trial.[104]

While impact of standard of care treatment for obstructive sleep apnea, continuous positive airway pressure (CPAP), on neurocognitive recovery in TBI patients has not been well-studied, treatment of obstructive sleep apnea can improve cognitive and executive function in patients without TBI.[2] While one study of CPAP treatment in TBI patients with obstructive sleep apnea showed it to correct apnea, hypopnea, and snoring symptoms, there was no demonstrable improvement in excessive daytime sleepiness as defined by the multiple sleep latency testing or Epworth Sleepiness Scale after treatment with CPAP.[105] However, obstructive sleep apnea treatment benefit requires therapy adherence for benefit, and many patients in the general population struggle with adherence—a problem that may be exacerbated among mTBI patients by insomnia or physical injuries that could limit proper device use.[106] Similarly, PTSD is a common comorbidity of mTBI and poor CPAP adherence is seen in patients with PTSD alone.[107]

One review by Bogdanov and colleagues showed that a number of nonpharmacologic sleep interventions were demonstrated to improve sleep outcomes among post-TBI individuals, seeking to promote nonpharmacologic therapies for use as first line treatment to avoid problems such as drug tolerance or dependency.[56] The authors noted limitations of the literature to date, such as varied study methodologies and lack of objective sleep measures, and varied TBI severity among subjects limiting ability to draw conclusions about response to nonpharmacologic intervention based on TBI severity. Nonetheless, potentially successful interventions they discussed included cognitive behavioral therapy, blue light therapy, problem solving treatment, and combination of sleep hygiene and prazosin, while mixed evidence was shown for the efficacy of exercise on sleep outcomes.

These interventions varied in target and efficacy; for instance, cognitive behavioral therapy was shown to be an effective treatment for post-TBI insomnia[108] and identified as treatment of choice for primary insomnia or insomnia comorbid to a medical or psychiatric condition,[69] while problem solving treatment only provided significant sleep treatment effect at six months, but not at 12 months. Blue light therapy was shown to be effective at reducing excessive daytime sleepiness among TBI patients—in fact, comparative studies found it more effective than modafinil treatment[56,79,103]—yet it had no significant impact on sleep quality, indicating blue light therapy may only be an effective treatment for certain types of sleep disturbance.

Sleep hygiene was also examined in one study, and found to be unsuccessful at promoting greater self-reported sleep duration when incorporated into routine care of hospitalized TBI patients.[109] Nonetheless, it has been suggested as first line treatment for sleeping difficulties in children with and without neurodevelopmental disability,[110,111] and advocated for incorporation into pediatric TBI care plan.[112] Sleep hygiene, along with other interventions, is indicated for patients with mTBI and comorbid sleep disturbance according to recent guidelines.[69]

Sleep hygiene counseling with and without prazosin (reported to improve sleep among patients with PTSD) was shown to reduce excessive daytime sleepiness among veterans.[113] However, confounding led Bogdanov and colleagues to conclude that it is unclear whether enhanced sleep outcome among the combined treatment group could be synergistic effects of sleep hygiene combined with pharmacologic intervention, noting evidence for synergism of pharmacologic and nonpharmacologic treatments.[114–116]

In terms of exercise, while in general improved sleep quality has been shown following moderate regular exercise,[117,118] and low level exercise for slow-recovering mTBI patients remains a clinical recommendation,[69,119] only one of three studies saw significant improvement in sleep quality among TBI patients through exercise.[120] However, authors of another study found improved sleep quality among those who exercised at least 90 minutes per week relative to less than 90, potentially supporting a dose–response relationship between exercise and sleep quality and warranting further study.[121]

Lastly, hyperbaric oxygen therapy was reported to improve sleep in two patients being treated for posttraumatic headaches.[122]

The older literature describes using stimulants and other drugs to treat the sleep disorders in the severe TBI. This significantly differs from the current more conservative approach for mild TBI. As noted above this likely represents a different severity of disease and population.

References

1. Mathias JL, Alvaro PK. Prevalence of sleep disturbances, disorders, and problems following traumatic brain injury: a meta-analysis. *Sleep Med* 2012;**13**(7):898–905.
2. Wickwire EM, Williams SG, Roth T, Capaldi VF, Jaffe M, Moline M, et al. Sleep, sleep disorders, and mild traumatic brain injury. What we know and what we need to know: findings from a National Working Group. *Neurotherapeutics* 2016;**13**(2):403–17.
3. Leo P, McCrea M. Epidemiology. In: Laskowitz D, Grant G, editors. *Translational research in traumatic brain injury*. Boca Raton, FL: CRC Press/Taylor and Francis Group; 2016. p. 1–12.
4. Anderson VA, Morse SA, Catroppa C, Haritou F, Rosenfeld JV. Thirty month outcome from early childhood head injury: a prospective analysis of neurobehavioural recovery. *Brain* 2004;**127**(Pt 12):2608–20.
5. Annoni JM, Beer S, Kesselring J. Severe traumatic brain injury—epidemiology and outcome after 3 years. *Disabil Rehabil* 1992;**14**(1):23–6.
6. Masson F, Maurette P, Salmi LR, Dartigues JF, Vecsey J, Destaillats JM, et al. Prevalence of impairments 5 years after a head injury, and their relationship with disabilities and outcome. *Brain Inj* 1996;**10**(7):487–97.
7. Plassman BL, Havlik RJ, Steffens DC, Helms MJ, Newman TN, Drosdick D, et al. Documented head injury in early adulthood and risk of Alzheimer's disease and other dementias. *Neurology* 2000;**55**(8):1158–66.
8. Schretlen DJ, Shapiro AM. A quantitative review of the effects of traumatic brain injury on cognitive functioning. *Int Rev Psychiatry* 2003;**15**(4):341–9.
9. Nakase-Richardson R, Sherer M, Barnett SD, Yablon SA, Evans CC, Kretzmer T, et al. Prospective evaluation of the nature, course, and impact of acute sleep abnormality after traumatic brain injury. *Arch Phys Med Rehabil* 2013;**94**(5):875–82.
10. Parcell DL, Ponsford JL, Redman JR, Rajaratnam SM. Poor sleep quality and changes in objectively recorded sleep after traumatic brain injury: a preliminary study. *Arch Phys Med Rehabil* 2008;**89**(5):843–50.
11. Collen J, Orr N, Lettieri CJ, Carter K, Holley AB. Sleep disturbances among soldiers with combat-related traumatic brain injury. *Chest* 2012;**142**(3):622–30.
12. Verma A, Anand V, Verma NP. Sleep disorders in chronic traumatic brain injury. *J Clin Sleep Med* 2007;**3**(4):357–62.
13. Kempf J, Werth E, Kaiser PR, Bassetti CL, Baumann CR. Sleep-wake disturbances 3 years after traumatic brain injury. *J Neurol Neurosurg Psychiatry* 2010;**81**(12):1402–5.
14. Ouellet MC, Beaulieu-Bonneau S, Morin CM. Sleep-wake disturbances after traumatic brain injury. *Lancet Neurol* 2015;**14**(7):746–57.

15. Castriotta RJ, Wilde MC, Lai JM, Atanasov S, Masel BE, Kuna ST. Prevalence and consequences of sleep disorders in traumatic brain injury. *J Clin Sleep Med* 2007;**3**(4):349–56.

16. Chaput G, Giguere JF, Chauny JM, Denis R, Lavigne G. Relationship among subjective sleep complaints, headaches, and mood alterations following a mild traumatic brain injury. *Sleep Med* 2009;**10**(7):713–16.

17. King NS, Crawford S, Wenden FJ, Moss NE, Wade DT. The Rivermead Post Concussion Symptoms Questionnaire: a measure of symptoms commonly experienced after head injury and its reliability. *J Neurol* 1995;**242**(9):587–92.

18. Haboubi NH, Long J, Koshy M, Ward AB. Short-term sequelae of minor head injury (6 years experience of minor head injury clinic). *Disabil Rehabil* 2001;**23**(14):635–8.

19. Walker JM, James NT, Campbell H, Wilson SH, Churchill S, Weaver LK. Sleep assessments for a mild traumatic brain injury trial in a military population. *Undersea Hyperb Med* 2016;**43**(5):549–66.

20. Towns SJ, Silva MA, Belanger HG. Subjective sleep quality and postconcussion symptoms following mild traumatic brain injury. *Brain Inj* 2015;**29**(11):1337–41.

21. Lew HL, Pogoda TK, Hsu PT, Cohen S, Amick MM, Baker E, et al. Impact of the "polytrauma clinical triad" on sleep disturbance in a department of veterans affairs outpatient rehabilitation setting. *Am J Phys Med Rehabil* 2010;**89**(6):437–41.

22. Baumann CR, Werth E, Stocker R, Ludwig S, Bassetti CL. Sleep-wake disturbances 6 months after traumatic brain injury: a prospective study. *Brain* 2007;**130**(Pt 7):1873–83.

23. Mahmood O, Rapport LJ, Hanks RA, Fichtenberg NL. Neuropsychological performance and sleep disturbance following traumatic brain injury. *J Head Trauma Rehabil* 2004;**19**(5):378–90.

24. Fogelberg DJ, Hoffman JM, Dikmen S, Temkin NR, Bell KR. Association of sleep and co-occurring psychological conditions at 1 year after traumatic brain injury. *Arch Phys Med Rehabil* 2012;**93**(8):1313–18.

25. Shekleton JA, Parcell DL, Redman JR, Phipps-Nelson J, Ponsford JL, Rajaratnam SM. Sleep disturbance and melatonin levels following traumatic brain injury. *Neurology* 2010;**74**(21):1732–8.

26. Gosselin N, Lassonde M, Petit D, Leclerc S, Mongrain V, Collie A, et al. Sleep following sport-related concussions. *Sleep Med* 2009;**10**(1):35–46.

27. Schulz MR, Marshall SW, Mueller FO, Yang J, Weaver NL, Kalsbeek WD, et al. Incidence and risk factors for concussion in high school athletes, North Carolina, 1996–1999. *Am J Epidemiol* 2004;**160**(10):937–44.

28. Gosselin N, Theriault M, Leclerc S, Montplaisir J, Lassonde M. Neurophysiological anomalies in symptomatic and asymptomatic concussed athletes. *Neurosurgery* 2006;**58**(6):1151–61.

29. Guskiewicz KM, Weaver NL, Padua DA, Garrett Jr. WE. Epidemiology of concussion in collegiate and high school football players. *Am J Sports Med* 2000;**28**(5):643–50.

30. Lovell MR, Iverson GL, Collins MW, Podell K, Johnston KM, Pardini D, et al. Measurement of symptoms following sports-related concussion: reliability and normative data for the post-concussion scale. *Appl Neuropsychol* 2006;**13**(3):166–74.

31. Osorio MB, Kurowski BG, Beebe D, Taylor HG, Brown TM, Kirkwood MW, et al. Association of daytime somnolence with executive functioning in the first 6 months after adolescent traumatic brain injury. *Phys Med Rehabil* 2013;**5**(7):554–62.

32. Imbach LL, Buchele F, Valko PO, Li T, Maric A, Stover JF, et al. Sleep-wake disorders persist 18 months after traumatic brain injury but remain underrecognized. *Neurology* 2016;**86**(21):1945–9.

33. Imbach LL, Valko PO, Li T, Maric A, Symeonidou ER, Stover JF, et al. Increased sleep need and daytime sleepiness 6 months after traumatic brain injury: a prospective controlled clinical trial. *Brain* 2015;**138**(Pt 3):726–35.

34. Hou L, Han X, Sheng P, Tong W, Li Z, Xu D, et al. Risk factors associated with sleep disturbance following traumatic brain injury: clinical findings and questionnaire based study. *PLoS One* 2013;**8**(10):e76087.

35. Baumann CR. Sleep and Traumatic Brain Injury. *Sleep Med Clin* 2016;**11**(1):19–23.

36. Pigeon WR, Sateia MJ, Ferguson RJ. Distinguishing between excessive daytime sleepiness and fatigue: toward improved detection and treatment. *J Psychosom Res* 2003;**54**(1):61–9.

37. Cantor JB, Ashman T, Gordon W, Ginsberg A, Engmann C, Egan M, et al. Fatigue after traumatic brain injury and its impact on participation and quality of life. *J Head Trauma Rehabil* 2008;**23**(1):41–51.

38. Ebrahim IO, Peacock KW, Williams AJ. Posttraumatic narcolepsy—two case reports and a mini review. *J Clin Sleep Med* 2005;**1**(2):153–6.

39. Longstreth Jr WT, Koepsell TD, Ton TG, Hendrickson AF, van Belle G. The epidemiology of narcolepsy. *Sleep* 2007;**30**(1):13−26.
40. Masel BE, Scheibel RS, Kimbark T, Kuna ST. Excessive daytime sleepiness in adults with brain injuries. *Arch Phys Med Rehabil* 2001;**82**(11):1526−32.
41. Parcell DL, Ponsford JL, Rajaratnam SM, Redman JR. Self-reported changes to nighttime sleep after traumatic brain injury. *Arch Phys Med Rehabil* 2006;**87**(2):278−85.
42. Beetar JT, Guilmette TJ, Sparadeo FR. Sleep and pain complaints in symptomatic traumatic brain injury and neurologic populations. *Arch Phys Med Rehabil* 1996;**77**(12):1298−302.
43. Bryan CJ. Repetitive traumatic brain injury (or concussion) increases severity of sleep disturbance among deployed military personnel. *Sleep* 2013;**36**(6):941−6.
44. Ouellet MC, Beaulieu-Bonneau S, Morin CM. Insomnia in patients with traumatic brain injury: frequency, characteristics, and risk factors. *J Head Trauma Rehabil* 2006;**21**(3):199−212.
45. Ouellet MC, Morin CM. Subjective and objective measures of insomnia in the context of traumatic brain injury: a preliminary study. *Sleep Med* 2006;**7**(6):486−97.
46. Jaffee MS, Winter WC, Jones CC, Ling G. Sleep disturbances in athletic concussion. *Brain Inj* 2015;**29**(2):221−7.
47. Rao V, Bergey A, Hill H, Efron D, McCann U. Sleep disturbance after mild traumatic brain injury: indicator of injury? *J Neuropsychiatry Clin Neurosci* 2011;**23**(2):201−5.
48. Cantor JB, Bushnik T, Cicerone K, Dijkers MP, Gordon W, Hammond FM, et al. Insomnia, fatigue, and sleepiness in the first 2 years after traumatic brain injury: an NIDRR TBI model system module study. *J Head Trauma Rehabil* 2012;**27**(6):E1−14.
49. Ayalon L, Borodkin K, Dishon L, Kanety H, Dagan Y. Circadian rhythm sleep disorders following mild traumatic brain injury. *Neurology* 2007;**68**(14):1136−40.
50. Duclos C, Dumont M, Blais H, Paquet J, Laflamme E, de Beaumont L, et al. Rest-activity cycle disturbances in the acute phase of moderate to severe traumatic brain injury. *Neurorehabil Neural Repair* 2014;**28**(5):472−82.
51. Ates O, Cayli S, Gurses I, Yucel N, Altinoz E, Iraz M, et al. Does pinealectomy affect the recovery rate after spinal cord injury? *Neurol Res* 2007;**29**(6):533−9.
52. Ates O, Cayli S, Gurses I, Yucel N, Iraz M, Altinoz E, et al. Effect of pinealectomy and melatonin replacement on morphological and biochemical recovery after traumatic brain injury. *Int J Dev Neurosci* 2006;**24**(6):357−63.
53. Carter KA, Lettieri CJ, Pena JM. An unusual cause of insomnia following IED-induced traumatic brain injury. *J Clin Sleep Med* 2010;**6**(2):205−6.
54. Kaufman Y, Tzischinsky O, Epstein R, Etzioni A, Lavie P, Pillar G. Long-term sleep disturbances in adolescents after minor head injury. *Pediatr Neurol* 2001;**24**(2):129−34.
55. Stores G, Stores R. Sleep disorders in children with traumatic brain injury: a case of serious neglect. *Dev Med Child Neurol* 2013;**55**(9):797−805.
56. Bogdanov S, Naismith S, Lah S. Sleep outcomes following sleep-hygiene-related interventions for individuals with traumatic brain injury: a systematic review. *Brain Inj* 2017;**31**(4):422−33.
57. Sumpter RE, Dorris L, Kelly T, McMillan TM. Pediatric sleep difficulties after moderate-severe traumatic brain injury. *J Int Neuropsychol Soc* 2013;**19**(7):829−34.
58. Milroy G, Dorris L, McMillan TM. Sleep disturbances following mild traumatic brain injury in childhood. *J Pediatr Psychol* 2008;**33**(3):242−7.
59. Van Dongen HP, Maislin G, Mullington JM, Dinges DF. The cumulative cost of additional wakefulness: dose-response effects on neurobehavioral functions and sleep physiology from chronic sleep restriction and total sleep deprivation. *Sleep* 2003;**26**(2):117−26.
60. Duclos C, Beauregard MP, Bottari C, Ouellet MC, Gosselin N. The impact of poor sleep on cognition and activities of daily living after traumatic brain injury: a review. *Aust Occup Ther J* 2015;**62**(1):2−12.
61. Goto F, Arai M, Kitamura M, Otomo T, Nagai R, Minami S, et al. A case of undiagnosed sleep disorder with hearing difficulty and dizziness. *Iran J Otorhinolaryngol* 2016;**28**(85):149−52.
62. Nakayama M, Kabaya K. Obstructive sleep apnea syndrome as a novel cause for Meniere's disease. *Curr Opin Otolaryngol Head Neck Surg* 2013;**21**(5):503−8.
63. Kayabasi S, Iriz A, Cayonu M, Cengiz B, Acar A, Boynuegri S, et al. Vestibular functions were found to be impaired in patients with moderate-to-severe obstructive sleep apnea. *Laryngoscope* 2015;**125**(5):1244−8.
64. Mihalik JP, Lengas E, Register-Mihalik JK, Oyama S, Begalle RL, Guskiewicz KM. The effects of sleep quality and sleep quantity on concussion baseline assessment. *Clin J Sport Med* 2013;**23**(5):343−8.

65. Carskadon MA, Wolfson AR, Acebo C, Tzischinsky O, Seifer R. Adolescent sleep patterns, circadian timing, and sleepiness at a transition to early school days. *Sleep* 1998;**21**(8):871–81.
66. Wilde MC, Castriotta RJ, Lai JM, Atanasov S, Masel BE, Kuna ST. Cognitive impairment in patients with traumatic brain injury and obstructive sleep apnea. *Arch Phys Med Rehabil* 2007;**88**(10):1284–8.
67. Makley MJ, English JB, Drubach DA, Kreuz AJ, Celnik PA, Tarwater PM. Prevalence of sleep disturbance in closed head injury patients in a rehabilitation unit. *Neurorehabil Neural Repair* 2008;**22**(4):341–7.
68. Lundin A, de Boussard C, Edman G, Borg J. Symptoms and disability until 3 months after mild TBI. *Brain Inj* 2006;**20**(8):799–806.
69. Marshall S, Bayley M, McCullagh S, Velikonja D, Berrigan L, Ouchterlony D, et al. Updated clinical practice guidelines for concussion/mild traumatic brain injury and persistent symptoms. *Brain Inj* 2015;**29**(6):688–700.
70. Mollayeva T, Colantonio A, Mollayeva S, Shapiro CM. Screening for sleep dysfunction after traumatic brain injury. *Sleep Med* 2013;**14**(12):1235–46.
71. Ownsworth T, Fleming J, Strong J, Radel M, Chan W, Clare L. Awareness typologies, long-term emotional adjustment and psychosocial outcomes following acquired brain injury. *Neuropsychol Rehabil* 2007;**17**(2):129–50.
72. Fictenberg NL, Putnam SH, Mann NR, Zafonte RD, Millard AE. Insomnia screening in postacute traumatic brain injury: utility and validity of the Pittsburgh Sleep Quality Index. *Am J Phys Med Rehabil* 2001;**80**(5):339–45.
73. Hoddes E, Zarcone V, Smythe H, Phillips R, Dement WC. Quantification of sleepiness: a new approach. *Psychophysiology* 1973;**10**(4):431–6.
74. Morin CM, Belleville G, Belanger L, Ivers H. The Insomnia Severity Index: psychometric indicators to detect insomnia cases and evaluate treatment response. *Sleep* 2011;**34**(5):601–8.
75. Horne JA, Ostberg O. A self-assessment questionnaire to determine morningness-eveningness in human circadian rhythms. *Int J Chronobiol* 1976;**4**(2):97–110.
76. Monk TH, Buysse DJ, Kennedy KS, Pods JM, DeGrazia JM, Miewald JM. Measuring sleep habits without using a diary: the sleep timing questionnaire. *Sleep* 2003;**26**(2):208–12.
77. Katz DI, Alexander MP. Traumatic brain injury. Predicting course of recovery and outcome for patients admitted to rehabilitation. *Arch Neurol* 1994;**51**(7):661–70.
78. Makley MJ, Johnson-Greene L, Tarwater PM, Kreuz AJ, Spiro J, Rao V, et al. Return of memory and sleep efficiency following moderate to severe closed head injury. *Neurorehabil Neural Repair* 2009;**23**(4):320–6.
79. Sinclair KL, Ponsford JL, Taffe J, Lockley SW, Rajaratnam SM. Randomized controlled trial of light therapy for fatigue following traumatic brain injury. *Neurorehabil Neural Repair* 2014;**28**(4):303–13.
80. Sommerauer M, Valko PO, Werth E, Baumann CR. Excessive sleep need following traumatic brain injury: a case-control study of 36 patients. *J Sleep Res* 2013;**22**(6):634–9.
81. Zollman FS, Cyborski C, Duraski SA. Actigraphy for assessment of sleep in traumatic brain injury: case series, review of the literature and proposed criteria for use. *Brain Inj* 2010;**24**(5):748–54.
82. Kushida CA, Littner MR, Morgenthaler T, Alessi CA, Bailey D, Coleman J, et al. Practice parameters for the indications for polysomnography and related procedures: an update for 2005. *Sleep* 2005;**28**(4):499–521.
83. Prigatano GP, Stahl ML, Orr WC, Zeiner HK. Sleep and dreaming disturbances in closed head injury patients. *J Neurol Neurosurg Psychiatry* 1982;**45**(1):78–80.
84. George B, Landau-Ferey J. Twelve months' follow-up by night sleep EEG after recovery from severe head trauma. *Neurochirurgia (Stuttg)* 1986;**29**(2):45–7.
85. George B, Landau-Ferey J, Benoit O, Dondey M, Cophignon J. Night sleep disorders during recovery of severe head injuries (author's transl). *Neurochirurgie* 1981;**27**(1):35–8.
86. Williams BR, Lazic SE, Ogilvie RD. Polysomnographic and quantitative EEG analysis of subjects with long-term insomnia complaints associated with mild traumatic brain injury. *Clin Neurophysiol* 2008;**119**(2):429–38.
87. Schreiber S, Barkai G, Gur-Hartman T, Peles E, Tov N, Dolberg OT, et al. Long-lasting sleep patterns of adult patients with minor traumatic brain injury (mTBI) and non-mTBI subjects. *Sleep Med* 2008;**9**(5):481–7.
88. Parsons LC, Crosby LJ, Perlis M, Britt T, Jones P. Longitudinal sleep EEG power spectral analysis studies in adolescents with minor head injury. *J Neurotrauma* 1997;**14**(8):549–59.
89. Marti I, Valko PO, Khatami R, Bassetti CL, Baumann CR. Multiple sleep latency measures in narcolepsy and behaviourally induced insufficient sleep syndrome. *Sleep Med* 2009;**10**(10):1146–50.

III. NEUROSENSORY DISORDERS IN CLINICAL PRACTICE

90. Baumann CR, Stocker R, Imhof HG, Trentz O, Hersberger M, Mignot E, et al. Hypocretin-1 (orexin A) deficiency in acute traumatic brain injury. *Neurology* 2005;**65**(1):147–9.

91. Baumann CR, Bassetti CL, Valko PO, Haybaeck J, Keller M, Clark E, et al. Loss of hypocretin (orexin) neurons with traumatic brain injury. *Ann Neurol* 2009;**66**(4):555–9.

92. Management of Concussion/m TBIWG. VA/DoD clinical practice guideline for management of concussion/mild traumatic brain injury. *J Rehabil Res Dev* 2009;**46**(6):CP1–P68.

93. Flanagan SR, Greenwald B, Wieber S. Pharmacological treatment of insomnia for individuals with brain injury. *J Head Trauma Rehabil* 2007;**22**(1):67–70.

94. Rao V, Rollings P. Sleep disturbances following traumatic brain injury. *Curr Treat Options Neurol* 2002;**4**(1):77–87.

95. Schallert T, Hernandez TD, Barth TM. Recovery of function after brain damage: severe and chronic disruption by diazepam. *Brain Res* 1986;**379**(1):104–11.

96. Chiu HY, Lin EY, Wei L, Lin JH, Lee HC, Fan YC, et al. Hypnotics use but not insomnia increased the risk of dementia in traumatic brain injury patients. *Eur Neuropsychopharmacol* 2015;**25**(12):2271–7.

97. Roth T, Walsh JK, Krystal A, Wessel T, Roehrs TA. An evaluation of the efficacy and safety of eszopiclone over 12 months in patients with chronic primary insomnia. *Sleep Med* 2005;**6**(6):487–95.

98. Li Pi, Shan RS, Ashworth NL. Comparison of lorazepam and zopiclone for insomnia in patients with stroke and brain injury: a randomized, crossover, double-blinded trial. *Am J Phys Med Rehabil* 2004;**83**(6):421–7.

99. Larson EB, Zollman FS. The effect of sleep medications on cognitive recovery from traumatic brain injury. *J Head Trauma Rehabil* 2010;**25**(1):61–7.

100. Buscemi N, Vandermeer B, Hooton N, Pandya R, Tjosvold L, Hartling L, et al. The efficacy and safety of exogenous melatonin for primary sleep disorders. A meta-analysis. *J Gen Intern Med* 2005;**20**(12):1151–8.

101. Paparrigopoulos T, Melissaki A, Tsekou H, Efthymiou A, Kribeni G, Baziotis N, et al. Melatonin secretion after head injury: a pilot study. *Brain Inj* 2006;**20**(8):873–8.

102. Kemp S, Biswas R, Neumann V, Coughlan A. The value of melatonin for sleep disorders occurring post-head injury: a pilot RCT. *Brain Inj* 2004;**18**(9):911–19.

103. Kaiser PR, Valko PO, Werth E, Thomann J, Meier J, Stocker R, et al. Modafinil ameliorates excessive daytime sleepiness after traumatic brain injury. *Neurology* 2010;**75**(20):1780–5.

104. Jha A, Weintraub A, Allshouse A, Morey C, Cusick C, Kittelson J, et al. A randomized trial of modafinil for the treatment of fatigue and excessive daytime sleepiness in individuals with chronic traumatic brain injury. *J Head Trauma Rehabil* 2008;**23**(1):52–63.

105. Castriotta RJ, Atanasov S, Wilde MC, Masel BE, Lai JM, Kuna ST. Treatment of sleep disorders after traumatic brain injury. *J Clin Sleep Med* 2009;**5**(2):137–44.

106. Wickwire EM, Smith MT, Birnbaum S, Collop NA. Sleep maintenance insomnia complaints predict poor CPAP adherence: a clinical case series. *Sleep Med* 2010;**11**(8):772–6.

107. Collen J, Holley A, Lettieri C, Shah A, Roop S. The impact of split-night versus traditional sleep studies on CPAP compliance. *Sleep Breath* 2010;**14**(2):93–9.

108. Ouellet MC, Morin CM. Efficacy of cognitive-behavioral therapy for insomnia associated with traumatic brain injury: a single-case experimental design. *Arch Phys Med Rehabil* 2007;**88**(12):1581–92.

109. De La Rue-Evans L, Nesbitt K, Oka RK. Sleep hygiene program implementation in patients with traumatic brain injury. *Rehabil Nurs* 2013;**38**(1):2–10.

110. Spruyt K, Curfs LM. Non-pharmacological management of problematic sleeping in children with developmental disabilities. *Dev Med Child Neurol* 2015;**57**(2):120–36.

111. Jan JE, Owens JA, Weiss MD, Johnson KP, Wasdell MB, Freeman RD, et al. Sleep hygiene for children with neurodevelopmental disabilities. *Pediatrics* 2008;**122**(6):1343–50.

112. Blinman TA, Houseknecht E, Snyder C, Wiebe DJ, Nance ML. Postconcussive symptoms in hospitalized pediatric patients after mild traumatic brain injury. *J Pediatr Surg* 2009;**44**(6):1223–8.

113. Ruff RL, Ruff SS, Wang XF. Improving sleep: initial headache treatment in OIF/OEF veterans with blast-induced mild traumatic brain injury. *J Rehabil Res Dev* 2009;**46**(9):1071–84.

114. Manber R, Buysse DJ, Edinger J, Krystal A, Luther JF, Wisniewski SR, et al. Efficacy of cognitive-behavioral therapy for insomnia combined with antidepressant pharmacotherapy in patients with comorbid depression and insomnia: a randomized controlled trial. *J Clin Psychiatry* 2016;**77**(10):e1316–23.

115. Manber R, Edinger JD, Gress JL, San Pedro-Salcedo MG, Kuo TF, Kalista T. Cognitive behavioral therapy for insomnia enhances depression outcome in patients with comorbid major depressive disorder and insomnia. *Sleep* 2008;**31**(4):489–95.
116. Holroyd KA, O'Donnell FJ, Stensland M, Lipchik GL, Cordingley GE, Carlson BW. Management of chronic tension-type headache with tricyclic antidepressant medication, stress management therapy, and their combination: a randomized controlled trial. *J Am Med Assoc* 2001;**285**(17):2208–15.
117. King AC, Pruitt LA, Woo S, Castro CM, Ahn DK, Vitiello MV, et al. Effects of moderate-intensity exercise on polysomnographic and subjective sleep quality in older adults with mild to moderate sleep complaints. *J Gerontol A Biol Sci Med Sci* 2008;**63**(9):997–1004.
118. King AC, Oman RF, Brassington GS, Bliwise DL, Haskell WL. Moderate-intensity exercise and self-rated quality of sleep in older adults. A randomized controlled trial. *J Am Med Assoc* 1997;**277**(1):32–7.
119. Silverberg ND, Iverson GL. Is rest after concussion "the best medicine?": recommendations for activity resumption following concussion in athletes, civilians, and military service members. *J Head Trauma Rehabil* 2013;**28**(4):250–9.
120. Damiano DL, Zampieri C, Ge J, Acevedo A, Dsurney J. Effects of a rapid-resisted elliptical training program on motor, cognitive and neurobehavioral functioning in adults with chronic traumatic brain injury. *Exp Brain Res* 2016;**234**(8):2245–52.
121. Hoffman JM, Bell KR, Powell JM, Behr J, Dunn EC, Dikmen S, et al. A randomized controlled trial of exercise to improve mood after traumatic brain injury. *Phys Med Rehabil* 2010;**2**(10):911–19.
122. Wright JK, Zant E, Groom K, Schlegel RE, Gilliland K. Case report: treatment of mild traumatic brain injury with hyperbaric oxygen. *Undersea Hyperb Med* 2009;**36**(6):391–9.

Vision Disorders in Mild Traumatic Brain Injury

Eric Singman, MD, PhD[1] and Patrick Quaid, Optometrist, MCOptom, FCOVD, PhD[2,3,4]

[1]Milton & Muriel Shurr Division Chief, General Eye Services Clinic of the Wilmer Eye Institute, Johns Hopkins Hospital, Baltimore, MD, United States [2]Vue-Cubed Vision Therapy Network, Guelph and North York, ON, Canada [3]Adjunct Faculty, School of Optometry and Vision Science, University of Waterloo, Waterloo, ON, Canada [4]Consultant Optometrist, David L. MacIntosh Sports Medicine Clinic and Faculty of Kinesiology, University of Toronto, Toronto, ON, Canada

OVERVIEW OF CONCUSSION AND VISUAL FUNCTION

Conservatively, it is estimated that at least 40% of the primate brain is primarily visual machinery.[1–5] Recognizing that accommodation, vergences, saccades, orbital sensation, eyelid function, visual fields/acuity, color vision, and pupillary function are subserved by 7 of the 12 cranial nerves, the importance of a detailed visuo-oculomotor examination in mTBI cases becomes apparent. It is therefore prudent to explore visual function carefully in mild traumatic brain injury (mTBI) beyond the ostensible reassurance offered when a patient sees with 20/20 acuity bilaterally. It is entirely appropriate to rule out pathology that might cause gross visual field/acuity and/or visuomotor defects, since these deficits are common in moderate to severe brain injury in which patients suffer loss of consciousness.[6] However, after mTBI, deficits in visual processing as reflected in abnormal eye teaming rather than those from direct injury to the afferent visual pathways or oculomotor nerves are far more common.[7–15] A difficulty that faces examiners in the emergency setting is the often subtle presentation of eye teaming issues, despite the fact they can cause significant symptomatology.[11,16] In addition, patients might not demonstrate certain deficits immediately after an injury due the later onset of inflammatory changes and cerebral perfusion deficits associated with concussion.[17–19] Patients themselves might not even notice certain visual deficits until they try to return to their normal routine with visual-intensive tasks such as reading, computer use and driving.

Visual symptoms commonly reported after mTBI include fluctuations in visual acuity at near, headaches with visual-intensive tasks and photophobia.[7,20,21] The prevalence of visual issues in mTBI patients between ages 11 and 17 has been estimated at 69% with overlapping issues including accommodative dysfunction (51%), convergence insufficiency (CI, 49%), and saccadic dysfunction (29%) being reported. Furthermore, 14% of patients were found to have significant dysfunction in all three domains.[22] Dual sensory damage such as vestibulo-ocular dysfunction in children after sport-related injuries was reported to be 63%.[23] Given that persistent (6 months or more after injury) visual symptoms are not uncommon in mTBI patients,[24–27] it is logical to suggest that we need to investigate the oculomotor system of patients with mTBI in more detail than what might be normally offered during a routine eye exam. This is even more vital if we consider that mTBI patients have approximately a $3\times$ higher suicide rate compared to the general population and that more than half saw their primary care physician less than a week before committing suicide.[28] This research speaks to the fact that these patients are reaching out to seek care, but are often underdiagnosed in terms of their underlying functional difficulties.[11]

It is appropriate, then, to refrain from assuming a normal visual status in the absence of appropriate visual testing. Areas vital to assess in mTBI patients include both subjective complaints and objective tests of visual function. Patients will often have difficulty verbalizing their complaints, not only because of cognitive difficulties such as impaired word-finding, memory, and complex attention,[12,29–31] but also because there are only vague terms available to the layperson for the subtle visual problems, such as *eyestrain*. The examiner must ask specific questions and may need to ask them in more than one way; a validated questionnaire is preferable.[32–34] Concerning the physical exam, saccadic testing, vergence amplitude/facility testing, accommodative amplitude/facility testing, and fixation disparity (FD) assessment [i.e., associated heterophoria (AH) testing] are all crucial.[35,36] If such tests are not performed, the assumption of normality might not only be incorrect, but can result in limited gains in other rehabilitative areas, such as vestibular rehabilitation therapy or physiotherapy. This is because patients with visual concerns after mTBI are less sure of their own positioning in space[37] and require correct visual cues to promote better balance.[38]

Once a patient has been shown to exhibit visual processing difficulties, therapy should be initiated in concert with a patient's other providers. As was so elegantly stated, "it takes a village and it begins with each of us."[39] There is a growing body of evidence demonstrating the efficacy of visual exercises for patients with visual concerns that might be seen after mTBI.[14,40–43] The Convergence Insufficiency Treatment Trial,[44,45] for example, proved that in-office therapy with home exercises can effectively resolve CI, albeit in children with no history of mTBI. Sports vision training has been shown to improve stereopsis in athletes,[46] visual search performance in students,[47] and even reduce concussion incidence when used on a team-wide basis;[48,49] these programs are not only likely translatable to mTBI patients, but are also germane, since concussion itself is a risk factor for a second concussion.[50,51] Other studies aimed specifically at mTBI patients have documented improvements in reading, accommodative responsivity,[52] and vergence facility.[53–57]

It should be noted that visuomotor training exercises are very similar to the visual tasks that produce symptoms in patients. Therefore, patients must be apprised with the caveat that visuomotor rehabilitation, like any other form of physical therapy or exercise program, is a process that starts gently, requires adequate engagement of the patient in terms of office visits and homework, and takes time.[58]

SPECIFIC OCULOMOTOR AND VISUAL PROCESSING DIFFICULTIES

Saccadic Dysfunction

Accurate saccadic eye movements underpin the ability to see in a moving environment and are crucial components of reading.[36] It is well-documented that difficulties with driving and reading, two tasks dependent upon saccades, are common complaints for patients suffering mTBI; there is often corresponding saccadic dysfunction demonstrable in these patients including hypometric saccades and reduced ability to inhibit saccades.[21,59-67] Excessive eye movements during reading have been linked to poorer reading skills and poor overall oculomotor function.[36] Notably, patients with reduced oculomotor function are far more likely to reveal a history of concussion.[35] A basic saccadic eye movement is a rapid refixation from one point to another.[68] In order to initiate a saccade, the visual system must not only release fixation from the point of regard, but also preplan where the next fixation will take hold, a process which ultimately requires peripheral awareness. Patients with mTBI demonstrate difficulties with both releasing and capturing objects of regard.[67,69-71] The preplanning phase is dependent upon the interaction between brain regions serving the bimodal vision processes, that is, *focal* (detailed information related to the macular cone-parvocellular ganglion cell pathways) and *ambient* [spatial awareness of the periphery (motion and luminance) related to the rod-magnocellular ganglion cell pathways].[69,72,73] To put this in terms that are likely too simplistic, focal vision is *where* one is looking, whereas ambient vision is the visual area *around* where one is looking. These vision processes appear to be subserved through ventral and dorsal anatomic streams in the brain.[74] In addition, both components ultimately integrate to achieve accurate saccadic performance.[68]

The neurophysiology underpinning oculomotor dysfunction after mTBI has only recently been explored. Studies employing magnetoencephalography (MEG)[75-77] and functional magnetic resonance imaging (fMRI)[78,79] have provided data suggesting aberrant functional connectivities in brains of patients with mTBI, both at rest and during visual tasks. In line with this approach, it has been proposed that mTBI leads to a decoupling of the ambient and focal visual pathways,[80] with subsequent dysfunction of the oculomotor system. Notably, subsequent studies employing diffusion tensor imaging (DTI) and fMRI suggest that human brain regions subserving the generation of saccades (right frontal eye fields, supplementary eye fields, and dorsal striatum) and their inhibition (dorsal striatum, right supplementary eye field, and right inferior frontal cortex) are not identical and even partly dissociable.[81] DTI studies have certainly demonstrated heretofore unknown structural damage after mTBI.[82,83] Therefore, it seems reasonable to suggest that this modality might serve to clarify the neurologic basis of saccadic dysfunction (and other visuomotor defects) seen in patients.

Screening for saccades can be performed in the office or the field by having a patient look quickly from central gaze to a peripheral target and also by passively rotating the patient's head rapidly to stimulate the vestibulo-ocular reflex (VOR); an excellent visual demonstration of this is provided in a video[84] attached to the review by Ventura et al.[67] Notably, more sophisticated tests of saccadic function such as the King-Devick and Developmental Eye Movement (DEM/DEM-A) tests are becoming standard equipment for providers.[70,85–87] Although clinic-based devices to measure ocular motility during saccades have been available for some time, it should be noted that newer portable devices that passively measure saccades, such as the Saccadometer™, have been introduced[88]; preliminary studies suggest this device might be useful to monitor patients in the field.[89] The available tests for evaluating saccades have age-matched normative data allowing a percentile score to be obtained post-mTBI. Ideally these tests would be offered to those at risk for concussion prior to play/deployment so that premorbid baseline data would be available for each individual where possible.[87] Data culled predeployment would not only be helpful in improving diagnosis of individuals but also in monitoring the progress of these patients through their rehabilitation/deployment.

The pattern of the saccadic dysfunction is important, with horizontal saccadic dysfunction being more suggestive of oculomotor impairment (DEM Type II result),[90] whereas reduction of both horizontal and vertical saccades is more suggestive of a generalized rapid automated naming (RAN) deficit.[90] A patient with a RAN deficit may have other concurrent nonoculomotor concerns such as reduced visual memory,[91] which has been linked to lower reading fluency rates.[92] While reduced saccadic performance has been studied in children with reading difficulties primarily employing DEM testing,[93] a similar evaluation of saccadic function (King-Devick) has been used in the context of concussion. In this case, it was demonstrated that horizontal saccades were impaired and this correlated with deficits in immediate memory recall.[65]

Our understanding of impaired visual processing leading to saccadic dysfunction in patients with mTBI may be supplemented by studies on patients with attention deficit/hyperactivity disorder (ADHD), since abnormal visual processing seems to underlie this disorder.[94–97] Notably, there is a growing body of evidence relating mTBI and ADHD; it is not uncommon for ADHD to develop in patients with mTBI,[98,99] with one study citing a hazard ratio of 1.32.[100] Additionally, a premorbid diagnosis of ADHD leads to poorer recovery in patients with mTBI.[101] Furthermore, a premorbid diagnosis of ADHD may be a risk factor to incur concussion.[102,103] Finally, patients with ADHD demonstrate saccadic dysfunction in ways qualitatively similar to patients with mTBI.[104–106]

Pursuit Dysfunction

A pursuit is a smooth, constant velocity eye movement from one point to another (as opposed to a saccade which is a ballistic jump). Smooth pursuits can be measured in the laboratory or clinic setting using electro-oculography,[107] although novel technologies that are portable, fieldable and relatively inexpensive have also been explored.[108,109] The upper limit of smooth pursuit velocity for normal humans is over 100°/sec,[110] although this rate declines with aging.[111] Pursuit disruption within the context of concussion has been examined in the past decade,[112–115] where reports suggest that patients with TBI demonstrated decreased target prediction, reduced tracking speed, and less accurate tracking. Smooth pursuits, like other oculomotor functions, are subserved by networks spanning much of the brain, including cortical (V5, frontal, and supplementary eye fields) and subcortical (basal ganglia, thalamus, and cerebellum) structures.[116] A subsequent fMRI study of athletes with acute/subacute concussion showed abnormal activity during tests of smooth pursuits, but did not specifically highlight any one area of the brain,[117] consistent with the idea that concussion causes a more global disruption of networks. MEG has been employed to study patients with concussion-related pursuit dysfunction.[76] These patients appeared to have normal function during visual pursuits until the object of regard was transiently blocked, after which the patients then showed deficits in resynchronizing their gaze when the object reappeared. Specifically, there was abnormal suppression of beta activity in the right parietal cortex and abnormally elevated activity in the left caudate and fronto-temporal cortex. This study highlights the important role that anticipatory control plays in oculomotor function. At present, there are no published studies employing DTI to explore dysfunction of pursuits in patients with mTBI. Notably, DTI has been employed to evaluate parkinsonian patients with disturbed smooth pursuits, and abnormalities in the middle cerebral peduncle (but not in cortical or subcortical white matter) were identified.[118]

Smooth eye movements not only permit tracking a target, but they also permit maintaining a fixed gaze upon a target when that target is stationary while the head is in motion, that is, the VOR, an integration of the oculomotor and vestibular systems. Patients with abnormal VOR screening demonstrate delayed recovery after concussion.[119] Furthermore, primates with lesions to the peripheral vestibular organs demonstrate poorer recovery if they also underwent lesioning of the primary visual cortex (V1).[120,121] Conversely, VOR recovery in monkeys post-labyrinthectomy is significantly better when the animal is in a more brightly lit environment.[121] DTI has demonstrated that the vestibular circuitry runs the length of the brain from brainstem to cortex, with multiple ladder-like crossings in the brainstem and corpus callosum.[122] While patients with mTBI and vestibular symptoms after blunt injury demonstrated abnormal findings in the fusiform gyri and cerebellum on DTI,[123] patients with blast injury and vestibular concerns showed more diffuse axonal injury,[124] highlighting the concern that the mechanism of injury causing mTBI must be a consideration.[125,126] That being said, it must be noted that visuomotor concerns and outcomes appear to be quite similar for patients with mTBI regardless of whether there was a history of blast exposure.[114,127] Concerning other novel imaging modalities, there is a dearth of published studies employing fMRI or MEG to evaluate patients with vestibulo-ocular dysfunction after mTBI.

It is interesting to note that there is significant overlap in the networks subserving saccades and smooth pursuits (e.g., dorsolateral prefrontal cortex, frontal eye fields, and posterior parietal cortex).[128] Despite this, it appears that visual smooth pursuits are not abnormal in patients with ADHD[129–131] in the way they are abnormal in patients with mTBI. If this finding proves to be consistent, one could hypothesize employing it to help differentiate patients with mTBI, ADHD and/or other causes of abnormal visual processing.

Vergence Dysfunction

Vergence function refers to how well the eyes team; this can be described in terms of convergence and divergence amplitude, vergence facility (converging and diverging in sequence) and vertical/torsional vergence ranges. Although, convergence and stereopsis have been shown to be present starting approximately 3–6 months of age,[132] peak normal vergence develops by age 4–5 years[133,134] and, in the absence of injury or disease, should remain stable until the 5th decade of life.[134,135] Isolated measurements of vergence can be accomplished employing graded prisms through which a subject looks from fixed distances; measuring vergence while changing the target distance simultaneously challenges the accommodation system and, therefore, should be avoided if only vergence measurements are sought. Vergence deficits (of amplitude and/or facility) have been shown to be quite common in mTBI,[20,35,136] with some forms of vergence deficit being reported in approximately 45% of adolescent concussions.[22] CI is the inability to move both eyes inwards without undue strain.[137] As with saccadic dysfunction, there is evidence connecting CI and ADHD. First, there is significant symptomatic overlap between the CI and ADHD (i.e., five out of the nine DSM-IV criteria are shared, namely symptoms 1, 2, 4, 6, and 8).[137] In addition, it has been reported that the incidence of CI in the general population is 1.8%–3.3% compared to 15.9% in the ADHD population,[137] although a later study did not support this finding.[138] Finally, children with CI who did not carry an official diagnosis of ADHD scored significantly higher on parental ratings of behavior consistent with ADHD.[139] Academic difficulties are common in children with visual complaints after concussion.[13] Since interventions for CI have been shown to result in academic gains post-mTBI,[140] it could be important to monitor particularly the trajectory of improvement in those mTBI patients who also suffer ADHD. Furthermore, since reduced vergence facility has also been linked to reading inefficiency[36] and training to improve vergence facility has been shown to improve saccadic function,[141] it appears reasonable to inquire about both reading and attentional problems in patients with mTBI.

The midbrain seems to be a key relay station of the pathways subserving vergences via networks to the cerebellum and pons,[142] area V1 (primary visual cortex),[143] middle superior temporal cortex,[144] and frontal eye fields.[142] It is likely that the diffuse axonal injury caused by concussion will affect multiple nodes along this extensive network[145] making the exact location of damage in patients with CI more difficult to pinpoint. One study employing DTI on concussed patients demonstrated abnormal fractional anisotropy values in the right anterior thalamic radiation and the right lateral geniculate nucleus.[123] Serendipitously, the diffuse nature of the vergence network (and therefore its susceptibility to injury) suggests that vergence dysfunction may prove to be a relatively sensitive marker for mTBI.

Accommodative Dysfunction

Accommodative function can be separated into amplitude and facility metrics. Accommodative amplitude can be defined as the monocular ability to sustain a clear image on the retina during fixation at a near target (closer than 20 m). Accommodative facility is the monocular ability to smoothly change focus quickly without undue strain or delay[36] as fixation targets approach or recede. Accommodative amplitude is measured in diopters [D] [i.e., the inverse of the distance (in meters) from viewer to target] while accommodative facility is measured in cycles per minute (cpm), usually with a ±2D lens monocularly.[36] While the neural network subserving accommodation spans the length of the human brain,[146] the endpoint is mediated via the third cranial nerve through innervation to the ciliary body of the eye, that is, a ring of muscle that controls the thickness of the crystalline lens. Accommodation naturally starts to decrease after age 40 years, a condition called presbyopia. Presbyopia is likely due to the hardening of the crystalline lens.[147–149]

Patients with mTBI commonly demonstrate a degradation of accommodation amplitude and facility; estimated prevalence rates range between 20% and 50% of patients.[20,22,52,61] These deficits might not only include reduced ability to focus at near but also a spasm of the near response.[15,20,22,59,60,67,86,150–153] Subsequently, vision-based rehabilitative strategies for accommodative dysfunction have been shown to be effective both in increasing accommodative function and improving objective VEP data in a small population of patients suffering concussion.[52,154] Positive results of vision-based rehabilitation from larger scale prospective randomized clinical trials studies on pediatric patients with accommodation dysfunction but without a history of mTBI (designed in a manner similar to the CITT study[155]) have also been reported.[156] It may be that mTBI somehow exacerbates the clinical significance of latent hyperopia, although there appear to be no published reports evaluating the prevalence of latent hyperopia in patients with accommodative dysfunction after mTBI. One published report evaluating children (without a history of mTBI) suggests that hyperopia as low as +1.50D in the presence of accommodative dysfunction can impair reading fluency, as assessed by objective infra-red eye-tracking devices.[36] In addition, patients with significant hypermetropia (>+4D) more commonly demonstrate accommodation lag.[157]

Accommodative facility can and should be tested monocularly using a ±2D flipper lens; testing binocularly will stimulate both accommodation and vergence and should be avoided if only accommodation facility is sought. Although the average normal monocular accommodative facility is approximately 11 cpm,[158,159] the range is wide, approximately ±6 cpm.[158] Accommodative amplitude is measured in diopters by first calculating the inverse of the distance of the near point for the emmetropized eye; this can then be compared to the age-adjusted normal amplitude of accommodation calculated with Hofstetter's formula (i.e., minimum monocular accommodative amplitude = 15D−0.25 × age).[160] As with vergence and saccadic dysfunction, accommodative abnormalities seem to have a link to ADHD; studies have shown that as little as 2D of excessive accommodative strain can induce symptoms akin to ADHD on the Connor's Rating Scale (CRS).[151] Given that accommodative dysfunction is relatively common in mTBI, it stands to reason that patients with any attention issues arising post-mTBI should be evaluated for accommodative dysfunction prior to diagnosing concomitant ADHD.

Fixation Disparity and Impaired Stereopsis

Recognizing that saccades, pursuits, vergences, and accommodation can be disrupted in mTBI, it is not surprising that visual fusion suffers as well.[161] In this context, deficits in visual fusion refer to FD slips, or AH.[162] FD slips represent a small misalignment of the visual axes of either eye under binocularly fused conditions such that there is a lack of bi-foveal fixation, but maintenance of normal retinal correspondence. This can occur because the disparity is still within Panum's area of fusion, which is approximately 10′ arc at fixation in normal subjects.[163] This small heterophoria, as low as 0.5PD, is too subtle to be measured by those tests use for dissociated heterophoria (DH), such as the cover-uncover test or Maddox-rod test. Whereas AH is a deviation from orthophoria that occurs when fusional contours are absent only from the central visual field, DH is a deviation that occurs when neither central nor peripheral fusional contours are offered,[164] such as during cover-uncover- or Maddox-rod testing. AH has been shown to be a much better indicator of symptomatology compared to DH[165] as the alignment of the visual axis under binocular conditions is more relevant to the habitual oculomotor status. In addition, AH is more useful in determining who might be uncomfortable using 3D-viewing technology.[166] It has been reported that patients with mTBI often demonstrate vertical heterophorias and that correction with prism aids in reducing symptomatology.[167,168] Devices to measure AH, that is, the minimum prismatic correction required to attain alignment recorded in arc minutes or prism diopters, include the Mallett unit, Sheedy Disparometer, and Wesson Fixation Disparity card.[163,169] These tests offer suppression checks, that is, polarized filters over either eye so that different targets can be viewed binocularly, allowing the examiner to determine whether patients are avoiding diplopia through suppression of one visual field, that is, becoming functionally monocular.

Another aspect of visual fusion is stereopsis (depth perception), which can be described as local or global in nature. Stereopsis is measured by standardized tests (e.g., see Refs.[170,171]) and reported in minutes/seconds of arc; normal values have been published.[172] Global stereoscopic targets (i.e., randot displays), which require a larger visual area in order to be seen, can better reveal symptomatology compared to local stereoscopic targets.[173] Notably, stereopsis normally declines as the visual target moves from the fovea to the retinal periphery.[174] In addition, perception of depth appears to require both retinal and extra-retinal inputs during motion of the scene or the observer. Finally, it is noteworthy that studies employing fMRI suggest that depth perception appears to be subserved by the dorsal visual stream in normal subjects, in particular to visual cortical areas V3A, V7, and MT +/V5.[175]

Patients with mTBI demonstrate reduced stereopsis at near[176] and, to a lesser degree, at distance.[177] However, these impairments seem insufficient to explain their relatively common complaint of reduced depth perception. Furthermore, patients suffering concussion report decreased tolerance to aniseikonia (different retinal image sizes due to differing refractive errors between the two eyes)[178] which may play some role in their reduced ability fuse. Although the primary visual cortex (V1) of adult patients suffering from blast-related mTBI demonstrate abnormalities with fMRI,[179] there are no published reports specifically exploring the changes in integrity or connectivity of the ventral and dorsal visual pathways.

Anecdotally, patients with mTBI frequently report intolerance to viewing 3D movies (personal experience, personal communications). Even in normal individuals, observing 3D movies is known to elicit symptoms of imbalance, headache, eyestrain, and motion sickness.[180–182] In addition, these symptoms tend to be more common and more severe in individuals with a history of susceptibility to motion sickness or migraine.[182] Although there are no studies of the responses of mTBI patients to watching 3D movies, it is likely they would fall into the category of susceptible patients. However, it is unclear whether their reduced stereopsis would play a role in that susceptibility; a large study of normal patients who reported untoward effects of watching 3D movies indicated that there was no correlation between degree of stereopsis and symptoms.[181]

Reduced stereoacuity also seems to a problem shared by patients with mTBI and those with ADHD,[183,184] further supporting the idea that mTBI is associated with abnormal vision information processing. While further research is certainly needed, it seems reasonable to hypothesize that reduced depth perception and binocular fusion may result from impaired integration of central (ventral) and peripheral visual (dorsal) information.

Deficits in Visual Information Processing

Visual information processing (VIP) is multifaceted and includes, among other things (*vide infra*) the ability to explore complex visual stimuli in which there are many equally salient targets of fixation (e.g., crowds of people). VIP appears to depend upon intact central-peripheral (i.e., ventral-dorsal visual stream) integration ability.[185] In addition, the activation of recruited neuronal areas requires a concomitant upregulation of cerebral perfusion pressure.[186] While there are no published reports evaluating the integrity of the dorsal-ventral visual networks after mTBI, it is known that patients with mTBI show measurable deficits with complex visual processing.[187–190] Notably, patients with ADHD also demonstrate abnormal cortical processing of salient visual information when examined with fMRI.[191,192] One could suggest a utility to employing fMRI in the evaluation of patients with mTBI as they scan targets of varying complexity, since they frequently voice complaints of being visually overwhelmed in environments such as a shopping mall.[193]

At present, the substrate for deficits in VIP after mTBI is unknown. There is a growing body of literature indicating that mTBI is associated with abnormal autonomic control of cortical perfusion, even long after the original injury.[194–197] However, it is unknown whether the reduced cerebral perfusion limits VIP or is a consequence of reduced recruitment by impaired visual networks. Concerning those visual processing networks, the dorsal stream is supported by fewer retinal ganglion cells than the ventral one; of approximately 1.2 million retinal ganglion cells, 200,000 are M-cells (motion and luminance detection) with most of the remaining 1 million retinal ganglion cells being P-cells (object identification).[198] The ratio of P-cells to M-cells by eccentricity changes from 15:1 at the fovea to 5:1 at 15 degrees eccentricity[198] reflecting the shift of increased magnocellular-type processing with increasing eccentricity.[199] One could hypothesize that the smaller size of the dorsal pathway is inherently less redundant and, therefore, more susceptible to damage after mTBI. Notably, M-cells also have a higher contrast/gain ratio (aside from increased sensitivity to motion) compared to P-cells.[200] This could support a hypothesis suggesting that defects in the M-cell mediated dorsal visual stream after mTBI contribute to the common complaint of photophobia.[201]

Another aspect of VIP is the figure-ground segregation ability, or the ability to recognize a salient visual target (i.e., figure) buried in a visually noisy background (i.e., ground).[202] An example would be a patient shopping in an aisle for a specific item. This visual task is arguably the crux of many other visual functions. For example, physiological diplopia (normal double vision from objects located outside the horopter) is a known cue for vergence and depends upon a subject's ability to discern "foreground" from "background" in order to ultimately control eye movements.[202] Given that saccades have been shown to be impaired after concussion and that figure-ground segregation skills are intimately associated with saccades,[203–206] it stands to reason that figure-ground segregation would be reduced after brain injury. Indeed, stroke patients demonstrate loss of figure-ground segregation and it has been suggested that loss of such skills were rooted in oculomotor dysfunction.[207] There are scattered case reports of patients with closed head injury demonstrating abnormal figure-ground perception,[208] but this aspect of VIP has not been systematically studied in patients with mTBI. It is worth mentioning that lesioning cortical area MT in primates (which has major inputs from the dorsal magnocellular stream) causes a persistent deficit in the ability to identify motion against a complex background.[209] This not only reinforces the importance of the M-system in figure-ground processing, but could support the notion that damage to the dorsal visual stream after mTBI contribute to patients' complaints of discomfiture with moving stimuli.[140]

Disturbance of the figure-ground segregation visual process has been observed in a recently described disorder dubbed "visual midline shift syndrome" (VMSS), in that the patient observes motion or tilting of a surface even in the absence of head or body motion (i.e., independent of vestibular involvement).[80,210] VMSS has been reported in patients with stroke,[211] TBI,[210] and other neurologic conditions[212] as a shift in the patient's sense of bodily midline, or egocenter, such that patients tend to bear weight nonorthogonally to the ground. Notably, it has been reported that patients suffering stroke (CVA)[213] and mTBI[214,215] demonstrate altered postural control, supporting the concept that sensorimotor integration processes for stance and balance are impaired. Stroke patients also demonstrate uneven weight-bearing during ambulation on pressure-sensitive treadmills and respond positively to yoked prisms that revert the visual midline to their body center.[212] VMSS is currently not a widely accepted nosologic entity outside the neuro-optometric community, although there is a case report in the sports medicine literature describing how prismatic correction of VMSS improved an athlete's posture and reduced his lower back pain.[216] Confirmation of the validity and etiology of VMSS is extremely important because this condition may be a significant cause of imbalance and falls after mTBI, independent of mTBI-related pathology to the vestibulo-ocular system.[217] As mentioned previously, the VOR stabilizes the visual scene perceived by a moving patient. Simultaneously, kinesthetic input from the vestibulospinal- and vestibulocollic reflexes steady the trunk and head, respectively.[217] If VMSS is a distinct vision processing disorder, one could hypothesize that it might impede physical rehabilitation directed toward balance disorders or even encourage maladaptive visual fixation techniques that can occur after brain injury.[218]

Clinically, the vestibular system can only be indirectly assessed via the visual system (e.g., saccadic eye movements and nystagmus).[219] Therefore, any oculomotor dysfunction can result in ambiguity as to the cause of abnormal eye movements demonstrated during VOR assessment. This supports the need for evaluating the oculomotor system prior to rendering a definitive diagnosis of vestibular dysfunction for patients with complaints often conflated by patients such as dizziness, vertigo, lightheadedness, imbalance, and disequilibrium; notably, true vertigo is usually caused by vestibular pathology.[220] Returning to the concept that "it takes a village" to evaluate and treat patients with mTBI, the oculomotor evaluation must be done in the context of a larger, more comprehensive assessment, including explorations of balance, vestibular-cognitive, and neurocognitive function. This suite of tests, called the vestibular-ocular-motor screening (VOMS) approach, appears to be validly sensitive in detecting concussion.[23,221–225] In addition, it has been reported that results of the VOMS may help predict outcomes after mTBI,[225] although conflicting data has been reported in this regard.[114,225]

THE GENERALIST'S APPROACH TO EVALUATING VISUAL DYSFUNCTION IN PATIENTS WITH MILD TRAUMATIC BRAIN INJURY

The subjective visual complaints expressed by patients with mTBI are legion. To guide a patient through this process and facilitate the provider's effort to document these complaints, it seems appropriate to offer a questionnaire for oculomotor dysfunction. One such instrument is the Convergence Insufficiency Symptom Survey (CISS).[226] Although this survey was designed to identify CI, it has also been reported to measure symptomatology in other oculomotor disorders such as accommodative dysfunction.[227] Indeed, this instrument may be more sensitive to global visual dysfunction rather than being specific to CI.[228,229] Given that patients with mTBI who complete vision rehabilitation show marked improvement in CISS scores,[40] it seems reasonable to offer the CISS to these patients early in the diagnostic process so as to proactively guide referrals. The CISS questionnaire is brief, being comprised of 15 questions with each answer being weighted from 0 to 4 (never = 0, infrequently = 1, sometimes = 2, fairly often = 3, always = 4) and scores ranging from 0 to 60; a score over 20 in adults should raise concerns. Notably, other vision-based surveys have been reported and deserve further efforts toward validation.[33,230]

A particular difficulty encountered when recording visual dysfunction after mTBI is that the list of ICD-10™[231] codes lags behind the science. For example, there are no codes for some of the proposed nosologic entities, such as VMSS or even confirmed ones such as indirect traumatic optic neuropathy[232] or central visual processing disorder. Notably, while there are assigned codes for both central and acquired *auditory* processing disorders, there are no codes for central *vestibular* processing disorder. Table 15.1 provides a list of diagnostic codes for conditions known to occur after TBI.

CONCLUSION

Visual dysfunction after mTBI is pervasive and long-lasting, albeit often amenable to treatment. It is the responsibility of the medical community to educate providers, offering better means of detection, and avenues of therapy. It is time to recognize that the term "mild TBI" is oxymoronic and a misnomer,[233,234] considering the fact that the impact on quality of life can be pervasive and chronic.

TABLE 15.1   Diagnoses of Visual Dysfunction After TBI

Diagnosis	ICD-10 Code
Strabismus (eso-, exo-, hyper-, hypo-, cyclo-tropias)	H50.xx
Monofixation syndrome	H50.42
Spasm of conjugate gaze	H51.0
Convergence insufficiency	H51.11
Convergence excess	H51.12
Other specified disorders of binocular movement	H51.8
Paresis of accommodation	H52.52
Spasm of accommodation	H52.53
Diplopia	H53.2
Anomalous retinal correspondence	H53.31
Fusion with defective stereopsis	H53.32
Simultaneous visual perception without fusion	H53.33
Suppression of binocular vision	H53.34
Visual field defects	H53.4x
Color vision deficiencies	H53.5x
Glare sensitivity	H53.71
Heterophoria (unspecified)	H55.50
Nystagmus	H55.50
Saccadic eye movements (deficiency)	H55.81
Other irregular eye movements	H55.89
Neurologic neglect syndrome (incl. visuospatial neglect)	R41.4
Visuospatial deficit	R41.842
Visual agnosia (incl. topograph-agnosia)	R48.3
Abnormal oculomotor study	R94.113
Injury of optic nerve and pathways	S04.0xxx
Injury of oculomotor nerve	S04.1xxx
Injury of trochlear nerve	S04.2xxx
Injury of abducens nerve	S04.4xxx

References

1. Felleman DJVED. Distributed hierarchal processing in the primate cerebral cortex. *Cerebral Cortex* 1991;**1**(1):1−47.
2. Drury HA, Van Essen DC. Functional specializations in human cerebral cortex analyzed using the visible man surface-based atlas. *Hum Brain Mapp* 1997;**5**(4):233−7.
3. Van Essen DC. Surface-based approaches to spatial localization and registration in primate cerebral cortex. *Neuroimage* 2004;**23**(Suppl 1):S97−107.
4. Van Essen DC. Towards a quantitative, probabilistic neuroanatomy of cerebral cortex. *Cortex* 2004;**40**(1):211−12.
5. Van Essen DC, Drury HA. Structural and functional analyses of human cerebral cortex using a surface-based atlas. *J Neurosci* 1997;**17**(18):7079−102.
6. Atkins EJ, Newman NJ, Biousse V. Post-traumatic visual loss. *Rev Neurol Dis* 2008;**5**(2):73−81.
7. Alvarez TL, Kim EH, Vicci VR, Dhar SK, Biswal BB, Barrett AM. Concurrent vision dysfunctions in convergence insufficiency with traumatic brain injury. *Optom Vis Sci* 2012;**89**(12):1740−51.
8. Goodrich GL, Kirby J, Cockerham G, Ingalla SP, Lew HL. Visual function in patients of a polytrauma rehabilitation center: a descriptive study. *J Rehabil Res Dev* 2007;**44**(7):929−36.
9. Tyler CW, Likova LT, Mineff KN, Elsaid AM, Nicholas SC. Consequences of traumatic brain injury for human vergence dynamics. *Front Neurol* 2014;**5**:282.
10. Kirkwood MW, Yeates KO, Taylor HG, Randolph C, McCrea M, Anderson VA:. Management of pediatric mild traumatic brain injury: a neuropsychological review from injury through recovery. *Clin Neuropsychol* 2008;**22**(5):769−800.
11. Mayer A, Wertz C, Ryman S, Storey E, Park G, Phillips J, et al. Neurosensory deficits vary as a function of point of care in pediatric mild traumatic brain injury. *J Neurotrauma* 2018;**35**(10):1178−84.
12. Tapper A, Gonzalez D, Roy E, Niechwiej-Szwedo E. Executive function deficits in team sport athletes with a history of concussion revealed by a visual-auditory dual task paradigm. *J Sports Sci* 2017;**35**(3):231−40.
13. Swanson MW, Weise KK, Dreer LE, Johnston J, Davis RD, Ferguson D, et al. Academic difficulty and vision symptoms in children with concussion. *Optom Vis Sci* 2017;**94**(1):60−7.
14. Storey EP, Master SR, Lockyer JE, Podolak OE, Grady MF, Master CL. Near point of convergence after concussion in children. *Optom Vis Sci* 2017;**94**(1):96−100.
15. Pillai C, Gittinger Jr. JW. Vision testing in the evaluation of concussion. *Semin Ophthalmol* 2017;**32**(1):144−52.
16. Schmid KE, Tortella FC. The diagnosis of traumatic brain injury on the battlefield. *Front Neurol* 2012;**3**:90.
17. Greve MW, Zink BJ. Pathophysiology of traumatic brain injury. *Mt Sinai J Med* 2009;**76**(2):97−104.
18. Katz DI, Cohen SI, Alexander MP. Mild traumatic brain injury. *Handbook Clin Neurol* 2015;**127**:131−56.
19. Werner C, Engelhard K. Pathophysiology of traumatic brain injury. *Br J Anaesth* 2007;**99**(1):4−9.
20. Barnett BP, Singman EL. Vision concerns after mild traumatic brain injury. *Curr Treat Options Neurol* 2015;**17**(2):329.
21. Singman E. Automating the assessment of visual dysfunction after traumatic brain injury. *Med Instrument* 2013;**1**:3. Available from: < https://doi.org/10.7243/2052-6962-1-3 >; [accessed 31.08.18].
22. Master CL, Scheiman M, Gallaway M, Goodman A, Robinson RL, Master SR, et al. Vision diagnoses are common after concussion in adolescents. *Clin Pediatr (Phila)* 2016;**55**(3):260−7.
23. Ellis MJ, Cordingley D, Vis S, Reimer K, Leiter J, Russell K. Vestibulo-ocular dysfunction in pediatric sports-related concussion. *J Neurosurg Pediatr* 2015;**16**(3):248−55.
24. Marshall S, Bayley M, McCullagh S, Velikonja D, Berrigan L, Ouchterlony D, et al. Group mEC: updated clinical practice guidelines for concussion/mild traumatic brain injury and persistent symptoms. *Brain Inj* 2015;**29**(6):688−700.
25. Serdarevic R. Disorders of accommodative convergence and accommodation (AC/A) relations at traumatic brain injury. *Med Arch* 2015;**69**(2):95−7.
26. Tokarz-Sawinska E, Lachowicz E. Conservative management of posttraumatic diplopia. *Klin Oczna* 2015;**117**(1):14−19.
27. Matuseviciene G, Johansson J, Moller M, Godbolt AK, Pansell T, Deboussard CN. Longitudinal changes in oculomotor function in young adults with mild traumatic brain injury in Sweden: an exploratory prospective observational study. *BMJ Open* 2018;**8**(2):e018734.

28. Fralick M, Thiruchelvam D, Tien HC, Redelmeier DA. Risk of suicide after a concussion. *Can Med Assoc J* 2016;**188**(7):497−504.
29. Barman A, Chatterjee A, Bhide R. Cognitive impairment and rehabilitation strategies after traumatic brain injury. *Indian J Psychol Med* 2016;**38**(3):172−81.
30. Dean PJ, Sterr A. Long-term effects of mild traumatic brain injury on cognitive performance. *Front Hum Neurosci* 2013;**7**:30.
31. Heitger MH, Jones RD, Macleod AD, Snell DL, Frampton CM, Anderson TJ. Impaired eye movements in post-concussion syndrome indicate suboptimal brain function beyond the influence of depression, malingering or intellectual ability. *Brain* 2009;**132**(Pt 10):2850−70.
32. Harris PGL. Changes in scores on the covd quality of life assessment before & after vision therapy: a multi-office study. *J Behav Optom* 2007;**18**:43−7.
33. Laukkanen H, Scheiman M, Hayes JR. Brain injury vision symptom survey (BIVSS) questionnaire. *Optom Vis Sci* 2017;**94**(1):43−50.
34. Politzer T, Berryman A, Rasavage K, Snell L, Weintraub A, Gerber DJ. The craig hospital eye evaluation rating scale (CHEERS). *Phys Med Rehabil* 2017;**9**(5):477−82.
35. Poltavski DV, Biberdorf D. Screening for lifetime concussion in athletes: importance of oculomotor measures. *Brain Inj* 2014;**28**(4):475−85.
36. Quaid P, Simpson T. Association between reading speed, cycloplegic refractive error, and oculomotor function in reading disabled children versus controls. *Graefes Arch Clin Exp Ophthalmol* 2013;**251**(1):169−87.
37. Chang ARS, Yu XX. *Neurovision Rehabilitation Guide*. Boca Raton, FL: CRC Press; 2016.
38. Asslander L, Hettich G, Mergner T. Visual contribution to human standing balance during support surface tilts. *Hum Mov Sci* 2015;**41**:147−64.
39. Driscoll PSC. *Hidden Battles on Unseen Fronts: Stories of American Soldiers With Traumatic Brain Injury and PTSD*. Havertown, PA: Casemate (for the Armed Forces Foundation); 2009.
40. Conrad JS, Mitchell GL, Kulp MT. Vision therapy for binocular dysfunction post brain injury. *Optom Vis Sci* 2017;**94**(1):101−7.
41. Scheiman MM, Talasan H, Mitchell GL, Alvarez TL. Objective assessment of vergence after treatment of concussion-related CI: a pilot study. *Optom Vis Sci* 2017;**94**(1):74−88.
42. Thiagarajan P, Ciuffreda KJ, Capo-Aponte JE, Ludlam DP, Kapoor N. Oculomotor neurorehabilitation for reading in mild traumatic brain injury (mTBI): an integrative approach. *NeuroRehabilitation* 2014;**34**(1):129−46.
43. Ciuffreda KJ, Yadav NK, Thiagarajan P, Ludlam DP, Novel A. Computer oculomotor rehabilitation (COR) program for mild traumatic brain injury (mTBI). *Brain Sci* 2017;**7**(8).
44. Convergence Insufficiency Treatment Trial Study G. Long-term effectiveness of treatments for symptomatic convergence insufficiency in children. *Optom Vis Sci* 2009;**86**(9):1096−103.
45. Group CITTS. Randomized clinical trial of treatments for symptomatic convergence insufficiency in children. *Arch Ophthalmol* 2008;**126**(10):1336−49.
46. Zwierko T, Puchalska-Niedbal L, Krzepota J, Markiewicz M, Wozniak J, Lubinski W. The effects of sports vision training on binocular vision function in female university athletes. *J Hum Kinet* 2015;**49**:287−96.
47. Krzepota J, Zwierko T, Puchalska-Niedbal L, Markiewicz M, Florkiewicz B, Lubinski W. The efficiency of a visual skills training program on visual search performance. *J Hum Kinet* 2015;**46**:231−40.
48. Clark JF, Colosimo A, Ellis JK, Mangine R, Bixenmann B, Hasselfeld K, et al. Vision training methods for sports concussion mitigation and management. *J Vis Exp* 2015;(99):e52648.
49. Clark JF, Graman P, Ellis JK, Mangine RE, Rauch JT, Bixenmann B, et al. An exploratory study of the potential effects of vision training on concussion incidence in football. *Optom Vis Perform* 2015;**3**(2):116−25.
50. Nordstrom A, Nordstrom P, Ekstrand J. Sports-related concussion increases the risk of subsequent injury by about 50% in elite male football players. *Br J Sports Med* 2014;**48**(19):1447−50.
51. Abrahams S, Fie SM, Patricios J, Posthumus M, September AV. Risk factors for sports concussion: an evidence-based systematic review. *Br J Sports Med* 2014;**48**(2):91−7.
52. Thiagarajan P, Ciuffreda KJ. Effect of oculomotor rehabilitation on accommodative responsivity in mild traumatic brain injury. *J Rehabil Res Dev* 2014;**51**(2):175−91.
53. Ciuffreda KJ, Han Y, Kapoor N, Ficarra AP. Oculomotor rehabilitation for reading in acquired brain injury. *NeuroRehabilitation* 2006;**21**(1):9−21.

54. Ciuffreda KJ, Rutner D, Kapoor N, Suchoff IB, Craig S, Han ME. Vision therapy for oculomotor dysfunctions in acquired brain injury: a retrospective analysis. *Optometry* 2008;**79**(1):18—22.
55. Thiagarajan P, Ciuffreda KJ. Effect of oculomotor rehabilitation on vergence responsivity in mild traumatic brain injury. *J Rehabil Res Dev* 2013;**50**(9):1223—40.
56. Thiagarajan P, Ciuffreda KJ. Versional eye tracking in mild traumatic brain injury (mTBI): effects of oculomotor training (OMT). *Brain Inj* 2014;**28**(7):930—43.
57. Scheiman M, Kulp MT, Cotter S, Mitchell GL, Gallaway M, Boas M, et al. Convergence insufficiency treatment trial study G: vision therapy/orthoptics for symptomatic convergence insufficiency in children: treatment kinetics. *Optom Vis Sci* 2010;**87**(8):593—603.
58. Seguin RAEJ, Buchner D, Block R, Nelson ME. Growing stronger: strength training for older adults. In: Boston, MA: Tufts University (for the US Dept. Health & Human Services, Centers for Disease Control & Prevention); 2002. p. 116. < http://dx.doi.org/10.7243/2052-6962-1-3 > ; 2018 [accessed 31.08.18].
59. Brahm KD, Wilgenburg HM, Kirby J, Ingalla S, Chang CY, Goodrich GL. Visual impairment and dysfunction in combat-injured servicemembers with traumatic brain injury. *Optom Vis Sci* 2009;**86**(7):817—25.
60. Capó-Aponte JE, Jorgensen-Wagers KL, Sosa JA, Walsh DV, Goodrich GL, Temme LA, et al. Visual dysfunctions at different stages after blast and non-blast mild traumatic brain injury. *Optom Vis Sci* 2017;**94**(1):7—15.
61. Capó-Aponte JE, Urosevich TG, Temme LA, Tarbett AK, Sanghera NK. Visual dysfunctions and symptoms during the subacute stage of blast-induced mild traumatic brain injury. *Mil Med* 2012;**177**(7):804—13.
62. Galetta KM, Barrett J, Allen M, Madda F, Delicata D, Tennant AT, et al. The King-Devick test as a determinant of head trauma and concussion in boxers and MMA fighters. *Neurology* 2011;**76**(17):1456—62.
63. Galetta KM, Brandes LE, Maki K, Dziemianowicz MS, Laudano E, Allen M, et al. The King-Devick test and sports-related concussion: study of a rapid visual screening tool in a collegiate cohort. *J Neurol Sci* 2011;**309**(1-2):34—9.
64. Galetta KM, Morganroth J, Moehringer N, Mueller B, Hasanaj L, Webb N, et al. Adding vision to concussion testing: a prospective study of sideline testing in youth and collegiate athletes. *J Neuroophthalmol* 2015;**35**(3):235—41.
65. Galetta MS, Galetta KM, McCrossin J, Wilson JA, Moster S, Galetta SL, et al. Saccades and memory: baseline associations of the King-Devick and SCAT2 SAC tests in professional ice hockey players. *J Neurol Sci* 2013;**328**(1-2):28—31.
66. Walsh DV, Capó-Aponte JE, Beltran T, Cole WR, Ballard A, Dumayas JY. Assessment of the King-Devick® (KD) test for screening acute mTBI/concussion in warfighters. *J Neurol Sci* 2016;**370**:305—9.
67. Ventura RE, Balcer LJ, Galetta SL. The neuro-ophthalmology of head trauma. *Lancet Neurol* 2014;**13**(10):1006—16.
68. Termsarasab P, Thammongkolchai T, Rucker JC, Frucht SJ. The diagnostic value of saccades in movement disorder patients: a practical guide and review. *J Clin Mov Disord* 2015;**2**:14.
69. Padula WVSE, Vicci V, Munitz R, Magrun WM. *Evaluating and treating visual dysfunction, Chapter 45. Brain Injury Medicine.* 2nd ed. New York: Demos Medical Publishing; 2013.
70. Ventura RE, Balcer LJ, Galetta SL. The concussion toolbox: the role of vision in the assessment of concussion. *Semin Neurol* 2015;**35**(5):599—606.
71. Ventura RE, Balcer LJ, Galetta SL, Rucker JC. Ocular motor assessment in concussion: current status and future directions. *J Neurol Sci* 2016;**361**:79—86.
72. Kravitz DJ, Saleem KS, Baker CI, Mishkin M. A new neural framework for visuospatial processing. *Nat Rev Neurosci* 2011;**12**(4):217—30.
73. Padula WV, Capo-Aponte JE, Padula WV, Singman EL, Jenness J. The consequence of spatial visual processing dysfunction caused by traumatic brain injury (TBI). *Brain Inj* 2017;**31**(5):589—600.
74. Sheth BR, Young R. Two visual pathways in primates based on sampling of space: exploitation and exploration of visual information. *Front Integr Neurosci* 2016;**10**:37.
75. Huang MX, Harrington DL, Robb Swan A, Angeles Quinto A, Nichols S, Drake A, et al. Resting-state magnetoencephalography reveals different patterns of aberrant functional connectivity in combat-related mild traumatic brain injury. *J Neurotrauma* 2017;**34**(7):1412—26.
76. Diwakar M, Harrington DL, Maruta J, Ghajar J, El-Gabalawy F, Muzzatti L, et al. Filling in the gaps: anticipatory control of eye movements in chronic mild traumatic brain injury. *Neuroimage Clin* 2015;**8**:210—23.

77. Dimitriadis SI, Zouridakis G, Rezaie R, Babajani-Feremi A, Papanicolaou AC. Functional connectivity changes detected with magnetoencephalography after mild traumatic brain injury. *Neuroimage Clin* 2015;**9**:519–31.

78. Laatsch L. The use of functional MRI in traumatic brain injury diagnosis and treatment. *Phys Med Rehabil Clin N Am* 2007;**18**(1):69–85.

79. Han KCS, Krawczyk DC. Disrupted intrinsic connectivity among default, dorsal attention, and frontoparietal control networks in individuals with chronic traumatic brain injury. *J Int Neuropsychol Soc* 2016;**22**(2):269–73.

80. Padula WV, Argyris S, Ray J. Visual evoked potentials (VEP) evaluating treatment for post-trauma vision syndrome (PTVS) in patients with traumatic brain injuries (TBI). *Brain Inj* 1994;**8**(2):125–33.

81. Thakkar KN, van den Heiligenberg FM, Kahn RS, Neggers SF. Speed of saccade execution and inhibition associated with fractional anisotropy in distinct fronto-frontal and fronto-striatal white matter pathways. *Hum Brain Mapp* 2016;**37**(8):2811–22.

82. Wallace EJ, Mathias JL, Ward L. Diffusion tensor imaging changes following mild, moderate and severe adult traumatic brain injury: a meta-analysis. *Brain Imaging Behav* 2018. Available from: < https://doi.org/ 10.1007/s11682-018-9823-2 >; [accessed 31.08.18].

83. Clough M, Mutimer S, Wright DK, Tsang A, Costello DM, Gardner AJ, et al. Oculomotor cognitive control abnormalities in australian rules football players with a history of concussion. *J Neurotrauma* 2018;**35** (5):730–8.

84. Supplementary video demonstrating testing of saccades; the neuro-ophthalmology of concussion. Provided in Ventura RE, Balcer LJ, Galetta SL. The neuro-ophthalmology of head trauma. *Lancet Neurol* 2014;**13**:1006–16.   <http://www.thelancet.com/cms/attachment/2018355895/2038564250/mmc1.mp4> [accessed 31.08.18].

85. Pillai C, Gittinger JW. Vision testing in the evaluation of concussion. *Semin Ophthalmol* 2017;**32**(1):144–52.

86. Ventura RE, Jancuska JM, Balcer LJ, Galetta SL. Diagnostic tests for concussion: is vision part of the puzzle? *J Neuroophthalmol* 2015;**35**(1):73–81.

87. Weise KK, Swanson MW, Penix K, Hale MH, Ferguson D. King-Devick and pre-season visual function in adolescent athletes. *Optom Vis Sci* 2017;**94**(1):89–95.

88. Saccadometer. <http://www.ober-consulting.com/11/lang/1/>.

89. Mullen SJ, Yucel YH, Cusimano M, Schweizer TA, Oentoro A, Gupta N. Saccadic eye movements in mild traumatic brain injury: a pilot study. *Can J Neurol Sci* 2014;**41**(1):58–65.

90. Tassinari JT, DeLand P. Developmental eye movement test: reliability and symptomatology. *Optometry* 2005;**76**(7):387–99.

91. Weaver MD, Hickey C, van Zoest W. The impact of salience and visual working memory on the monitoring and control of saccadic behavior: an eye-tracking and EEG study. *Psychophysiology* 2017;**54**(4):544–54.

92. Kulp MT, Edwards KE, Mitchell GL. Is visual memory predictive of below-average academic achievement in second through fourth graders? *Optom Vis Sci* 2002;**79**(7):431–4.

93. Palomo-Alvarez C, Puell MC. Relationship between oculomotor scanning determined by the DEM test and a contextual reading test in schoolchildren with reading difficulties. *Graefes Arch Clin Exp Ophthalmol* 2009;**247** (9):1243–9.

94. Raz S, Dan O. Behavioral and neural correlates of facial versus nonfacial stimuli processing in adults with ADHD: an ERP study. *Neuropsychology* 2015;**29**(5):726–38.

95. Hale TS, Kane AM, Kaminsky O, Tung KL, Wiley JF, McGough JJ, et al. Visual network asymmetry and default mode network function in ADHD: an fMRI study. *Front Psychiatry* 2014;**5**:81.

96. Koller HP. Visual processing and learning disorders. *Curr Opin Ophthalmol* 2012;**23**(5):377–83.

97. Marzinzik F, Wahl M, Kruger D, Gentschow L, Colla M, Klostermann F. Abnormal distracter processing in adults with attention-deficit-hyperactivity disorder. *PLoS One* 2012;**7**(3):e33691.

98. Adeyemo BO, Biederman J, Zafonte R, Kagan E, Spencer TJ, Uchida M, et al. Mild traumatic brain injury and ADHD: a systematic review of the literature and meta-analysis. *J Atten Disord* 2014;**18**(7):576–84.

99. Keenan HT, Clark AE, Holubkov R, Cox CS, Ewing-Cobbs L. Psychosocial and executive function recovery trajectories one year after pediatric traumatic brain injury: the influence of age and injury severity. *J Neurotrauma* 2018;**35**(2):286–96.

100. Yang LY, Huang CC, Chiu WT, Huang LT, Lo WC, Wang JY. Association of traumatic brain injury in childhood and attention-deficit/hyperactivity disorder: a population-based study. *Pediatr Res* 2016;**80**(3):356–62.

101. Bonfield CM, Lam S, Lin Y, Greene S. The impact of attention deficit hyperactivity disorder on recovery from mild traumatic brain injury. *J Neurosurg Pediatr* 2013;**12**(2):97–102.

102. Biederman J, Feinberg L, Chan J, Adeyemo BO, Woodworth KY, Panis W, et al. Mild traumatic brain injury and attention-deficit hyperactivity disorder in young student athletes. *J Nerv Ment Dis* 2015;**203**(11):813–19.

103. Alosco ML, Fedor AF, Gunstad J. Attention deficit hyperactivity disorder as a risk factor for concussions in NCAA division-I athletes. *Brain Inj* 2014;**28**(4):472–4.

104. Lee YJ, Lee S, Chang M, Kwak HW. Saccadic movement deficiencies in adults with ADHD tendencies. *Atten Defic Hyperact Disord* 2015;**7**(4):271–80.

105. Fried M, Tsitsiashvili E, Bonneh YS, Sterkin A, Wygnanski-Jaffe T, Epstein T, et al. ADHD subjects fail to suppress eye blinks and microsaccades while anticipating visual stimuli but recover with medication. *Vision Res* 2014;**101**:62–72.

106. Damyanovich EV, Baziyan B, Sagalov MV, Kumskova GA. Saccadic movements of the eyes in children with attention deficit and hyperactivity syndrome. *Bull Exp Biol Med* 2013;**156**(1):25–8.

107. Versino M, Cosi V. Quantitative evaluation of smooth pursuit eye movements by personal computer. (I) Normative data and effect of aging. *Boll Soc Ital Biol Sper* 1990;**66**(7):701–8.

108. Gibaldi A, Vanegas M, Bex PJ, Maiello G. Evaluation of the Tobii EyeX Eye tracking controller and Matlab toolkit for research. *Behav Res Methods* 2017;**49**(3):923–46.

109. Mele ML, Federici S. Gaze and eye-tracking solutions for psychological research. *Cogn Process* 2012;**13**(Suppl 1):S261–5.

110. Meyer CH, Lasker AG, Robinson DA. The upper limit of human smooth pursuit velocity. *Vision Res* 1985;**25**(4):561–3.

111. Seferlis F, Chimona TS, Papadakis CE, Bizakis J, Triaridis S, Skoulakis C. Age related changes in ocular motor testing in healthy subjects. *J Vestib Res* 2015;**25**(2):57–66.

112. Suh M, Kolster R, Sarkar R, McCandliss B, Ghajar J. Cognitive, neurobiological research C: deficits in predictive smooth pursuit after mild traumatic brain injury. *Neurosci Lett* 2006;**401**(1–2):108–13.

113. Cifu DX, Wares JR, Hoke KW, Wetzel PA, Gitchel G, Carne W. Differential eye movements in mild traumatic brain injury versus normal controls. *J Head Trauma Rehabil* 2015;**30**(1):21–8.

114. Liston DB, Wong LR, Stone LS. Oculometric assessment of sensorimotor impairment associated with TBI. *Optom Vis Sci* 2017;**94**(1):51–9.

115. DiCesare CA, Kiefer AW, Nalepka P, Myer GD. Quantification and analysis of saccadic and smooth pursuit eye movements and fixations to detect oculomotor deficits. *Behav Res Methods* 2017;**49**(1):258–66.

116. Lencer R, Trillenberg P. Neurophysiology and neuroanatomy of smooth pursuit in humans. *Brain Cogn* 2008;**68**(3):219–28.

117. Johnson B, Zhang K, Hallett M, Slobounov S. Functional neuroimaging of acute oculomotor deficits in concussed athletes. *Brain Imaging Behav* 2015;**9**(3):564–73.

118. Gorges M, Maier MN, Rosskopf J, Vintonyak O, Pinkhardt EH, Ludolph AC, et al. Regional microstructural damage and patterns of eye movement impairment: a DTI and video-oculography study in neurodegenerative parkinsonian syndromes. *J Neurol* 2017;**264**(9):1919–28.

119. Anzalone AJ, Blueitt D, Case T, McGuffin T, Pollard K, Garrison JC, et al. A positive vestibular/ocular motor screening (VOMS) is associated with increased recovery time after sports-related concussion in youth and adolescent athletes. *Am J Sports Med* 2017;**45**(2):474–9.

120. Paige GD. Vestibuloocular reflex and its interactions with visual following mechanisms in the squirrel monkey. II. Response characteristics and plasticity following unilateral inactivation of horizontal canal. *J Neurophysiol* 1983;**49**(1):152–68.

121. Fetter M, Zee DS, Proctor LR. Effect of lack of vision and of occipital lobectomy upon recovery from unilateral labyrinthectomy in rhesus monkey. *J Neurophysiol* 1988;**59**(2):394–407.

122. Kirsch V, Keeser D, Hergenroeder T, Erat O, Ertl-Wagner B, Brandt T, et al. Structural and functional connectivity mapping of the vestibular circuitry from human brainstem to cortex. *Brain Struct Funct* 2016;**221**(3):1291–308.

123. Alhilali LM, Yaeger K, Collins M, Fakhran S. Detection of central white matter injury underlying vestibulopathy after mild traumatic brain injury. *Radiology* 2014;**272**(1):224–32.

124. Gattu R, Akin FW, Cacace AT, Hall CD, Murnane OD, Haacke EM. Vestibular, balance, microvascular and white matter neuroimaging characteristics of blast injuries and mild traumatic brain injury: four case reports. *Brain Inj* 2016;**30**(12):1501—14.

125. Mendez MF, Owens EM, Reza Berenji G, Peppers DC, Liang LJ, Licht EA. Mild traumatic brain injury from primary blast vs. blunt forces: post-concussion consequences and functional neuroimaging. *Neuro Rehabilitation* 2013;**32**(2):397—407.

126. Mu W, Catenaccio E, Lipton ML. Neuroimaging in blast-related mild traumatic brain injury. *J Head Trauma Rehabil* 2017;**32**(1):55—69.

127. Greer N, Sayer N, Koeller E, Velasquez T, Wilt TJ. Outcomes associated with blast versus nonblast-related traumatic brain injury in us military service members and veterans: a systematic review. *J Head Trauma Rehabil* 2018;**33**(2):E16—29.

128. Gonzalez CC, Billington J, Burke MR. The involvement of the fronto-parietal brain network in oculomotor sequence learning using fMRI. *Neuropsychologia* 2016;**87**:1—11.

129. Gargouri-Berrechid A, Lanouar L, Kacem I, Ben Djebara M, Hizem Y, Zaouchi N, et al. Eye movement recordings in children with attention deficit hyperactivity disorder. *J Fr Ophtalmol* 2012;**35**(7):503—7.

130. Ross RG, Olincy A, Harris JG, Sullivan B, Radant A. Smooth pursuit eye movements in schizophrenia and attentional dysfunction: adults with schizophrenia, ADHD, and a normal comparison group. *Biol Psychiatry* 2000;**48**(3):197—203.

131. Jacobsen LK, Hong WL, Hommer DW, Hamburger SD, Castellanos FX, Frazier JA, et al. Smooth pursuit eye movements in childhood-onset schizophrenia: comparison with attention-deficit hyperactivity disorder and normal controls. *Biol Psychiatry* 1996;**40**(11):1144—54.

132. Weinacht S, Kind C, Monting JS, Gottlob I. Visual development in preterm and full-term infants: a prospective masked study. *Invest Ophthalmol Vis Sci* 1999;**40**(2):346—53.

133. Jimenez R, Perez MA, Garcia JA, Gonzalez MD. Statistical normal values of visual parameters that characterize binocular function in children. *Ophthalmic Physiol Opt* 2004;**24**(6):528—42.

134. Qing Y, Kapoula Z. Saccade-vergence dynamics and interaction in children and in adults. *Exp Brain Res* 2004;**156**(2):212—23.

135. Winn B, Gilmartin B, Sculfor DL, Bamford JC. Vergence adaptation and senescence. *Optom Vis Sci* 1994;**71**(12):797—800.

136. Vernau BT, Grady MF, Goodman A, Wiebe DJ, Basta L, Park Y, et al. Oculomotor and neurocognitive assessment of youth ice hockey players: baseline associations and observations after concussion. *Dev Neuropsychol* 2015;**40**(1):7—11.

137. Granet DB, Gomi CF, Ventura R, Miller-Scholte A. The relationship between convergence insufficiency and ADHD. *Strabismus* 2005;**13**(4):163—8.

138. Mezer E, Wygnanski-Jaffe T. Do children and adolescents with attention deficit hyperactivity disorder have ocular abnormalities? *Eur J Ophthalmol* 2012;**22**(6):931—5.

139. Borsting E, Rouse M, Chu R. Measuring ADHD behaviors in children with symptomatic accommodative dysfunction or convergence insufficiency: a preliminary study. *Optometry* 2005;**76**(10):588—92.

140. Lovell M, Collins M, Bradley J. Return to play following sports-related concussion. *Clin Sports Med* 2004;**23**(3):421—41.

141. Daniel F, Morize A, Bremond-Gignac D, Kapoula Z. Benefits from vergence rehabilitation: evidence for improvement of reading saccades and fixations. *Front Integr Neurosci* 2016;**10**:33.

142. Gamlin PD. Neural mechanisms for the control of vergence eye movements. *Ann N Y Acad Sci* 2002;**956**:264—72.

143. Trotter Y, Celebrini S, Stricanne B, Thorpe S, Imbert M. Neural processing of stereopsis as a function of viewing distance in primate visual cortical area V1. *J Neurophysiol* 1996;**76**(5):2872—85.

144. Takemura A, Inoue Y, Kawano K, Quaia C, Miles FA. Single-unit activity in cortical area MST associated with disparity-vergence eye movements: evidence for population coding. *J Neurophysiol* 2001;**85**(5):2245—66.

145. Thiagarajan P, Ciuffreda KJ, Ludlam DP. Vergence dysfunction in mild traumatic brain injury (mTBI): a review. *Ophthalmic Physiol Opt* 2011;**31**(5):456—68.

146. Richter HO, Costello P, Sponheim SR, Lee JT, Pardo JV. Functional neuroanatomy of the human near/far response to blur cues: eye-lens accommodation/vergence to point targets varying in depth. *Eur J Neurosci* 2004;**20**(10):2722—32.

147. Hickenbotham A, Roorda A, Steinmaus C, Glasser A. Meta-analysis of sex differences in presbyopia. *Invest Ophthalmol Vis Sci* 2012;**53**(6):3215−20.

148. Charman WN. The eye in focus: accommodation and presbyopia. *Clin Exp Optom* 2008;**91**(3):207−25.

149. Richdale K, Sinnott LT, Bullimore MA, Wassenaar PA, Schmalbrock P, Kao CY, et al. Quantification of age-related and per diopter accommodative changes of the lens and ciliary muscle in the emmetropic human eye. *Invest Ophthalmol Vis Sci* 2013;**54**(2):1095−105.

150. Green W, Ciuffreda KJ, Thiagarajan P, Szymanowicz D, Ludlam DP, Kapoor N. Accommodation in mild traumatic brain injury. *J Rehabil Res Dev* 2010;**47**(3):183−99.

151. Poltavski DV, Biberdorf D, Petros TV. Accommodative response and cortical activity during sustained attention. *Vision Res* 2012;**63**:1−8.

152. Chan RV, Trobe JD. Spasm of accommodation associated with closed head trauma. *J Neuroophthalmol* 2002;**22**(1):15−17.

153. Bohlmann BJ, France TD. Persistent accommodative spasm nine years after head trauma. *J Clin Neuroophthalmol* 1987;**7**(3):129−34.

154. Yadav NK, Thiagarajan P, Ciuffreda KJ. Effect of oculomotor vision rehabilitation on the visual-evoked potential and visual attention in mild traumatic brain injury. *Brain Inj* 2014;**28**(7):922−9.

155. Convergence Insufficiency Treatment Trial Study G. The convergence insufficiency treatment trial: design, methods, and baseline data. *Ophthalmic Epidemiol* 2008;**15**(1):24−36.

156. Scheiman M, Cotter S, Kulp MT, Mitchell GL, Cooper J, Gallaway M, et al. Convergence insufficiency treatment trial study G: treatment of accommodative dysfunction in children: results from a randomized clinical trial. *Optom Vis Sci* 2011;**88**(11):1343−52.

157. Candy TR, Gray KH, Hohenbary CC, Lyon DW. The accommodative lag of the young hyperopic patient. *Invest Ophthalmol Vis Sci* 2012;**53**(1):143−9.

158. Yekta A, Khabazkhoob M, Hashemi H, Ostadimoghaddam H, Ghasemi-Moghaddam S, Heravian J, et al. Binocular and accommodative characteristics in a normal population. *Strabismus* 2017;**25**(1):5−11.

159. Zellers JA, Alpert TL, Rouse MW. A review of the literature and a normative study of accommodative facility. *J Am Optom Assoc* 1984;**55**(1):31 7.

160. Hofstetter HW. A longitudinal study of amplitude changes in presbyopia. *Am J Optom Arch Am Acad Optom* 1965;**42**:3−8.

161. Schmidtmann G, Ruiz T, Reynaud A, Spiegel DP, Lague-Beauvais M, Hess RF, et al. Sensitivity to binocular disparity is reduced by mild traumatic brain injury. *Invest Ophthalmol Vis Sci* 2017;**58**(5):2630−5.

162. Jaschinski W. Individual objective and subjective fixation disparity in near vision. *PLoS One* 2017;**12**(1): e0170190.

163. Pickwell LD, Gilchrist JM, Hesler J. Comparison of associated heterophoria measurements using the Mallett test for near vision and the Sheedy Disparometer. *Ophthalmic Physiol Opt* 1988;**8**(1):19−25.

164. Kromeier M, Schmitt C, Bach M, Kommerell G. Comparison between dissociated and associated heterophoria. *Ophthalmologe* 2002;**99**(7):549−54.

165. Pickwell LD, Kaye NA, Jenkins TC. Distance and near readings of associated heterophoria taken on 500 patients. *Ophthalmic Physiol Opt* 1991;**11**(4):291−6.

166. Park J, Oh H, Lee S, Bovik AC. 3D visual discomfort predictor: analysis of horizontal disparity and neural activity statistics. *IEEE Trans Image Process* 2015;**24**(3):1101−14.

167. Doble JE, Feinberg DL, Rosner MS, Rosner AJ. Identification of binocular vision dysfunction (vertical heterophoria) in traumatic brain injury patients and effects of individualized prismatic spectacle lenses in the treatment of postconcussive symptoms: a retrospective analysis. *Phys Med Rehabil* 2010;**2**(4):244−53.

168. Rosner MS, Feinberg DL, Doble JE, Rosner AJ. Treatment of vertical heterophoria ameliorates persistent post-concussive symptoms: a retrospective analysis utilizing a multi-faceted assessment battery. *Brain Inj* 2016;**30**(3):311−17.

169. van Haeringen R, McClurg P, Cameron KD. Comparison of Wesson and modified Sheedy fixation disparity tests. Do fixation disparity measures relate to normal binocular status? *Ophthalmic Physiol Opt* 1986;**6** (4):397−400.

170. Howard IPRB. *Binocular vision and stereopsis*. New York: Oxford University Press; 1995.

171. A comparison of three tests of stereoacuity. <http://www.paulharrisod.com/sites/default/files/2015_ AAO_Harris_3.pdf>.

172. Piano ME, Tidbury LP, O'Connor AR. Normative values for near and distance clinical tests of stereoacuity. *Strabismus* 2016;**24**(4):169–72.
173. Momeni-Moghaddam H, Goss DA, Dehvari A. Vergence facility with stereoscopic and nonstereoscopic targets. *Optom Vis Sci* 2014;**91**(5):522–7.
174. Wardle SG, Bex PJ, Cass J, Alais D. Stereoacuity in the periphery is limited by internal noise. *J Vis* 2012;**12**(6):12.
175. Wang F, Yang W, Zhang L, Gundran A, Zhu X, Liu J, et al. Brain activation difference evoked by different binocular disparities of stereograms: an fMRI study. *Phys Med* 2016;**32**(10):1308–13.
176. Hellerstein LF, Freed S, Maples WC. Vision profile of patients with mild brain injury. *J Am Optom Assoc* 1995;**66**(10):634–9.
177. Ciuffreda KJ, Yadav NK, Han E, Ludlam DP, Peddle A, Hulse P, et al. Distance perception in mild traumatic brain injury (mTBI). *Optometry* 2012;**83**(4):127–36.
178. Steinhorst U, Haase W, Alten C. Post-concussion decrease in aniseikonia tolerance. *Klin Monbl Augenheilkd* 1990;**197**(5):436–7.
179. Gilmore CS, Camchong J, Davenport ND, Nelson NW, Kardon RH, Lim KO, et al. Deficits in visual system functional connectivity after blast-related mild TBI are associated with injury severity and executive dysfunction. *Brain Behav* 2016;**6**(5):e00454.
180. Yang SN, Schlieski T, Selmins B, Cooper SC, Doherty RA, Corriveau PJ, et al. Stereoscopic viewing and reported perceived immersion and symptoms. *Optom Vis Sci* 2012;**89**(7):1068–80.
181. Read JC, Bohr I. User experience while viewing stereoscopic 3D television. *Ergonomics* 2014;**57**(8):1140–53.
182. Solimini AG. Are there side effects to watching 3D movies? A prospective crossover observational study on visually induced motion sickness. *PLoS One* 2013;**8**(2):e56160.
183. Kim S, Chen S, Tannock R. Visual function and color vision in adults with attention-deficit/hyperactivity disorder. *J Optom* 2014;**7**(1):22–36.
184. Gronlund MA, Aring E, Landgren M, Hellstrom A. Visual function and ocular features in children and adolescents with attention deficit hyperactivity disorder, with and without treatment with stimulants. *Eye (Lond)* 2007;**21**(4):494–502.
185. Chang HC, Grossberg S, Cao Y. Where's Waldo? How perceptual, cognitive, and emotional brain processes cooperate during learning to categorize and find desired objects in a cluttered scene. *Front Integr Neurosci* 2014;**8**:43.
186. Smirl JD, Wright AD, Bryk K, van Donkelaar P. Where's Waldo? The utility of a complicated visual search paradigm for transcranial Doppler-based assessments of neurovascular coupling. *J Neurosci Methods* 2016;**270**:92–101.
187. Konigs M, Heij HA, van der Sluijs JA, Vermeulen RJ, Goslings JC, Luitse JS, et al. Pediatric traumatic brain injury and attention deficit. *Pediatrics* 2015;**136**(3):534–41.
188. Konigs M, Weeda WD, van Heurn LW, Vermeulen RJ, Goslings JC, Luitse JS, et al. Pediatric traumatic brain injury affects multisensory integration. *Neuropsychology* 2017;**31**(2):137–48.
189. Lachapelle J, Bolduc-Teasdale J, Ptito A, McKerral M. Deficits in complex visual information processing after mild TBI: electrophysiological markers and vocational outcome prognosis. *Brain Inj* 2008;**22**(3):265–74.
190. McKay A, Liew C, Schonberger M, Ross P, Ponsford J. Predictors of the on-road driving assessment after traumatic brain injury: comparing cognitive tests, injury factors, and demographics. *J Head Trauma Rehabil* 2016;**31**(6):E44–52.
191. Tegelbeckers J, Bunzeck N, Duzel E, Bonath B, Flechtner HH, Krauel K. Altered salience processing in attention deficit hyperactivity disorder. *Hum Brain Mapp* 2015;**36**(6):2049–60.
192. Leroy A, Petit G, Zarka D, Cebolla AM, Palmero-Soler E, Strul J, et al. EEG dynamics and neural generators in implicit navigational image processing in adults with ADHD. *Neuroscience* 2018;**373**:92–105.
193. Webster B. Lost & Found: A survivor's guide for reconstructing life after brain injury. Lash & Associates/Training, Inc.; 2011. ISBN#978-1-931117-61-6.
194. Wang Y, West JD, Bailey JN, Westfall DR, Xiao H, Arnold TW, et al. Decreased cerebral blood flow in chronic pediatric mild TBI: an MRI perfusion study. *Dev Neuropsychol* 2015;**40**(1):40–4.
195. Romero K, Lobaugh NJ, Black SE, Ehrlich L, Feinstein A. Old wine in new bottles: validating the clinical utility of SPECT in predicting cognitive performance in mild traumatic brain injury. *Psychiatry Res* 2015;**231**(1):15–24.

196. Bartnik-Olson BL, Holshouser B, Wang H, Grube M, Tong K, Wong V, et al. Impaired neurovascular unit function contributes to persistent symptoms after concussion: a pilot study. *J Neurotrauma* 2014;**31** (17):1497−506.

197. Liu W, Wang B, Wolfowitz R, Yeh PH, Nathan DE, Graner J, et al. Perfusion deficits in patients with mild traumatic brain injury characterized by dynamic susceptibility contrast MRI. *NMR Biomed* 2013;**26**(6):651−63.

198. Azzopardi P, Jones KE, Cowey A. Uneven mapping of magnocellular and parvocellular projections from the lateral geniculate nucleus to the striate cortex in the macaque monkey. *Vision Res* 1999;**39**(13):2179−89.

199. Koch C, Wang HT, Mathur B. Computing motion in the primate's visual system. *J Exp Biol* 1989;**146**:115−39.

200. Purpura K, Kaplan E, Shapley RM. Background light and the contrast gain of primate P and M retinal ganglion cells. *Proc Natl Acad Sci USA* 1988;**85**(12):4534−7.

201. Digre KB, Brennan KC. Shedding light on photophobia. *J Neuroophthalmol* 2012;**32**(1):68−81.

202. Layton OW, Mingolla E, Yazdanbakhsh A. Neural dynamics of feedforward and feedback processing in figure-ground segregation. *Front Psychol* 2014;**5**:972.

203. von der Heydt R. Figure-ground organization and the emergence of proto-objects in the visual cortex. *Front Psychol* 2015;**6**:1695.

204. Gilad A, Pesoa Y, Ayzenshtat I, Slovin H. Figure-ground processing during fixational saccades in V1: indication for higher-order stability. *J Neurosci* 2014;**34**(9):3247−52.

205. Cha O, Chong SC. The background is remapped across saccades. *Exp Brain Res* 2014;**232**(2):609−18.

206. Super H. Figure-ground activity in V1 and guidance of saccadic eye movements. *J Physiol Paris* 2006;**100** (1−3):63−9.

207. Cate Y, Richards L. Relationship between performance on tests of basic visual functions and visual-perceptual processing in persons after brain injury. *Am J Occup Ther* 2000;**54**(3):326−34.

208. Baylis GC, Baylis LL. Deficit in figure-ground segmentation following closed head injury. *Neuropsychologia* 1997;**35**(8):1133−8.

209. Rudolph K, Pasternak T. Transient and permanent deficits in motion perception after lesions of cortical areas MT and MST in the macaque monkey. *Cereb Cortex* 1999;**9**(1):90−100.

210. Padula WV, Argyris S. Post trauma vision syndrome and visual midline shift syndrome. *NeuroRehabilitation* 1996;**6**(3):165−71.

211. Padula WV, Nelson CA, Padula WV, Benabib R, Yilmaz T, Krevisky S. Modifying postural adaptation following a CVA through prismatic shift of visuo-spatial egocenter. *Brain Inj* 2009;**23**(6):566−76.

212. Padula WV, Subramanian P, Spurling A, Jenness J. Risk of fall (RoF) intervention by affecting visual egocenter through gait analysis and yoked prisms. *NeuroRehabilitation* 2015;**37**(2):305−14.

213. Lamontagne A, Paquet N, Fung J. Postural adjustments to voluntary head motions during standing are modified following stroke. *Clin Biomech (Bristol, Avon)* 2003;**18**(9):832−42.

214. Sosnoff JJ, Broglio SP, Shin S, Ferrara MS. Previous mild traumatic brain injury and postural-control dynamics. *J Athl Train* 2011;**46**(1):85−91.

215. Wares JR, Hoke KW, Walker W, Franke LM, Cifu DX, Carne W, et al. Characterizing effects of mild traumatic brain injury and posttraumatic stress disorder on balance impairments in blast-exposed servicemembers and Veterans using computerized posturography. *J Rehabil Res Dev* 2015;**52**(5):591−603.

216. Robey JH, Boyle K. The role of prism glass and postural restoration in managing a collegiate baseball player with bilateral sacroiliac joint dysfunction: a case report. *Int J Sports Phys Ther* 2013;**8**(5):716−28.

217. Balaban CD, Hoffer ME, Gottshall KR. Top-down approach to vestibular compensation: translational lessons from vestibular rehabilitation. *Brain Res* 2012;**1482**:101−11.

218. Kaski D, Buttell J, Greenwood R. Targeted rehabilitation reduces visual dependency and improves balance in severe traumatic brain injury: a case study. *Disabil Rehabil* 2018;**40**(7):856−8.

219. Mantokoudis G, Saber Tehrani AS, Wozniak A, Eibenberger K, Kattah JC, Guede CI, et al. Impact of artifacts on VOR gain measures by video-oculography in the acute vestibular syndrome. *J Vestib Res* 2016;**26** (4):375−85.

220. Herdman SJCR. *Vestibular rehabilitation*. 4th ed. Philadelphia, PA: FA Davis Company; 2014.

221. Mucha A, Collins MW, Elbin RJ, Furman JM, Troutman-Enseki C, DeWolf RM, et al. A Brief Vestibular/Ocular Motor Screening (VOMS) assessment to evaluate concussions: preliminary findings. *Am J Sports Med* 2014;**42**(10):2479−86.

222. Anderson M, Anderson M, Dobbs E, Elbin RJ, Shatz P. Baseline normative data of the vestibular/ocular motor screening (voms) assessment for high school athletes: 1909 Board #61 June 2, 2: 00 PM - 3: 30 PM. *Med Sci Sports Exerc* 2016;**48**(5 Suppl 1):526.
223. Kontos AP, Sufrinko A, Elbin RJ, Puskar A, Collins MW. Reliability and associated risk factors for performance on the vestibular/ocular motor screening (VOMS) tool in healthy collegiate athletes. *Am J Sports Med* 2016;**44**(6):1400−6.
224. Yorke AM, Smith L, Babcock M, Alsalaheen B. Validity and reliability of the vestibular/ocular motor screening and associations with common concussion screening tools. *Sports Health* 2017;**9**(2):174−80.
225. Sufrinko AM, Marchetti GF, Cohen PE, Elbin RJ, Re V, Kontos AP. Using acute performance on a comprehensive neurocognitive, vestibular, and ocular motor assessment battery to predict recovery duration after sport-related concussions. *Am J Sports Med* 2017;**45**(5):1187−94.
226. Rouse M, Borsting E, Mitchell GL, Cotter SA, Kulp M, Scheiman M, et al. Convergence insufficiency treatment trial investigator G: validity of the convergence insufficiency symptom survey: a confirmatory study. *Optom Vis Sci* 2009;**86**(4):357−63.
227. Momeni-Moghaddam H, Goss DA, Sobhani M. Accommodative response under monocular and binocular conditions as a function of phoria in symptomatic and asymptomatic subjects. *Clin Exp Optom* 2014;**97**(1):36−42.
228. Horan LA, Ticho BH, Khammar AJ, Allen MS, Shah BA. Is the convergence insufficiency symptom survey specific for convergence insufficiency? A prospective, randomized study. *Am Orthopt J* 2015;**65**:99−103.
229. Horwood AM, Toor S, Riddell PM. Screening for convergence insufficiency using the CISS is not indicated in young adults. *Br J Ophthalmol* 2014;**98**(5):679−83.
230. Goodrich GL, Martinsen GL, Flyg HM, Kirby J, Asch SM, Brahm KD, et al. Development of a mild traumatic brain injury-specific vision screening protocol: a Delphi study. *J Rehabil Res Dev* 2013;**50**(6):757−68.
231. ICD-10 Version 2016. <http://apps.who.int/classifications/icd10/browse/2016/en>.
232. Singman EL, Daphalapurkar N, White H, Nguyen TD, Panghat L, Chang J, et al. Indirect traumatic optic neuropathy. *Mil Med Res* 2016;**3**:2.
233. Papa L, Edwards D, Ramia M. Exploring serum biomarkers for mild traumatic brain injury. In: Kobeissy FH, editor. Brain neurotrauma: molecular, neuropsychological, and rehabilitation *aspects*. Boca Raton, FL: CRC Press; 2015.
234. McMahon P, Hricik A, Yue JK, Puccio AM, Inoue T, Lingsma HF, et al. Symptomatology and functional outcome in mild traumatic brain injury: results from the prospective TRACK-TBI study. *J Neurotrauma* 2014;**31**(1):26−33.

DIAGNOSIS
AND TREATMENT

Diagnostic Approaches Techniques in Concussion/Mild Traumatic Brain Injury: Where are we?

Rebecca Smith, Mariya Chepisheva,
Thomas Cronin, PhD and Barry M. Seemungal

Department of Medicine, Imperial College, London, United Kingdom

INTRODUCTION

Currently, sporting body consensus criteria consider concussion to be a mild traumatic brain injury (mTBI), which is indicated by a transient mental obtundation.[1] Acute concussion diagnosis, thus, relies upon first-hand observation of the impact and the effect upon the patient (or recorded video), and clinical assessment including clinical history and examination. The diagnosis of a concussion can be difficult if there are no witnesses. Additionally, the inability of the patient to provide a clear account of the circumstances of the injury can make the diagnostic process more challenging, and on the other hand, is suggestive of a retrospective amnesia and, hence, supportive of a concussion. However, the converse may not be true, since some patients may provide a clear history of no concussion, but display objective signs of momentary mental obtundation, not recalled by the patient. Thus, since a concussion diagnosis by patient history is problematic, diagnosis should rely upon objective measures, including third-person witness account, clinical examination, and laboratory testing. We review the different means to make a diagnosis of concussion.

The Clinical Approach

Clinical testing is a vital tool in establishing new or ongoing impairments secondary to concussion. There are a plethora of bedside diagnostic techniques, some of which

Neurosensory Disorders in Mild Traumatic Brain Injury
DOI: https://doi.org/10.1016/B978-0-12-812344-7.00016-9

require little or no equipment and can provide helpful clues detail regarding potential areas of injury.[2,3]

How Important is a Subjective History?

Typically, diagnosis in related fields of neurology and neuro-otology rely heavily upon a detailed subjective history to define symptoms and, hence, explore differential diagnoses. Particular attention is given to the frequency, nature and severity of symptoms. However, in acute concussion, paying close attention to symptoms may confuse the clinician. For example, the patient may not complain of symptoms such as imbalance or dizziness, yet objectively may score poorly on clinical vestibular or balance tests. It is, therefore, important that clinicians do not rely solely on patients' subjective complaints. Asking family members or carers separately may help to corroborate any functional deficits.

Subjective Measures: "Symptom Scales"

To provide further detail on the severity and impact of symptoms, patient reported outcome measures (PROMs) can evaluate the impact of impairments on physical and mental health, and patients' ability to carry out activities of daily living. PROMs evaluating specific impairments such as imbalance or dizziness, may include for example, the Activities-specific Balance Confidence Scale (ABC) or Dizziness handicap inventory (DHI), while those evaluating function or the ability to carry out activities of daily living include the Functional Independence Measure (FIM) or Disability Rating Scale (DRS). It is important to consider the psychometric properties of the measure as well as more practical factors including time to administer and ease of use.

More holistic patient reported outcomes include those evaluating quality of life (QOL) or health-related quality of life (HRQOL). Such measures can be useful in monitoring recovery or progress with rehabilitation. Measures of QOL or HRQOL specific to the TBI population include Quality of Life after Brain Injury (QOLIBRI), the European Brain Injury Questionnaire (EBIQ), and the TBI quality of life measurement system (TBI-QOL). Despite relative rigorous evaluation of the psychometric properties of each measure,[4,5] there appears to be no current consensus regarding the most appropriate tool to use. Although a systematic review indicated further work is required to establish the most relevant measure for this population, the authors did recommend the use of a TBI specific measure such as the QOLIBRI in conjunction with a more robust tool such as the Short Form 36 (SF-36).[6]

Bedside Clinical (Objective) Tests

EYE MOVEMENT EXAMINATION

A physical eye movement examination is a critical tool in the assessment of mTBI patients. It serves to evaluate and highlight peripheral and/or central injuries and, thus, acts as an important diagnostic tool.[7] Essential components of the eye movement examination include the cover test, which is performed to ascertain failure of binocular gaze mechanisms including any skew deviation, and gaze assessment for nystagmus in primary and lateral gaze. Smooth pursuit, vergence and extra ocular range of movement can then also be evaluated. Deficits noted in smooth pursuit indicate abnormal brain function ipsilesionally, that is, in the direction of the pursuit deficit, but localizes poorly since lesions from the cerebellum to the cortex can produce impaired smooth pursuit.[8,9] Saccadic hypo- or hypermetria and/or latency should be examined during vertical and horizontal saccades and indicate central dysfunction. Increased latency and/or error rates with antisaccades indicate frontal cortical deficits.

BEDSIDE VESTIBULAR OCULAR REFLEX TESTING

A proportion of patients with acute TBI will display signs of temporal bone transection with injury to the vestibular (and auditory) system; however, this level of injury is not usually found in acute concussion/mTBI, unless a chronic case was misclassified.[10] Hence, it is always sensible to routinely evaluate the vestibular ocular reflex (VOR) using the head thrust test, a high acceleration but low amplitude single jerk movement of the head in a horizontal plane. The patient is instructed to keep their gaze fixed on the clinician. A refixation saccade back to the focus point (lost because of the deficient VOR) indicates a positive result. This test shows high sensitivity in detecting VOR deficits.[11,12] The video head impulse test (vHIT) is able to quantify any high frequency VOR dysfunction. A head mounted camera and inertial sensors simultaneously collect data on head and eye motion, and hence can provide a VOR slow-phase velocity gain with respect to the head motion. Evidence demonstrates high specificity and sensitivity of the vHIT,[13,14] while additional benefits include the ability to measure covert saccades (eye movements not observable to the clinician) and short testing times.[15]

BENIGN PAROXYSMAL POSITIONAL VERTIGO

BBPV is common in acute TBI, causing dizziness, imbalance, and falls, especially in older adults. Posttraumatic benign paroxysmal positional vertigo (BPPV) is thought to be due to mechanical displacement of the otoconia caused by the head trauma itself. Current evidence from retrospective and nonacute cases extrapolate a BPPV incidence in acute TBI patients of 10%−28%[16−18]; however, our experience in acute TBI (patients admitted to a major trauma unit with a moderate-severe brain injury) shows a true BPPV incidence of nearer 50%. TBI patients also appear to have a propensity for more complex variants of the condition, that is, those with multi canal BPPV, requiring multiple treatment sessions with higher rates of recurrence.[19] The Dix Hallpike test is the gold standard test for diagnosis of BPPV,[20] while particle repositioning maneuvers, depending on the BPPV variant, are utilized to treat a positive diagnosis.[20] The incidence of BPPV in mTBI (as opposed to moderate to severe TBI) is, however, unclear.

GAIT AND BALANCE ASSESSMENT

Problems with walking and balance are often detected long after injury. Indeed, the majority of patients with chronic TBI report problems with mobility and balance,[21] unsurprising given higher levels of societal participation and QOL are associated with improved mobility.[22] It is, therefore, vital to assess any deficits in mobility or balance thoroughly.

Bedside examination of mobility can be assessed using simple measures such as gait velocity using a pre-measured walkway and timed using a stopwatch. Indeed, evidence suggests walking speed can be measured accurately and reliably in this manner within the TBI population.[23−25] Deficits in walking speed have been noted previously in the TBI population,[24,26] although the ability to predict recovery or its relationship with functional outcomes such as falls, is currently unknown. Observation of other gait abnormalities, such as kinematic parameters, may be more difficult to quantify at the bedside. In a study by Williams et al., researchers demonstrated low reliability between clinicians when looking for gait kinematics following TBI.[27] However, such gait abnormalities may well be more relevant for those with more severe brain injury.

Measures of mobility and dynamic balance, typically including walking and concurrent tasks such as head movements or changes in gait speed or direction, may also be useful when considering rehabilitation options, and for evaluating patients' safety in accessing the community or returning to work. Such measures can be undertaken with relatively little equipment and take minimal time. Examiners may observe deficiencies in speed, fluidity, or ability to maintain direction, with total scores reflecting risk of falls. The Berg Balance Scale,[28] High level Mobility Assessment Tool,[29–31] and Community Balance and Mobility Scale[31,32] are commonly used in TBI and have undergone psychometric evaluation. The Berg Balance Scale is relatively easy to administer, but may be susceptible to ceiling effects in some individuals.[33,34] The High level mobility assessment tool and Community Balance and Mobility Scale demonstrate good reliability and validity in the TBI population and appear most commonly used in high functioning patients. Other theoretically promising measures include the modified Dynamic Gait Index and the Functional Gait Assessment, although their psychometric properties have yet to be studied in the TBI population. Further work in this area is indicated, particularly focusing on consensus agreement of which measures are most appropriate for specific groups of TBI patients.

Simple static balance measures requiring minimal equipment include the modified clinical test of sensory interaction in balance (mCTSIB) which, albeit somewhat crudely, aims to categorize balance deficits into either proprioceptive, visual or vestibular system impairments. Surprisingly, there is little evidence concerning the psychometric properties of this measure within the TBI population. The Balance Error Scoring System (BESS) is also a frequently administered measure, with previous studies in mTBI and moderate-severe TBI demonstrating moderate to good reliability.[35] However, there is inherent subjectivity within its scoring system and it is unable to discern more subtle balance deficits.

Other simple measures of balance include timed tandem or single-leg stance and tandem walking. Timed tandem or single-leg stance tests have demonstrated moderate test retest reliability in the TBI population.[36] Tandem walking has been used widely in TBI and in general neurology although little evidence exists regarding its validity or reliability. Data in elderly populations shows moderate interreliability scores[37] and excellent scores in healthy adults.[38] Evidence in TBI is more sparse although Howe et al.[31] did demonstrate reasonable intra- and interrater reliability of tandem walking as a component of a wider dynamic balance assessment. Ceiling effects were noted in 60% of TBI patients in this study, indicating tandem walking may not adequately probe balance function in sufficient depth.

COGNITION

mTBI can result in a variety of neuropsychological deficits. Indeed, assessing mTBI is the second most frequent diagnostic activity in clinical neuropsychology. Domains which are typically affected include[39]:

- attention,
- memory,
- executive functioning, and
- information processing.

A degree of controversy exists regarding whether to assess cognition using a fixed battery of tests or specific tests based on the symptoms reported by the patient. Short, easy to administer measures include the Mini Mental State Examination (MMSE) or Montreal Cognitive Assessment (MoCA) which have been used as screening tools for those with mTBI.[40,41] However, these measures they have been criticized for providing only a gross estimate of cognitive capacity and therefore may be relevant for inpatient screening where the emphasis is focused on discharge and rehabilitation planning.

More comprehensive neuropsychological tests are also commonly used. Fixed battery tests such as The Halstead-Reitan Neuropsychological Battery (HRNB) or the Repeatable Battery for the Assessment of Neuropsychological Status (RBANS) have been utilized in TBI.[39,42] These fixed batteries of tests have the advantage of providing detailed assessments and having standardized formats allowing rigorous analysis.[43] However, this approach may not always be time efficient and may be considered somewhat rigid. An alternative may be to select specific tests based on the symptoms the patient reports, or to use a screening tool to ascertain the particular domain affected. This approach has been used in several studies in TBI.[44,45] Podell et al. usefully documented neuropsychological tests relevant to each cognitive domain.[43] For example, a patient complaining of poor attention or concentration may be best provided with a test such as the Stroop, Trail making, or Cancellation test. Such tests have been demonstrated to predict psychosocial outcome in the TBI population.[46]

Clinical Laboratory Tests

For some patients, where facilities and equipment are available, further evaluation of suspected or potential impairments is appropriate in a laboratory. Such additional testing needs to be considered in light of a patient's reserve especially in the acute stage, but may have important and insightful results which could impact treatment and recovery. An overview of some relevant laboratory tests is laid out in the following section.

VESTIBULAR SYSTEM EVALUATION

Electronystamography (ENG) or other means of eye movement recording (e.g., infrared video-oculography—similar to ENG but with higher cost, and the need for a higher level of technical experience[47]) can record subtle abnormalities in both volitional and reflex eye movements such as gaze, saccades, optokinetic nystagmus, and smooth pursuit.[48] On its own, ENG does not provide much more information about absolute deficits than clinical examination by an experienced clinician (especially if Frenzels glasses or ophthalmoscopy is used). However, it is noninvasive, quick and provides a quantification of any deficits which can then be used to monitor patients' recovery.[49] When combined with whole-body velocity steps, ENG records the evoked VOR responses either to whole-body sinusoids or velocity steps which elicit a post rotation nystagmus in the opposite direction to the movement of the chair.[48,50] Rotational chair testing is usually better tolerated than caloric irrigation and is quick, reproducible and has the ability to produce sensitive data.

Bithermal caloric irrigation allows the quantification of responses from the left or right labyrinth independently. Caloric irrigation provides a very low frequency stimulus and primarily interrogates the horizontal semicircular canals.[51] Warm or cool water irrigation is used to create a temperature difference in the endolymph within the semicircular canal, generating a convection current that deflects the cupula. The resulting nystagmus can then be recorded by ENG. Other techniques can be used to ascertain full labyrinth function such as testing of the otoliths via vestibular evoked myogenic potentials (VEMP), discussed later in the chapter.

BALANCE AND GAIT: POSTUROGRAPHY

Static balance can be quantified in the laboratory using computerized dynamic posturography or sway platforms. A variety of protocols to assess static balance using such equipment exist, although most commonly participants stand on a static or movable platform under different conditions. These typically include eyes open or closed and standing on firm or soft surfaces. Using these conditions, clinicians can interrogate, albeit somewhat crudely, the three aspects of balance (visual, somatosensory, and vestibular). Outputs from posturography tests vary, but can be categorized into kinetics (center of pressure velocity or displacement) or kinematics (center of mass and postural compensatory strategies). Currently, there is no consensus on the most clinically relevant parameter to examine, although in a review Visser et al. remarked velocity related rather than displacement measures may be more appropriate, particularly for patients with neurodegenerative conditions.[51]

Studies examining posturography in TBI patients report differences between healthy controls and TBI patients, with the latter demonstrating more impaired balance.[52–55] However, the clinical application of such data is somewhat controversial. Some authors argue such methods of balance testing are unable to predict or assess changes in function or balance. Further, there is currently no prospective data in acute TBI or data which explores the relationship between posturography and falls. Therefore, the use of posturography in isolation may not be advised and it may be pertinent to use additional objective and subjective measures.

GAIT ANALYSIS

Gait analysis using three dimensional (3D) systems is currently the gold standard for measuring parameters including spatiotemporal variables and joint kinematics.[56] Such information may be useful when considering rehabilitation options or during complex clinical decision making. In a study by Ochi et al., 172 TBI patients completed gait analysis measures. Analysis of gait parameters demonstrated reduced walking speed, with a prolonged stance phase and shorter step length for the unaffected limb.[24] Additionally, a systematic review of biomechanical abnormalities during gait following TBI identified 38 studies of relevance. All included studies demonstrated participants had reduced gait speed seemingly secondary to a smaller step length.[56] Data on gait kinematics remains sparse, although this may be more relevant to those with a more severe brain injury. Although such data may be useful to guide rehabilitation, there remains no prospective data regarding the predictive ability of 3D gait systems and long-term recovery, or functional outcomes such as falls.

AUDITION

A comprehensive and standardized battery of tests can be utilized including otoscopy, air and bone conduction thresholds, audiometry, and speech reception/intelligibility. Brainstem auditory evoked potentials (BAEPs) and auditory steady-state response testing (ASSR) can be completed if behavioral responses cannot be obtained.[57] Protocols and processes may have to be altered to take into account the complexity of head injuries, for example, skull fractures and bone conduction.

BIOMARKERS FOR CONCUSSION AND MILD TRAUMATIC BRAIN INJURY IN BLOOD AND OTHER BODY FLUIDS

The correct identification of a brain injury and the monitoring of its progress by means of a biomarker can help with patient management as well as the development of new treatments.

A biomarker can be defined as some feature that can objectively be assessed and interpreted as an indicator of biological processes and/or responses.[58] During the past 20 years, there has been an exponential increase in publications investigating biomarkers in concussion and mTBI (Fig. 16.1).

In 1983, Bakay and Ward[59] proposed the criteria for an ideal biomarker for a brain injury. These included: high specificity for brain tissue; high sensitivity for brain injury; rapid appearance in serum; reliable assays for immediate analysis; release after irreversible destruction of brain tissue and in time-locked sequence with injury; a low age and gender variability; and certain clinical relevance.[59] However, there is yet no biomarker that satisfies all these criteria. One of the key reasons is the poor biomarker specificity, for example, brain-specific biomarkers released in response to TBI may be released in response to many different stimuli: for example, oxidative stress, inflammation, cerebral blood flow dysregulation, excitotoxicity, regeneration and repair, apoptosis, and cell death.[60] The current consensus is that a combination of markers—that is, a "biomarker panel"—will provide a more robust measure of concussion than any single biomarker.[61]

As patients with mTBI are diagnostically challenging, neuroimaging may visualize brain injury (see next section), but is relatively expensive, time-consuming, and impractical for a daily use in an environment where decisions need to be taken quickly. In order for the correct diagnosis to be made and for prompt and appropriate treatment to be initiated, a set of biomarkers with high level of sensitivity and specificity are needed as they may allow the clinician to confirm or reject the hypothesis of a mild brain injury in concussion patients. In this chapter section, we discuss different biomarkers obtained from blood, cerebrospinal fluid (CSF), or other biological fluids (i.e., urine, saliva) for concussion/mTBI and their usage for diagnostic purposes, severity assessment or recovery monitoring.

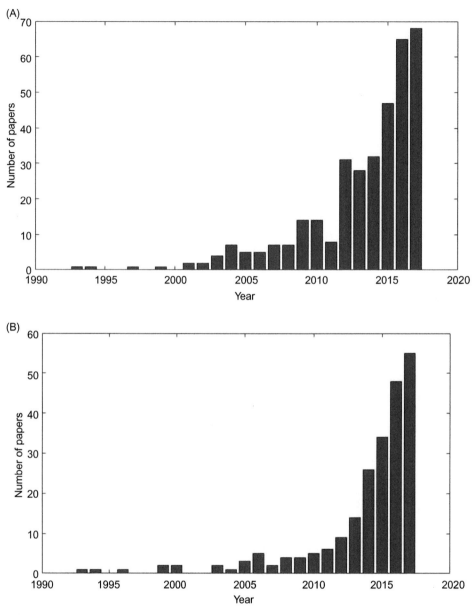

FIGURE 16.1   Number of papers discussing biomarkers for mTBI (A) and concussion (B) (1993—2017). Pubmed search.

Blood

Blood-based biomarkers (serum and plasma) for brain damage have long been used as a potential measure of mTBI. At present however, no single biomarker is able to provide a quick, sensitive, and specific diagnosis for concussion/mTBI. The main reasons for this include the rapid flux in their plasma concentrations or poor specificity as related to mTBI. In general, a higher serum biomarker concentration was usually associated with worse outcome.[62] The poor understanding of the biomarkers' dependence on variables other than the medical condition itself, makes it even more difficult to find that one universal blood biomarker. These variables include the molecular weight, marker specific biophysical properties, half-life time in blood, glomerular filtration effects, age, gender, and ethnicity.[63] To address this issue, Dadas et al. developed a multi-compartment, pharmacokinetic model that integrated the properties of a given brain molecule and was able to predict its behavior and concentration over time in the blood.[63]

Further difficulty to mention is connected to the half-life time of the biomarkers. As its length depends on many factors from the in vivo environment, its value is no constant that one can depend on. Often, if the patients do not present during the postacute phase, some of these markers cannot even be detected anymore. Based on our literature review, it became obvious that authors often do not specify the exact half-life of the biomarkers used, but sometimes mention approximations. Consequently, we will provide an overview of the half-life time for the most popular biomarkers in their specific sections.

Overall, although encouraging, research into blood biomarkers in mTBI requires studies with larger sample sizes, similar outcome measures, increased homogeneity in study design and sample collection (allowing between-study comparisons).[64]

Calcium Binding Protein B-S100β

First described in 1965, the S100β—calcium binding protein B—is the most studied mTBI biomarker,[65] some authors calling it "the CRP of the brain."[66] In the nervous system, S100β is concentrated in astrocytes and other glial cells (including oligodendrocytes, Schwann cells, ependymal cells, enteric glial cells, and retinal Muller cells) and is a marker for astroglial injury. Notably S100β is also found in nonneural tissues including melanocytes, Langerhans cells, chondrocytes, and dendritic cells in lymphoid organs.[67] S100β acts via autocrine, paracrine, or even endocrine manner with trophic effects at physiological (nanomolar) concentrations, but toxic at higher (micromolar) concentrations.[67]

A review article from 2017 checked the biological half-life time ($t_{1/2}$) of the calcium binding protein B in adults and pediatrics and it turned out to be quite a various variable.[68] Based on their observations from 66 TBI articles, the authors concluded that $t_{1/2}$ for S100β had a cut-off of approximately 4–6 hours after mTBI; in moderate to severe cases was 24–48 hours, 49–72 hours and to be around 24 hours, even reaching 6 days after severe TBI[68]; an article discussing perinatal medicine mentions a half-life time of about 1 hour after brain injury (brain injury because of insult).[69]

Most studies evaluating S100β assays for mTBI have assessed S100β in blood serum, less commonly in CSF and the urine and rarely in saliva. S100β has been assessed for use in diagnosis, severity, and prognosis scoring in moderate to severe TBI[65,70–73] for distinguishing mTBI from non-TBI cases S100β.[74] It was also suggested that it is important to combine S100β with proper imaging techniques to visualize the location of the injury.[75]

As S100β has a short half-life[61] its use is limited to the moderate and severe TBI cases as lesser severity cases will have a raised level beyond an hour following injury and hence its use for measurements as a marker for mTBI is problematic if cases are not assessed hyperacutely.[76]

Another problem with S100β is its poor specificity.[71,77-80] S100β is elevated in other neurological conditions including brain tumors, neuro-inflammation and neurodegenerative disorders,[67] stroke, trauma without head injury,[81] and even physical exercise.[82,83] Other extracerebral sources of serum S100β include fat, muscle, and bone marrow,[81,84] hence, the use of S100β levels as a biomarker of concussion should also consider the clinical context. The poor specificity of S100β for mTBI when used in the wrong clinical context may in part explain the inconsistency between published studies.[85]

S100β may, however, be useful as a strong negative predictor of mTBI if assessed within 6 hours of head injury. A S100β level of less than 0.10 μg/L is a strong indicator of the absence of computed tomography (CT) abnormalities.[86] Subsequently, the Scandinavian Neurotrauma Committee incorporated serum S100β analysis into their guidelines for deciding whether or not to CT scan individuals with a low-risk mTBI.[87] This has the potential to reduce unnecessary CT scans, patients' exposure to radiation,[88] as well as admissions in patients with mild head injuries, which in turn leads to significant cost savings.

Glial Fibrillary Acidic Protein

Glial fibrillary acidic protein (GFAP) was first isolated in 1971 and is only found in glial cells of the CNS, constituting the major part of the cytoskeleton of astrocytes. GFAP is a biomarker for astroglial injury, as is S100β. Unlike S100β, GFAP is a brain-specific protein released after any brain injury, from stroke to TBI.[89]

Consistent with its brain-specific expression, GFAP levels are normal in polytrauma patients without brain injury.[90,91] Furthermore, GFAP is conveniently detectable in serum within 1 hour of mTBI allowing the clinician to rapidly distinguish TBI cases from other non-TBI trauma cases.[92] In general, Thelin et al.[68] discusses the biological half-life time ($t_{1/2}$) of the GFAP in 18 articles to be between 24 and 48 hours in severe TBI and quite variable for cases of mild to severe TBI: <6 hours, around or >24, 32, 24-48 hours in patients who survived and 61-84 hours in patients who did not survive. Serum GFAP may also be a surrogate marker for neuroimaging abnormalities, with significantly higher levels in mTBI patients with intracranial lesions on CT compared with those without lesions.[92] GFAP may also be useful for predicting outcome; for example, GFAP levels predicted patients who required neurosurgical intervention[92] and a high serum level (GFAP >1.5 μg/L) strongly predicted death or poor outcome both acutely[93] and at 6 months.[94]

In summary, GFAP shows good potential to predict outcome after severe TBI, but although promising, more data is required to comment upon its utility in mTBI diagnosis.[65]

Neuron-Specific Enolase

Neuron-specific enolase (NSE) was first described in 1965 and is part of the group of the glycolytic enzymes. It is found in the cytoplasm of the neurons (isoenzyme γγ) and neuroendocrine cells (isoenzyme αγ) and is considered a biomarker for neuronal injury. NSE is the only biomarker that can directly assess functional damage to neurons[95] and it was also found that high level concentrations in TBI correspond with injury severity.[96] One of the main problems associated with the use of NSE as a marker of brain damage is hemolysis. Erythrocytes contain a large amount of NSE and hemolysis may, therefore, cause a marked increase of NSE in the blood.[95] This makes acute levels difficult to interpret and might not reflect "real time" pathological processes when measured alone.[61]

Normally, NSE is already detectable within 6 hours of brain injury, increases in the first 12 hours[95] after the traumatic event and after that decreases with a possible secondary peak in the lethal cases. NSE has an average half-life time ($t_{1/2}$) of 24 hours in mild to severe TBI, but can also vary to 48−73−96 hours in severe TBI and up to 10−14 days (review on 27 articles).[68] Further, NSE levels of more than 10 µg/L are considered to be pathological. Studies in pediatric population found that NSE levels >15 ng/mL within 24 hours of TBI were associated with intracranial lesions.[64] Another characteristic of NSE is its slow elimination from the plasma leading to difficulties in distinguishing between primary and secondary insults to the brain.[97]

Clinical studies in mTBI show both increased NSE levels after brain injury[98] or no difference in NSE levels between injured people and controls.[99] Used in isolation, higher levels of NSE do not necessarily account for TBI as NSE is also an indicator for different tumors and ischemic stroke. However, very often S100β and NSE are used together. Żurek et al. argue that although further prospective studies are needed, the findings suggesting that S100β and NSE levels correlate with mortality, may definitely be useful as predictors of outcome in children with (not specified/general) TBI.[76] On the contrary, Geyer et al. did not manage to discriminate between S100β and NSE for symptomatic and asymptomatic children with minor head injury and concluded that these two biomarkers are not good estimation tools for pediatrics with mTBI.[100] However, another successful example shows that a set of preclinical and clinical parameters combined with S100β and NSE could serve as a reliable guidance for accurate diagnosis[101] or just for successful early diagnosis of TBI.[102]

Overall, inadequate sensitivity and poor specificity limits the use of NSE in mTBI. In contrast, given its relatively long half-life, it may be useful for patients presenting late. Most likely, NSE will be of use as part of a panel of biomarkers and not in isolation.

Ubiquitin C-Terminal Hydrolase L1

Ubiquitin C-terminal hydrolase L1 (UCH-L1) is a protein found in the neuronal cell body. It is involved in the addition or removal of ubiquitin from abnormal proteins including misfolded proteins and proteins damaged by oxidation or denatured by other means destined for proteasomal degradation and has previously been used as a neuronal cell soma marker.[95] This biomarker is considered as an indicator for neuronal injury. There is increasing evidence that UCH-L1 is one of only a few markers that has been found to identify minor TBI as well as more severe injury and also appears to be able to distinguish between patients with TBI and uninjured patients at 6 hours when Glasgow Coma Scale (GCS) is altered secondary to drugs and alcohol.[97] A review by Thelin et al., as already mentioned in the previous sections, identified nine articles about UCH-L1 and concluded that the half-life time ($t_{1/2}$) for mTBI is around 7 hours, whereas for severe TBI it is around 10 hours.[68]

In patients with mTBI, Papa et al. detected serum UCH-L1 within 1 hour of injury that not only discriminated patients with mTBI from uninjured controls, but also patients with a GCS score of 15 from uninjured controls (both with AUC of 0.87).[103] In addition, UCH-L1 distinguished patients with CT lesions from CT-negative TBI patients with an AUC of

0.73. Further, increases in serum UCH-L1 have also been found in children with moderate and severe TBI,[104] but there was no increase after mTBI. UCH-L1 was also correlated with the Glasgow Outcome Score (GOS), and this correlation was stronger than the correlations with NSE, S100β, or myelin basic protein (MBP).[104] Another successful example provides prospective evidence of significant increases in serum levels of UCH-L1 and S100β during the early acute period following sport related concussion.[105]

Myelin Basic Protein

MBP is one of the two most abundant proteins in myelin expressed by oligodendrocytes. Normal serum levels of MBP are "low, typically less than 0.3 ng/mL"[90] and so when MBP is released into the serum, it is because of a brain damage or demyelination. Shearing of brain white matter leading to diffuse axonal injury can trigger release of MBP into the CSF and blood serum, where it has been found to remain elevated for up to 2 weeks after a traumatic event.[106] MBP can trigger opening of the blood−brain barrier (BBB) and so facilitate its own entry (and possibly other CNS-derived biomarkers) into the circulation.[107]

Although there are abundant data in severe TBI where MBP levels correlate with the severity of injury, the data for mTBI are sparse. In a study of pediatric brain injury, high serum MBP levels were found to correlate with poor outcome with a sensitivity of 73% and specificity of 61%.[108] Although circulating levels of MBP in people who have sustained an mTBI have not been measured, the ability of this protein to open the BBB suggests that it may be detectable in mTBI in which axonal injury is a feature.[90] Even though reports have demonstrated excellent specificity for TBI, MBP has limited sensitivity[109] and has more potential when measured alongside NSE levels.[110]

Very often MBP is used together with other biomarkers to establish a diagnosis or predict severity and outcome of the trauma. In a small series of 25 patients, Yamazaki et al. found that serum NSE and MBP levels give a reliable laboratory indicator of the degree of brain damage and allow the early prediction of the prognosis in patients with acute head injury.[111]

Discussing abusive and nonabusive head trauma in children, Berger et al. concluded that serum NSE, S100β, or MBP rose in the majority of the children with acute noninflicted TBI and inflicted TBI, including children with normal outer appearance and inflicted TBI in whom the correct diagnosis might otherwise have been missed.[109] It is because of the lack of clinical validity that popularity of MBP as a biomarker has decreased more recently in comparison with NSE, S100β, and GFAP.[74]

Neurofilaments

Neurofilaments are heteropolymeric components of the axonal cytoskeleton that consist of a light neurofilament subunit (NF-L) backbone with either a medium (NF-M) or a heavy subunit (NF-H) side arms.[112] Following axonal injury, the influx of calcium alters the phosphorylation state and there is a loss of cytoskeletal structure, leading to impaired transport and swelling and subsequent proteolysis.[61,113] A study from 2008 discussed the use of the heavily phosphorylated axonal form of the neurofilament subunit NF-H (pNF-H) as a biomarker for TBI in rats subjected to an experimental cortical contusion.[114] Considering that neurofilaments are located exclusively in neurons, their presence in blood is indicative of damage to the neurons following brain injury. Further, using enzyme-linked immunosorbent assay (ELISA), this research team detected the presence of pNF-H as early as 6 hour post-injury, with levels increasing at 24–48 hours, and then slowly decreasing to baseline over several days post-injury. The levels of serum pNF-H detected were linked with the severity of the brain injury. Previous studies using a similar injury model reported that a mTBI injury without extensive neuronal loss resulted in significant behavioral changes.[115] However, ELISA appears capable of detecting moderate and severe axonal injury in the cerebral cortex.[114] Since blood collection is faster and safer than collection of CSF, and the ELISA assay is rapid and fairly simple, this suggests that analysis of blood for pNF-H could prove to be a useful research and clinical tool to conveniently assess axonal damage.[114] In 2011, Zurek et al. also demonstrated that levels of hyperphosphorylated neurofilament NF-H correlate with mortality and may be useful as predictors of outcome in children with TBI.[116] In another study, Gatson et al. compares the blood serum pNF-H in patients suffering from mTBI with positive and negative CT findings on Days 1 and 3 after the traumatic event.[117] Compared with healthy controls, the mTBI patients exhibited an increase in the serum levels of pNF-H on Days 1 and 3. However, pNF-H serum levels were only significantly higher on Day 1 in mTBI patients from the group with positive CT findings compared with the group with negative CT findings. The results suggest that with certain limitation the detection of pNF-H may be useful in determining which individuals require CT imaging to assess the severity of their injury.

Tau (τ) (T-Tau and c-Tau)

Tau is an intracellular, microtubule-associated protein that is mainly localized in the axons. As already mentioned, T-tau (total tau) protein is highly expressed in thin, nonmyelinated axons of cortical interneurons[118] and so might be indicative of axonal damage in gray matter neurons. Axons are the structures most vulnerable to damage from mTBI, and thus the identification of peripheral blood biomarkers there could give valuable information about the brain injury.

However, standard immunoassay techniques very often lack precision of biomarker detection because of the low concentration of the potential biomarkers in the peripheral blood (compared to CSF). In addition, their accuracy can also be affected by the binding of the potential biomarkers to carrier proteins, and by extracerebral sources of possible biomarkers.[78] A review article of Zetterberg et al. from 2013 suggests that tau protein and neurofilament proteins are promising biomarkers, but analytical techniques for assessing these two classes of biomarkers in blood need to have better sensitivity than that usually achieved utilizing the traditional immunoassays (such as f.ex. ELISA, etc.).[78]

Blood plasma T-tau is another promising biomarker for diagnosing concussion and in deciding when an athlete can be declared fit to return to playing.[119,120] Elevated plasma tau concentrations within 6 hours postconcussion predicts a prolonged return to play. However, a study in pediatrics showed elevated serum tau protein after mild head trauma mTBI, but did not distinguish between patients with intracranial lesions and such without intracranial lesions demonstrable on brain CT scanning.[121]

C-TAU

A further interesting biomarker is the c-tau (cleaved τ protein = τc = c-tau) which is a secondary structure of the cleaved-form of MAP-tau. When an axonal injury such as trauma or hypoxia occurs, tau (τ) is released from the CNS neurons into the extracellular space, cleaves proteolytically at the N- and C-terminals, and diffuses into the CSF and plasma.[122] Monoclonal antibodies that recognize this cleaved form of τ-protein have been used in an ELISA format to quantify CSF and plasma levels of the cleaved τ protein.[123] The study demonstrated an elevation of CSF c-tau levels in a comatose head-injured patient with an unremarkable CT scan which indicated that CSF c-tau levels are a more sensitive measure of axonal damage than CT.[123] So, the CSF c-tau levels were suggested to be a good predictor of severity of head injury and patient outcome.

In a study by Shaw et al., blood levels of c-tau were significantly elevated in patients with closed head injury compared with controls and c-tau levels of more than zero were associated with a greater chance of an actual intracranial injury and poor outcome after discharge.[122] However, using blood samples, Ma et al. concluded that C-tau is a poor predictor of postconcussion syndrome after mTBI regardless of whether CT scan findings were negative or positive.[124] Even when used together with S100β to determine the relationship of serum S100β and c-tau levels to long-term outcome after mTBI, it turned out that the initial serum S100β and c-tau levels appeared to be poor predictors of 3-month outcome after mTBI.[80]

Cerebrospinal Fluid

CSF is a clear fluid that surrounds the brain and provides mechanical support. It carries nutrients and signaling molecules to neurons and helps in disposing metabolites. The total CSF volume is around 150 mL and the production and clearance rates are around 20 mL/h.[125] Standard procedure to obtain CSF is the lumbar puncture which, although considered safe, is highly invasive. CSF provides a window into changes in the CNS, and contains low protein levels relative to volume, making detection of released proteins or fragments easier than with serum.[126] Whereas patients with severe TBI receive a ventriculostomy catheter for collection of CSF, obtaining CSF from individuals with a mTBI and from healthy controls is more complicated as CSF samples are not typically obtained following mTBI.[127]

Given the invasive nature of a lumbar puncture, any CSF biomarker for concussion should demonstrate significant advantages for this approach to be clinically acceptable. However, even then, it is likely that CSF sampling would only be used in the research domain as a gold standard by which less invasive markers of brain injury could not be assessed. One study[128] assessed CSF levels of T-tau, NF-L, GFAP, and S100β in Olympic boxers with head injury finding increased CSF levels for all markers in >80% of the boxers. Furthermore, the biomarker levels were raised both acutely and in a cumulative fashion according to head trauma in Olympic boxing. The lack of normalization of NF-L and GFAP after a rest period in some boxers may indicate some ongoing degeneration, and so the recurrent head trauma in boxing might be linked with an increased risk of chronic

TBI.[128] The fact that the finding was not ubiquitous might indicate that some individuals may be at more risk for cumulative effects of head trauma.

Considering CSF limited use in mTBI, it is an advantage that most of the frequently used biomarkers for mTBI/ concussion are detectable in both: the blood (plasma and serum) and the CSF—"S100β, protein breakdown products, UCHL-1, MBP, miRNA."[90] However, NSE and GFAP are mostly considered as blood biomarkers. In the past, levels of NSE in CSF were also obtained and have been suggested as a possible screening tool for inflicted TBI in children,[110] but studies on the level of NSE in CSF obtained by lumbar puncture in patients with mTBI are generally lacking. The main limitation of using NSE levels in CSF as a biomarker of neuronal injury is its high sensitivity to haemolysis[78] which led to a decreased interest for this method.

However, when used, CSF biomarkers are, similarly to blood biomarkers, obtained for diagnostic purposes, establishing the severity of injury and outcome of the trauma event.

Neurofilaments

Further to its use in blood samples, research in neurofilaments from CSF has also been conducted. In cases of severe TBI the amount of phosphorylated NF-H was measured and found to be elevated in the CSF of adult patients.[129] However, studies about the expression of neurofilaments as biomarkers for mTBI are not so many.

An interesting study discussing the severity and outcome in boxers, based on CSF obtained NF-L, T-tau, GFAP, phosphorylated tau, β-amyloid protein 1−40, and β-amyloid protein 1−42 was performed by Zetterberg et al.[129] As amateur boxing is associated with acute neuronal and astroglial injury, it was important to determine whether severity and number of hits are associated with elevated levels of biochemical markers for neuronal injury in CSF. The two best-established CSF biomarkers of axonal injury are T-tau and neurofilament light polypeptide (NF-L).[78] These two proteins have different regional distributions in the brain, which might be useful in determining which areas of the brain have been affected by TBI: T-tau protein is highly expressed in thin, nonmyelinated axons of cortical interneurons,[118] whereas NF-L is most abundant in the large-caliber myelinated axons that project into deeper brain layers and the spinal cord.[130] So, when the researchers found that the amount of rise for NF-L was larger than that for T-tau protein, it was suggested that mTBI affects the long myelinated axons in white matter to a greater extent than it affects the short nonmyelinated axons in the cortex.[129] In addition, the level of NF-L in CSF correlates positively with the exposure to head trauma, such as the number of blows to the head received, and subjective and objective estimates of the intensity of the fight.[127,129]

Tau (τ) (T-tau)

Total tau (T-tau) levels in ventricular CSF were often discussed in severe TBI patients, but there is hardly any data about mTBI. Studies in patients with mTBI, such as amateur, showed elevated levels of total tau in CSF 4−10 days after the trauma, and similar results were found in boxers who were knocked out.[127,129] In addition, total tau protein levels in these athletes normalized 8−12 weeks after the event, provided that the boxers didn't participate in any further boxing matches.

Other Potential Sources for Biomarkers

Saliva, urine, sweat, and tears are further examples of possible biological markers and can be noninvasively sampled making them a desirable option for mTBI biomarkers. However, the lack to produce a clear link to changes in the brain, given the many barriers and compartments these markers would have to cross on their way to the sampling site, has led to significant skepticism among researchers about their use and biological plausibility.[124]

Saliva

Saliva is an easily obtainable, but a rarely used biomarker for TBI. However, there are articles reviewing its use and one successful example is a research from 2015 discussing the development of a nanoparticle-enabled protein biomarker and its implementation for saliva-based TBI detection.[131]

Another use of saliva as a biomarker is explored with the help of microRNAs (miRNAs) which are small, noncoding molecules that are transported through the extracellular space protected in exosomes and microvesicles, which allows them to be easily measured in biofluids, including serum, CSF, and saliva.[132,133] Because of their abundance, stability in fluctuating pH levels and resistance to enzymatic degradation the miRNAs are good candidates for biomarkers.[134]. Johnson et al. were able to evaluate the efficacy of salivary miRNAs for identifying children with concussion who are at risk for developing long-term symptoms.[135] The concentrations of miRNA determined a positive postconcussion status in 42 of 50 participants. Although the results were promising, further studies are needed to establish the validity of salivary miRNA for the duration and character of concussion symptoms.

Urine

Urine is easily obtained, particularly in the postacute phase where it could be self-collected by the patient. However, quantitation of urinary biomarkers is problematic as they are also dependent upon urine flow rates.[136]

In 2006, Berger and Kochanek investigated levels of S100β in serum and urine and showed that S100β was detectable in the urine of the majority of the patients with elevated serum S100β and that all subjects with undetectable urine S100β had a favorable outcome.[137] Due to the renal excretion pathway, the S100β peak in the urine occurs later than in the serum (mean 55.3 vs 14.6 hour after the injury)—a fact which could help to recognize injuries, even in patients with delayed referral. Measuring S100β in the urine is noninvasive—a clear benefit in pediatric patients. Unfortunately, up to now, no reference ranges for S100β in the urine have been published in the literature.[138] Despite detecting measurable S100β levels in urine following head injury, the same levels were measured following extracranial trauma. Urinary S100β is, therefore, not useful as an early biochemical marker following head injury in children.[139] In another study urine S100β measurements that were reported as an early predictor of short-term mortality perform generally worse than previously determined serum measurements.[140] Furthermore, patients tested had all incurred severe TBI, so it is unlikely that similar results would be found in less severe injuries.

Other Less Studied Biomarkers

Many biomarkers of TBI have been assessed for diagnosis, severity classification and prognosis including: (1) metabolites of lipids, neurotransmitters and glycolytic intermediates; (2) microtubule-associated proteins; (3) neuroinflammatory cytokine markers; (4) soluble urokinase plasminogen activator receptors; (5) creatine kinase brain isoenzymes; (6) plasma desoxyribonucleic acid; (7) brain-derived neurotrophic factor; (8) CSF αII-spectrin breakdown products;[141] (9) a customized set of copeptin; (10) galectin 3 (LGALS3), matrix metalloproteinase 9, and occludin.[142] In a 2017 review, McCrea et al.[143] discuss the more or less successful use of the following fluid biomarkers in clinical assessment of sport related concussion: α-amino-3-hydroxy-5-methyl-4-isoxazolepropionic acid receptor peptide, S100β, total tau, marinobufagenin, plasma soluble cellular prion protein, GFAP, NSE, calpain-derived αII-spectrin N-terminal fragment (SNTF), tau-C, and metabolomics profiling. In addition, NSE, visinin-like protein-1, total tau, tau-A, and salivary cortisol did not distinguish concussed athletes from nonconcussed athletes.[143] Nevertheless, the authors conclude that this information can contribute to our scientific understanding of the underlying pathophysiology of concussion in humans.

NEUROPHYSIOLOGICAL TESTING AND NEUROIMAGING IN MILD TRAUMATIC BRAIN INJURY

Given the multifocal impact of head trauma, multimodal assessment in acute concussion patients is required. Despite this need, there are currently no objective biomarkers of mTBI in concussion. There is, thus, the requirement for sensitive state-of-the-art testing to enable the effective and safe triage of patients who present to acute services. As well as triage, objective monitoring of patients' recovery over time, and separate from clinical features that patients may develop following the injury (e.g., depression and migraine) is also required.

Since concussion can be considered an event with an associated clinical syndrome rather than a diagnosis, diagnostic testing of the whole neuroaxis is critical in assessing concussion patients. Neuroimaging alongside neurophysiological testing is likely to be a crucial component in this assessment.

Neurophysiological testing can interrogate the functional and anatomical integrity of neural systems as a whole and be of potential diagnostic utility in mTBI patients. This does not apply to patients with severe brain injury and coma, where neurophysiology has an undoubted clinical application—for example, in excluding underlying subclinical epilepsy or providing initial insight into the prognosis of brain functional recovery. In contrast, it is unclear whether neurophysiological testing can provide a similar insight into patients with concussion with or without mild brain injury. Current clinical evaluation methods solely focusing on assessing the functional deficits caused by brain injury often also fail to monitor the physiology underlying the functional abnormality. Ideally the assessment should include function and physiology. Electrophysiology can provide important information in understanding questions such as the therapeutic benefits of rest during acute recovery. At the moment, there are no consensus guidelines or well-accepted criteria available about retiring young athletes from contact sports after frequent or severe concussions, and electrophysiology may provide the criteria needed. Furthermore, in contrast, to neuroimaging, electrophysiology is readily available, cheap, and there are internationally recognized standardized methodologies.

Nonetheless, neuroimaging is widely used in concussion, and most typically employed to exclude severe TBI. Magnetic resonance imaging (MRI), particularly diffusion weighted and T2 star weighted imaging, is far more sensitive than CT for the identification of subtle abnormalities such as microhemorrhages. However, although diffusion tensor imaging (DTI) metrics are potential biomarkers of mild brain injury, inconsistencies across studies in the direction of altered diffusion, between center variations in imaging protocols, quality assurance and analysis techniques, and the scarcity of normative data applicable across centers have to be resolved before clinical application is an option.

This section focuses on the evidence supporting the use of neurophysiological techniques in concussion. Additionally, evidence for the use of structural and functional neuroimaging in concussion and mTBI are also discussed. Ultimately, the necessity for multimodal assessment of patients with mTBI that bridges the link between neurophysiology and neuroimaging is set forth.

Neurophysiology Testing in Mild Traumatic Brain Injury

Visual System—Visual Evoked Potentials

Visual evoked potentials (VEPs) also known as visual evoked responses (VERs) provide an objective method of measuring abnormalities in the afferent visual system. It was developed after it was shown that regularly repeated flashes of light before the eyes produced evoked responses in the electroencephalogram (EEG) recorded over the occipital cortex. However, in only a small number of people was there a VEP because usually the response was so small it was lost in the random noise of the EEG. It was not until early in the 1960s that computers were developed that permitted averaging of an evoked response that was time locked to the stimulus. Thus, if a light flash repeated rapidly 100 times before the eyes and the occipital EEG was recorded by a computer-averager, the common time-locked evoked response was added together to produce a clear wave form while the random EEG noise was slowly approximated to zero. The stimulus often used to produce VEPs are one hundred white flashes of light from a photostimulator. However, other investigators find that a more reproducible response is produced to a rapidly reversing black and white checkerboard pattern. Still other investigators use a straight pattern flash without pattern reversal. Thus, one of the problems when reading VEP literature is to know what stimulus is used (i.e., flash, pattern reversal, or pattern flash) and what that laboratory considers normal response.[144]

Its use in concussion and mTBI has been put forward since 1970s.[145] Despite this, published literature has produced mixed results on its ability to distinguish mTBI. Werner and Vanderzant found no difference in the P100 value (the large positive peak wave that occurs at about 100 ms in healthy individuals) beyond three standard deviations of normality.[146] In this particular group, 18 head-injured subjects, defined as a period of unconsciousness as less than 20 minutes and GCS on admission of >13, had VEPs recorded within 2 weeks of the injury.

Similarly, Papathanasopoulos and colleagues observed no differences in VEPs compared with normal controls; however, they found a significant within-subject decrease in P100 latency over a period of 30 days.[147] Nonetheless, it has been shown for subjects with persistent postconcussion syndrome, 30% had latencies beyond a 2.5 standard deviation of the normal limit[148] and significant improvements in VEP latency and amplitude of concussed individuals has been reported after optometric rehabilitation.[149]

More recently, possible magnocellular deficits have been reported for individuals with a history of mTBI compared with visually normal control subjects based on their P100 visually evoked potential responses to a high-contrast (85%) checkerboard stimulus (1.49-cycle/degree check size) at a very low luminance level (0.3% transmittance; greater P100 latency and smaller amplitude),[150] as well as to low-contrast (20%) checkerboard stimuli of varying sizes (smaller P100 amplitude).[151]

Interestingly, by analyzing low-level VEPs evoked by stimuli with a homogenous motion or orientation pattern in comparison to stimuli of greater complexity (i.e., textured stimuli), Lachapelle et al. observed that VEP peak times to homogenous stimuli did not differ between TBI patients and controls but peak times were longer to textured stimuli in TBI patients than controls.[152] These findings may indicate that TBI patients show spared first-order visual processing (restricted to area V1 of visual cortex) but impaired higher order visual processing mechanisms that may originate from second-order antero–posterior cortical processes higher in the visual processing chain.

Poltavski and colleagues investigated a subset of patients with a history of concussion and subsequent convergence abnormalities, on the basis that this particular visual disorder was a frequent finding in mTBI patients.[153] They compared VEP latencies in this group, and subjects with a convergence abnormality and no history of concussion, finding a significant prolonged difference in the P100 measurement.

Auditory System: Brainstem Auditory Evoked Potentials

The role of BAEPs has been little evaluated in mTBI, although its potential use is suggested by findings in moderate and severe traumatic head injury where the wave I–V is prolonged.[154,155] Additionally, a previous study found that BAEPs can detect brainstem lesions even in the absence of MRI findings.[156] All patients within the study had brainstem trauma as revealed by early MRI or electrophysiological studies. Of the 35 included cases, seven had brainstem lesions detected by MRI only, whereas in 10 patients, BAEP examination disclosed impairment of brainstem function with normal MRI, with the remainder of cases having impairment in both diagnostic techniques.

Vestibular System: Vestibular Evoked Myogenic Potentials

The VEMP provides a noninvasive complementary method for assessing peripheral vestibular function—specifically otolith function[157]—and can be used at the bedside. The VEMP test involves delivering acoustic energy to the vestibular system via headphones or a bone vibrator and short latency myogenic responses are recorded, either via electromyographic electrodes on the ipsilateral sternocleidomastoid muscle, the cervical VEMP (cVEMP), or the inferior oblique muscle over the contralateral eye, the ocular VEMP (oVEMP). The generator sites for the cVEMP and oVEMP are now recognized as being the saccule and utricle respectively and as such these tests offer a unique objective methodology to probe these structures. Given that the link between head injury and BPPV has been established it seems highly likely that the source for this pathology is disruption to the structure of the otolith organs. Therefore VEMPs could potentially be a highly sensitive objective marker in this patient cohort.

Transcranial Magnetic Stimulation and Somatosensory Evoked Potentials

The neurophysiology of the primary motor cortex (M1) can be probed using noninvasive stimulation techniques such as TMS. Given the consistent topography of motor representations in M1, TMS can be used to generate cortically mediated myogenic potentials in a target muscle (e.g., the first dorsal interosseous).

Upper limb somatosensory evoked potentials (SEPs) and central motor conduction time with respect to TMS were found to be unaltered in asymptomatic concussed athletes.[158] However, when TMS was performed immediately and following a sport-related concussion (acute), the abductor digiti minimi motor evoked potential (MEP) amplitude ratio was found to be reduced 3 and 5 days after the injury.[159] Also in the same study, the MEP latency with cortical stimulation was found to be prolonged on Day 10 with recording from the abductor pollicis brevis muscle (APB). Two weeks after mild to moderate head injury, a reduction in the amplitude ratio was noted (APB recording), with a significant amplitude difference in the majority of patient.[160] In these same patients, central motor conduction time was prolonged in those of the mild type, and tended to correlate with the presence of diffuse or combined (diffuse axonal injury and contusions) brain injury. The prolonged latencies from the same muscle were also noted in patients with diffuse axonal injury.[161]

Evaluated SEP amplitudes are difficult to perform on an individual basis, probably due to variability in this parameter.[162] There are no reported studies with SEPs in mild head injury or concussion. The data from studies in more severely affected TBI cases are conflicting in terms of its ability to predict acute brain injury severity and long-term prognosis. For example, in severe TBI, short latency SEPs did not correlate with clinical disability,[163] whereas a normal central conduction time (the time with cervical and cortical waveforms with reference to the median nerves) or normal cortical time correlated with better survival and less disability.[164–167] In addition, SEPs were found to be better predictors of outcome than motor or papillary responses.[167]

Electroencephalogram

There are a large number of EEG studies in concussion with large heterogeneity in their methods including defining concussion, time of testing, patient groups and medical comorbidities. EEG recording during a working memory task showed lower amplitudes for frontal N350 and parietal P300 for concussed subjects. Comparatively, in one study of auditory oddball and Go/No-go tasks event-related potentials could not be differentiated between concussed athletes and controls.[168] An additional study suggests that ERPs are only useful with a preconcussion baseline.[169]

Structural Neuroimaging Techniques

Computed Tomography

By definition, concussion does not involve any abnormality on standard structural neuro-imaging studies.[170] Nonetheless, CT imaging is widely used in head injured patients and can be completed in seconds. Indeed, it remains the modality of choice in emergency departments to look for macroscopic injuries of the brain in trauma.[171] Outside of excluding intracranial hemorrhage or contusion, it has no utility in diagnosing or assessing concussion per se.[172]

Magnetic Resonance Imaging

Conventional MRI includes T_1-weighted, T_2-weighted, and fluid attenuated inversion recovery images. These images provide extensive detail of intracranial and cerebral structure, and can indicate occult lesions not demonstrated on CT, such as small cerebral contusions, as well as detecting structural abnormalities earlier. Limitations may include claustrophobia, with patients requiring sedation or even general anesthesia when undergoing an MRI, availability of machines and incompatibility with certain life-support equipment within the scanner. Nevertheless, over the past decade these limitations are being addressed, with scan times shorter and MRI-compatible technology being developed.

A number of publications have evaluated the sensitivity of MRI in mTBI[173–175]; however, these were small number studies, with varying definitions of mTBI, as well as commenting on potentially nonspecific MRI findings unrelated to trauma, such as mild cortical atrophy. In many countries, routine use of MRI for mTBI is not practical or feasible, given the number of available machines, waiting lists and costs.

Diffusion Tensor Imaging

DTI is an MRI-based imaging technique that can produce structural images of brain white matter tracts. It utilizes the physiology of the myelin sheaths and cell membranes of white matter tracts, which restricts the movement of water molecules. Water molecules diffuse in various directions in the brain, but often travel along the length of axons which enables this technique to create images of axons by analyzing the direction of water diffusion.[176] Fractional anisotropy, a measurement of the relative position of water diffusion in axons, is used as a marker of white matter integrity, and has been shown to be sensitive to white matter abnormalities following mTBI.[173,177,178] These abnormalities have been correlated with increased reaction time and persistent concussive symptoms in patients with a history of mTBI compared to controls.

DTI can also give useful intelligence for gray matter integrity, with particular reference to gliosis and necrosis, which may be markers of brain injury from concussion.[179] Although DTI is being used more commonly, its utility in adults has not yet reached the level of diagnostic capabilities, and therefore remains a research tool.

Functional Neuroimaging Techniques

Single Photon Emission Computerized Tomography

Single photon emission computerized tomography (SPECT) involves intravenous injection of a radioisotope (e.g., technetium 99 m) followed by acquisition of brain images from a scintillation camera, enabling a proxy measure of regional cerebral blood flow. In adults and children with mTBI and postconcussion syndrome, abnormalities have been detected in the medial temporal lobe on SPECT.[180,181]

Nevertheless, the American Academy of Neurology has cautioned against the routine use of SPECT for the evaluation of patients with mTBI or postconcussion syndrome.[182] It exposes individuals to radiation and SPECT is considered more helpful in assessing focal injuries (e.g., stroke/brain tumor) rather than diffuse injuries like mTBI.

Positron Emission Tomography

Positron emission tomography (PET) can be used to measure aspects of cerebral metabolism, including blood flow and metabolic rate for oxygen. PET relies on intravenous administration of radionuclides—for example, 2(F-18) fluoro-2-deoxyglucose (FDG)—that have very short half-lives, and are taken up by brain cells.[175] In a study employing SPECT in adults with mTBI, PET was also shown to demonstrate medial temporal hypometablism.[181] However, Chen et al. found normal cerebral FDG uptake at rest in five adults with mTBI, although minor differences emerged during a visuo-spatial memory task.[183] PET is limited by exposure to radio-labeled tracers, cost, and being time-intensive.

Functional Magnetic Resonance Imaging

Functional MRI (fMRI) can offer insight into patterns of brain activation during specific cognitive or behavioral events. fMRI studies have the benefit of being noninvasive and not requiring the use of a radioactive tracer. fMRI assumes neuronal activity based on hemoglobin oxygenation changes, with the signal contrast generated, termed BOLD (blood oxygenation-level dependent).[184]

Abnormalities on fMRI have been linked with the presence of postconcussion symptoms and the severity of these symptoms.[183,185–187] Typically, research subjects are examined on working memory tasks, with abnormal activation patterns of the right parietal and dorsolateral prefrontal cortex being identified in concussion subjects.[188] It has been suggested the disruption working memory may explain certain behavior and decisions in mTBI individuals.[171]

The working memory tasks employed often differs in the published literature, as well as whether the activation of the dorsolateral prefrontal cortex is increased and decreased.[171] Further problems associated with this technique include the interpretation of scans requiring considerable expertise, while the lack of standardization in activation tasks presents a further issue before fMRI can be utilized in routine clinical use.

Magnetoencephalography

Magnetoencephalography (MEG) is a noninvasive technique used to measure the magnetic fields produced by electrical activity in the brain via the use of super conducting quantum interference devices. MEG abnormalities have been detected in adults with persistent postconcussive symptoms suggestive of neuronal injury.[171] In conjunction with other modalities, it has been put forward as a measurement of mTBI. The limitations of MEG include its limited availability and high cost.[172]

Magnetic Resonance Spectroscopy

Magnetic resonance spectroscopy (MRS) is a noninvasive technique used to measure concentrations of various compounds in the brain within a sampled region. This compares to MRI which detects signal from water and lipids. It enables the determination of a range of neurometabolites including creatine, N-acetyl aspartate (NAA), and glutamine.[171]

MRS has been used in the assessment of patients with mTBI, identifying abnormal levels of glutamine in gray matter, and higher levels of creatine in white matter, compared to healthy controls.[189] Furthermore, NAA to creatine ratio has been used to determine outcome in patients with sports-related concussion, with a decreased ratio, indicating a longer recovery time.[190]

Despite the current published literature, the evidence for MRS is not yet sufficient for routine clinical practice. There are few, well-controlled studies, especially those with prospective data linking neurophysiological parameters and clinical outcome. Thus, at present we cannot recommend neurophysiological assessments in the standard clinical testing for postconcussion patients simply because there is insufficient data to do so. Nevertheless, the wide plethora of available neuro-electrophysiological testing suggest that at least some of these tools will be useful in the clinical evaluation of such patients. Furthermore, demonstrable abnormalities in electrophysiological testing in moderate-to-severe TBI is supportive that clinical application in mTBI may also be relevant. Future studies should aim to link neurophysiology and neuroimaging to help bridge the gap in literature that link these two parameters in the assessment of TBI.

Emerging neuroimaging, particularly functional neuroimaging, presents exciting opportunities to develop an improved assessment of concussion. However, standardization of technique and larger prospective studies are required before these methods can move from the research environment to clinical application.

CONCLUSION

mTBI, or concussion, is a commonly occurring and potentially life-changing injury. Whereas severe brain injury is easy to diagnose, mTBI is challenging to diagnose even for experienced professionals. Consequently, very often such patients get discharged from the emergency unit and remain with a hidden brain injury that can cause long-term cognitive, neurological, and behavioral abnormalities. Therefore, it is crucial that new tools, apart from imaging and standard clinical testing, are developed in order to facilitate rapid and correct diagnosis to start appropriate treatment in the acute phase. Given the pace of research, it is likely that sensitive and specific biomarkers for concussion will be widely available in the next 5–10 years.

References

1. Arciniegas DB, Anderson CA, Topkoff J, et al. Mild traumatic brain injury: a neuropsychiatric approach to diagnosis, evaluation, and treatment. *Neuropsychiatr Dis Treat* 2005;1:311–27.
2. Patricios J, Fuller GW, Ellenbogen R, et al. What are the critical elements of sideline screening that can be used to establish the diagnosis of concussion? A systematic review. *Br J Sports Med* 2017;51:888–94.

3. Feddermann-Demont N, Echemendia RJ, Schneider KJ, et al. What domains of clinical function should be assessed after sport-related concussion? A systematic review. *Br J Sports Med* 2017;**51**:903–18.
4. Tulsky DS, Kisala PA, Victorson D, et al. TBI-QOL: development and calibration of item banks to measure patient reported outcomes following traumatic brain injury. *J Head Trauma Rehabil* 2016;**31**:40–51.
5. Steinbuchel N, Covic A, Polinder S, et al. Assessment of health-related quality of life after TBI: comparison of a disease-specific (QOLIBRI) with a Generic (SF-36) Instrument. *Behav Neurol* 2016;**1**:1–14.
6. Polinder S, Haagsma JA, van Klaveren D, et al. Health-related quality of life after TBI: a systematic review of study design, instruments, measurement properties, and outcome. *Popul Health Metr* 2015;**13**:4.
7. Leigh J, Zee D. *The neurology of eye movements*. Oxford: Oxford University Press; 2015.
8. Cifu D, Wares J, Hoke K, et al. Differential eye movements in mild traumatic brain injury versus normal controls. *J Head Trauma Rehabil* 2015;**30**:21–8.
9. DiCesare CA, Kiefer AW, Nalepka P, et al. Quantification and analysis of saccadic and smooth pursuit eye movements and fixations to detect oculomotor deficits. *Behav Res Methods* 2017;**49**:258–66.
10. Alshehri M, Sparto P, Furman J, et al. The usefulness of of the video head impulse test in children and adults post concussion. *J Vestib Res* 2017;**26**:439–46.
11. Yip CW, Glaser M, Frenzel C, et al. Comparison of the bedside head-impulse test with the video head-impulse test in a clinical practice setting: a prospective study of 500 outpatients. *Front Neurol* 2016;**7**. Available from: https://doi.org/10.3389/fneur.2016.00058. Epub ahead of print.
12. Schubert MC, Tusa RJ, Grine LE, et al. Optimizing the sensitivity of the head thrust test for identifying vestibular hypofunction. *Phys Ther* 2004;**84**:151–8.
13. Burston A, Mossman S, Mossman B, et al. Comparison of the video head impulse test with the caloric test in patients with sub-acute and chronic vestibular disorders. *J Clin Neurosci* 2018;**47**:294–8.
14. Bartolomeo M, Biboulet R, Pierre G, et al. Value of the video head impulse test in assessing vestibular deficits following vestibular neuritis. *Eur Arch Otorhinolaryngol* 2014;**271**:681–8.
15. Halmagyi GM, Chen L, MacDougall HG, et al. The video head impulse test. *Front Neurol* 2017;**8**:258. Available from: https://doi.org/10.3389/fneur.2017.00258. Epub ahead of print.
16. Hoffer M, Gottshall K, Moore R, et al. Characterizing and treating dizziness after mild head trauma. *Otol Neurotol* 2004;**25**:135–8.
17. Motin M, Keren O, Groswasser Z, et al. Benign paroxysmal positional vertigo as the cause of dizziness in patients after severe traumatic brain injury: diagnosis and treatment. *Brain Inj* 2005;**19**:693–7.
18. Ahn S-K, Jeon S-Y, Kim J-P, et al. Clinical characteristics and treatment of benign paroxysmal positional vertigo after traumatic brain injury. *J Trauma* 2011;**70**:442–6.
19. Balatsouras D, Koukoutsis G, Aspris G, et al. Benign paroxysmal positional vertigo secondary to mild head trauma. *Ann Otol Rhinol Laryngol* 2016;**126**:54–60.
20. Bhattacharyya N, Gubbels SP, Schwartz SR, et al. Clinical practice guideline: benign paroxysmal positional vertigo (update). *Otolaryngol Neck Surg* 2017;**156**:S1–47.
21. Dean S, Colantonio A, Ratcliff G, et al. Clients' perspectives on problems many years after traumatic brain injury. *Psychol Rep* 2000;**86**:653–8.
22. Williams G, Willmott C. Higher levels of mobility are associated with greater societal participation and better quality-of-life. *Brain Inj* 2012;**26**:1065–71.
23. Hirsch MA, Williams K, Norton HJ, et al. Reliability of the timed 10-metre walk test during inpatient rehabilitation in ambulatory adults with traumatic brain injury. *Brain Inj* 2014;**28**:1115–20.
24. Ochi F, Esquenazi A, Hirai B, et al. Temporal-spatial feature of gait after traumatic brain injury. *J Head Trauma Rehabil* 1999;**14**:105–15.
25. van Loo MA, Moseley AM, Bosman JM, et al. Test–re-test reliability of walking speed, step length and step width measurement after traumatic brain injury: a pilot study. *Brain Inj* 2004;**18**:1041–8.
26. Niechwiej-Szwedo E, Inness EL, Howe JA, et al. Changes in gait variability during different challenges to mobility in patients with traumatic brain injury. *Gait Posture* 2018;**25**:70–7.
27. Williams G, Morris ME, Schache A, et al. Observational gait analysis in traumatic brain injury: accuracy of clinical judgment. *Gait Posture* 2009;**29**:454–9.
28. Newstead A, Hinman M, Ann Tomberlin J. *Reliability of the berg balance scale and balance master limits of stability tests for individuals with brain injury* 2005. Available from: https://doi.org/10.1097/01.NPT.0000282258.74325. cf. 2005. Epub ahead of print.

29. Williams GP, Robertson V, Greenwood KM, et al. The high-level mobility assessment tool (HiMAT) for traumatic brain injury. Part 2: content validity and discriminability. *Brain Inj* 2005;**19**:833–43.
30. Williams GP, Greenwood KM, Robertson VJ, et al. High-Level Mobility Assessment Tool (HiMAT): interrater reliability, retest reliability, and internal consistency. *Phys Ther* 2006;**86**:395–400.
31. Howe J, Inness E, Venturini A, et al. The Community Balance and Mobility Scale—a balance measure for individuals with traumatic brain injury. *Clin Rehabil* 2006;**20**:885–95.
32. Inness J, Howe J, Niechwiej-Szwedo E, et al. Measuring balance and mobility after traumatic brain injury: validation of the community balance and mobility scale (CB& M). *Physiother Can* 2011;**63**:199–203.
33. Salbach NM, Mayo NE, Higgins J, et al. Responsiveness and predictability of gait speed and other disability measures in acute stroke. *Arch Phys Med Rehabil* 2001;**82**:1204–12.
34. Lemay JF, Nadeau S. Standing balance assessment in ASIA D paraplegic and tetraplegic participants: concurrent validity of the Berg Balance Scale. *Spinal Cord* 2009;**48**:245.
35. Bell DR, Guskiewicz KM, Clark MA, et al. Systematic review of the balance error scoring system. *Sports Health* 2011;**3**:287–95.
36. Vartiainen MV, Rinne MB, Lehto TM, et al. The test–retest reliability of motor performance measures after traumatic brain injury. *Adv Physiother* 2006;**8**:50–9.
37. Giorgetti M, Harris B, Jette A. Reliability of clinical balance outcome measures in the elderly. *Physiother Res Int* 1998;**3**:274–83.
38. Koyama S, Tanabe S, Itoh N, et al. Intra- and inter-rater reliability and validity of the tandem gait test for the assessment of dynamic gait balance. *Eur J Physiother* 2017;1–6.
39. Kosaka B. Neuropsychological assessment in mild traumatic brain injury: a clinical overview. *Br Columbia Med J* 2006;**48**:447–52.
40. Kumar S, Jawahar A, Shah P, et al. Montreal Cognitive Assessment, a screening tool for Mild TraumaticBrain Injury (P7.185). *Neurology*; 84. http://n.neurology.org/content/84/14_Supplement/P7.185.abstract (2015).
41. de Guise E, Alturki AY, LeBlanc J, et al. The montreal cognitive assessment in persons with traumatic brain injury. *Appl Neuropsychol Adult* 2014;**21**:128–35.
42. McKay C, Wertheimer JC, Fichtenberg NL, et al. The repeatable battery for the assessment of neuropsychological status (RBANS): clinical utility in a traumatic brain injury sample. *Clin Neuropsychol* 2008;**22**:228–41.
43. Podell K, Gifford K, Bougakov D, et al. Neuropsychological assessment in traumatic brain injury. *Psychiatr Clin North Am* 2010;**33**:855–76.
44. Leininger BE, Gramling SE, Farrell AD, et al. Neuropsychological deficits in symptomatic minor head injury patients after concussion and mild concussion. *J Neurol Neurosurg Psychiatry* 1990;**53**:293.
45. Echemendia R, Putukian M, Mackin R, et al. Neuropsychological test performance prior to and following sports-related mild traumatic brain injury. *Clin J Sport Med* 2001;**11**:23–31.
46. Ross SR, Millis SR, Rosenthal M. Neuropsychological prediction of psychosocial outcome after traumatic brain injury. *Appl Neuropsychol* 1997;**4**:165–70.
47. Bhansali S, Honrubia V. Current status of electronystagmography testing. *Otolaryngol Head Neck Surg* 1999;**120**:419–26.
48. Ashley M. *Traumatic brain injury: rehabilitation, treatment and case management.* Boca Raton, FL: CRC Press; 2016.
49. Baloh W, Honrubia V. *Clinical neurophysiology of the vestibular system.* New York: Oxford University Press; 2001.
50. Jacobsen G, Shepherd N. *Balance function assessment and management.* San Diego, CA: Plural Publishing; 2016.
51. Visser JE, Carpenter MG, van der Kooij H, et al. The clinical utility of posturography. *Clin Neurophysiol* 2008;**119**:2424–36.
52. Sosnoff JJ, Broglio SP, Shin S, et al. Previous mild traumatic brain injury and postural-control dynamics. *J Athl Train* 2011;**46**:85–91.
53. Basford JR, Chou L-S, Kaufman KR, et al. An assessment of gait and balance deficits after traumatic brain injury. *Arch Phys Med Rehabil* 2003;**84**:343–9.
54. Buster TW, Chernyavskiy P, Harms NR, et al. Computerized dynamic posturography detects balance deficits in individuals with a history of chronic severe traumatic brain injury. *Brain Inj* 2016;**30**:1249–55.
55. Kaufman KR, Brey RH, Chou L-S, et al. Comparison of subjective and objective measurements of balance disorders following traumatic brain injury. *Med Eng Phys* 2006;**28**:234–9.

IV. DIAGNOSIS AND TREATMENT

56. Williams G, Galna B, Morris M, et al. Spatiotemporal deficits and kinematic classification of gait following a traumatic brain injury: a systematic review. *J Head Trauma Rehabil* 2010;**25**:366–74.
57. Fausti S, Wilmington D, Gallun F, et al. Auditory and vestibular dysfunction associated with blast-related traumatic brain injury. *J Rehabil Res Dev* 2009;**46**:797–810.
58. Arthur J, Atkinson Jr MD, Wayne A, Colburn M, ScD VGD, et al. Biomarkers and surrogate endpoints: preferred definitions and conceptual framework. *Clin Pharmacol Ther* 2001;**69**:89–95.
59. Bakay R, Ward A. Enzymatic changes in serum and cerebrospinal fluid in neurological injury. *J Neurosurg* 2012;**116**:27–37.
60. Rothermundt M, Peters M, Prehn JH, et al. S100B in brain damage and neurodegeneration. *Microsc Res Tech* 2003;**60**:614–32.
61. Toman E, Harrisson S, Belli T. Biomarkers in traumatic brain injury: a review. *J R Army Med Corps* 2016;**162**:103–8.
62. Berger RP, Beers SR, Richichi R, et al. Serum biomarker concentrations and outcome after pediatric traumatic brain Injury. *J Neurotrauma* 2007;**24**:1793–801.
63. Dadas A, Washington J, Marchi N, Janigro D. Improving the clinical management of traumatic brain injury through the pharmacokinetic modeling of peripheral blood biomarkers. *Fluids and Barriers of the CNS* 2016;**13**:21. Available from: https://doi.org/10.1186/s12987-016-0045-y.
64. Papa L, Ramia MM, Kelly JM, et al. Systematic review of clinical research on biomarkers for pediatric traumatic brain injury. *J Neurotrauma* 2013;**30**:324–38.
65. Svetlov S, Larner S, Kirk D, et al. Biomarkers of blast-induced neurotrauma: profiling molecular and cellular mechanisms of blast brain injury. *J Neurotrauma* 2009;913–21.
66. Sen J, Belli A. S100B in neuropathologic states: the CRP of the brain? *J Neurosci Res* 2007;1373–80.
67. Michetti F, Corvino V, Geloso MC, et al. The S100B protein in biological fluids: more than a lifelong biomarker of brain distress. *J Neurochem* 2012;**120**:644–59.
68. Thelin EP, Zeiler FA, Ercole A, et al. Serial sampling of serum protein biomarkers for monitoring human traumatic brain injury dynamics: a systematic review. *Front Neurol* 2017;**8**:1–23.
69. Michetti F, Gazzolo D. S100B protein in biological fluids: a tool for perinatal medicine. *Clin Chem* 2002;**48**:2097–104.
70. Pelinka LE, Kroepfl A, Leixnering M, et al. GFAP versus S100B in serum after traumatic brain injury: relationship to brain damage and outcome. *J Neurotrauma* 2004;**21**:1553–61.
71. Korfias S, Stranjalis G, Boviatsis E, et al. Serum S-100B protein monitoring in patients with severe traumatic brain injury. *Intens. Care Med* 2007;**33**:255–60.
72. Kövesdi E, Lückl J, Bukovics P, et al. Update on protein biomarkers in traumatic brain injury with emphasis on clinical use in adults and pediatrics. *Acta Neurochir (Wien)* 2010;**152**:1–17.
73. Berger RP, Adelson PD, Pierce MC, et al. Serum neuron-specific enolase, S100B, and myelin basic protein concentrations after inflicted and noninflicted traumatic brain injury in children. *J Neurosurg* 2005;**103**:61–8.
74. Strathmann FG, Schulte S, Goerl K, et al. Blood-based biomarkers for traumatic brain injury: evaluation of research approaches, available methods and potential utility from the clinician and clinical laboratory perspectives. *Clin Biochem* 2014;**47**:876–88.
75. Thelin EP, Nelson DW, Bellander B-M. A review of the clinical utility of serum S100B protein levels in the assessment of traumatic brain injury. *Acta Neurochir (Wien)* 2016;**159**:209–25.
76. Žurek J, Fedora M. The usefulness of S100B, NSE, GFAP, NF-H, secretagogin and Hsp70 as a predictive biomarker of outcome in children with traumatic brain injury. *Acta Neurochir (Wien)* 2012;**154**:93–103.
77. Pham N, Fazio V, Cucullo L, et al. Extracranial sources of S100B do not affect serum levels. *PLoS One* 2010;**5**:1–9.
78. Zetterberg H, Smith DH, Blennow K. Biomarkers of mild traumatic brain injury in cerebrospinal fluid and blood. *Nat Rev Neurol* 2013;**9**:201–10.
79. Mercier E, Tardif P-A, Cameron P, et al. Prognostic value of S-100ßprotein for prediction of post-concussion symptoms following a mild traumatic brain injury: systematic review and meta-analysis. *J Neurotrauma* 2017;**622** neu.2017.5013.
80. Bazarian J, Zemlan F, Mookerjee S. Serum S-100B and cleaved-tau are poor predictors of long-term outcome after mild traumatic brain injury. *Brain Inj* 2006;**20**:759–65.

81. Anderson R, Hansson L, Nilsson O. High serum S100B levels for trauma patients without head injuries. *Neurosurgery* 2001;**48**:1255–60.

82. Stocchero C, Oses J, Cunha G. Serum S100B level increases after running but not cycling exercise. *Appl Physiol Nutr Metab* 2014;**39**:340–4.

83. Dietrich MO, Tort AB, Schaf DV, et al. Increase in serum S100B protein level after a swimming race. *Can J Appl Physiol* 2003;**28**:710–16.

84. Missler U, Orlowski N, Nötzold A, et al. Early elevation of S-100B protein in blood after cardiac surgery is not a predictor of ischemic cerebral injury. *Clin Chim Acta* 2002;**321**:29–33.

85. O'Connell B, Kelly Áine M, Mockler D, et al. Use of blood biomarkers in the assessment of sports-related concussion—a systematic review in the context of their biological significance. *Clin J Sport Med* 2017;**0**:1–11.

86. Zongo D, Ribéreau-Gayon R, Masson F. S100-B protein as a screening tool for the early assessment of minor head injury. *Ann Emerg Med* 2012;209–18.

87. Undén J, Ingebrigtsen T, Romner B. Scandinavian guidelines for initial management of minimal, mild and moderate head injuries in adults: an evidence and consensus-based update. *BMC Med* 2013;**11**:50.

88. Undén L, Calcagnile O, Undén J. Validation of the Scandinavian guidelines for initial management of minimal, mild and moderate traumatic brain injury in adults. *BMC Med* 2015;**13**:292.

89. Papa L., Edwards D., Ramia M. Exploring serum biomarkers for mild traumatic brain injury. In: Brain neurotrauma: molecular, neuropsychological, and rehabilitation aspects Taylor & Francis. 2015.

90. Jeter CB, Hergenroeder GW, Hylin MJ, et al. Biomarkers for the diagnosis and prognosis of mild traumatic brain injury/concussion. *J Neurotrauma* 2013;**30**:657–70.

91. Pelinka LE, Kroepfl A, Schmidhammer R. Glial fibrillary acidic protein in serum after traumatic brain injury and multiple trauma. *J Trauma* 2004;**57**:1006–12.

92. Papa L, Lewis LM, Falk JL, et al. Elevated levels of serum glial fibrillary acidic protein breakdown products in mild and moderate traumatic brain injury are associated with intracranial lesions and neurosurgical intervention. *Ann Emerg Med* 2012;**59**:3–24.

93. Vos PE, Lamers KJ, Hendriks JC, et al. Glial and neuronal proteins in serum predict outcome after severe traumatic brain injury. *Neurology* 2004;**62**:1303–10.

94. Vos PE, Jacobs B, Andriessen TM, et al. GFAP and S100B are biomarkers of traumatic brain injury: an observational cohort study. *Neurology* 2010;**75**:1786–93.

95. Giacoppo S, Bramanti P, Barresi M, et al. Predictive biomarkers of recovery in traumatic brain injury. *Neurocrit Care* 2012;**16**:470–7.

96. Herrmann M. Release of biochemical markers of damage to neuronal and glial brain tissue is associated with short and long term neuropsychological outcome after traumatic brain injury. *J Neurol Neurosurg Psychiatry* 2001;**70**:95–100.

97. Mrozek S, Geeraerts T, Dumurgier J. Biomarkers and acute brain injuries: interest and limits. *Crit Care* 2014;**220**:220.

98. Ergün R, Bostanci U, Akdemir G, et al. Prognostic value of serum neuron-specific enolase levels after head injury. *Neurol Res* 1998;418–20.

99. Ross SA, Cunningham RT, Johnston CF, et al. Neuronspecific enolase as an aid to outcome prediction in head injury. *Br J Neurosurg* 1996;471–6.

100. Geyer C, Ulrich A, Gräfe G, et al. Diagnostic value of S100B and neuron-specific enolase in mild pediatric traumatic brain injury. *J Neurosurg Pediatr* 2009;**4**:339–44.

101. Wolf H, Frantal S, Pajenda GS, et al. Predictive value of neuromarkers supported by a set of clinical criteria in patients with mild traumatic brain injury: S100B protein and neuron-specific enolase on trial. *J Neurosurg* 2013;**118**:1298–303.

102. Topolovec-Vranic J, Pollmann-Mudryj M-A, Ouchterlony D. The value of serum biomarkers in prediction models of outcome after mild traumatic brain injury. *J Trauma* 2011;**71**:478–86.

103. Papa L, Lewis LM, Silvestri S, et al. Serum levels of ubiquitin C-terminal hydrolase distinguish mild traumatic brain injury from trauma controls and are elevated in mild and moderate traumatic brain injury patients with intracranial lesions and neurosurgical intervention. *J Trauma Acute Care Surg* 2012;**72**:1335–44.

104. Berger RP, Hayes RL, Richichi R, et al. Serum concentrations of ubiquitin C-terminal hydrolase-L1 and αII-spectrin breakdown product 145 kDa correlate with outcome after pediatric TBI. *J Neurotrauma* 2012;**29**:162–7.

105. Meier TB, Nelson LD, Huber DL, et al. Prospective assessment of acute blood markers of brain injury in sport-related concussion. *J Neurotrauma* 2017;3142 neu.2017.5046.
106. Kochanek PM, Berger RP, Bayir H, et al. Biomarkers of primary and evolving damage in traumatic and ischemic brain injury: diagnosis, prognosis, probing mechanisms, and therapeutic decision making. *Curr Opin Crit Care* 2008;**14**:135−41.
107. D'Aversa TG, Eugenin EA, Lopez L, et al. Myelin basic protein induces inflammatory mediators from primary human endothelial cells and blood-brain-barrier disruption: implications for the pathogenesis of multiple sclerosis. *Neuropathol Appl Neurobiol* 2013;**39**:270−83.
108. Berger RP, Bazaco MC, Wagner AK, et al. Trajectory analysis of serum biomarker concentrations facilitates outcome prediction after pediatric traumatic and hypoxemic brain injury. *Dev Neurosci* 2010;**32**:396−405.
109. Berger RP, Adelson PD, Pierce MC, et al. Serum neuron-specific enolase, S100B, and myelin basic protein concentrations after inflicted and noninflicted traumatic brain injury in children. *J Neurosurg Pediatr* 2005;**103**:61−8.
110. Berger RP. Identification of inflicted traumatic brain injury in well-appearing infants using serum and cerebrospinal markers: a possible screening tool. *Pediatrics* 2006;**117**:325−32.
111. Yamazaki Y, Yada K, Morii S, et al. Diagnostic significance of serum neuron-specific enolase and myelin basic proteinassay in patients with acute head injury. *Surg Neurol* 1995;**43**:267−71.
112. Julien J, Mushynski W. Neurofilaments in health and disease. *Prog Nucleic Acid Res Mol Biol* 1998;**6**:1−23.
113. Rostami E, Davidsson J, Chye Ng K, et al. A model for mild traumatic brain injury that induces limited transient memory impairment and increased levels of axon related serum biomarkers. *Front Neurol* 2012;1−9.
114. Anderson KJ, Scheff SW, Miller KM, et al. The phosphorylated axonal form of the neurofilament subunit NF-H (pNF-H) as a blood biomarker of traumatic brain injury. *J Neurotrauma* 2008;**25**:1079−85.
115. Scheff SW, Sullivan PG. Cyclosporin A significantly ameliorates cortical damage following experimental traumatic brain injury in rodents. *J Neurotrauma* 1999;**16**:783−92.
116. Zurek J, Bartlová L, Fedora M. Hyperphosphorylated neurofilament NF-H as a predictor of mortality after brain injury in children. *Brain Inj* 2011;**25**:221−6.
117. Gatson JW, Barillas J, Hynan LS, et al. Detection of neurofilament-H in serum as a diagnostic tool to predict injury severity in patients who have suffered mild traumatic brain injury. *J Neurosurg* 2014;**121**:1232−8.
118. Trojanowski JQ, Schuck T, Schmidt ML, et al. Distribution of tau proteins in the normal human central and peripheral nervous system. *Histochem Cytochem* 1989;209−15.
119. Shahim P, Tegner Y, Wilson DH, et al. Blood biomarkers for brain injury in concussed professional ice hockey players. *JAMA Neurol* 2014;**71**:684−92.
120. Guzel A, Karasalihoglu S, Aylanç H, et al. Validity of serum tau protein levels in pediatric patients with minor head trauma. *Am J Emerg Med* 2010;**28**:399−403.
121. Shaw GJ, Jauch EC, Zemlan FP. Serum cleaved Tau protein levels and clinical outcome in adult patients with closed head injury. *Ann Emerg Med* 2002;**39**:254−7.
122. Zemlan FP, Rosenberg WS, Luebbe PA, et al. Quantification of axonal damage in traumatic brain injury: affinity purification and characterization of cerebrospinal fluid tau proteins. *J Neurochem* 1999;**72**:741−50.
123. Ma M, Lindsell CJ, Rosenberry CM, et al. Serum cleaved-tau does not predict postconcussion syndrome after mild traumatic brain injury. *Am J Emerg Med* 2009;**26**:763−8.
124. Zetterberg H, Blennow K. Fluid markers of traumatic brain injury. *Mol Cell Neurosci* 2015;**66**:99−102.
125. Romeo MJ, Espina V, Lowenthal M, et al. CSF proteome: a protein repository for potential biomarker identification. *Expert Rev Proteomics* 2005;**2**:57−70.
126. Good DM, Thongboonkerd V, Novak J, et al. Body fluid proteomics for biomarker discovery: lessons from the past hold the key to success in the future. *J Proteome Res* 2007;**6**:4549−55.
127. Neselius S, Brisby H, Theodorsson A, et al. Csf-biomarkers in olympic boxing: diagnosis and effects of repetitive head trauma. *PLoS One* 2012;**7**:1−8.
128. Siman R, Toraskar N, Dang A, et al. A panel of neuron-enriched proteins as markers for traumatic brain injury in humans. *J Neurotrauma* 2009;**26**:1867−77.
129. Zetterberg H, et al. Neurochemical aftermath of amateur boxing. *Arch Neurol* 2006;**63**:1277−80.
130. Friede RL, Samorajski T. Axon caliber related to neurofilaments and microtubules in sciatic nerve fibers of rats and mice. *Anat Rec* 1970;379−87.

IV. DIAGNOSIS AND TREATMENT

131. Caswell SV, Cortes N, Mitchell K, et al. Development of nanoparticle-enabled protein biomarker discovery: implementation for saliva-based traumatic brain injury detection. *Advances in Salivary Diagnostics Springer* 2015;121−9.

132. Bhomia M, Balakathiresan NS, Wang KK, et al. A panel of serum MiRNA biomarkers for the diagnosis of severe to mild traumatic brain injury in humans. *Sci Rep* 2016;**6**:1−12.

133. Valadi H, Ekström K, Bossios A, et al. Exosome-mediated transfer of mRNAs and microRNAs is a novel mechanism of genetic exchange between cells. *Nat Cell Biol* 2007;**9**:654−9.

134. Gilad S, Meiri E, Yogev Y. Serum microRNAs are promising novel biomarkers. *PLoS One* 2008;**3**:e3148.

135. Johnson JJ, Loeffert AC, Stokes J, et al. Association of salivary microRNA changes with prolonged concussion symptoms. *JAMA Pediatr* 2018;**172**:65−73.

136. Kulbe JR, Geddes JW. Current status of fluid biomarkers in mild traumatic brain injury. *Exp Neurol* 2016;**275**:334−52.

137. Berger R, Kochanek P. Urinary S100B concentrations are increased after brain injury in children: a preliminary study. *Pediatr Crit Care Med* 2006;**7**:557−61.

138. Weinberg AM, Castellani C. Role of neuroprotein S-100B in the diagnostic of pediatric mild brain injury. *Eur J Trauma Emerg Surg* 2010;**36**:318−24.

139. Pickering A, Carter J, Hanning I, et al. Emergency department measurement of urinary s100B in children following head injury: can extracranial injury confound findings? *Emerg Med J* 2008;**25**:88−9.

140. Rodríguez-Rodríguez A, Egea-Guerrero JJ, León-Justel A, et al. Role of S100B protein in urine and serum as an early predictor of mortality after severe traumatic brain injury in adults. *Clin Chim Acta* 2012;**414**:228−33.

141. Ringger NC, O'steen BE, Brabham JG, et al. A novel marker for traumatic brain injury: CSF αII-spectrin breakdown product levels. *J Neurotrauma* 2004;**21**:1443−56.

142. Shan R, Szmydynger-Chodobska J, Warren OU, et al. A new panel of blood biomarkers for the diagnosis of mild traumatic brain injury/concussion in adults. *J Neurotrauma* 2016;**33**:49−57.

143. McCrea M, Meier T, Huber D, et al. Role of advanced neuroimaging, fluid biomarkers and genetic testing in the assessment of sport-related concussion: a systematic review. *Br J Sports Med* 2017;**51**:919−29.

144. Keltner J. Visual evoked response. *West J Med* 1977;**126**:130.

145. Feinsod M, Hoyt WF, Wilson WB, et al. Visually evoked response: use in neurologic evaluation of posttraumatic subjective visual complaints. *Arch Ophthalmol* 1976;**94**:237−40.

146. Werner R, Vanderzant CW. Multimodality evoked potential testing in acute mild closed head injury. *Arch Phys Med Rehabil* 1991;**72**:31−4.

147. Papathanasopoulos P, Konstantinou D, Flaburiari K, et al. Pattern reversal visual evoked potentials in minor head injury. *Eur Neurol* 1994;**34**:268−71.

148. Gaetz M, Weinberg H. Electrophysiological indices of persistent post-concussion symptoms. *Brain Inj* 2000;**14**:815−32.

149. Freed S, Fishman-Hellerstein L. Visual electrodiagnostic findings in mild traumatic brain injury. *Brain Inj* 1997;**11**:25−36.

150. Fimreite V, Ciuffreda KJ, Yadav NK. Effect of luminance on the visually-evoked potential in visually-normal individuals and in mTBI/concussion. *Brain Inj* 2015;**29**:1199−210.

151. Yadav N, Ciuffreda K. Objective assessment of visual attention in mild traumatic brain injury (mTBI) using visual-evoked potentials (VEP). *Brain Inj* 2015;**29**:352−65.

152. Lachapelle J, Ouimet C, Bach M, et al. Texture segregation in traumatic brain injury−−a VEP study. *Vision Res* 2004;**44**:2835−42.

153. Poltavski D, Lederer P, Cox LK. Visually evoked potential markers of concussion history in patients with convergence insufficiency. *Vis Optom* 2017;**94**:742.

154. Munjal S, Panda N, Pathak A. Relationship between severity of traumatic brain injury (TBI) and extent of auditory dysfunction. *Brain Inj* 2010;**24**:525−32.

155. Theilen H, Ragaller M, von Kummer R, et al. Functional recovery despite prolonged bilateral loss of somatosensory evoked potentials: report on two patients. *J Neurol Neurosurg Psychiatry* 2000;**68**:657−60.

156. Wedekind C, Hesselmann V, Klug N. Comparison of MRI and electrophysiological studies for detecting brainstem lesions in traumatic brain injury. *Muscle Nerve* 2002;**26**:270−3.

157. Christyakov A, Soustiel J, Hafner H, et al. Excitatory and inhibitory corticospinal responses to transcranial magnetic stimulation in patients with minor to moderate head injury. *J Neurol Neurosurg Psychiatry* 2001;**70**:580−7.

IV. DIAGNOSIS AND TREATMENT

158. Jang S, Cho S-H, Kim Y-H, et al. Motor recovery mechanism of diffuse axonal injury: a combined study of transcranial magnetic stimulation and functional MRI. *Restorat Neurol Neurosci* 2005;**23**:51−6.
159. Takeuchi N, Ikoma K, Chuma T, et al. Measurement of transcallosal inhibition in traumatic brain injury by transcranial magnetic stimulation. *Brain Inj* 2006;**20**:991−6.
160. Di Virgilio T, Hunter A, Wilson L, et al. Evidence for acute electrophysiological and cognitive changes following routine soccer heading. *EBioMed* 2016;**13**:66−71.
161. Wolters A, Ziemann U, Benecke R, et al. *The Oxford handbook of transcranial stimulation*. Oxford: Oxford University Press; 2008.
162. Schalamon J, Singer G, Kurschel S, et al. Somatosensory evoked potentials in children with severe head trauma. *Eur J Pediatr* 2005;**164**:417−20.
163. Carter B, Butt W. A prospective study of outcome predictors after severe brain injury in children. *Int Care Med* 2005;**31**:840−5.
164. Crossley M, Shiel A, Wilson B, et al. Monitoring emergence from coma following severe brain injury in an octogenarian using behavioural indicators, electrophysiological measures and metabolic studies: a demonstration of the potential for good recovery in older adults. *Brain Inj* 2005;**19**:729−37.
165. Schwarz S, Schwab S, Aschoff A, et al. Favourable outcome from bilateral loss of somatosensory evoked potentials. *Crit Care Med* 1999;**27**:182−7.
166. Carter B, Taylor A, Butt W. Severe brain injury in children: long-term outcome and its prediction using somatosensory evoked potentials. *Snt Care Med* 1999;**25**:722−8.
167. Robe P, Dubuisson A, Bartsch S, et al. Favourable outcome of a brain trauma patient despite bilateral loss of cortical somatosensory evoked potential during thiopental sedation. *J Neurol Neurosurg Psychiatry* 2003;**74**:1157−8.
168. Castriotta R, Atanasov S, Wilde M, et al. Treatment of sleep disorders after traumatic brain injury. *J Clin Sleep Med* 2009;**5**:137−44.
169. Shekleton J, Parcell D, Redman J, et al. Sleep disturbance and melatonin levels following traumatic brain injury. *Neurology* 2010;**74**:1732−8.
170. McCrory P, Meeuwisse WH, Aubry M, et al. Consensus statement on concussion in sport: the 4th International Conference on Concussion in Sport. *Br J Sport Med* 2013;**47**:250−8.
171. Prabhu S. The role of neuroimaging in sport-related concussion. *Clin Sport Med* 2011;**30**:103−14.
172. Davis G, Iverson G, Guskiewicz K, et al. Contributions of neuroimaging, balance testing, electrophysiology and blood markers to the assessment of sport-related concussion. *Br J Sports Med* 2009;**43**:36−45.
173. Hughes D, Jackson A, Mason D, et al. Abnormalities on magnetic resonance imaging seen acutely following mild traumatic brain injury: correlation with neuropsychological tests and delayed recovery. *Neuroradiology* 2004;**46**:550−8.
174. Doezema D, King JN, Tandberg D, et al. Magnetic resonance imaging in minor head injury. *Ann Emerg Med* 1991;**20**:1281−5.
175. Lewine J, Davis J, Bigler E, et al. Objective documentation of traumatic brain injury subsequent to mild head trauma: multimodal brain imaging with MEG, SPECT, and MRI. *J Head Trauma Rehabil* 2007;**22**:141−55.
176. Basser P, Jones D. Diffusion-tensor MRI: theory, experimental design and data analysis—a technical review. *NMR Biomed* 2002;**15**:456−67.
177. Le Bihan D, Mangin J, Poupon C. Diffusion tensor imaging: concepts and applications. *J Magn Reson Imaging* 2001;**13**:534−46.
178. Wilde E, McCauley S, Hunter J. Diffusion tensor imaging of acute mild traumatic brain injury in adolescents. *Neurology* 2008;**70**:948−55.
179. Mukherjee P, Miller JH, Shimony JS. Diffusion-tensor MR imaging of gray and white matter development during normal human brain maturation. *Am J Neuroradiol* 2002;**23**:144−56.
180. Agrawal D, Gowda NK, Bal CS. Is medial temporal injury responsible for pediatric postconcussion syndrome? A prospective controlled study with singlephoton emission computerized tomography. *J Neurosurg* 2005;**102**:167−71.
181. Umile E, Sandel M, Alavi A. Dynamic imaging in mild traumatic brain injury: support for the theory of medial temporal vulnerability. *Arch Phys Med Rehabil* 2002;**83**:1506−13.
182. Neurology R of the T and TAS of the AA of *Assessment of brain SPECT*. 1996.

183. Chen J, Johnston K, Collie A. A validation of the post concussion symptom scale in the assessment of complex concussion using cognitive testing and functional MRI. *J Neurol Neurosurg Psychiatry* 2007;**78**:1231−8.

184. Ogawa S, Lee TM, Kay AR. Brain magnetic resonance imaging with contrast dependent on blood oxygenation. *Proc Natl Acad Sci* 1990;**87**:9869−72.

185. Lovell M, Pardini J, Welling J. Functional brain abnormalities are related to clinical recovery and time to return-to-play in athletes. *Neurosurgery* 2007;**61**:359−60.

186. Chen S, Kareken D, Fastenau P. A study of persistent post-concussion symptoms in mild head trauma using positron emission tomography. *J Neurol Neurosurg Psychiatry* 2003;**74**:326−32.

187. Jantzen K, Anderson B, Steinberg F. A prospective functional MR imaging study of mild traumatic brain injury in college football players. *Am J Neuroradiol* 2004;**25**:738−45.

188. McAllister TW, Saykin AJ, Flashman LA, et al. Brain activation during working memory 1 month after mild traumatic brain injury A functional MRI study. *Neurology* 1999;**53**:1300.

189. Gasparovic C, Yeo R, Mannell M, et al. Neurometabolite concentrations in gray and white matter in mild traumatic brain injury: an 1H−magnetic resonance spectroscopy study. *J Neurotrauma* 2009;**26**:1635−43.

190. Tollard E, Galanaud D, Perlbarg V, et al. Experience of diffusion tensor imaging and 1H spectroscopy for outcome prediction in severe traumatic brain injury: preliminary results. *Crit Care Med* 2009;**37**:1448−55.

Neurosensory Diagnostic Techniques for Mild Traumatic Brain Injury

Joo Hyun Park, MD, PhD[1] and Ja-Won Koo, MD, PhD[2]

[1]Department of Otorhinolaryngology-Head and Neck Surgery, Dongguk University Ilsan Hospital, Goyang, South Korea [2]Department of Otorhinolaryngology-Head and Neck Surgery, Seoul National University Bundang Hospital, Seongnam, South Korea

INTRODUCTION

Mild traumatic brain injury (mTBI) and concussion are interchangeable terms that refer to mild brain injuries arising from external forces.[1] mTBI is an acute condition characterized by transient alterations in mental status and memory disorders based on various events that occur directly following the insult,[2] including loss of consciousness (LOC), posttraumatic amnesia (PTA), and/or other neurosensory problems. If an individual sustains head trauma, but does not exhibit these accompanying signs or symptoms, a diagnosis of mTBI will not be made.

One of the major challenges associated with the management of mTBI is the lack of a "gold standard" for assessing and diagnosing mTBI after injury. The diagnosis of mTBI remains a clinical diagnosis based on a combination of the patient's self-reported symptoms (somatic, cognitive, and neurobehavioral), physical examination findings, and impairments in cognitive function. To further complicate matters, the clinical features of mTBI vary among individuals and can present in a delayed fashion following trauma. Despite evolving brain imaging techniques, mTBI is still considered to be a functional injury and not one that can be structurally identified on imaging scans. Thus, a variety of diagnostic tools have been studied and developed to properly assess and manage mTBI, especially in sports and the military.

Previously, mTBI (concussion) severity scales have utilized classical injury characteristics such as LOC and/or PTA to establish the diagnosis and prognosis. The diagnosis of mTBI typically requires a recent history of head trauma and one or more of the following: a Glasgow Coma Scale (GCS)[3] score of 13–15 (best value within initial 24 hours), the loss of or decreased consciousness lasting less than 30 minutes, a loss of memory for events immediately after the event and PTA lasting less than 24 hours, and/or any alteration of mental state immediately following the event.[4,5] Structural imaging techniques such as computed tomography and magnetic resonance imaging (MRI) do not usually show associated abnormalities in patients suspected of mTBI.[6]

Patients with mTBI report heterogeneous and complex neurocognitive and neuropsychological symptoms as well as physical symptoms (e.g., headache, dizziness, balance problem, nausea, fatigue, sleep disturbance, blurred vision, sensitivity to light or noise, hearing difficulties, seizure, transient neurological abnormalities, numbness, and tingling), cognitive symptoms (e.g., attention, concentration, memory, speed of processing, judgment, and executive control), and behavioral/emotional symptoms (e.g., depression, anxiety, agitation, irritability, impulsivity, and aggression).[7] The cardinal features of mTBI are acute alterations in one's level of consciousness and memory function that are resolved within 30 minutes. However, deficits in cognitive function and other symptoms may persist for hours, days, or even weeks following the injury. Therefore, clinicians have attempted to visualize and quantify patient discomfort to evaluate the severity of mTBI and to facilitate customized management for each patient; neurosensory tests are not essential for the diagnosis of mTBI itself.

Studies and recommendations have indicated that previous approaches focusing on LOC and PTA may not be the most appropriate markers with which to diagnose mTBI.[8] Instead, a multifaceted approach that emphasizes the use of objective assessment tools that can capture the spectrum of clinical symptoms, signs, cognitive dysfunction, and physical problems associated with mTBI has been proposed for its diagnosis and management.[8-12] Further studies have concluded that these multifaceted assessments are more sensitive to head trauma than any one evaluation tool alone.[13-16] It is essential for clinicians to fully understand the necessary components of a multifaceted evaluation for mTBI.

The establishment of standardized tests that can measure the effects of mTBI has been implemented in sports medicine[12]; however, these tools can also assist in the evaluation of civilian mTBI by refining the processes involved in the diagnosis, prognosis, and clinical decision-making of these injuries. According to a recent consensus statement on concussion in sports, mTBI (concussion) should be suspected and the appropriate management instituted if one or more of the following clinical components is present: (1) various somatic, cognitive, and/or emotional symptoms; (2) physical signs (e.g., LOC and PTA); (3) behavioral changes (e.g., irritability); (4) cognitive impairments (e.g., slowed reaction times); and/or (5) sleep disturbances.[12] Medical assessments of mTBI typically include a comprehensive history and detailed neurological examination that incorporates a thorough assessment of mental status, cognitive functioning, gait, and balance. Furthermore, mTBI evaluation tools should determine whether the symptoms and signs have improved or deteriorated since the time of injury; this may involve seeking additional information from parents, accompanying guardians, and/or eyewitnesses to the injury.[12] Regardless of the recent progress that has been made in terms of clinical assessments, the needs for emergent neuroimaging to exclude a more severe brain injury and checklists for the initial evaluation remain.

In this chapter, several clinical assessment tools that have been accepted and practically used for the assessment of mTBI by international experts or related groups will be introduced.

EVALUATION OF CONSCIOUSNESS

Glasgow Coma Scale

The GCS is commonly used to provide an initial assessment score for patients with TBI and has been widely accepted in the fields of neurosurgery, emergency medicine, and acute trauma as a marker of the severity of head injury in adults[17–20]; GCS scores range from 3 to 15 (Table 17.1). These scores are often not included in mTBI studies because the very nature of a mild injury would result in a GCS score of at least 14 or 15, which is frequently normal. Nonetheless, the GCS is widely accepted as one of the best predictors of outcome following more moderate to severe injuries and, as such, is appropriate for the identification of more severe injuries.[21] Some authors have reported the efficacy of the GCS-Extended (GCS-E; Table 17.1), which includes duration of PTA along with the traditional GCS, for the prediction of symptoms in mTBI patients.[17] The use of the GCS-E in mTBI patients has shown that longer lengths of amnesia following injury are associated with greater incidences of dizziness, depression, and cognitive impairments during the first weeks after the injury.[17] Thus, it is important to assess PTA multiple times beginning with an initial assessment and then at documented intervals throughout the stages of recovery.

TABLE 17.1   Glasgow Coma Scale and Extended Version

Eye Response (E)	Verbal Response (V)	Motor Response (M)	Duration of Amnesia (A)	
No eye opening	No verbal response	No motor response	31–90 days	1
Eye opening in response to pain	Eyes opening spontaneously	Extension (decerebrate response) on painful stimuli	8–30 days	2
Eye opening to speech	Inappropriate words	Abnormal flexion (decorticate response) on painful stimuli	1–7 days	3
Eyes opening spontaneously	Confused	Withdrawal from pain	3–24 h	4
–	Oriented	Localizes to pain	30 min to 3 h	5
–	–	Obeys commands	<30 min	6
–	–	–	None	7
Glasgow Coma Score (E + V + M)				of 15
Glasgow Coma-Extended score (E + V + M + A)				of 22

SYMPTOM ASSESSMENT

Several postconcussion symptom questionnaires are widely used to evaluate mTBI. Symptom inventories allow patients to self-report their current symptoms with severity ratings for each endorsed symptom.[22,23] Although there are slight differences in the number and content of question items among these questionnaires, they are essentially the same and can be used to assess the presence and severity of postconcussion symptoms.

Rivermead Post-Concussion Symptoms Questionnaire

The Rivermead Post-Concussion Symptoms Questionnaire (RPQ) is used to determine the presence and severity of postconcussion syndrome and is thought to reflect somatic/physical, cognitive, and emotional symptoms following TBI.[24] The RPQ consists of 16 items that represent the most frequently reported symptoms in the literature: headache, dizziness, nausea and/or vomiting, noise sensitivity, sleep disturbance, fatigue, being irritable, feeling depressed, feeling frustrated, forgetfulness, poor concentration, taking longer time to think, blurred vision, light sensitivity, double vision, and restlessness.[25] The RPQ is a reliable measure of postconcussion symptoms and a valid tool for the measurement of postconcussion syndrome.[26] Patients are asked to rate the degree to which each item has been more of a problem during the last 24 hours compared to before the TBI using a 5-point Likert scale: 0 = not experienced at all; 1 = no more of a problem; 2 = a mild problem; 3 = a moderate problem; and 4 = a severe problem.

Post-Concussion Symptom Scale

The Post-Concussion Symptom Scale (PCSS) is a self-report symptom checklist on which participants rate 22 items using a seven-point Likert scale. The PCSS is reliable and valid for the assessment of both symptom presence and severity[16,27–31] and has been used in a variety of settings to assess concussion.[32–34] A graded symptom checklist is the most commonly used type of postconcussion assessment tool[35] and, accordingly, the PCSS is included in the Sport Concussion Assessment Tool, version 3 (SCAT3).[12] Symptom assessment is important initially as well as during serial evaluations following concussion to understand the courses of symptom presentation and resolution after an injury. The maximum number of symptom items on this scale is 22 and the maximal symptom severity score is 132, which is obtained by summing the rated symptom scores from 0 (none) to 6 (severe) for each symptom as follows: 0 = none; 1–2 = mild; 3–4 = moderate; and 5–6 = severe. Two other "yes/no" questions are posed and rated as to whether the symptoms are exacerbated by either physical or mental activity.[12]

Post-Concussion Symptom Scale-Revised

Similar to the PCSS, the Post-Concussion Symptom Scale-Revised (PCS-R) is a self-report concussion symptom checklist that rates 21 symptoms (e.g., headache, nausea, fatigue, and irritability) using a seven-point Likert scale ranging from 0 (none) to 6 (severe); higher scores indicate greater symptom severity (Fig. 17.1). This scale has been

Symptom	Rating						
	None		Moderate			Severe	
Headache	0	1	2	3	4	5	6
Nausea	0	1	2	3	4	5	6
Vomiting	0	1	2	3	4	5	6
Balance problems	0	1	2	3	4	5	6
Dizziness	0	1	2	3	4	5	6
Fatigue	0	1	2	3	4	5	6
Trouble falling asleep	0	1	2	3	4	5	6
Excessive sleep	0	1	2	3	4	5	6
Loss of sleep	0	1	2	3	4	5	6
Drowsiness	0	1	2	3	4	5	6
Light sensitivity	0	1	2	3	4	5	6
Noise sensitivity	0	1	2	3	4	5	6
Irritability	0	1	2	3	4	5	6
Sadness	0	1	2	3	4	5	6
Nervousness	0	1	2	3	4	5	6
More emotional	0	1	2	3	4	5	6
Numbness	0	1	2	3	4	5	6
Feeling slowed down	0	1	2	3	4	5	6
Feeling "foggy"	0	1	2	3	4	5	6
Difficulty concentrating	0	1	2	3	4	5	6
Difficulty remembering	0	1	2	3	4	5	6
Total score							

FIGURE 17.1 Post-Concussion Symptom Scale-Revised. *Source: Permission was obtained for use of figure (Lovell and Collins, J Head Trauma Rehab, 1998).*[36]

used for the sideline assessment of players in the National Football League and National Hockey League.[36]

Concussion Symptom Inventory

The Concussion Symptom Inventory (CSI) is a list of 12 symptoms that are graded by the patient in terms of severity using a seven-point Likert scale.[37] The CSI was developed by analyzing a large set of data from sports-related concussion patients to derive a sensitive and efficient scale. The assessed symptoms include headache, nausea, balance problems/dizziness, fatigue, drowsiness, feeling like one is "in a fog," difficulty concentrating, difficulty remembering, sensitivity to light, sensitivity to noise, blurred vision, and feeling slowed down. This scale has a maximum symptom number score of 12 and a maximum severity score of 72, where lower scores indicate lower severity.

Maddocks Score/Questions

Maddocks questions assess the orientation of a patient, particularly their recall of recently acquired events. These questions are more sensitive to concussion than standard

Maddocks score

(1 point for each correct answer)

What venue are we at today?	0	1
Which half is it now?	0	1
Who scored last in this match?	0	1
What team did you play last week/game?	0	1
Did your team win the last game?	0	1
Maddocks score	of 5	

FIGURE 17.2   Modified Maddocks questions. *Source: McCrory et al., J Athl Train, 2012.*[12]

orientation questions and can provide important clinical information at the time of injury, especially on the field of sports games.[38] The SCAT3 includes modified Maddocks questions and has been validated only for the sideline diagnosis of concussion; it is not used for serial testing (see Fig. 17.2).[12]

COGNITIVE ASSESSMENTS

Standardized Assessment of Concussion

General cognitive function and sustained concentration have also been assessed using bedside cognitive screening tests.[39–42] The Standardized Assessment of Concussion (SAC) has been extensively used in research related to TBI and has accepted degrees of diagnostic and predictive validity in this type of injury setting.[14,41–46] The SAC provides an objective, reproducible, and standardized report of the consequences of concussion.[40] This measure is a paper-and-pencil assessment that consists of four domains: orientation, immediate memory, concentration, and delayed recall (Fig. 17.3). Total SAC scores range from 0 to 30, where higher scores indicate better neurocognitive function. This procedure also includes a standard neurological screening to examine strength, sensation, and coordination (description of occurrence and duration of LOC and pre- and posttraumatic amnesia) and an assessment of exertional maneuvers when appropriate (five jumping jacks, push-ups, sit-ups, and knee-bends). The SAC takes 10 minutes or less to complete and has been extensively validated for use in sports-related concussed populations.[40,43]

This tool is sensitive to sports concussions if administered within the first 48 hours[14,41,43,45,46]; concussed players score significantly lower than nonconcussed controls as well as their own baseline performance.[40,46,47] Decreased scores tend to normalize within 2–3 days[46] or show a gradual slope of recovery later after injury.[47] SAC scores that are three points lower represent a statistically reliable and clinically significant change in performance.[43] Several studies have reported the sensitivity and specificity of the SAC for detecting concussions. For example, a one-point drop on the SAC is 94% sensitive and 76% specific for football players,[43] and has 95% sensitivity and 76% specificity for diagnosing sideline sports-related concussions immediately after head injury.[48] However, it is notable that these studies exclusively assessed male high school and college football players. Additionally, subsequent studies have reported markedly lower degrees of sensitivity and specificity than previous studies[49] and found no differences between posttrauma and baseline SAC scores (0.52 ± 1.18) when tested after injury.[50]

1. Orientation (one point for each correct answer)

	0	1
Month	0	1
Date	0	1
Day of week	0	1
Year	0	1
Time (within 1 h)	0	1
Orientation total score		of 5

2. Immediate memory (all three trials are completed regardless of score on trials 1 & 2; total score equals sum across all three trials)

List	Trial 1		Trial 2		Trial 3	
Word 1	0	1	0	1	0	1
Word 2	0	1	0	1	0	1
Word 3	0	1	0	1	0	1
Word 4	0	1	0	1	0	1
Word 5	0	1	0	1	0	1
Immediate memory total score						of 15

(Note: Subject is not informed of Delayed Recall testing of memory)

Neurological screening

Loss of consciousness: (occurrence, duration)

Pre- & Posttraumatic Amnesia: (recollection of events pre- & postinjury)

Strength:

Sensation:

Coordination:

Exertional maneuvers (when appropriate)

5 jumping jacks	5 push-ups
5 sit-ups	5 knee-bends

3. Concentration

Digits backward (If correct, go to next string length. If incorrect, read trial 2. Stop after incorrect on both trials.)

		0	1
4-9-3	6-2-9	0	1
3-8-1-4	3-2-7-9	0	1
6-2-9-7-1	1-5-2-8-6	0	1
7-1-8-4-6-2	5-3-9-1-4-8	0	1

Months in reverse order (entire sequence correct for 1 point)

	0	1
Dec-Nov-Oct-Sep-Aug-Jul-Jun-May-Apr-Mar-Feb-Jan	0	1
Concentration total score		of 5

4. Delayed recall

	0	1
Word 1	0	1
Word 2	0	1
Word 3	0	1
Word 4	0	1
Word 5	0	1
Delayed recall total score		of 5
Overall total score		**of 30**

Summary of total score

Orientation	———	/5
Immediate memory	———	/15
Concentration	———	/5
Delayed recall	———	/5
Overall total score	———	/30

FIGURE 17.3 Standardized Assessment of Concussion. *Source: Permission was obtained for use of figure (MacCrea et al., Neurology, 1997).[40]*

Regarding mTBI in nonathletic populations, a baseline SAC score generally cannot be obtained. A study of mTBI patients in an emergency department showed that SAC scores significantly improve over time (assessed immediately and 3 and 6 hours after arrival), but that the symptoms do not correlate with improvement as many of the subjects complained of headache or nausea after their scores improved.[42] The SAC appears to be sensitive to acute changes following mTBI whereas GCS scores and radiological findings are usually normal in mTBI patients. The average initial score on the SAC in emergency room mTBI patients is approximately 21 ± 5.4,[42] which is lower than the score of 26 reported for concussed patients in a study of 1313 high school athletes.[43] Studies investigating the use of the SAC in civilian mTBI populations are limited; however, emergency department patients may exhibit lower scores because many of them likely sustained more severe trauma than high school students.[42]

The effects of age and sex on SAC scores have been reported by several studies that investigated only young athletes. Despite initial findings showing no effect of age on the

SAC,[41,51] increasing age has recently been associated with significant increases in SAC scores.[52] Findings from athletes have been inconsistent in terms of the relationship between sex and SAC scores[40,46,53–55]; however, there is a decrease in mental status immediately after mTBI according to the SAC.[43,48]

King–Devick Test

The King–Devick Test (K-D)[56] is a brief measure that assesses cognitive processing speed, visual tracking, and saccadic eye movements and also includes oculomotor-based measurements (described below). This test may be a useful adjunct for the assessment of mTBI and is typically used for sports-related concussions and civilian trauma patients.[57–59] The K-D is based on measurements of speed during rapid number naming[56] and involves the reading aloud of a series of single-digit numbers that are displayed on the extreme left and right columns of three test cards from left to right (Fig. 17.4); good performance requires rapid gaze shifts. Standardized instructions are used, one demonstration

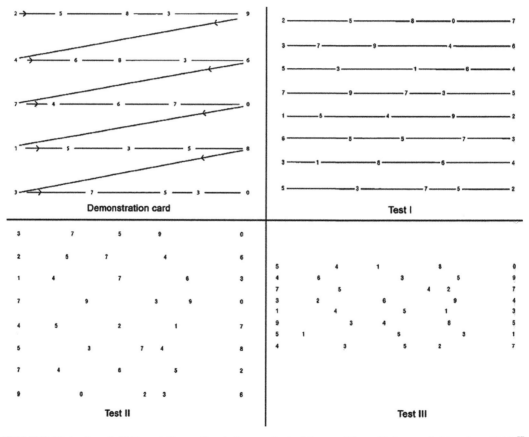

FIGURE 17.4   Sample K-D card. *Source: Permission was obtained for use of figure (Galetta et al., Neurology, 2011).*[57]

card and three test cards are included, and the test requires less than 2 minutes to be performed. Subjects are asked to read the numbers on each card from left to right as quickly as possible without making any errors. Following completion of the demonstration card, the subjects are asked to read each of the three test cards in the same manner. The sum of the time scores from the three test cards constitutes the summary score for the entire test (K-D time score). The number of errors made reading the test cards is recorded; immediate self-corrections are not counted as errors.[52]

Multiple oculomotor and cognitive skills are necessary to complete the K-D and, thus, abnormalities in test performance are not specific to saccades and may be reflective of impairments in other oculomotor (e.g., vergence or accommodation) or cognitive (e.g., attention) functions.[51] Results from sports-related studies indicate that performance on the K-D is significantly poorer following mTBI compared with baseline performance and that test scores improve to baseline levels within 2–3 weeks post-injury.[52,58–62] An evaluation of boxers and fighters revealed that postfight scores are significantly worse for those experiencing head trauma during the match and that those with LOC show the greatest score decreases from pre- to postfight. Reductions in K-D scores by ≥ 5 s are a distinguishing characteristic that are evident only among participants with head trauma. A study of concussed athletes demonstrated that the K-D has 75% sensitivity and is more sensitive than either the tandem gait test or the SAC alone.[63]

Current evidence suggests that the K-D can serve as a complementary test to increase the sensitivity of other screening tools. For example, a combination of the SAC and the Balance Error Scoring System (BESS) has 90% sensitivity for concussions and this rate increases to 100% with the addition of the K-D.[64] A recent narrative review[58] suggested that the K-D is an efficient sideline assessment tool for sports-related concussions, but not a concussion diagnosis tool. Additionally, proper baseline scores, including results from multiple tests, are necessary to exclude the learning effect and to have a reliable baseline level with which to measure from for future reference. A difference of 3 seconds appears to be appropriate to identify the possibility of concussion and to remove an athlete from play.[58] Although these studies were performed using small sample numbers and a detailed description of the assessments has yet to be established, the consistency of the results encourages further investigation of the K-D as an objective indicator of mTBI following head trauma.[65]

Computerized Neurocognitive Tests

Computerized neurocognitive tests have been utilized to assess the effects of mTBI in athletes and have become very popular in recent years due to the numerous benefits of these tests versus traditional paper-and-pencil tests.[66] An increasing number of studies have focused on the purpose and validity of baseline testing, the performance of special populations on computer-based tests, the psychometric properties of different computerized neurocognitive tools, and considerations for the valid and reliable administration of these tools.[67,68] A number of computerized reaction time tests are commercially available, including Immediate Post-Concussion and Cognitive Testing (ImPACT®), Automated Neuropsychological Assessment Metrics (ANAM), and the Axon Sports CNT, which was derived from CogState.[16,69–71] These programs are advantageous because they are widely accessible internet-based platforms and utilize highly standardized test administration and scoring procedures.[66] Additionally, these programs include numerous alternate test forms useful for repeat testing and the performance data can be stored in centralized data repositories for the benefit of users and ongoing test development efforts.[66,67,72]

The online version of ImPACT® (ImPACT Applications, Inc.; San Diego, CA, United States) was developed for baseline and post-injury assessments of concussed athletes and has been used neurocognitive testing concussion assessment tool since its inception in the 1990s.[73] This tool includes six tasks (Word Memory, Design Memory, X's and O's, Symbol Match, Color Match, and Three Letters) that yield composite scores for verbal memory, visual memory, visual-motor processing speed, reaction time, and impulse control.[74] Although ImPACT® demonstrates convergent validity as a cognitive measure after concussion, a recent review article demonstrated that its discriminant and predictive validities, diagnostic accuracy, and utility after symptom resolution are inconclusive.[68] Although several studies have examined the diagnostic accuracy of ImPACT® within the first 72 hours of an injury against different reference standards,[16,70,75,76] the diagnostic accuracy of the test beyond this time point remains unclear.

A reliable change in at least one of the four composite scores was used as a positive finding in two studies[16,76] and provided a sensitivity of 62.5%–83%. The sensitivity of the individual composite scores ranges from 29.3% to 75.6%[75]; however, the inclusion of the PCSS raises the overall sensitivity to 79.2%–81.9%.[16,70] The diagnostic accuracy of ImPACT® within 72 hours of a concussion appears to be supported when postconcussion symptoms are evaluated simultaneously. A reliable change was identified in 33%–38% of concussed subjects despite the absence of concussion symptoms.[77,78] Data regarding diagnostic sensitivity and specificity beyond the resolution of symptoms are sparse[79] and factors such as a young age, the testing environment, exertion, invalid baseline scores, and sandbagging appear to influence the validity and utility of ImPACT scores.[68,80–83] Younger individuals, individuals with learning disability/attention deficit hyperactivity disorder, and individuals who complete the test in a group setting appear to have a higher proportion of invalid baseline scores.[84,85] Thus, clinicians must consider factors that can influence the validity of ImPACT scores and the psychometric properties of the test when interpreting results in the clinical practice of mTBI patients.[68]

BALANCE EXAMINATION

Balance Error Scoring System/modified Balance Error Scoring System

The BESS is a clinical test battery that utilizes modified Romberg tests on different surfaces to evaluate the postural stability of a subject. The BESS[86] consists of three balance assessments on both firm and foam surfaces for a total of six trials that last 20 seconds each. Subjects perform double-leg, single-leg, and tandem (heel-to-toe) stances on the floor and then again on medium-density foam (approximately $50 \times 40 \times 46$ cm) for 20 seconds each while standing with the hands on the iliac crests, head up, and eyes closed. Investigators record the number of balance errors, or times that foot placement was

TABLE 17.2   Balance Error Scoring System

No. of Errors	Firm Surface	Foam Surface
Double-leg stance		
Single-leg stance		
Tandem stance		
Total errors		
Total score		

changed according to the particular balance test, which are defined as: (1) opening the eyes; (2) taking a step, stumbling, or falling out of the position; (3) removing the hands from the hips; (4) moving the hip to more than 30 degrees of flexion or abduction; (5) lifting the toes or heels; and/or (6) remaining out of the test position for longer than 5 seconds. Subjects perform the stances in the following order: double-leg, single-leg using the nondominant foot, and tandem with the nondominant foot in the rear; the maximum total number of errors for any single condition is 10. If a subject commits multiple errors simultaneously, only one error is recorded but the subject should quickly return to the testing position and counting should resume once the subject is set. Subjects that are unable to perform the testing procedure for a minimum of 5 seconds at the start are assigned the highest possible score[10] for that testing condition. The total number of errors on each of the six tests is calculated and summed for the total BESS score (Table 17.2).

The BESS has been widely studied in terms of sports-related mTBI. Studies using the BESS to evaluate postural stability after mTBI in athletes have reported decreased stability on the foam surfaces through Day 3 after injury, which indicates that the BESS is sensitive to postural instability after mTBI.[87] In most cases, athletic trainers reevaluate the athlete with the BESS on several occasions after mTBI to assess recovery and aid return-to-play decision-making.[41,87,88] However, one should be cautious when interpreting changes in BESS scores for clinical purposes because there can be significant variability in scoring due to poor interrater and even intrarater reliability.[89] Furthermore, an individual's score on the BESS may fluctuate during the course of an athletic season independent of concussion status[90] and may be influenced by lower extremity injuries and fatigue.[91,92] During the readministration of the BESS to monitor recovery or aid in return-to-play decision-making, clinicians should be cautious because repeated administrations of this test can elicit a practice effect,[88,93,94] especially with the single-leg stance on foam.[86] A modified version of BESS (mBESS, except for the foam component)[38] has been included in the SCAT3 with a timed tandem gait test to examine balance[12]; it has been shown that mBESS scores decline from baseline following concussion.[50] An updated version of the SCAT (SCAT5) included a more sensitive foam component compared with the full BESS.[95]

Although several studies of young athletes have suggested that females perform better than males on the mBESS, these sex differences are not definite. Furthermore, age appears to have a variable association with scores in young athletes.[96] The use of additional instrumentation in the mBESS in the form of an inertial sensor (accelerometer and gyroscope) was implemented to improve concussion detection.[97]

Tandem Gait/Timed Tandem Gait

Tandem gait is a method of walking in a straight line where the toes of the back foot touch the heel of the front foot at each step. This technique has been used in neurology departments to aid in the diagnosis of ataxia but the tandem gait procedure exacerbates all gait problems, including those associated with cerebellar disease, vision difficulties, and vestibular and motor problems, and many disorders can cause an unsteady tandem gait. The timed tandem gait test[41,98] is also included in the SCAT3.[12] For this test, subjects stand with their feet together behind a starting line and then walk in a forward direction as quickly and accurately as possible along a 3 m line using a tandem gait. Once they cross the end of the line, they turn around and return to the starting point using the same tandem gait. A total of four identical trials are performed and the best time is recorded as the official score.[49] Athletes should complete the test in 14 seconds and fail the test if they step off the line, show separation between the heel and toe, or touch or grab the examiner or an object. Timed tandem gait performance can be affected by exercise and fatigue, but less so than with the BESS.[99,100]

Sport Concussion Assessment Tool

At the 2004 International Conference on Concussion in Sport, the Concussion in Sport Group (CSIG) proposed the use of the SCAT based on an expert consensus of the best measures for assessing concussion available at that time.[11] It includes a test battery to assess symptoms and a detailed neurological examination that incorporates a thorough assessment of mental status, cognitive function, gait, and balance within a short period of time. The first iteration of the SCAT was comprised of the SAC combined with the PCSS, Maddocks questions, on-field markers of concussion (e.g., PTA and LOC), and guidelines for a systematic stepwise return-to-play.[11] The second and third international meetings of this group included discussions of the current literature to identify the most sensitive and reliable concussion assessment components.[8,12] Subsequently, the GCS and mBESS were added to SCAT version 2 (SCAT2)[8]; the subscales can be scored independently and then summed for a maximum total score of 100.

The CSIG proposed another revised version of the SCAT (SCAT3) based on the deliberations at the fourth international meeting in Zurich, November 2012; this version aimed to standardize assessments across sports internationally.[8,12] The SCAT3 removed the total score of the SCAT2 because there was no evidence for its validity, but retained scoring of the individual subscales. In the SCAT3, additional physical signs (e.g., blank/vacant look and cervical stability assessment) were added with the option of using either foam stances or a timed tandem gait task for the postural stability assessment. Additionally, a version of SCAT3 tailored to children younger than 13 years of age (Child-SCAT3) was introduced. Revisions of the SCAT3 culminated in the fifth edition of the SCAT (SCAT5), which is the most recent version that was proposed at the fifth International Consensus Concussion in Sport Group in Berlin in 2016.[95] The SCAT5 revised the immediate and delayed word recall lists of the SAC and includes an option to use 10 words instead of 5 words to minimize ceiling effects.

Several researchers have attempted to correlate test scores and outcomes after concussion in young athletes with sports-related head trauma. A lower total SCAT2 score at the time of injury is correlated with more days until one is free of symptoms and can return to usual activity.[50,101,102] A greater number of symptoms is correlated with more days until being free of symptoms and returning to restricted activity and play whereas neither the SAC nor mBESS scores are predictive of a longer recovery.[101,103] The symptom checklist also demonstrates clinical utility for tracking recovery.[95,96]

A systematic review of studies assessing the SCAT5[104] concluded that utilizing the SCAT (all forms) or its components is generally associated with low-to-moderate levels of bias and is generalizable to the larger population, although variability was noted in terms of methodology, risk of bias, quality of evidence, and presentation of data review.[95,104] Immediately posttrauma, the SAC and the BESS/mBESS are the most useful tools for differentiating concussed athletes from nonconcussed athletes when using either intraindividual or normative baseline/posttrauma comparisons.[63] The diagnostic utility of the SCAT and its components appears to decrease significantly 3–5 days post-injury. Thus, the SCAT is clinically useful for screening evaluations and making a diagnosis, but has a more limited role in tracking recovery and assisting return-to-play decision-making.[63] A significant amount of research has investigated the SCAT; however, evaluations of its utility across different cultural and linguistic groups remain limited.[95]

OCULOMOTOR ASSESSMENT

Although concussion screening has historically focused on a broad range of neurological functions, a majority of individuals with TBI also manifest oculomotor dysfunction.[105] The incidence of visual dysfunction following TBI is considerable and has been reported to be as high as 90% in adults.[65,105] In the mTBI population, impaired eye movement can be identified in the first 2 weeks following an injury as well as during prolonged recovery.[106–108] The visual system is particularly vulnerable to the effects of brain injury due to its expansive neural network that involves multiple areas of the brain.[109] Given the diffuse and nonspecific nature of neurological injury in concussion, it follows that the integrity of a diffuse neuronal network, such as that related to visual function, can be affected.[110] Attention impairments are also a key feature of both the immediate, and delayed symptoms of concussion[111,112] and the gaze and attention networks overlap on functional imaging scans.[113] Thus, vision and oculomotor function have been targeted as practical and reliable surrogates for attention when diagnosing concussion.

Nonetheless, the diagnosis and management of mTBI may be challenging for clinicians due to a lack of objective measures and a resultant reliance on self-reported symptom scales. As a result, researchers have proposed oculomotor-based vision assessments as objective methods of identifying impairments following brain injury[105,114–116] because the severity of oculokinetic dysfunction is correlated with the severity of neurological dysfunction in mTBI.[117] Oculomotor-based vision impairment refers to deficits in version (e.g., fixation, saccade, and pursuit), vergence (e.g., convergence and divergence), and accommodation.[65] Measurements of oculomotor function, including assessments of saccades, smooth pursuit, and vergence, have been used to evaluate mTBI patients and have shown that abnormalities in eye movements are correlated to the severity of postconcussion syndromes and mTBI.[65,117,118] Previous studies that employed eye tracker protocols, optometric assessments, and the K-D test demonstrated that vision and oculomotor testing are practical and reliable surrogates for attention when evaluating mTBI patients,[110] as is the K-D as described above. However, a recent review of oculomotor-based vision assessments for mTBI patients indicated that the evidence supporting the use of these tools is not yet sufficient to warrant clinical recommendations. Research using rigorous methods will be required to develop reliable and clinically useful assessment protocols for mTBI.[65]

Saccadic Eye Movements

Saccadic eye movements are the most frequently studied oculomotor measure in relation to mTBI[65] because they are thought to be related to frontal lobe function and cognitive processing that can be impacted by mTBI.[119] Saccades are relatively easily measured using eye-tracking technology and can be studied as a reflexive movement based on reaction times,[107] component parts such as acceleration, amplitudes, and velocity,[117,120] and in conjunction with tasks requiring cognitive control (e.g., antisaccades or memory-guided saccades).[65,121−124]

Saccades in mTBI patients are significantly slower than those in controls[117,120] and commonly reported findings across studies of mTBI patients using eye-tracking technology include greater amplitudes, smaller peak accelerations, slower velocities, and less accurate target prediction responses compared with controls.[65,117,120] These changes in saccadic eye movements may be associated with functional problems in daily life (e.g., locating items in one's environment[125]; as well as symptoms such as fatigue, headache, and blurred vision[126]). A study of saccades related to recovery from mTBI demonstrated that saccadic eye movements are significantly prolonged during the acute post-injury phase (from 3 hours to 6 days) relative to controls and, in fact, some issues remained after 3 weeks.[107]

Smooth Pursuit Eye Movement

Several studies have utilized video-oculographic techniques and devices to evaluate visual tracking in the context of mTBI diagnosis and management.[110] The tracking of a circular target trajectory is well-suited for measuring predictive visual tracking given its highly predictable trajectory and quantification with parameters such as smooth pursuit velocity gain, phase error, root-mean-square error, and gaze position error variability.[110,127] Changes in visual tracking identified by video-oculography in mTBI patients are correlated with reduced attention and working memory scores on neurocognitive testing as well as white matter tract damage in the corona radiate and genu of the corpus callosum identified using diffusion tensor imaging (DTI) scans.[128] These authors also reported a significant decline in oculomotor abnormality scores within 2 weeks of a concussive injury, but these changes eventually recovered to normal.[129] Another study used a nonspatially calibrated, binocular, eye movement-tracking algorithm to detect differences in dysconjugate gaze in concussion patients relative to healthy controls.[115] Measures of horizontal dysconjugacy significantly increased in concussion patients and were correlated with SCAT3 and SAC scores; these same metrics improved back to baseline at follow-up testing. In a subsequent expanded investigation of the same group, the eye-tracking technology had 88% sensitivity and 87% specificity for the concussion diagnosis.[130] Studies investigating smooth pursuit in patients with mTBI have identified changes in at least one measure of visual pursuit, including large saccades, uneven gaze trajectory, decreased target prediction, increased eye position error, and eye position variability, during smooth pursuit eye movement.[65,118,121,122,128,131] However, the findings were not consistent between studies; clinical and easily reproducible protocols for the assessment of smooth pursuit are needed.

Vergence and Accommodation

Several studies evaluated convergence and accommodation using optometrist assessments and found significant deficits in the near point of convergence and accommodation (e.g., deficits in static and dynamic accommodation) in patients with mTBI compared with controls[131–136]; a receded near point of convergence is a common impairment.[131,132,134,135] Furthermore, research investigating oculomotor-based vision rehabilitation for vergence has demonstrated that improvements in objective abnormal optometric findings are associated with reductions in self-reported symptoms (e.g., fatigue and headache) and improvements in function (e.g., visual attention and reading rate and ability).[137,138] Because vergence is easily assessed and may be relatively easily correctable with glasses or improved with ocular rehabilitation, further study of the utility of vergence in relation to the clinical identification of mTBI may be worthwhile.[65]

NEUROIMAGING AND FLUID BIOMARKERS

Due to advances in functional imaging and molecular genetic technologies, more attention has been placed on diagnostic biomarkers as objective tools to assess the presence and severity of mTBI.[139–141] Beyond the potential diagnostic utility of these tools, there is great interest in the development of prognostic biomarkers of recovery after mTBI.

Neuroimaging Studies

Over the past 20 years, advanced technologies have allowed researchers to use various neuroimaging and electrophysiological measures, including DTI, task-based or resting-state functional MRI (fMRI), electroencephalography (EEG), and magnetic resonance spectroscopy (MRS), to assess mTBI. However, the limited number of studies, lack of investigations for any specific marker, use of various time frames, lack of standardization, and different analysis techniques have made it difficult to determine consistent patterns in mTBI patients.[140] Nevertheless, MRS studies have consistently identified reductions in N-acetylaspartate (NAA; relative to creatine and/or choline) predominately in white matter[142–148] and have shown that there are acute decreases in NAA in conjunction with recovery by 30 days post-injury.[142,143] On the other hand, other studies have reported more chronic decreases in NAA levels.[148,149] The majority of DTI studies have identified decreases in mean diffusivity and/or increases in fractional anisotropy in white matter within 6 months post-injury,[150–154] although opposite or null results have also been reported.[155,156]

The findings of task-based fMRI studies are more variable. The majority utilized working memory paradigms that have produced varying and seemingly contradictory findings with reports of both increased and decreased activity in task-related networks, such as the dorsolateral prefrontal cortex.[140,157,158] Several studies have demonstrated the effects of concussion on EEG/quantitative EEG at rest or during different task conditions by assessing electrophysiological changes following injury relative to a baseline measure.[159–161] Fewer studies have employed measures of cerebrovascular reactivity, arterial spin labeling, transcranial magnetic stimulation, or susceptibility weighted imaging.[140] Furthermore, consistent findings across other modalities are difficult to assess due to the limited number of studies. Magnetoencephalography (MEG) studies have shown that abnormal slow delta waves (1–4 Hz) in the brain can be measured and localized in mTBI patients[162]; this may represent a sensitive and objective test and has a positive finding rate of 87% with no false positives when detecting symptomatic mTBI. Additionally, previous studies revealed abnormal low-frequency magnetic fields using MEG[163,164] and showed that MEG is more sensitive than conventional MRI or EEG for detecting abnormalities in mTBI patients.[163,164]

Although the majority of neuroimaging studies are of high quality and informative, the level of evidence for the clinical application of these techniques is low due to small sample sizes, varied study designs, a lack of consistency in the timing of post-injury data collection, and very limited generalizability.[140] Thus, imaging modalities cannot yet be endorsed as clinical diagnostic tools for mTBI and considerable additional research will be required to determine their ultimate utility in a clinical setting. Nonetheless, advanced neuroimaging is sure to play a critical role in the future of mTBI diagnosis and management.

Fluid Biomarker Studies

Most recently, a number of studies have analyzed blood (plasma or serum), salivary cortisol, or cerebrospinal fluid levels to determine biomarkers that can aid in the diagnosis of mTBI. Significant alterations in several blood biomarkers were identified including α-amino-3-hydroxy-5-methyl-4-isoxazolepropionic acid receptor peptide, S100 calcium binding protein B, total tau, marinobufagenin, plasma soluble cellular prion protein, glial fibrillary acidic protein, neuron-specific enolase, calpain-derived αII-spectrin N-terminal fragment (SNTF), and tau-C.[140,165–170] However, possible candidates are limited due to a small number of young male athletes assessed in the studies and the lack of control data for comparison. Thus, to date, the use of fluid biomarkers for the clinical assessment of mTBI has little supporting evidence, but may advance current scientific understanding of the pathophysiologies underlying concussion in humans.[140]

Genetic Testing Studies

Genetic influences have also received attention as a possible factor that can affect outcomes after mTBI. Individual outcomes vary among patients with mTBI and researchers have considered host genotype as a possible modulator of outcomes after TBI. Emerging evidence on the genetic predictors of TBI has highlighted their relevance[171] and several studies have tested hypotheses related to specific candidate genes, including SLC17A7

APOEe4, and GRIN2A, a gene coding an NMDA glutamate receptor subunit.[172–175] However, the overall level of evidence supporting genetic assessments remains low and cannot yet be endorsed as a clinical tool for mTBI management.[140] Nevertheless, it certainly warrants future research.

The use of various neurocognitive and neurosensory tests has become popular for the assessment of mTBI. However, some skepticism remains regarding the validity and clinical utility of these measures for the diagnosis and management of mTBI, despite emerging evidence. To date, there is no single established assessment that is accepted as a diagnostic test for mTBI but it is generally agreed upon that no single measure should be the sole basis for evaluating mTBI patients. Many studies recommend the use of a multifaceted approach that includes neurosensory testing in conjunction with clinical examinations, a symptom checklist, and other tests. However, considerable research will be required in the future to determine the ultimate utility of these tools in a clinical setting. When evaluating the utility of mTBI tests, it is important to distinguish between sideline screening assessments and evaluations that are more suitable for a definitive diagnosis or the monitoring of postconcussive symptoms. Additionally, advanced neuroimaging techniques, the assessment of various fluid biomarkers related to brain damage, and genetic tests for mTBI show significant promise as research tools for mTBI.

References

1. Bigler ED. Neuropsychology and clinical neuroscience of persistent post-concussive syndrome. *J Int Neuropsychol Soc* 2008;**14**(1):1–22.
2. Holm L, Cassidy JD, Carroll LJ, Borg J. Summary of the WHO Collaborating Centre for neurotrauma task force on mild traumatic brain injury. *J Rehabil Med* 2005;**37**(3):137–41.
3. Teasdale G, Jennett B. Assessment of coma and impaired consciousness. A practical scale. *Lancet* 1974;**2**(7872):81–4.
4. Ruff RM, Iverson GL, Barth JT, Bush SS, Broshek DK. Recommendations for diagnosing a mild traumatic brain injury: a National Academy of Neuropsychology education paper. *Arch Clin Neuropsychol* 2009;**24**(1):3–10.
5. Powell JM, Ferraro JV, Dikmen SS, Temkin NR, Bell KR. Accuracy of mild traumatic brain injury diagnosis. *Arch Phys Med Rehabil* 2008;**89**(8):1550–5.
6. Belanger HG, Vanderploeg RD, Curtiss G, Warden DL. Recent neuroimaging techniques in mild traumatic brain injury. *J Neuropsyc Clin Neurosci* 2007;**19**(1):5–20.
7. Cifu D, Hurley R, Peterson M, Cornis-Pop M, Rikli P.A, Ruff RL, et al., VA/DoD clinical practice guideline for Management of Concussion/Mild Traumatic Brain Injury. *J Rehabil Res Dev* 2009;**46**(6):CP1–68.
8. McCrory P, Meeuwisse W, Johnston K, Dvorak J, Aubry M, Molloy M, et al. Consensus statement on Concussion in Sport 3rd International Conference on Concussion in Sport held in Zurich, November 2008. *Clin J Sport Med* 2009;**19**(3):185–200.
9. Aubry M, Cantu R, Dvorak J, Graf-Baumann T, Johnston K, Kelly J, et al. Summary and agreement statement of the First International Conference on Concussion in Sport, Vienna 2001. Recommendations for the improvement of safety and health of athletes who may suffer concussive injuries. *Br J Sports Med* 2002;**36**(1):6–10.
10. Herring SA, Cantu RC, Guskiewicz KM, Putukian M, Kibler WB, Bergfeld JA, et al. Concussion (mild traumatic brain injury) and the team physician: a consensus statement—2011 update. *Med Sci Sports Exerc* 2011;**43**(12):2412–22.
11. McCrory P, Johnston K, Meeuwisse W, Aubry M, Cantu R, Dvorak J, et al. Summary and agreement statement of the 2nd International Conference on Concussion in Sport, Prague 2004. *Br J Sports Med* 2005;**39**(4):196–204.

12. McCrory P, Meeuwisse WH, Aubry M, Cantu RC, Dvorak J, Echemendia RJ, et al. Consensus statement on concussion in sport: the 4th International Conference on Concussion in Sport, Zurich, November 2012. *J Athl Train* 2013;**48**(4):554–75.

13. Register-Mihalik JK, Guskiewicz KM, Mihalik JP, Schmidt JD, Kerr ZY, McCrea MA. Reliable change, sensitivity, and specificity of a multidimensional concussion assessment battery: implications for caution in clinical practice. *J Head Trauma Rehabil* 2013;**28**(4):274–83.

14. McCrea M, Barr WB, Guskiewicz K, Randolph C, Marshall SW, Cantu R, et al. Standard regression-based methods for measuring recovery after sport-related concussion. *J Int Neuropsychol Soc* 2005;**11**(1):58–69.

15. Guskiewicz KM, Register-Mihalik JK. Postconcussive impairment differences across a multifaceted concussion assessment protocol. *Phys Med Rehabil* 2011;**3**(10Suppl 2):S445–51.

16. Broglio SP, Macciocchi SN, Ferrara MS. Sensitivity of the concussion assessment battery. *Neurosurgery* 2007;**60**(6):1050–7 discussion7-8.

17. Drake AI, McDonald EC, Magnus NE, Gray N, Gottshall K. Utility of Glasgow Coma Scale-Extended in symptom prediction following mild traumatic brain injury. *Brain Inj* 2006;**20**(5):469–75.

18. Ono K, Wada K, Takahara T, Shirotani T. Indications for computed tomography in patients with mild head injury. *Neurol Med Chir (Tokyo)* 2007;**47**(7):291–7 discussion7-8.

19. Catroppa C, Anderson VA, Morse SA, Haritou F, Rosenfeld JV. Outcome and predictors of functional recovery 5 years following pediatric traumatic brain injury (TBI). *J Pediatr Psychol* 2008;**33**(7):707–18.

20. Cunningham J, Brison RJ, Pickett W. Concussive symptoms in emergency department patients diagnosed with minor head injury. *J Emerg Med* 2011;**40**(3):262–6.

21. Yeates KO, Taylor HG, Rusin J, Bangert B, Dietrich A, Nuss K, et al. Longitudinal trajectories of postconcussive symptoms in children with mild traumatic brain injuries and their relationship to acute clinical status. *Pediatrics* 2009;**123**(3):735–43.

22. Lundin A, de Boussard C, Edman G, Borg J. Symptoms and disability until 3 months after mild TBI. *Brain Inj* 2006;**20**(8):799–806.

23. McLean SA, Kirsch NL, Tan-Schriner CU, Sen A, Frederiksen S, Harris RE, et al. Health status, not head injury, predicts concussion symptoms after minor injury. *Am J Emerg Med* 2009;**27**(2):182–90.

24. Potter S, Leigh E, Wade D, Fleminger S. The Rivermead Post Concussion Symptoms Questionnaire: a confirmatory factor analysis. *J Neurol* 2006;**253**(12):1603–14.

25. King NS, Crawford S, Wenden FJ, Moss NE, Wade DT. The Rivermead Post Concussion Symptoms Questionnaire: a measure of symptoms commonly experienced after head injury and its reliability. *J Neurol* 1995;**242**(9):587–92.

26. Ingebrigtsen T, Waterloo K, Marup-Jensen S, Attner E, Romner B. Quantification of post-concussion symptoms 3 months after minor head injury in 100 consecutive patients. *J Neurol* 1998;**245**(9):609–12.

27. McLeod TC, Leach C. Psychometric properties of self-report concussion scales and checklists. *J Athl Train* 2012;**47**(2):221–3.

28. Mailer BJ, Valovich-McLeod TC, Bay RC. Healthy youth are reliable in reporting symptoms on a graded symptom scale. *J Sport Rehabil* 2008;**17**(1):11–20 PubMed PMID: 18270383. Epub 2008/02/14. eng.

29. Alla S, Sullivan SJ, Hale L, McCrory P. Self-report scales/checklists for the measurement of concussion symptoms: a systematic review. *Br J Sports Med* 2009;**43**(Suppl 1). i3-12.

30. Lau BC, Collins MW, Lovell MR. Sensitivity and specificity of subacute computerized neurocognitive testing and symptom evaluation in predicting outcomes after sports-related concussion. *Am J Sports Med* 2011;**39**(6):1209–16.

31. Lovell MR, Iverson GL, Collins MW, Podell K, Johnston KM, Pardini D, et al. Measurement of symptoms following sports-related concussion: reliability and normative data for the post-concussion scale. *Appl Neuropsychol* 2006;**13**(3):166–74.

32. Covassin T, Elbin 3rd RJ, Larson E, Kontos AP. Sex and age differences in depression and baseline sport-related concussion neurocognitive performance and symptoms. *Clin J Sport Med* 2012;**22**(2):98–104.

33. Covassin T, Elbin RJ, Harris W, Parker T, Kontos A. The role of age and sex in symptoms, neurocognitive performance, and postural stability in athletes after concussion. *Am J Sports Med* 2012;**40**(6):1303–12.

34. Roe C, Sveen U, Alvsaker K, Bautz-Holter E. Post-concussion symptoms after mild traumatic brain injury: influence of demographic factors and injury severity in a 1-year cohort study. *Disabil Rehabil* 2009;**31**(15):1235–43.

35. Notebaert AJ, Guskiewicz KM. Current trends in athletic training practice for concussion assessment and management. *J Athl Train* 2005;**40**(4):320–5.
36. Lovell MR, Collins MW. Neuropsychological assessment of the college football player. *J Head Trauma Rehabil* 1998;**13**(2):9–26.
37. Randolph C, Millis S, Barr WB, McCrea M, Guskiewicz KM, Hammeke TA, et al. Concussion symptom inventory: an empirically derived scale for monitoring resolution of symptoms following sport-related concussion. *Arch Clin Neuropsychol* 2009;**24**(3):219–29.
38. Maddocks DL, Dicker GD, Saling MM. The assessment of orientation following concussion in athletes. *Clin J Sport Med* 1995;**5**(1):32–5.
39. Grubenhoff JA, Kirkwood M, Gao D, Deakyne S, Wathen J. Evaluation of the standardized assessment of concussion in a pediatric emergency department. *Pediatrics* 2010;**126**(4):688–95.
40. McCrea M, Kelly JP, Kluge J, Ackley B, Randolph C. Standardized assessment of concussion in football players. *Neurology* 1997;**48**(3):586–8.
41. McCrea M, Kelly JP, Randolph C, Kluge J, Bartolic E, Finn G, et al. Standardized assessment of concussion (SAC): on-site mental status evaluation of the athlete. *J Head Trauma Rehabil* 1998;**13**(2):27–35.
42. Naunheim RS, Matero D, Fucetola R. Assessment of patients with mild concussion in the emergency department. *J Head Trauma Rehabil* 2008;**23**(2):116–22.
43. Barr WB, McCrea M. Sensitivity and specificity of standardized neurocognitive testing immediately following sports concussion. *J Int Neuropsychol Soc* 2001;**7**(6):693–702.
44. Iverson GL, Lovell MR, Collins MW. Validity of ImPACT for measuring processing speed following sports-related concussion. *J Clin Exp Neuropsychol* 2005;**27**(6):683–9.
45. Bloom BM, Kinsella K, Pott J, Patel HC, Harris T, Lecky F, et al. Short-term neurocognitive and symptomatic outcomes following mild traumatic brain injury: a prospective multi-centre observational cohort study. *Brain Inj* 2017;**31**(3):304–11.
46. McCrea M, Guskiewicz KM, Marshall SW, Barr W, Randolph C, Cantu RC, et al. Acute effects and recovery time following concussion in collegiate football players: the NCAA Concussion Study. *J Am Med Assoc* 2003;**290**(19):2556–63.
47. McCrea M, Kelly JP, Randolph C, Cisler R, Berger L. Immediate neurocognitive effects of concussion. *Neurosurgery* 2002;**50**(5):1032–40 discussion40-2.
48. McCrea M. Standardized mental status testing on the sideline after sport-related concussion. *J Athl Train* 2001;**36**(3):274–9.
49. Galetta KM, Morganroth J, Moehringer N, Mueller B, Hasanaj L, Webb N, et al. Adding vision to concussion testing: a prospective study of sideline testing in youth and collegiate athletes. *J Neuroophthalmol* 2015;**35**(3):235–41 PubMed PMID: 25742059. Epub 2015/03/06. eng.
50. Putukian M, Echemendia R, Dettwiler-Danspeckgruber A, Duliba T, Bruce J, Furtado JL, et al. Prospective clinical assessment using Sideline Concussion Assessment Tool-2 testing in the evaluation of sport-related concussion in college athletes. *Clin J Sport Med* 2015;**25**(1):36–42.
51. Hunt TN, Ferrara MS. Age-related differences in neuropsychological testing among high school athletes. *J Athl Train* 2009;**44**(4):405–9.
52. Galetta MS, Galetta KM, McCrossin J, Wilson JA, Moster S, Galetta SL, et al. Saccades and memory: baseline associations of the King-Devick and SCAT2 SAC tests in professional ice hockey players. *J Neurol Sci* 2013;**328**(1-2):28–31.
53. Jinguji TM, Bompadre V, Harmon KG, Satchell EK, Gilbert K, Wild J, et al. Sport Concussion Assessment Tool-2: baseline values for high school athletes. *Br J Sports Med* 2012;**46**(5):365–70.
54. Zimmer A, Marcinak J, Hibyan S, Webbe F. Normative values of major SCAT2 and SCAT3 components for a college athlete population. *Appl Neuropsychol Adult* 2015;**22**(2):132–40.
55. Zimmer A, Piecora K, Schuster D, Webbe F. Sport and team differences on baseline measures of sport-related concussion. *J Athl Train* 2013;**48**(5):659–67.
56. Oride MK, Marutani JK, Rouse MW, DeLand PN. Reliability study of the Pierce and King-Devick saccade tests. *Am J Optom Physiol Opt* 1986;**63**(6):419–24.
57. Galetta KM, Barrett J, Allen M, Madda F, Delicata D, Tennant AT, et al. The King-Devick test as a determinant of head trauma and concussion in boxers and MMA fighters. *Neurology* 2011;**76**(17):1456–62.
58. Howitt S, Brommer R, Fowler J, Gerwing L, Payne J, DeGraauw C. The utility of the King-Devick test as a sideline assessment tool for sport-related concussions: a narrative review. *J Can Chiropr Assoc* 2016;**60**(4):322–9.

59. Galetta KM, Brandes LE, Maki K, Dziemianowicz MS, Laudano E, Allen M, et al. The King-Devick test and sports-related concussion: study of a rapid visual screening tool in a collegiate cohort. *J Neurol Sci* 2011;**309** (1–2):34–9.
60. Tjarks BJ, Dorman JC, Valentine VD, Munce TA, Thompson PA, Kindt SL, et al. Comparison and utility of King-Devick and ImPACT(R) composite scores in adolescent concussion patients. *J Neurol Sci* 2013;**334** (1–2):148–53.
61. King D, Clark T, Gissane C. Use of a rapid visual screening tool for the assessment of concussion in amateur rugby league: a pilot study. *J Neurol Sci* 2012;**320**(1–2):16–21.
62. King D, Brughelli M, Hume P, Gissane C. Concussions in amateur rugby union identified with the use of a rapid visual screening tool. *J Neurol Sci* 2013;**326**(1–2):59–63.
63. Patricios J, Fuller GW, Ellenbogen R, Herring S, Kutcher JS, Loosemore M, et al. What are the critical elements of sideline screening that can be used to establish the diagnosis of concussion? A systematic review. *Br J Sports Med* 2017;**51**(11):888–94.
64. Ventura RE, Jancuska JM, Balcer LJ, Galetta SL. Diagnostic tests for concussion: is vision part of the puzzle? *J Neuroophthalmol* 2015;**35**(1):73–81.
65. Hunt AW, Mah K, Reed N, Engel L, Keightley M. Oculomotor-based vision assessment in mild traumatic brain injury: a systematic review. *J Head Trauma Rehabil* 2016;**31**(4):252–61.
66. Nelson LD, Pfaller AY, Rein LE, McCrea MA. Rates and predictors of invalid baseline test performance in high school and collegiate athletes for 3 computerized neurocognitive tests: ANAM, Axon Sports, and ImPACT. *Am J Sports Med* 2015;**43**(8):2018–26.
67. Rahman-Filipiak AA, Woodard JL. Administration and environment considerations in computer-based sports-concussion assessment. *Neuropsychol Rev* 2013;**23**(4):314–34.
68. Alsalaheen B, Stockdale K, Pechumer D, Broglio SP. Validity of the Immediate Post Concussion Assessment and Cognitive Testing (ImPACT). *Sports Med* 2016;**46**(10):1487–501.
69. Bleiberg J, Kane RL, Reeves DL, Garmoe WS, Halpern E. Factor analysis of computerized and traditional tests used in mild brain injury research. *Clin Neuropsychol* 2000;**14**(3):287–94.
70. Schatz P, Pardini JE, Lovell MR, Collins MW, Podell K. Sensitivity and specificity of the ImPACT Test Battery for concussion in athletes. *Arch Clin Neuropsychol* 2006;**21**(1):91–9.
71. Erlanger D, Feldman D, Kutner K, Kaushik T, Kroger H, Festa J, et al. Development and validation of a web-based neuropsychological test protocol for sports-related return-to-play decision-making. *Arch Clin Neuropsychol* 2003;**18**(3):293–316.
72. Collie A, Darby D, Maruff P. Computerised cognitive assessment of athletes with sports related head injury. *Br J Sports Med* 2001;**35**(5):297–302.
73. Maroon JC, Lovell MR, Norwig J, Podell K, Powell JW, Hartl R. Cerebral concussion in athletes: evaluation and neuropsychological testing. *Neurosurgery* 2000;**47**(3):659–69 discussion69-72.
74. Maroon JC, Field M, Lovell M, Collins M, Bost J. The evaluation of athletes with cerebral concussion. *Clin Neurosurg* 2002;**49**:319–32.
75. Gardner A, Shores EA, Batchelor J, Honan CA. Diagnostic efficiency of ImPACT and CogSport in concussed rugby union players who have not undergone baseline neurocognitive testing. *Appl Neuropsychol Adult* 2012;**19**(2):90–7.
76. Van Kampen DA, Lovell MR, Pardini JE, Collins MW, Fu FH. The "value added" of neurocognitive testing after sports-related concussion. *Am J Sports Med* 2006;**34**(10):1630–5.
77. Broglio SP, Macciocchi SN, Ferrara MS. Neurocognitive performance of concussed athletes when symptom free. *J Athl Train* 2007;**42**(4):504–8.
78. Fazio VC, Lovell MR, Pardini JE, Collins MW. The relation between post concussion symptoms and neurocognitive performance in concussed athletes. *NeuroRehabilitation* 2007;**22**(3):207–16.
79. Nelson LD, LaRoche AA, Pfaller AY, Lerner EB, Hammeke TA, Randolph C, et al. Prospective, head-to-head study of three Computerized Neurocognitive Assessment Tools (CNTs): reliability and validity for the assessment of sport-related concussion. *J Int Neuropsychol Soc* 2016;**22**(1):24–37.
80. Broglio SP, Sosnoff JJ, Ferrara MS. The relationship of athlete-reported concussion symptoms and objective measures of neurocognitive function and postural control. *Clin J Sport Med* 2009;**19**(5):377–82.
81. Lichtenstein JD, Moser RS, Schatz P. Age and test setting affect the prevalence of invalid baseline scores on neurocognitive tests. *Am J Sports Med* 2014;**42**(2):479–84.

82. Szabo AJ, Alosco ML, Fedor A, Gunstad J. Invalid performance and the ImPACT in national collegiate athletic association division I football players. *J Athl Train* 2013;**48**(6):851–5.

83. Schatz P, Kelley T, Ott SD, Solomon GS, Elbin RJ, Higgins K, et al. Utility of repeated assessment after invalid baseline neurocognitive test performance. *J Athl Train* 2014;**49**(5):659–64.

84. Zuckerman SL, Lee YM, Odom MJ, Solomon GS, Sills AK. Baseline neurocognitive scores in athletes with attention deficit-spectrum disorders and/or learning disability. *J Neurosurg Pediatr* 2013;**12**(2):103–9.

85. Elbin RJ, Kontos AP, Kegel N, Johnson E, Burkhart S, Schatz P. Individual and combined effects of LD and ADHD on computerized neurocognitive concussion test performance: evidence for separate norms. *Arch Clin Neuropsychol* 2013;**28**(5):476–84.

86. Valovich TC, Perrin DH, Gansneder BM. Repeat administration elicits a practice effect with the balance error scoring system but not with the standardized assessment of concussion in high school athletes. *J Athl Train* 2003;**38**(1):51–6.

87. Riemann BL, Guskiewicz KM. Effects of mild head injury on postural stability as measured through clinical balance testing. *J Athl Train* 2000;**35**(1):19–25.

88. Onate JA, Guskiewicz KM, Riemann BL, Prentice WE. A comparison of sideline versus clinical cognitive test performance in collegiate athletes. *J Athl Train* 2000;**35**(2):155–60.

89. Finnoff JT, Peterson VJ, Hollman JH, Smith J. Intrarater and interrater reliability of the Balance Error Scoring System (BESS). *Phys Med Rehabil* 2009;**1**(1):50–4.

90. Burk JM, Munkasy BA, Joyner AB, Buckley TA. Balance error scoring system performance changes after a competitive athletic season. *Clin J Sport Med* 2013;**23**(4):312–17.

91. Wilkins JC, Valovich McLeod TC, Perrin DH, Gansneder BM. Performance on the balance error scoring system decreases after fatigue. *J Athl Train* 2004;**39**(2):156–61.

92. Docherty CL, Valovich McLeod TC, Shultz SJ. Postural control deficits in participants with functional ankle instability as measured by the balance error scoring system. *Clin J Sport Med* 2006;**16**(3):203–8.

93. Oliaro SM, Guskiewicz KM, Prentice WE. Establishment of normative data on cognitive tests for comparison with athletes sustaining mild head injury. *J Athl Train* 1998;**33**(1):36–40.

94. Macciocchi SN. "Practice makes perfect:" retest effects in college athletes. *J Clin Psychol* 1990;**46**(5):628–31.

95. Echemendia RJ, Meeuwisse W, McCrory P, Davis GA, Putukian M, Leddy J, et al. The Sport Concussion Assessment Tool 5th Edition (SCAT5). *Br J Sports Med* 2017;**51**(11):851–85.

96. Yengo-Kahn AM, Hale AT, Zalneraitis BH, Zuckerman SL, Sills AK, Solomon GS. The Sport Concussion Assessment Tool: a systematic review. *Neurosurg Focus* 2016;**40**(4):E6.

97. King LA, Horak FB, Mancini M, Pierce D, Priest KC, Chesnutt J, et al. Instrumenting the balance error scoring system for use with patients reporting persistent balance problems after mild traumatic brain injury. *Arch Phys Med Rehabil* 2014;**95**(2):353–9.

98. McCrea M. Standardized mental status assessment of sports concussion. *Clin J Sport Med* 2001;**11**(3):176–81.

99. King D, Brughelli M, Hume P, Gissane C. Assessment, management and knowledge of sport-related concussion: systematic review. *Sports Med* 2014;**44**(4):449–71.

100. Schneiders AG, Sullivan SJ, Handcock P, Gray A, McCrory PR. Sports concussion assessment: the effect of exercise on dynamic and static balance. *Scand J Med Sci Sports* 2012;**22**(1):85–90.

101. Schmitt DM, Hertel J, Evans TA, Olmsted LC, Putukian M. Effect of an acute bout of soccer heading on postural control and self-reported concussion symptoms. *Int J Sports Med* 2004;**25**(5):326–31.

102. Baker JG, Leddy JJ, Darling SR, Rieger BP, Mashtare TL, Sharma T, et al. Factors associated with problems for adolescents returning to the classroom after sport-related concussion. *Clin Pediatr (Phila)* 2015;**54**(10):961–8.

103. McCrea M, Guskiewicz K, Randolph C, Barr WB, Hammeke TA, Marshall SW, et al. Incidence, clinical course, and predictors of prolonged recovery time following sport-related concussion in high school and college athletes. *J Int Neuropsychol Soc* 2013;**19**(1):22–33.

104. Davis GA, Purcell L, Schneider KJ, Yeates KO, Gioia GA, Anderson V, et al. The Child Sport Concussion Assessment Tool 5th Edition (Child SCAT5). *Br J Sports Med* 2017;**51**(11):859–61.

105. Ciuffreda KJ, Kapoor N, Rutner D, Suchoff IB, Han ME, Craig S. Occurrence of oculomotor dysfunctions in acquired brain injury: a retrospective analysis. *Optometry* 2007;**78**(4):155–61.

106. Heitger MH, Jones RD, Macleod AD, Snell DL, Frampton CM, Anderson TJ. Impaired eye movements in post-concussion syndrome indicate suboptimal brain function beyond the influence of depression, malingering or intellectual ability. *Brain* 2009;**132**(Pt 10):2850–70.

107. Mullen SJ, Yucel YH, Cusimano M, Schweizer TA, Oentoro A, Gupta N. Saccadic eye movements in mild traumatic brain injury: a pilot study. *Can J Neurol Sci* 2014;**41**(1):58—65 PubMed PMID: 24384339. Epub 2014/01/05. eng.
108. Riggs RV, Andrews K, Roberts P, Gilewski M. Visual deficit interventions in adult stroke and brain injury: a systematic review. *Am J Phys Med Rehabil* 2007;**86**(10):853—60.
109. Kelts EA. Traumatic brain injury and visual dysfunction: a limited overview. *NeuroRehabilitation* 2010;**27**(3):223—9.
110. Sussman ES, Ho AL, Pendharkar AV, Ghajar J. Clinical evaluation of concussion: the evolving role of oculomotor assessments. *Neurosurg Focus* 2016;**40**(4):E7.
111. Bernstein DM. Recovery from mild head injury. *Brain Inj* 1999;**13**(3):151—72.
112. Binder LM, Rohling ML, Larrabee GJ. A review of mild head trauma. Part I: Meta-analytic review of neuropsychological studies. *J Clin Exp Neuropsychol* 1997;**19**(3):421—31.
113. Corbetta M, Akbudak E, Conturo TE, Snyder AZ, Ollinger JM, Drury HA, et al. A common network of functional areas for attention and eye movements. *Neuron* 1998;**21**(4):761—73.
114. Ciuffreda KJ, Ludlam DP, Thiagarajan P, Yadav NK, Capo-Aponte J. Proposed objective visual system biomarkers for mild traumatic brain injury. *Mil Med* 2014;**179**(11):1212—17.
115. Samadani U, Ritlop R, Reyes M, Nehrbass E, Li M, Lamm E, et al. Eye tracking detects disconjugate eye movements associated with structural traumatic brain injury and concussion. *J Neurotrauma* 2015;**32**(8):548—56.
116. Kraus MF, Little DM, Wojtowicz SM, Sweeney JA. Procedural learning impairments identified via predictive saccades in chronic traumatic brain injury. *Cogn Behav Neurol* 2010;**23**(4):210—17.
117. Heitger MH, Jones RD, Dalrymple-Alford JC, Frampton CM, Ardagh MW, Anderson TJ. Motor deficits and recovery during the first year following mild closed head injury. *Brain Inj* 2006;**20**(8):807—24.
118. Cifu DX, Wares JR, Hoke KW, Wetzel PA, Gitchel G, Carne W. Differential eye movements in mild traumatic brain injury versus normal controls. *J Head Trauma Rehabil* 2015;**30**(1):21—8.
119. Stuss DT. Frontal lobes and attention: processes and networks, fractionation and integration. *J Int Neuropsychol Soc* 2006;**12**(2):261—71.
120. Heitger MH, Anderson TJ, Jones RD, Dalrymple-Alford JC, Frampton CM, Ardagh MW. Eye movement and visuomotor arm movement deficits following mild closed head injury. *Brain* 2004;**127**(Pt 3):575—90.
121. Suh M, Kolster R, Sarkar R, McCandliss B, Ghajar J. Deficits in predictive smooth pursuit after mild traumatic brain injury. *Neurosci Lett* 2006;**401**(1—2):108—13.
122. Suh M, Basu S, Kolster R, Sarkar R, McCandliss B, Ghajar J. Increased oculomotor deficits during target blanking as an indicator of mild traumatic brain injury. *Neurosci Lett* 2006;**410**(3):203—7.
123. Crevits L, Hanse MC, Tummers P, Van Maele G. Antisaccades and remembered saccades in mild traumatic brain injury. *J Neurol* 2000;**247**(3):179—82.
124. Kraus MF, Little DM, Donnell AJ, Reilly JL, Simonian N, Sweeney JA. Oculomotor function in chronic traumatic brain injury. *Cogn Behav Neurol* 2007;**20**(3):170—8.
125. Gillen G. *Cognitive and perceptual rehabilitation optimizing function.* St Louis, MO: Mosby Elsevier; 2009.
126. Kapoor N, Ciuffreda KJ. Vision disturbances following traumatic brain injury. *Curr Treat Options Neurol* 2002;**4**(4):271—80.
127. Maruta J, Ghajar J. Detecting eye movement abnormalities from concussion. *Prog Neurol Surg* 2014;**28**:226—33.
128. Maruta J, Suh M, Niogi SN, Mukherjee P, Ghajar J. Visual tracking synchronization as a metric for concussion screening. *J Head Trauma Rehabil* 2010;**25**(4):293—305.
129. Maruta J, Heaton KJ, Kryskow EM, Maule AL, Ghajar J. Dynamic visuomotor synchronization: quantification of predictive timing. *Behav Res Methods* 2013;**45**(1):289—300.
130. Samadani U, Li M, Qian M, Laska E, Ritlop R. Sensitivity and specificity of an eye movement tracking-based biomarker for concussion. *Concussion* 2015;**1**(1):CNC3.
131. Brahm KD, Wilgenburg HM, Kirby J, Ingalla S, Chang CY, Goodrich GL. Visual impairment and dysfunction in combat-injured servicemembers with traumatic brain injury. *Optom Vis Sci* 2009;**86**(7):817—25.
132. Capo-Aponte JE, Urosevich TG, Temme LA, Tarbett AK, Sanghera NK. Visual dysfunctions and symptoms during the subacute stage of blast-induced mild traumatic brain injury. *Mil Med* 2012;**177**(7):804—13.
133. Hellerstein LF, Freed S, Maples WC. Vision profile of patients with mild brain injury. *J Am Optom Assoc* 1995;**66**(10):634—9.
134. Szymanowicz D, Ciuffreda KJ, Thiagarajan P, Ludlam DP, Green W, Kapoor N. Vergence in mild traumatic brain injury: a pilot study. *J Rehabil Res Dev* 2012;**49**(7):1083—100.

135. Poltavski DV, Biberdorf D. Screening for lifetime concussion in athletes: importance of oculomotor measures. *Brain Inj* 2014;**28**(4):475–85.
136. Green W, Ciuffreda KJ, Thiagarajan P, Szymanowicz D, Ludlam DP, Kapoor N. Accommodation in mild traumatic brain injury. *J Rehabil Res Dev* 2010;**47**(3):183–99.
137. Thiagarajan P, Ciuffreda KJ, Capo-Aponte JE, Ludlam DP, Kapoor N. Oculomotor neurorehabilitation for reading in mild traumatic brain injury (mTBI): an integrative approach. *NeuroRehabilitation* 2014;**34**(1):129–46.
138. Thiagarajan P, Ciuffreda KJ. Effect of oculomotor rehabilitation on vergence responsivity in mild traumatic brain injury. *J Rehabil Res Dev* 2013;**50**(9):1223–40.
139. Peters ME, Rao V, Bechtold KT, Roy D, Sair HI, Leoutsakos JM, et al. Head injury serum markers for assessing response to trauma: design of the HeadSMART study. *Brain Inj* 2017;**31**(3):370–8.
140. McCrea M, Meier T, Huber D, Ptito A, Bigler E, Debert CT, et al. Role of advanced neuroimaging, fluid biomarkers and genetic testing in the assessment of sport-related concussion: a systematic review. *Br J Sports Med* 2017;**51**(12):919–29.
141. Eierud C, Craddock RC, Fletcher S, Aulakh M, King-Casas B, Kuehl D, et al. Neuroimaging after mild traumatic brain injury: review and meta-analysis. *Neuroimage Clin* 2014;**4**:283–94.
142. Vagnozzi R, Signoretti S, Tavazzi B, Floris R, Ludovici A, Marziali S, et al. Temporal window of metabolic brain vulnerability to concussion: a pilot 1H-magnetic resonance spectroscopic study in concussed athletes—part III. *Neurosurgery* 2008;**62**(6):1286–95 discussion95-6.
143. Vagnozzi R, Signoretti S, Cristofori L, Alessandrini F, Floris R, Isgro E, et al. Assessment of metabolic brain damage and recovery following mild traumatic brain injury: a multicentre, proton magnetic resonance spectroscopic study in concussed patients. *Brain* 2010;**133**(11):3232–42.
144. Johnson B, Gay M, Zhang K, Neuberger T, Horovitz SG, Hallett M, et al. The use of magnetic resonance spectroscopy in the subacute evaluation of athletes recovering from single and multiple mild traumatic brain injury. *J Neurotrauma* 2012;**29**(13):2297–304.
145. Henry LC, Tremblay S, Boulanger Y, Ellemberg D, Lassonde M. Neurometabolic changes in the acute phase after sports concussions correlate with symptom severity. *J Neurotrauma* 2010;**27**(1):65–76.
146. Vagnozzi R, Signoretti S, Floris R, Marziali S, Manara M, Amorini AM, et al. Decrease in N-acetylaspartate following concussion may be coupled to decrease in creatine. *J Head Trauma Rehabil* 2013;**28**(4):284–92.
147. Cimatti M. Assessment of metabolic cerebral damage using proton magnetic resonance spectroscopy in mild traumatic brain injury. *J Neurosurg Sci* 2006;**50**(4):83–8.
148. Bartnik-Olson BL, Holshouser B, Wang H, Grube M, Tong K, Wong V, et al. Impaired neurovascular unit function contributes to persistent symptoms after concussion: a pilot study. *J Neurotrauma* 2014;**31**(17):1497–506.
149. Henry LC, Tremblay S, Leclerc S, Khiat A, Boulanger Y, Ellemberg D, et al. Metabolic changes in concussed American football players during the acute and chronic post-injury phases. *BMC Neurol* 2011;**11**:105.
150. Meier TB, Bergamino M, Bellgowan PS, Teague TK, Ling JM, Jeromin A, et al. Longitudinal assessment of white matter abnormalities following sports-related concussion. *Hum Brain Mapp* 2016;**37**(2):833–45.
151. Lancaster MA, Olson DV, McCrea MA, Nelson LD, LaRoche AA, Muftuler LT. Acute white matter changes following sport-related concussion: a serial diffusion tensor and diffusion kurtosis tensor imaging study. *Hum Brain Mapp* 2016;**37**(11):3821–34.
152. Sasaki T, Pasternak O, Mayinger M, Muehlmann M, Savadjiev P, Bouix S, et al. Hockey Concussion Education Project, Part 3. White matter microstructure in ice hockey players with a history of concussion: a diffusion tensor imaging study. *J Neurosurg* 2014;**120**(4):882–90.
153. Henry LC, Tremblay J, Tremblay S, Lee A, Brun C, Lepore N, et al. Acute and chronic changes in diffusivity measures after sports concussion. *J Neurotrauma* 2011;**28**(10):2049–59.
154. Borich M, Makan N, Boyd L, Virji-Babul N. Combining whole-brain voxel-wise analysis with in vivo tractography of diffusion behavior after sports-related concussion in adolescents: a preliminary report. *J Neurotrauma* 2013;**30**(14):1243–9.
155. Murugavel M, Cubon V, Putukian M, Echemendia R, Cabrera J, Osherson D, et al. A longitudinal diffusion tensor imaging study assessing white matter fiber tracts after sports-related concussion. *J Neurotrauma* 2014;**31**(22):1860–71.
156. Zhu DC, Covassin T, Nogle S, Doyle S, Russell D, Pearson RL, et al. A potential biomarker in sports-related concussion: brain functional connectivity alteration of the default-mode network measured with longitudinal resting-state fMRI over thirty days. *J Neurotrauma* 2015;**32**(5):327–41.

157. Dettwiler A, Murugavel M, Putukian M, Cubon V, Furtado J, Osherson D. Persistent differences in patterns of brain activation after sports-related concussion: a longitudinal functional magnetic resonance imaging study. *J Neurotrauma* 2014;**31**(2):180—8.
158. Keightley ML, Saluja RS, Chen JK, Gagnon I, Leonard G, Petrides M, et al. A functional magnetic resonance imaging study of working memory in youth after sports-related concussion: is it still working? *J Neurotrauma* 2014;**31**(5):437—51.
159. Cao C, Slobounov S. Application of a novel measure of EEG non-stationarity as 'Shannon- entropy of the peak frequency shifting' for detecting residual abnormalities in concussed individuals. *Clin Neurophysiol* 2011;**122**(7):1314—21.
160. Slobounov S, Sebastianelli W, Hallett M. Residual brain dysfunction observed one year post-mild traumatic brain injury: combined EEG and balance study. *Clin Neurophysiol* 2012;**123**(9):1755—61.
161. Cao C, Slobounov S. Alteration of cortical functional connectivity as a result of traumatic brain injury revealed by graph theory, ICA, and sLORETA analyses of EEG signals. *IEEE Trans Neural Syst Rehabil Eng* 2010;**18**(1):11—19.
162. Lee RR, Huang M. Magnetoencephalography in the diagnosis of concussion. *Prog Neurol Surg* 2014;**28**:94—111.
163. Lewine JD, Davis JT, Sloan JH, Kodituwakku PW, Orrison Jr. WW. Neuromagnetic assessment of pathophysiologic brain activity induced by minor head trauma. *Am J Neuroradiol* 1999;**20**(5):857—66.
164. Lewine JD, Davis JT, Bigler ED, Thoma R, Hill D, Funke M, et al. Objective documentation of traumatic brain injury subsequent to mild head trauma: multimodal brain imaging with MEG, SPECT, and MRI. *J Head Trauma Rehabil* 2007;**22**(3):141—55.
165. Dambinova SA, Shikuev AV, Weissman JD, Mullins JD. AMPAR peptide values in blood of nonathletes and club sport athletes with concussions. *Mil Med* 2013;**178**(3):285—90.
166. Kiechle K, Bazarian JJ, Merchant-Borna K, Stoecklein V, Rozen E, Blyth B, et al. Subject-specific increases in serum S-100B distinguish sports-related concussion from sports-related exertion. *PLoS One* 2014;**9**(1):e84977.
167. Shahim P, Tegner Y, Wilson DH, Randall J, Skillback T, Pazooki D, et al. Blood biomarkers for brain injury in concussed professional ice hockey players. *JAMA Neurol* 2014;**71**(6):684—92.
168. Oliver J, Abbas K, Lightfoot JT, Baskin K, Collins B, Wier D, et al. Comparison of neurocognitive testing and the measurement of marinobufagenin in mild traumatic brain injury: a preliminary report. *J Exp Neurosci* 2015;**9**:67—72.
169. Schulte S, Rasmussen NN, McBeth JW, Richards PQ, Yochem E, Petron DJ, et al. Utilization of the clinical laboratory for the implementation of concussion biomarkers in collegiate football and the necessity of personalized and predictive athlete specific reference intervals. *EPMA J* 2015;**7**:1.
170. Siman R, Shahim P, Tegner Y, Blennow K, Zetterberg H, Smith DH. Serum SNTF increases in concussed professional ice hockey players and relates to the severity of postconcussion symptoms. *J Neurotrauma* 2015;**32**(17):1294—300.
171. McAllister TW. Genetic factors in traumatic brain injury. *Handb Clin Neurol* 2015;**128**:723—39.
172. Madura SA, McDevitt JK, Tierney RT, Mansell JL, Hayes DJ, Gaughan JP, et al. Genetic variation in SLC17A7 promoter associated with response to sport-related concussions. *Brain Inj* 2016;**30**(7):908—13.
173. Merritt VC, Ukueberuwa DM, Arnett PA. Relationship between the apolipoprotein E gene and headache following sports-related concussion. *J Clin Exp Neuropsychol* 2016;**38**(9):941—9.
174. McDevitt J, Tierney RT, Phillips J, Gaughan JP, Torg JS, Krynetskiy E. Association between GRIN2A promoter polymorphism and recovery from concussion. *Brain Inj* 2015;**29**(13—14):1674—81.
175. Merritt VC, Arnett PA. Apolipoprotein E (APOE) 4 allele is associated with increased symptom reporting following sports concussion. *J Int Neuropsychol Soc* 2016;**22**(1):89—94.

Perfusion and Susceptibility Weighted Imaging in Traumatic Brain Injury

*Natalie M. Wiseman[1], Kiarash Ghassaban, MS[2],
David T. Utriainen, BS[2,3], Sagar Buch, PhD[4],
Zhifeng Kou, PhD[5,6] and E. Mark Haacke, PhD[2,3,4,5,6]*

[1]Department of Psychiatry and Behavioral Neurosciences, Wayne State University School
of Medicine, Detroit, MI, United States [2]Magnetic Resonance Innovations, Inc., Detroit, MI,
United States [3]The MRI Institute for Biomedical Research, Detroit, MI, United States
[4]The MRI Institute for Biomedical Research, Waterloo, ON, Canada [5]Department of
Biomedical Engineering, Wayne State University College of Engineering, Detroit, MI,
United States [6]Department of Radiology, Wayne State University School of Medicine,
Detroit, MI, United States

INTRODUCTION

Traumatic brain injury (TBI) affects over 1.7 million people each year in the United States alone and costs the nation over $68 billion in direct health care.[1] In recent years, soldiers suffering blast-induced TBI in the wars in Iraq and Afghanistan drew a great deal of attention.[2] More recently, sports injuries have drawn the most attention, especially as they relate to concussion.[3,4] In closed head injury, which represents most cases of civilian TBI, there are two major subtypes.[5,6] The first is focal contusion of the brain,[6] evidenced by focal hemorrhages and edema at the inferior frontal, temporal, or occipital lobes. This usually happens during a direct blow to the head and causes the brain surface to impact the bony structure of the inner table of the skull directly. Because focal contusion is confined to limited regions of the brain, these patients usually have favorable long-term outcomes.[6] The other subtype is diffuse axonal injury (DAI),[7] which manifests as a multifoci pathology in major white matter (WM) regions and in the upper part of brain stem in autopsy findings. However, DAI is nearly invisible in conventional clinical imaging and difficult to diagnose in patients.[8] DAI is usually associated with inertial forces, acceleration

Neurosensory Disorders in Mild Traumatic Brain Injury
DOI: https://doi.org/10.1016/B978-0-12-812344-7.00018-2

or deceleration of the brain, and particularly rotational movements of the head. It has been reported as shearing or stretching of the WM of the brain in autopsy.[9,10] Despite the fact that our brain is well protected by a thick skull, it is not designed to withstand inertial and rotational forces. Because WM tracts serve as the major communication infrastructure to allow signals to pass between different brain regions, damage to WM could result in more wide-spread deficits in patients' functional and neurocognitive performance. Significant attention has been invested in the past decades to understand axonal pathology and WM injury and major progress has been made in this area. However, there is little evidence as to why axonal injury leads to prolonged functional deficits.[11] This suggests that there may be more happening at the microscopic level that we have not yet been able to image.

During the moment of head injury, both the brain tissue and vasculature are vulnerable to injury. Despite progress in the investigation of brain cellular and axonal injury, very limited effort has been reported on the investigation of vascular injury and its consequences. In neurosurgery, protection of major blood vessels is considered higher priority than the protection of brain tissue itself because damage to a major blood vessel could have devastating consequences, including hemorrhages and later infarction of brain regions perfused by that vessel. Similarly, injury to brain vasculature during TBI could have far reaching consequences over and above neuronal or axonal injury. While arteries receive more attention generally, veins are more vulnerable to injury than arteries because they have a thinner vessel wall.[12] From a biomechanical perspective, arteries are five times stronger than veins.[12] Acute computed tomography (CT) can detect rupture of bigger arteries or veins in a major blow to the head could result in significant hemorrhages, making CT an important part of standard of care for acute TBI patients, especially those with moderate to severe injuries.[13] Smaller impacts, such as those that occur in mild TBI (mTBI), can still cause damage to small vessels, particularly veins, and may lead to local cerebral microbleeds (CMBs) which are also referred to as microhemorrhages. In diagnostic radiology, petechial hemorrhages at the major white and gray matter junctions are major diagnostic biomarkers for DAI,[8] despite the fact that they are direct evidence of blood vessel injury rather than WM axonal injury. This effect is likely quite distinct from WM damage. However, due to their small size, usually on the order of a millimeter or less, conventional clinical imaging cannot effectively detect these CMBs.[14] A novel magnetic resonance imaging (MRI) sequence called susceptibility weighted imaging (SWI) has been shown to be 3–6 times more sensitive to CMBs than conventional gradient echo (GRE) sequence.[14] SWI has now been widely accepted in clinical settings as the gold standard for CMB detection.[15] As the major developers of SWI,[16] this chapter will give an overview of how to detect CMBs in the brain.

Although moderate to severe TBI patients suffer from significant tissue damage such as DAI and hemorrhages or lower levels of impact can still lead to disruption of the blood–brain barrier, which will result in deposition of hemosiderin along the outside of the vessel wall during the extravasation process. The resulting damage to the veins can also lead to medullary vein thrombosis which may be treatable.[17] Alternatively, the vessel wall may lose its smooth muscle tone in response to changes in brain metabolic demand,[18] leading to a decoupling between cerebral blood supply, or perfusion, and brain tissue metabolic demand. Local perfusion can be assessed with two major MRI methods, dynamic susceptibility contrast (DSC) enhanced perfusion-weighted imaging (PWI) and arterial spin labeling (ASL). Combined with oxygen saturation measurements, one could then use cerebral metabolic oxygen consumption ($CMRO_2$) to probe local tissue damage or dysfunction in TBI. The latter can be imaged today with the next generation of SWI referred to as susceptibility weighted imaging and mapping (SWIM), a quantitative susceptibility mapping (QSM) method.[19,20] In this chapter, we will review the use of SWI, SWIM, PWI, and ASL in studying the role of these vascular imaging techniques in assessing tissue damage and dysfunction in TBI. We will introduce the utility of imaging microbleeds and venous damage, imaging perfusion, and estimating oxygen extraction fraction (OEF) changes in the brain. In the future, we expect more and more of these methods will become quantifiable not just on a relative basis but on an absolute basis.

CEREBRAL MICROBLEEDS IN MILD TRAUMATIC BRAIN INJURY

This section will focus on the current understanding of CMBs and their involvement in assessing mTBI. This includes imaging CMBs using MRI, prevalence of CMBs in mTBI cohorts, and a review of correlations of how CMBs impact motor physical and neuropsychological/cognitive testing following mTBI. Over 75% of all TBI cases are mild, and while 80%–90% will make a favorable recovery, the remaining 10%–20%, defined by Ruff et al. as the "miserable minority," continue to experience persistent cognitive, behavioral or neurological symptoms 6–12 months posttrauma.[21–23] Some of these symptoms are both common and nonspecific (e.g., anxiety, fatigue, loss of concentration, dizziness, irritability) making it difficult to differentiate mTBI-induced symptoms from symptoms resulting from other etiologies. Persistent neurologic impairment may impair quality of life[22,24–27] and may even prevent return to work, leading to claims for lost wages, costs of medical treatment, and disability benefits.[28] Therefore, being able to determine problems associated with chronic mTBI patients would be a major contribution to the field.

CMBs are chronic, focal deposits of hemosiderin, resulting from vascular damage which allows blood products to leak into the surrounding perivascular space and nearby tissues. This damage can be caused by weakened or hardened arterial walls due to aging or plaque build-up, and is typically associated with aging individuals who are at risk for dementia. However, CMBs can also be caused by impact in mTBI. Studies have indicated that an increased prevalence of CMBs is seen in a variety of cohorts including: neurologically healthy elderly populations; patients with neurovascular diseases such as mild cognitive impairment, dementia, and AD; patients receiving antithrombotic medications or chemotherapy; patients with hypertension or cardiovascular risks; and patients with stroke. CMBs can also be seen as a risk factor for developing dementia and stroke.

Once vascular damage has occurred, the extravasated blood products evolve through the hemorrhagic transformation process, which includes the initial hemoglobin changing to methemoglobin and then to hemosiderin. This progression and its final stage suggests that the finding we see in MRI using SWI is the iron that has been sequestered in the iron storage protein hemosiderin. Other iron in the brain is typically in the form of ferritin, which is a highly paramagnetic protein. Ferritin is soluble while hemosiderin is not; hence,

CMBs tend to remain stable over time, depending on their size. Practically, most CMBs tend to remain in the brain and they can also be associated with further bleeding.

The most common approach to imaging CMBs today is using MRI, specifically with SWI as the sequence of choice. While the magnitude component from the sequence can be used to detect CMBs and rule out some potential CMB mimics, the increased sensitivity and specificity for CMBs in SWI comes from the phase information being included, which increases the contrast in the final images. CMBs are visible in GRE and SWI for two reasons: first, because the iron creates a local magnetic field effect which increases proportional to the echo time and field strength, known as the blooming effect; and, second, due to the susceptibility enhancement from the phase. Due to their paramagnetic properties, CMBs appear as focal, round or elliptical hypo-intensities on GRE imaging. While many CMBs are likely very small sub-voxel events of blood leakage, they may grow to appear several pixels across in-plane due to the blooming effect. Today, a multi-echo version of SWI is available that makes it possible to remove the usual venous contribution and better visualize just CMBs. Due to their intermediate susceptibility, veins will be shown best at long echo times (17.5 ms or more), but disappear on short echo time images (7.5 ms or less), leaving just the high susceptibility objects visible such as thrombi or CMBs.

Another approach to visualizing iron content is the use of QSM, and in our case, using SWIM. These methods image the source of the magnetic field disturbance by inverse transforming the phase information. With SWIM, we can measure the susceptibility of a CMB and use that susceptibility to estimate the iron content.[29] Using susceptibility maps, CMBs can be easily identified from veins based on their shape and susceptibility as described below.[20] Alternatively, T2* mapping may be used, but it cannot be used to accurately quantify high iron content objects. When the microbleed is very small, SWIM will underestimate the iron content because of partial volume effects.[18] An example of a CMB viewed with several SWI modalities is shown in Fig. 18.1.

When reviewing an MRI, there are certain properties that an object must demonstrate to conclude a true positive identification of a CMB. Greenberg et al. has defined some initial guidelines for CMB detection,[30] but with the recent use of phase information directly or after postprocessing with SWIM, further recommendations can be made to differentiate CMBs from potential mimics. The following guidelines to detect CMBs are designed to augment those of Greenberg et al.[30] by including SWIM and phase information. We can classify an object as a putative CMB if it: (1) has a round or ovoid in-plane and through-plane appearance; (2) is dark on T2*W MRI with blooming; (3) shows a dipole effect in SWI phase images; (4) appears bright (paramagnetic) on SWIM images; (5) is isolated; (6) is at least half surrounded by brain parenchyma or CSF and not air; (7) is not continuous with venous structures; and (8) is distinct from other potential CMB mimics. Mimics which may be misinterpreted as CMBs without these guidelines include calcifications, flow voids, and vascular structures.

Another form of vascular damage is thrombosis in, or extravasation of, blood from medullary veins.[17] This occurs when smaller veins in the WM of the brain are ruptured do to sheering forces following injury. This results in profuse blood leakage into the parenchyma and surrounding perivascular space or thrombosis inside the vein. These damaged medullary veins are often seen in mTBI in the frontal WM where the medullary veins

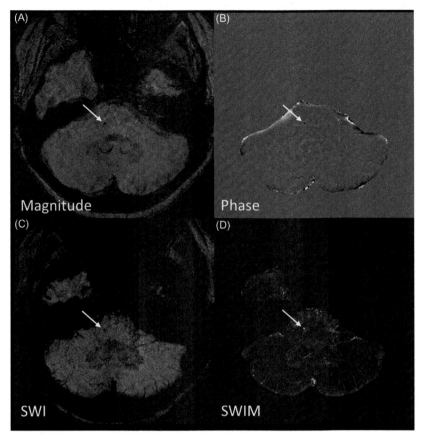

FIGURE 18.1   Appearance of a CMB (white arrow) across SWI-derived images. The CMB appears as a focal hypo-intensity in (A) the SWI magnitude. A clear hypo-intensity with a bright dipole phase behavior is seen through the equatorial plane of the CMB in (B) the SWI high pass filtered phase image. High CMB contrast can be seen as a focal hypo-intensity without a clear connection to surrounding vascular structures as seen in (C) the SWI-composite image. Finally, the CMB appears as a focal hyper-intensity (representing its paramagnetic nature) in the quantitative susceptibility map (D).

drain into the septal veins, but this type of damage can be seen anywhere in the brain depending on the severity and location of the impact. The same rules used in CMB detection do not apply here, but both SWI and SWIM are useful in detecting damaged medullary veins. This effect is rarely, if ever, seen in normal subjects unless it is in the form of a deep venous anomaly. Fig. 18.2 shows an example of CMBs as well as medullary vein lesions in mTBI subjects.

CMBs can occur in the unimpaired healthy population as well, but their prevalence is low, at around 2%−5% for subjects under age 50 years and increasing after this. However, even for older individuals, when a CMB is detected it is usually very small (about 4 mm or less) and there is usually only one. For subjects above the age of 70 years, the prevalence increases to above 20%.[17] When reviewing lesions following mTBI it is important to

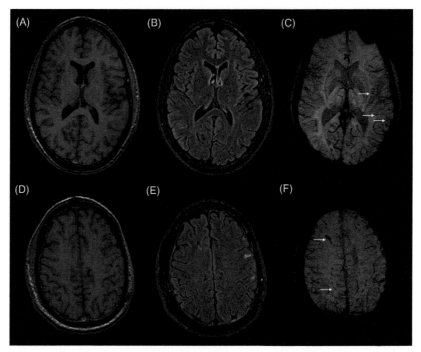

FIGURE 18.2   Two mTBI cases are presented. The first (A–C) shows a lack of lesions in both the T1WI (A) and T2 FLAIR (B). In the SWI projection image (C), multiple CMBs are shown in the subcortical parietal lobe (white arrows). The second case (D–F) shows lesions in both the T1WI (D) and T2 FLAIR (E). The (C) SWI minimum intensity projection (F) shows many lesions which were not evident in the conventional imaging. The linear course of the lesions (white arrows in (F)) likely indicates medullary vein thrombosis.

keep these normal rates of prevalence in mind, as well as noting the size, count, and location of CMB and medullary vein damage. Other studies have shown that for persons 45–50 years old, CMB prevalence is 6.5% and increases to 35.7% for persons 80 years old and above.[31] When persons with major cardiovascular risk factors (HTN, DM, hyperlipidemia) are excluded, the CMB prevalence is lower, from 1% for controls below 60 years old, to 4% for persons above 60 years old.[32] Along with location, the size of the CMB also gives an indication of its severity. Fig. 18.3 shows varying CMB size in the same location across two mTBI subjects.

Overall, the literature reveals a prevalence of CMBs of 3%–24%,[33–35] depending on the MRI protocol applied and the age of the subjects. We report on a few of the more recent interesting studies. (1) Huang et al.[36] looked at a cohort of 111 mTBI subjects and 111 healthy volunteers. Of these, 26 mTBI subjects (37±13 years) and 12 healthy volunteers (40±9 years) were found to have CMBs using SWI. This yields a prevalence of 23% for the mTBI group and 11% for the control group. In this case, 87% of the CMBs in the mTBI group were located in the cortex/subcortical regions, while for controls, 60% of CMBs were located in the central brain. Also, there were 60 CMBs in the 26 mTBI cases, and 15 in the healthy controls. (2) Of 150 chronic mTBI cases and 94 HC, Trifan et al.[37] found SWI

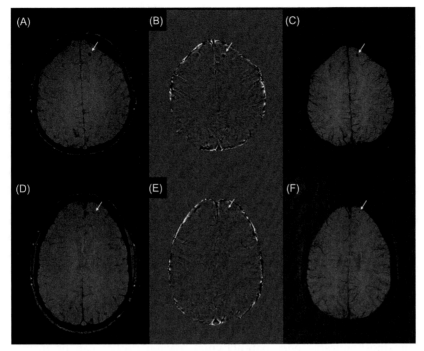

FIGURE 18.3   Example of two subjects, each with a CMB located in the left frontal lobe. The first subject (top row) shows a large CMB (white arrow) which is visible across (A) SWI magnitude, (B) SWI phase, and (C) SWI minimum intensity projection. The second subject (bottom row) shows a smaller CMB (white arrow) in the same location which is also visible across (D) SWI magnitude, (E) SWI phase, and (F) SWI minimum intensity projection. Identification of CMBs is important following injury and quantification of these CMBs includes their count, location, and size.

lesions in 28% versus 3%, respectively. When divided into subjects under 45 years of age, the number with CMBs was 9% versus 0%, respectively. Of these 150 mTBI cases, 17% showed hemorrhage: 9% showed CMBs, 6% showed contusions, and 1% showed both. (3) Wang et al.[38] studied 165 mTBI patients using SWI and found an overall prevalence of CMBs at 1 year posttrauma to be 19.4% compared with 9% in healthy controls. Their subjects were further divided in two groups, based on the presence or absence of major depressive-like episodes at 1 year posttrauma. Among the 17% of patients who reported depressive-like episodes, 71% showed CMBs on SWI compared with 9% in the nondepressed group. Spitz et al.[39] looked at 12 mTBI cases and found that SWI showed greater lesion volume than FLAIR showed, and that SWI was able to identify TBI-related lesions in almost a third of patients for whom FLAIR was negative. (4) Imaizumi et al. showed that increasing clinical severity is associated with an increase in hemorrhagic pathology. They studied 312 acute TBI patients with a mean GCS of 10 using T2*-weighted GRE imaging (which is not as sensitive to small CMBs as SWI) and found CMBs in 7% of cases.[40] Clearly, CMBs are an important imaging biomarker that appear to be associated with worse clinical outcome.[33,41]

OXYGEN SATURATION

Perfusion and oxygen saturation are of particular interest for assessing brain function after injury, as almost all neuronal energy production is through aerobic metabolism. Neurons and glia of the normal, uninjured brain closely regulate local blood flow to match metabolic activity, but in the injured brain, damage to the vasculature, dysfunction of mitochondria, or abnormal function of glia can lead to an uncoupling of blood flow and neuronal activity.[42,43] Under normal circumstances, even challenges with caffeine or acetazolamide cause changes in blood flow which are not coupled to changes in $CMRO_2$, so measurement of blood flow alone may not reveal the functional status of the neurons unless oxygen saturation is also measured. Combining information about blood flow and oxygen saturation gives us a better chance to identify abnormal brain metabolism after TBI.

Under normal conditions, the brain extracts about 30%−40% of the oxygen delivered to it, resulting in a venous oxygen saturation (SvO_2) of about 60%[44,45]−70%,[46] respectively. However, when oxygen supply is reduced or oxygen demand is increased, the percentage of oxygen extracted, or the OEF increases. In conditions like stroke, this mismatch of demand and supply results in a decrease in both local parenchymal and venous oxygenation (SvO_2). By assessing either parenchymal oxygenation, SvO_2, or $CMRO_2$ directly, we can then better identify areas of abnormal activity or metabolism in the brain.

Cerebral oxygen saturation can be estimated by several invasive and noninvasive methods.[47] On the most invasive end, parenchymal oxygen probes can be inserted into the injured brain to detect local tissue oxygenation with good temporal resolution. However, due to the invasiveness, these are only used in severe TBI patients. Methods like near-infrared spectroscopy offer similar regional measurements with less invasiveness, but rely on assumptions of arterial to venous blood volume ratios and oxygenation ratios to estimate oxygen saturation. Alternatively, one can use ^{15}O positron emission tomography (PET) to assess $CMRO_2$, which is less invasive and offers better spatial resolution. However, PET has poorer temporal resolution and cannot be performed repeatedly during assessment and treatment due to the radiation involved. Another approach is to use jugular venous oxygen saturation monitoring to observe SvO_2, which offers better temporal resolution but represents global rather than regional oxygen saturation.

MRI offers a variety of less invasive methods that can be performed repeatedly to measure OEF. Although MRI has more limited temporal resolution, there are a variety of regional and global imaging approaches. These include QSM, T2 relaxation under spin tagging,[48] calibrated functional magnetic resonance imaging (fMRI), and others. QSM in particular can provide SvO_2 estimates for veins across the brain by utilizing phase information, unlike some of the other methods that provide global estimates. Because the SWI MRI sequence can be performed repeatedly, unlike a ^{15}O PET scan, SvO_2 can be estimated before and after administration of vasoactive compounds like caffeine, a vasoconstrictor which reduces blood flow and correspondingly increases OEF (Fig. 18.4), or acetazolamide, a vasodilator which increases blood flow and correspondingly reduces OEF.[49] Fig. 18.4A,D shows SWI-composite magnitude images, whereas Fig. 18.4B,E represents the SWIM results, on a healthy volunteer, before and after the administration of 200 mg NoDoz caffeine pill (Novartis Consumer Health, Inc, Parsippany, NJ,

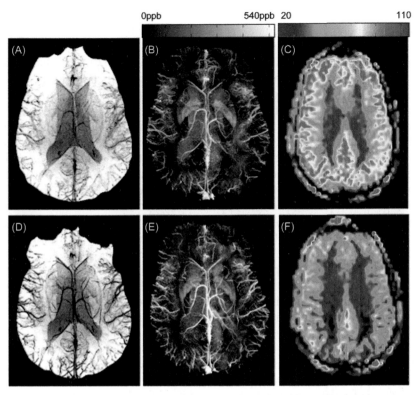

FIGURE 18.4 Brain MRI scans showing the effect of caffeine consumption on CBF and venous oxygen saturation of a healthy volunteer precaffeine (A, B, C) and postcaffeine (D, E, F). SWI data were acquired using the following parameters: TE = 15 ms, TR = 24, FA = 15, bandwidth (BW) = 119 Hz/pixel and voxel resolution = $0.5 \times 0.5 \times 0.5$ mm^3. (A, D) mIP of SWI-composite data and (B, E) MIP of SWIM data projected over 32 mm. Respective CBF maps (C and F) were generated from PCASL data with TE/TR = 22.7/3500 ms, TI = 1500 ms, FA = 180°, BW = 2003 Hz/pixel and $3.5 \times 3.5 \times 3.5$ mm^3 resolution. The scale bar values for the CBF maps (C and F) are expressed in mL/100 g of tissue/min.

United States), respectively. Susceptibility maps were produced using a truncated k-space method along with the geometry constrained iterative algorithm to improve the unreliable k-space elements, thereby reducing the streaking artifacts on the final susceptibility mapping result.[19] The images are maximum intensity projected (MIP) over 64 slices with an effective slice thickness of 32 mm. The venous contrast shows a marked increase in amplitude after caffeine administration, signifying an increase in susceptibility, which is due to the reduced SvO$_2$. Using this technique, the SvO$_2$ level inside the internal cerebral veins (ICVs) showed a decrease from 69.9% to 59.8% after caffeine administration (assuming a hematocrit level of 44% and a susceptibility difference ($\Delta\chi_{do}$) between fully deoxygenated blood and fully oxygenated blood of 0.27 ppm). This offers us the opportunity to probe the vasculature's ability, locally, to facilitate changes in CBF, as well, which is particularly important given the possibility of shearing injury to blood vessels in TBI.

Finally, in animal models, there are a variety of even more invasive techniques that provide information about the molecular processes underlying changes in SvO_2 or $CMRO_2$. Animal work in TBI also affords us the opportunity to study the brain on time scales not available in human brain injury studies. In particular, rodent TBI work has demonstrated that injury leads to multiple alterations to neuronal and glial metabolic activity that develops and resolve along a wide range of time scales.[50] TBI induces impairments in oxidative metabolism in the acute phase after injury by a few mechanisms.[50, 51] Calcium flows into the cells at greater rates due to axonal stretching or posttraumatic depolarization, neurotransmitter release, and N-methyl-D-aspartate receptor activation. This gets sequestered in mitochondria and reduces oxidative metabolism. Over the course of several days, mitochondrial dysfunction leads to a reduction in oxidative ATP production and an increase in ATP production through glycolysis, which has been seen in animal studies to resolve within about 10 days.[50] This represents a period of hypometabolism for the injured brain that largely resolves and has been hypothesized as being either a period of relative protection due to decreased oxidative stress or a period of increased susceptibility to secondary injury due to decreased ability to respond to further changes in energy demands.[50] Experiments on posttraumatic hypoxia and hyperoxia, in hypobaric, normobaric, or hyperbaric environments, do not fully answer this question but do shed some light on it. In experiments meant to test the time-dependent effects of medivac conditions on injury severity, hypobaric hypoxic conditions caused worsening of a marker of injury severity in mice exposed 3 hours after injury but not 12 hours after injury, suggesting that the sensitive period for hypoxia-induced worsening of injury is short.[52] Similarly, normobaric hyperoxia only had helpful effects on dopamine levels or morphology at 3 hours after injury, but not at later timepoints, supporting this short window of sensitivity to oxygen changes.[53,54] However, other groups have reported worsening of injury with hyperoxia in the hour immediately following injury.[55]

In humans, these early timepoints after injury are difficult or impossible to assess, due to delays between injury and hospital arrival and the need to prioritize treatment over research. However, later timepoints do offer some insight into oxygenation status that parallels some of what we see in the animal work. In a study of excised brain tissue removed between 2 and 60 hours after injury, isolated mitochondria showed decreased ATP production and a decrease in calcium transport, which fits the expectations of calcium-induced mitochondrial dysfunction derived from the animal model experiments.[56] At a mean of just over 2 days after injury, mTBI patients were found to have increased oxygenation of the major deep veins of the brain (Fig. 18.5), indicating a decreased OEF,[57] which could correspond to the period of decreased mitochondrial function and hypometabolism seen in the rodent work. At the same time, increases in CBF may indicate that the CBF exceeds the oxygen demand of the tissue, thus producing decreases in OEF if $CMRO_2$ is unchanged. In more severe cases, regions of increased OEF surround the central contusion of the injury, indicating a region that is under-perfused and hypoxic.[58] In pediatric cases, decreased OEF at 2 weeks after injury was found to correlate with worse 3-month outcomes,[59] though timepoints this late are missing from the animal work, keeping us from making a direct comparison to time-matched pathophysiology seen in experimental TBI. As such, it is possible that this represents ongoing metabolic dysfunction while the non-reduced OEF group has mostly recovered by 2 weeks after, but it is difficult to say for certain without animal research to assess such late timepoints.

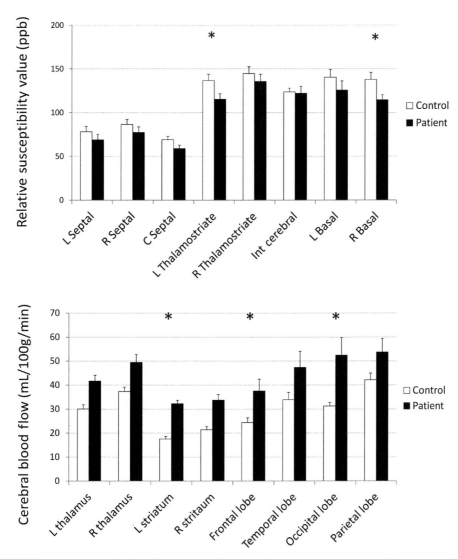

FIGURE 18.5 Mean susceptibility values and standard error bars in major veins in mTBI patients and controls (top) and mean CBF and standard error bars of deep brain structures (bottom). Decreases in magnetic susceptibility in patients correspond to decreased deoxyhemoglobin content, or increased oxygenation. This corresponds with increased CBF in patients as compared to controls, and may reflect CBF exceeding the oxygen demands of the tissue, or a decoupling of oxygen metabolism and CBF. * Indicates significance at $p < 0.05$. *Source: Reprinted with permission from Doshi et al.[57]*

In the normal, uninjured brain, neuronal activity is supported by blood flow that increases to meet increasing metabolic demands and reduces again as demand reduces. However, in the injured brain, this coupling is disturbed. So, in addition to understanding the changes in oxygen saturation of the veins of the brain and OEF, we must also consider the changes in cerebral blood flow to fully understand the changes in brain metabolism.

PERFUSION IMAGING

There are a few studies that have evaluated perfusion of the brain in TBI, using a variety of noninvasive medical imaging techniques.[60] Although some methodologies such as single-photon emission computed tomography (SPECT), PET, and Doppler ultrasonography have been used to investigate perfusion abnormalities,[60,61] the preferred imaging modalities routinely utilized by researchers and clinicians are usually CT and MRI techniques. Generally, in both perfusion CT (CTP) and DSC PWI MR applications, the conventional way to evaluate CBF and subsequent postprocessed parameters is through administering specific doses of contrast agents. Monitoring the concentration of such molecules inside the vascular system can give an estimate of hemodynamic changes and, hence, qualitative if not quantitative measurements of cerebral perfusion. Some of these quantitative parametric maps include: CBF, cerebral blood volume (CBV) and mean transit time (MTT).

CTP and DSC-MRI have been used to assess both focal and diffuse perfusion in acute and chronic stages of TBI. Vascular autoregulation and pseudo-autoregulation can be monitored using PWI methods and there is usually a clear association between CBF, CBV and MTT changes that represent abnormal perfusion.[60] Moreover, CTP has been shown to provide additional diagnostic information compared to noncontrast CT in severe TBI patients.[62,63] On the other hand, MR PWI studies have shown that relative CBF measurements can be used to map changes in mTBI patients.[64]

However, in many circumstances, giving a contrast agent is not possible or not desirable, and in these cases, noncontrast MR methods are preferred. One such approach is ASL, an advanced noncontrast MRI technique which spin-tags inflowing arterial blood feeding the brain tissue to reconstruct perfusion-weighted images and parametric maps. Pseudo-continuous ASL (PCASL) in particular has found its place among perfusion studies, especially in TBI research. Hemodynamic variations following cognitive impairment can be detected in order to more efficiently predict mTBI outcome.[65] From an fMRI perspective, resting state and task-evoked ASL-CBF measurements have demonstrated correlations between perfusion abnormalities and performance of different brain regions compared to healthy subjects.[66]

On the venous side and in conjunction with SWI postprocessing techniques, vascular abnormalities have been found to be correlated with CBF changes in TBI patients, indicating that perfusion could serve as a biomarker for TBI prognosis. A study of 23 moderate to severe TBI patients and 18 healthy controls has shown that moderate to severe TBI patients have significantly lower CBF than normal controls in brain regions drained by several major veins (Fig. 18.6).[67] This decrease in CBF was accompanied by a significant increase in magnetic susceptibility in those same veins, implying lower SvO_2 and higher deoxyhemoglobin content.[67] However, these changes are in the opposite directions of those seen in the mTBI patients in the previously mentioned study (Fig. 18.5), who were seen to have increased regional CBF and decreased venous susceptibility.[57] This phenomenon may suggest a neuroprotective mechanism following mTBI which is not seen or not effective in more severe injuries, or a difference in the predominant pathology and pathophysiology between mTBI and more severe TBI. Because mTBI does not involve the extensive tissue damage that moderate to severe TBI includes, the metabolic changes in

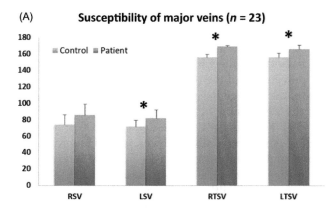

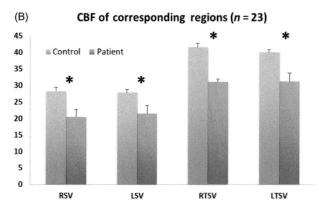

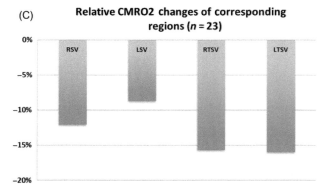

FIGURE 18.6 Susceptibility, CBF, and relative $CMRO_2$ measurements in the brain regions drained by major veins in 23 moderate to severe TBI patients as compared to 18 healthy controls. (A) Patients with moderate to severe TBI showed increases in susceptibility of major veins, indicating decreases in oxygenation. (B) Patients also showed decreases in average ASL-CBF in the draining regions of those veins. (C) Patients showed relative decreases in $CMRO_2$ of the same drainage territories, based on a calculation using both susceptibility and CBF. RSV, right septal vein; LSV, left septal vein; RTSV, right thalamostriatal vein; LTSV, left thalamostriatal vein. Asterisks indicate t-test P-value <.05. *Source: Reprinted with permission from Kou et al.*[67]

mTBI may reflect increases in cellular activity after injury while severe TBI may induce decreases in cellular activity due to cell death or overwhelming damage.

Finally, these changes in CBF and OEF can be used to calculate the $CMRO_2$ of their corresponding brain regions, which tends to vary little across the brain or in response to hemodynamically active stimuli. For the susceptibility and CBF maps shown in Fig. 18.4, measurement of the average magnetic susceptibility of the ICVs and the average global

CBF yielded $\Delta\chi = 0.45 \pm 0.06$ ppm and 67.7 mL/100 g/min for precaffeine, and $\Delta\chi = 0.61 \pm 0.07$ ppm and CBF = 47.9 mL/100 g/min for postcaffeine, respectively. In other words, the drop in venous oxygen saturation after caffeine consumption accompanies a decrease in the average CBF, which are balanced if the $CMRO_2$ is unchanged; a reduction in CBF would lead to an increase in the percentage of the oxygen extracted, if oxygen consumption remained constant. Furthermore, the change in SvO_2 has been previously shown to be related to the CBF changes using the expression: $|\Delta Y/(1 - Y)| \approx |\Delta CBF/CBF|$.[68] The data from the healthy volunteer in Fig. 18.4 suggest that the decrease in CBF is sufficiently compensated by increased OEF, leaving the $CMRO_2$ unchanged. However, this may not be the case for an injured or abnormal region of tissue, as seen in the moderate to severe TBI patients in Fig. 18.6. These measurements yield a reduction of 12%−16% in $CMRO_2$ in TBI patients implying that, unlike a healthy brain, oxygen consumption is affected post-TBI. Therefore, both CBF and venous susceptibility should be measured to investigate if they show appropriately balanced changes after TBI or if they may reveal changes in $CMRO_2$. Additionally, a challenge of the vascular system with caffeine or other vasoactive stimuli, like carbon dioxide, could be used to assess the ability of the blood vessels to autoregulate appropriately after TBI.

CONCLUSIONS

In summary, MRI offers a powerful means to detect vascular abnormalities after TBI. Structurally, using SWI, we can see the presence of CMBs and medullary vein thrombosis even in mTBI on the order of 10%−20% of cases. Using PWI, mTBI exhibits a different effect in that perfusion increases and then returns to normal in the subacute stage, whereas the opposite occurs in moderate to severe TBI. In the future, we can envision that combining flow from PWI and oxygen saturation estimates from SWI, it may be possible to estimate $CMRO_2$, or at least changes in $CMRO_2$, over time.

References

1. Seifert J. Incidence and economic burden of injuries in the United States. *J Epidemiol Community Health* 2007;**61**:926.
2. Department of Defense. *U.S. Casualty status for operation iraqi freedom (oif) and operation enduring freedom (oef).* <http://www.defenselink.mil/news/casualty.pdf>; 2007 [accessed 12.09.07].
3. McCrory P, Johnston K, Meeuwisse W, Aubry M, Cantu R, Dvorak J, et al. Summary and agreement statement of the 2nd international conference on concussion in sport, Prague 2004. *Br J Sports Med* 2005;**39**:i78.
4. Harmon KG, Drezner JA, Gammons M, Guskiewicz KM, Halstead M, Herring SA, et al. American medical society for sports medicine position statement: concussion in sport. *Br J Sports Med* 2012;**47**:15.
5. Gennarelli TA, Graham DI. Neuropathology of the head injuries. *Semin Clin Neuropsych* 1998;**3**:160−75.
6. Gennarelli TA. Mechanisms of brain injury. *J Emerg Med* 1993;**11**(Suppl 1):5−11.
7. Adams JH, Doyle D, Ford I, Gennarelli TA, Graham DI, McLellan DR. Diffuse axonal injury in head injury: definition, diagnosis and grading. *Histopathology* 1989;**15**:49−59.
8. Grossman RI, David Y. *Neuroradiology.* Philadelphia, PA: Mosby; 2003.
9. Gennarelli TA, Thibault LE, Tipperman R, Tomei G, Sergot R, Brown M, et al. Axonal injury in the optic nerve: a model simulating diffuse axonal injury in the brain. *J Neurosurg* 1989;**71**:244−53.

10. Gennarelli TA, Thibault LE, Adams JH, Graham DI, Thompson CJ, Marcincin RP. Diffuse axonal injury and traumatic coma in the primate. *Ann Neurol* 1982;**12**:564–74.

11. Gean AD. *Imaging of head trauma*. New York: Raven Press; 1994.

12. Monson KL, Goldsmith W, Barbaro NM, Manley GT. Axial mechanical properties of fresh human cerebral blood vessels. *J Biomech Eng* 2003;**125**:288–94.

13. Stiell IG, Wells GA, Vandemheen K, Clement C, Lesiuk H, Laupacis A, et al. The canadian ct head rule for patients with minor head injury. *Lancet* 2001;**357**:1391–6.

14. Tong KA, Ashwal S, Holshouser BA, Shutter LA, Herigault G, Haacke EM, et al. Hemorrhagic shearing lesions in children and adolescents with posttraumatic diffuse axonal injury: Improved detection and initial results. *Radiology* 2003;**227**:332–9.

15. Kou Z, Wu Z, Tong KA, Holshouser B, Benson RR, Hu J, et al. The role of advanced mr imaging findings as biomarkers of traumatic brain injury. *J Head Trauma Rehabil* 2010;**25**:267–82.

16. Haacke EM, Xu Y, Cheng YC, Reichenbach JR. Susceptibility weighted imaging (swi). *Magn Reson Med* 2004;**52**:612–18.

17. Jamjoom AA, Jamjoom AB. Safety and efficacy of early pharmacological thromboprophylaxis in traumatic brain injury: systematic review and meta-analysis. *J Neurotrauma* 2013;**30**:503–11.

18. Zauner A, Muizelaar JP. *Brain metabolism and cerebral blood flow, in head injury*. London: Chapman & Hall; 1997.

19. Tang J, Liu S, Neelavalli J, Cheng YC, Buch S, Haacke EM. Improving susceptibility mapping using a threshold-based k-space/image domain iterative reconstruction approach. *Magn Reson Med* 2013;**69**:1396–407.

20. Liu J, Xia S, Hanks R, Wiseman N, Peng C, Zhou S, et al. Susceptibility weighted imaging and mapping of micro-hemorrhages and major deep veins after traumatic brain injury. *J Neurotrauma* 2016;**33**:10–21.

21. Ruff RM, Camenzuli L, Mueller J. Miserable minority: Emotional risk factors that influence the outcome of a mild traumatic brain injury. *Brain Inj* 1996;**10**:551–65.

22. McMahon P, Hricik A, Yue JK, Puccio AM, Inoue T, Lingsma HF, et al. Symptomatology and functional outcome in mild traumatic brain injury: Results from the prospective track-tbi study. *J Neurotrauma* 2014;**31**:26–33.

23. Ruff R. Two decades of advances in understanding of mild traumatic brain injury. *J Head Trauma Rehabil* 2005;**20**:5–18.

24. Benedictus MR, Spikman JM, van der Naalt J. Cognitive and behavioral impairment in traumatic brain injury related to outcome and return to work. *Arch Phys Med Rehabil* 2010;**91**:1436–41.

25. Zumstein MA, Moser M, Mottini M, Ott SR, Sadowski-Cron C, Radanov BP, et al. Long-term outcome in patients with mild traumatic brain injury: a prospective observational study. *J Trauma* 2011;**71**:120–7.

26. Pierallini A, Pantano P, Fantozzi LM, Bonamini M, Vichi R, Zylberman R, et al. Correlation between MRI findings and long-term outcome in patients with severe brain trauma. *Neuroradiology* 2000;**42**:860–7.

27. Sasse N, Gibbons H, Wilson L, Martinez-Olivera R, Schmidt H, Hasselhorn M, et al. Self-awareness and health-related quality of life after traumatic brain injury. *J Head Trauma Rehabil* 2013;**28**:464–72.

28. Shukla D, Devi BI. Mild traumatic brain injuries in adults. *J Neurosci Rural Pract* 2010;**1**:82–8.

29. Buch S, Cheng YN, Hu J, Liu S, Beaver J, Rajagovindan R, et al. Determination of detection sensitivity for cerebral microbleeds using susceptibility-weighted imaging. *NMR Biomed* 2017;30.

30. Greenberg SM, Vernooij MW, Cordonnier C, Viswanathan A, Al-Shahi Salman R, Warach S, et al. Cerebral microbleeds: a guide to detection and interpretation. *Lancet Neurol* 2009;**8**:165–74.

31. Poels MM, Vernooij MW, Ikram MA, Hofman A, Krestin GP, van der Lugt A, et al. Prevalence and risk factors of cerebral microbleeds: an update of the rotterdam scan study. *Stroke* 2010;**41**:S103–6.

32. Chowdhury MH, Nagai A, Bokura H, Nakamura E, Kobayashi S, Yamaguchi S. Age-related changes in white matter lesions, hippocampal atrophy, and cerebral microbleeds in healthy subjects without major cerebrovascular risk factors. *J Stroke Cerebrovasc Dis* 2011;**20**:302–9.

33. Sharp DJ, Ham TE. Investigating white matter injury after mild traumatic brain injury. *Curr Opin Neurol* 2011;**24**:558–63.

34. Loitfelder M, Seiler S, Schwingenschuh P, Schmidt R. Cerebral microbleeds: a review. *Panminerva Med* 2012;**54**:149–60.

35. Stehling C, Wersching H, Kloska SP, Kirchhof P, Ring J, Nassenstein I, et al. Detection of asymptomatic cerebral microbleeds: a comparative study at 1.5 and 3.0 t. *Acad Radiol* 2008;**15**:895–900.

36. Huang YL, Kuo YS, Tseng YC, Chen DY, Chiu WT, Chen CJ. Susceptibility-weighted MRI in mild traumatic brain injury. *Neurology* 2015;**84**:580–5.
37. Trifan G, Gattu R, Haacke EM, Kou Z, Benson RR. Mr imaging findings in mild traumatic brain injury with persistent neurological impairment. *Magn Reson Imaging* 2017;**37**:243–51.
38. Wang X, Wei XE, Li MH, Li WB, Zhou YJ, Zhang B, et al. Microbleeds on susceptibility-weighted MRI in depressive and non-depressive patients after mild traumatic brain injury. *Neurol Sci* 2014;**35**:1533–9.
39. Spitz G, Maller JJ, Ng A, O'Sullivan R, Ferris NJ, Ponsford JL. Detecting lesions after traumatic brain injury using susceptibility weighted imaging: a comparison with fluid-attenuated inversion recovery and correlation with clinical outcome. *J Neurotrauma* 2013;**30**:2038–50.
40. Imaizumi T, Miyata K, Inamura S, Kohama I, Nyon KS, Nomura T. The difference in location between traumatic cerebral microbleeds and microangiopathic microbleeds associated with stroke. *J Neuroimaging* 2011;**21**:359–64.
41. Geurts BH, Andriessen TM, Goraj BM, Vos PE. The reliability of magnetic resonance imaging in traumatic brain injury lesion detection. *Brain Inj* 2012;**26**:1439–50.
42. Venkat P, Chopp M, Chen J. New insights into coupling and uncoupling of cerebral blood flow and metabolism in the brain. *Croat Med J* 2016;**57**:223–8.
43. Bergsneider M, Hovda DA, Shalmon E, Kelly DF, Vespa PM, Martin NA, et al. Cerebral hyperglycolysis following severe traumatic brain injury in humans: a positron emission tomography study. *J Neurosurg* 1997;**86**:241–51.
44. Ito H, Kanno I, Kato C, Sasaki T, Ishii K, Ouchi Y, et al. Database of normal human cerebral blood flow, cerebral blood volume, cerebral oxygen extraction fraction and cerebral metabolic rate of oxygen measured by positron emission tomography with 15o-labelled carbon dioxide or water, carbon monoxide and oxygen: A multicentre study in japan. *Eur J Nucl Med Mol Imaging* 2004;**31**:635–43.
45. An H, Lin W. Cerebral oxygen extraction fraction and cerebral venous blood volume measurements using MRI: effects of magnetic field variation. *Magn Reson Med* 2002;**47**:958–66.
46. Haacke EM, Reichenbach JR. *Susceptibility weighted imaging in MRI: basic concepts and clinical applications*. Hoboken, NJ: Wiley-Blackwell; 2011.
47. Weigl W, Milej D, Janusek D, Wojtkiewicz S, Sawosz P, Kacprzak M, et al. Application of optical methods in the monitoring of traumatic brain injury: a review. *J Cereb Blood Flow Metab* 2016;**36**:1825–43.
48. Lu H, Ge Y. Quantitative evaluation of oxygenation in venous vessels using t2-relaxation-under-spin-tagging MRI. *Magn Reson Med* 2008;**60**:357–63.
49. Buch S, Ye Y, Haacke EM. Quantifying the changes in oxygen extraction fraction and cerebral activity caused by caffeine and acetazolamide. *J Cereb Blood Flow Metab* 2016. 0271678X16641129.
50. Giza CC, Hovda DA. The neurometabolic cascade of concussion. *J Athl Train* 2001;**36**:228–35.
51. Giza CC, Hovda DA. The new neurometabolic cascade of concussion. *Neurosurgery* 2014;**75**(Suppl 4):S24–33.
52. Goodman MD, Makley AT, Huber NL, Clarke CN, Friend LA, Schuster RM, et al. Hypobaric hypoxia exacerbates the neuroinflammatory response to traumatic brain injury. *J Surg Res* 2011;**165**:30–7.
53. Muthuraju S, Islam MR, Pati S, Jaafar H, Abdullah JM, Yusoff KM. Normobaric hyperoxia treatment prevents early alteration in dopamine level in mice striatum after fluid percussion injury: a biochemical approach. *Int J Neurosci* 2015;**125**:686–92.
54. Muthuraju S, Pati S, Rafiqul M, Abdullah JM, Jaafar H. Effect of normabaric hyperoxia treatment on neuronal damage following fluid percussion injury in the striatum of mice: a morphological approach. *J Biosci* 2013;**38**:93–103.
55. Ahn ES, Robertson CL, Vereczki V, Hoffman GE, Fiskum G. Normoxic ventilatory resuscitation following controlled cortical impact reduces peroxynitrite-mediated protein nitration in the hippocampus. *J Neurosurg* 2008;**108**:124–31.
56. Verweij BH, Muizelaar JP, Vinas FC, Peterson PL, Xiong Y, Lee CP. Impaired cerebral mitochondrial function after traumatic brain injury in humans. *J Neurosurg* 2000;**93**:815–20.
57. Doshi H, Wiseman N, Liu J, Wang W, Welch RD, O'Neil BJ, et al. Cerebral hemodynamic changes of mild traumatic brain injury at the acute stage. *PLoS One* 2015;**10**:e0118061.
58. Wu HM, Huang SC, Vespa P, Hovda DA, Bergsneider M. Redefining the pericontusional penumbra following traumatic brain injury: Evidence of deteriorating metabolic derangements based on positron emission tomography. *J Neurotrauma* 2013;**30**:352–60.

59. Ragan DK, McKinstry R, Benzinger T, Leonard J, Pineda JA. Depression of whole-brain oxygen extraction fraction is associated with poor outcome in pediatric traumatic brain injury. *Pediatr Res* 2012;**71**:199–204.
60. Haacke EM, Duhaime AC, Gean AD, Riedy G, Wintermark M, Mukherjee P, et al. Common data elements in radiologic imaging of traumatic brain injury. *J Magn Reson Imaging* 2010;**32**:516–43.
61. Gura M, Silav G, Isik N, Elmaci I. Noninvasive estimation of cerebral perfusion pressure with transcranial doppler ultrasonography in traumatic brain injury. *Turk Neurosurg* 2012;**22**:411–15.
62. Bendinelli C, Bivard A, Nebauer S, Parsons MW, Balogh ZJ. Brain CT perfusion provides additional useful information in severe traumatic brain injury. *Injury* 2013;**44**:1208–12.
63. Rostami E, Engquist H, Enblad P. Imaging of cerebral blood flow in patients with severe traumatic brain injury in the neurointensive care. *Front Neurol* 2014;**5**:114.
64. Liu W, Wang B, Wolfowitz R, Yeh PH, Nathan DE, Graner J, et al. Perfusion deficits in patients with mild traumatic brain injury characterized by dynamic susceptibility contrast MRI. *NMR Biomed* 2013;**26**:651–63.
65. Grossman EJ, Jensen JH, Babb JS, Chen Q, Tabesh A, Fieremans E, et al. Cognitive impairment in mild traumatic brain injury: A longitudinal diffusional kurtosis and perfusion imaging study. *Am J Neuroradiol* 2013;**34**:951–7 S1-3.
66. Kim J, Whyte J, Patel S, Europa E, Slattery J, Coslett HB, et al. A perfusion fMRI study of the neural correlates of sustained-attention and working-memory deficits in chronic traumatic brain injury. *Neurorehabil Neural Repair* 2012;**26**:870–80.
67. Kou Z, Ye Y, Haacke EM. Evaluating the role of reduced oxygen saturation and vascular damage in traumatic brain injury using magnetic resonance perfusion-weighted imaging and susceptibility-weighted imaging and mapping. *Top Magn Reson Imaging* 2015;**24**:253–65.
68. Haacke EM, Lai S, Reichenbach JR, Kuppusamy K, Hoogenraad FG, Takeichi H, et al. In vivo measurement of blood oxygen saturation using magnetic resonance imaging: a direct validation of the blood oxygen level-dependent concept in functional brain imaging. *Hum Brain Mapp* 1997;**5**:341–6.

Current Treatment Modalities for mTBI: An Interdisciplinary Model[*]

Michael S. Jaffee, MD[1], Stephen Z. Sutton, PT, DPT[2], Kyle Platek[3], Molly Sullan, MS[4] and Russell M. Bauer, PhD, ABPP[4]

[1]Department of Neurology, University of Florida, Gainesville, FL, United States
[2]UF Health Rehabilitation Center, University of Florida, Gainesville, FL, United States
[3]UF Health Fixel Center for Neurological Diseases, University of Florida, Gainesville, FL, United States [4]Department of Clinical & Health Psychology, University of Florida, Gainesville, FL, United States

INTRODUCTION

The heterogeneous symptom presentations and recovery patterns observed following mTBI make management and treatment complex. While pathophysiological brain changes contribute directly to many post-mTBI symptoms, recovery is often complicated further by both preexisting and ongoing medical, neurological, psychological, and social aspects of the injured person's unique circumstances. Indeed, conceptualizing symptoms and outcomes after concussion/mTBI from a broad neurobiopsychocial framework is emerging as a useful approach to understanding the individual differences in concussion symptoms and recovery.[1] Adopting a perspective of this breadth requires multiple sources of input. Toward this end, results of a recent systematic review of sports-related concussion recommends treatment by a multidisciplinary collaborative team with healthcare providers experienced in post-TBI symptoms and problems.[2] This chapter, authored by such a team, outlines useful interventions that target post-TBI symptoms from the viewpoint of the following disciplines: neurology, neuropsychology/clinical psychology, physical therapy,

---

[*]From the UF Health Trauma, Concussion, and Sports Neuromediicne (TRACS) Program, Department of Neurology, University of Florida, Gainesville, FL, United States.

and occupational therapy (OT). Combined and integrated treatments by two or more of the disciplines are often needed to assist patients with complicated symptoms to achieve full recovery after injury.

NEUROLOGICAL INTERVENTIONS AFTER TBI

Pharmacological Management

Other chapters dealing with specific symptoms will address specific pharmacological treatment regimens of these conditions. Here we will discuss basic and common principles of pharmacological management of postconcussive symptoms.

Basic Principles

Pharmacological management of postconcussive symptoms follows several principles. First, it is important to recognize that there are very few medication choices that are FDA approved for postconcussive symptoms. Therefore, like other aspects of neuropsychiatry, a target symptom approach is favored. This means that after identifying symptoms that contribute to functional impairment or distress, medications used to treat those symptoms, irrespective of their etiologic connection to concussion, are used. In general, dosing is done in a "start low and go slow" manner due to the fact that in the postconcussion period, some patients may be more sensitive to adverse effects from medications. One important factor to consider is that, when using medications that require a titration schedule, that the schedule be arranged so that the patient can avoid a prolonged period at a subtherapeutic dose. When selecting the specific agent to be used, consideration should include known side-effect profiles to avoid exacerbation of other associated symptoms and premorbid medical conditions. For example, if a patient has cognitive complaints as part of their symptom profile, and a prescription for headache prophylaxis is being considered, the physician may favor a medication with fewer adverse cognitive side-effects.[3] Additional attention for selection should be paid to the avoidance of agents that have been found to impair plasticity and neuronal recovery such as benzodiazepines and first-generation (typical) neuroleptics.[3] The fundamental principle is to select medications and schedules of administration with consideration for the total symptom profile with which a patient presents.

Short-Term Versus Prophylactic Medications

Some medication regimens are intended for a brief period of time in order to alleviate a sustained exacerbation, or flare, of symptoms. This strategy has been most fully articulated in procotols for headache management. Some professionals refer to this short-term strategy as "bridging."[4] In headache management, a first-tier approach to managing an acute symptom flare would be the use of scheduled nonsteroidal antiinflammatory agents. More aggressive options include: several days of steroids, atypical neuroleptics, or long half-life triptans.[5]

Conversely, if a patient has a prior history of symptoms such as headache that has been exacerbated by the injury, they may require longer-term prophylactic medication. In this case, an additional consideration in medication selection may be to select a medication targeting both acute symptomatology and longer-term comorbidities affecting the patient.[5] For instance, if mood symptom is a comorbidity of headaches, an antidepressant that could target both pain and mood, such as an serotonin and norepinephrine reuptake inhibitor (SNR) I, may be considered as an option for headache prophylaxis.

Baseline Medications

If a patient is on medication for a baseline condition at the time of injury, it is important that these medications be at least maintained at baseline dosages. A pre-injury condition that was in remission due to the efficacy from pharmacological management would be a significant risk factor for prolonged recovery if these medications were not continued. It is important to consider baseline medications and potential drug–drug interactions when considering medication selection for post-injury symptom management.

Follow-Up and Maintenance

One of the most important aspects of clinical follow-up is to determine if a previously prescribed medication is effective for the individual patient, and to decide whether to continue with the prescribed regimen, to consider changing to another agent, or to add an augmenting agent. In general, if there is partial efficacy and the medication is well-tolerated without adverse effects, a dose titration may be considered. If the target symptom is in remission, but the patient has adverse effects, a dose reduction may be tried in order to determine the lowest dose that is effective and minimizes adverse effects. If there is limited efficacy and adverse effects, then discontinuation and consideration of another agent may be considered.[6]

Discontinuation

There is limited evidence as to how long symptoms should be in remission before discontinuing medications. Some practitioners use anywhere from 3 to 6 months of remission as a guideline for discontinuation. When it is time to discontinue, it is recommended that this be in done with a gradual taper.

Topical Medications

In the case of headache management, there is some anecdotal evidence for using topical nonsteroidal agents over affected areas of focal pain, such as nummular headache or pain limited to the area of impact on the head. The targeting of strained muscles, such as with cervicalgia, can also be augmented with a patch over the affected muscles, which releases lidocaine superficially into the muscle.

Injections or Nerve Blocks

Injections are sometimes considered as part of an overall management strategy for headaches and focal muscle pain following injury. These procedures are typically considered as part of a pain management program. Some of these procedures are intended to provide relief in the subacute phase whereas others are part of a more chronic management program.

Subacute Procedures

Occipital nerve blocks are sometimes incorporated into the management of headaches with an occipital neuralgia component. Sometimes this occipital neuralgia component may be conceptualized as occurring secondary to posterior cervical muscle strain and trigger points of the muscles may be a consideration. For older individuals who may have underlying degenerative disc disease of the cervical spine with neuroforaminal involvement, there may be some evidence for epidural steroid injections. These injections are typically done with a local anesthetic, such as lidocaine, a local steroid, or a combination of the two. Some practitioners have described success with dry needling for associated myofascial pain.

Head trauma of a severity greater than concussion may be associated with extremity trauma that could have a delayed complication of complex regional pain syndrome (formerly known as reflex sympathetic dystrophy). This complication is sometimes diagnosed with a sympathetic nerve block.

Chronic Procedures

For chronic headaches lasting for more than 15 days a month for at least 3 hours and having persisted for at least 3 months, the FDA has approved management with Botulinim Toxin A. Insurance companies may have additional requirements such as previous failure of prophylactic medication therapy. The administration sequence approved by the FDA includes a pattern of 31 subcutaneous injections in a specified pattern around the head. Repeat injections are required every 90 days to maintain efficacy.[7]

Another intervention used for the migraine component of headache disorders is sphenopalatine ganglion blocks. One study in migraine patients showed a reduced frequency and severity over a 6-month period if the procedure was performed twice a week for 6 weeks for a total of 12 treatments.[8]

Neurostimulation

There is emerging experience with neurostimulation as a modality for several symptoms that are part of a postconcussive syndrome, such as headaches, cognition, mood and anxiety, and vertigo, but there are limited studies evaluating the efficacy of these modalities specifically for management of postconcussive symptoms. These devices have emerged primarily in the management of headaches. The main underlying theory is that these neuromodulation devices work by inhibiting central pathways that are underlying clinical symptoms. However, preliminary studies suggest some symptom improvement with neurostimulation.

Headaches

There are currently three devices approved by the FDA for the use in primary headache syndromes. One is a transcutaneous supraorbital nerve stimulator (tSNS).[9] The patient uses electrode pads wrapped around the forehead placing the electrodes over the procerus. The initial studies showed that 3 months of treatment was needed to achieve symptom relief.[10] Another FDA approved device is single-pulse transcranial magnetic stimulation (sTMS).[11] This is a device that is held up to the back of the head over the occipital area, and was found to work best in patients who have migraine with aura and when administered at the time of the aura.[12] Further studies have demonstrated a prophylactic effect when used daily.[13] It is hypothesized that the sTMS devices may be targeting thalamocortical pathways that are considered migraine integration pathways. The third FDA approved device is a noninvasive vagal neve stimulator (nVNS).[14] It is placed on the neck over the vagus nerve and stimulated for 90 seconds to two minutes. These have been studied primarily in the management of cluster headaches, one of the autonomic cephalgias.[15,16] There is also ongoing investigation of a sphenopalatine ganglion stimulation device.[8]

Cognition

Most of the preliminary work on cognitive effects of neurostimulation has been done with transcutaneous direct current stimulation (tDCS).[17,18] This treatment has been used to mitigate cognitive decline of aging.[19] There have been some limited pilot trials in the use of cognitive sequelae following concussion which suggested promise.

Mood and Anxiety

There has been some evaluation using transcutaneous vagal nerve stimulation in reducing the symptoms of posttraumatic stress disorder (PTSD) given the significant autonomic contribution of this disorder.[20] Past studies suggest that vagal nerve stimulation reduces the severity of anxiety symptoms in PTSD patients,[21] but more work needs to be done in postconcussion patients to prove efficacy of this treatment in this population.

Vertigo

Under development is a caloric vestibular stimulation device. This is being investigated for both symptoms of vertigo and headache.[22]

Neuropsychological Interventions After TBI

The heterogeneous behavioral and emotional symptom presentations and recovery patterns observed following mTBI make management complex. Lishman contends that indirect effects of mTBI, such as psychosocial stressors and poor reaction or coping strategies, are the driving force maintaining symptom expression.[23] From a treatment standpoint, these indirect effects can be targeted for intervention and previous research has demonstrated some success. One important dimension worthy of assessment and intervention is the patient's knowledge of TBI and their expectations for recovery.[24] Such expectations affect the degree to which patients attribute, and react to, nonspecific problems or symptoms as sequelae of their injury. Expectations that exaggerate the severity of the concussion or that elongate its likely recovery timeline should be addressed early in the post-injury period. Patients who catastrophize the impact of their injury, and patients who minimize its impact, can suffer different but equally detrimental consequences. The former are at risk for developing depression-related symptoms (e.g., hopelessness about the future, low self-esteem, etc.) and the latter are at risk for more stress- and anxiety-related symptoms with growing worry that their injury is more serious than they initially believed. This section briefly addresses psychological interventions that may be useful in the management of concussion. While such interventions may be useful clinically, it should be noted that, at this point, the evidence base in support of such treatments is quite limited. For example, a Cochrane review on post-TBI interventions for depression[25] found only six studies that were generally of poor quality, showed small effect sizes, and differed significantly in their definition and measurement of depression. Despite this, there is general clinical consensus that behavioral interventions can be effective treatment options for addressing the symptoms suffered by many mTBI patients, and can be useful in preventing protracted postconcussion syndrome and in reducing long-term disability.[26]

Cognitive Behavioral Therapy

The primary goal of psychotherapeutic intervention following mTBI is to establish early recognition and treatment of potentially maladaptive thinking and behavior patterns and their impact on the patient's emotional state. Cognitive-behavioral therapy (CBT) is a psychotherapeutic approach aimed at altering these maladaptive patterns and is well-established as an effective treatment for numerous medical and psychological disorders.[27] CBT has been shown to be effective in treating patients with persistent postconcussion syndrome (PPCS[24,28,29]), with significant benefits observed after as few as six 50-minute sessions.[30] Emerging evidence suggests that intervention soon (within the first week or two) after mTBI may be useful in reducing risk of PPCS.[24,30] Some PPCS symptoms (e.g., anxiety, fatigue, overall quality of life) may be more responsive to treatment than others (e.g., depression, PTSD).[28] Most CBT protocols involve both therapeutic work during the treatment visit coupled with homework that requires the patient to apply principles learned in session to problems encountered in everyday life. The real-life (ecological) application of these techniques with regular homework may be an important active ingredient of the CBT approach.

Mindfulness-Based Stress Reduction

While originally designed to treat patients with chronic pain, mindfulness-based stress-reduction (MBSR) is now widely implemented for many medical and psychological conditions. MBSR is a technique that incorporates "mindfulness" (being in the moment; diverting attention nonjudgmentally to experience in an effort to more directly and effectively process stress-inducing stimuli).[31] In addition to being an effective means of symptom management, studies have demonstrated structural and functional neuroplastic changes associated with these attention-control-based treatments. Further evidence suggests association between mindfulness meditation and improved sustained attention and working memory,[32] and it is hypothesized that mindfulness interventions improve behavioral and emotional self-regulation.[33] Specific to mTBI patients, MBSR has been shown to be effective in improving subjective quality-of-life and self-efficacy measures, and in improving cognitive functioning.[34] A subsequent meta-analysis indicated that MBSR-based interventions may have moderate usefulness for treatment of fatigue in TBI patients.[35]

Cognitive-Behavioral Treatment for Insomnia

Cognitive-behavioral therapy for insomnia (CBT-I) includes a 7−8 session treatment protocol targeting areas such as sleep hygiene (establishing sleep-related routines), stimulus control (managing interfering stimuli such as TV or smartphone use, lighting, and sound), sleep restriction (limiting the amount of sleep and relegating it to certain times of the day as a way to improve sleep efficiency), relaxation practices (to produce autonomic quieting), and cognitions contributing to poor sleep.[36] CBT-I has been shown to be highly effective in the treatment of symptoms of insomnia and, when compared to pharmacological interventions, is often more successful at treating sleep-onset symptoms with reduced potential for side-effects.[37] Past literature regarding the treatment of sleep disorders suggests that CBT-I is effective at reducing symptoms of insomnia in severe TBI populations.[38,39]

CBT-I is also very effective at alleviating sleep-related symptoms associated with psychological disorders that are often comorbid with TBI, such as PTSD, depression and anxiety.[40] Talbot et al.[41] performed a randomized control trial to determine the efficacy of CBT-I in veterans with PTSD. They found full symptom remission in subjective sleep complaints in 41% of the intervention group versus 0% of the control group, as well as improved work and interpersonal functioning, which were noted at the 6-month follow-up.[41] Monitoring sleep patterns in athletes with TBI may also help to alleviate detrimental effects of TBI and sleep dysfunction on athletic performance.[42] These results suggest that, in addition to current protocols for reduced activity following TBI until full symptom resolution, CBT-I may be helpful in treating TBI-related sleep symptoms, and in improving overall psychosocial functioning, which, if untreated, are associated with poorer outcome after mTBI.[43]

CBT-I protocols may be tailored to specific patient needs, and coordinated care with neurology is recommended if medications are proposed in addition to behavioral therapy. For example, Ponsford et al.[44] proposed the addition of light therapy to decrease daytime fatigue, pharmacologic treatment with melatonin supplements or modafinil, and a more general cognitive-behavioral therapy to support lifestyle modifications needed for better sleep cycle maintenance and reduced daytime fatigue to CBT-I treatment in TBI patients. Other available additions and modifications to the individual treatment plan include strategies to target nightmares in PTSD patients (such as combined pharmacotherapy and imagery rehearsal therapy),[45] or online therapies for athlete populations, who might not be able to attend weekly CBT-I sessions due to rigorous travel schedules.[46]

Physical Therapy Interventions After TBI

Physical therapists (PT) specialize in the diagnosis and management of mobility, balance, and pain, each of which can be significantly impaired by mTBI. PTs use a variety of treatment strategies to address symptoms that are common after mTBI, including headaches, neck pain, dizziness, blurred vision, impaired balance, fatigue, and decreased activity tolerance. Interventions may include symptom-limited controlled aerobic exercise, vestibular rehabilitation techniques (VRT), spinal mobilization and therapeutic exercise for cervical spine dysfunction. While large scale randomized control trials are currently lacking, there is growing support for an active approach to mTBI treatment.[47]

Physical Activity

Questions regarding "when" to initiate physical activity, and "how much" physical activity should be prescribed after mTBI have been recent topics of debate. Recent publications have challenged the widely accepted notion that complete physical rest until a patient is asymptomatic is the most effective means of treatment. The fifth International Conference on Concussion in Sport held in Berlin concluded that there is "insufficient evidence to support the use of complete physical and cognitive rest to reduce postconcussion symptoms" and to "promote recovery to minimizing brain energy demands."[48] A recent systematic review by Schneider and colleagues concluded that a "brief period (24–48 hours) of cognitive and physical rest is appropriate for most patients."[49] After acute symptoms have begun to subside individuals may begin to gradually increase activity. In fact, Grool et al., in 2016, found that early physical activity was associated with reduced incidence of persistent symptoms at 28 days.[50]

While there is no "gold standard" protocol for the most effective mode of activity following injury, moderate intensity activities are shown to reduce symptom duration compared to complete rest or high-intensity activity.[51] Leddy et al., in 2010, achieved a moderate activity approach by utilizing a graded treadmill test to establish a baseline threshold for symptom exacerbation.[52] Other recommendations based in part on anecdotal evidence suggest the use of a stationary bike to limit perturbations from ground impact that could exacerbate headaches or vestibular symptoms. When determining a treatment protocol for each patient, several factors should be considered prior to initiating exercise including pre-injury fitness levels, presence of cardiovascular disease, orthopedic injury, focal neurologic deficit, or significant visual or balance deficits. During exercise, patients should be closely monitored for symptom exacerbation or abnormal cardiac response.

This type of individualized protocol was outlined in a 2009 case series in which a multi-faceted model for controlled active rehabilitation in children slow to recover from a sports-related concussion was proposed.[53] Interventions included aerobic exercise (60%–80% of age predicted max heart rate), coordination exercises (sport specific), visualization and a home program consisting of the same interventions performed in the clinic. In addition to visualization techniques, patients and their parents were provided education, reassurance, and motivation to address self-efficacy and limit disruption of normal daily life. While Gagnon's case series did not include a control group, all participants were reported to have shown improvement and returned to prior activities.[54]

Vestibular and Balance Therapy

Second to headache, dizziness is the most common symptom after mTBI and its presence is associated with prolonged recovery.[54–56] Dizziness can result from dysfunction of the peripheral vestibular apparatus, central vestibular pathways, injury to the cervical spine, disruption of the autonomic nervous system and/or anxiety. It is important to clearly determine the type of dizziness the patient is experiencing when considering the proper intervention modality for each patient. Dizziness described as "lightheaded" or presyncope may indicate a dysfunction in the autonomic nervous system that would be managed differently than true vertigo or imbalance, which are more consistent with vestibular impairment.

The primary role of the vestibular system is to stabilize gaze during head or body movements, postural control, balance, and provide spatial orientation. As such, in addition to dizziness, patients with vestibular dysfunction often complain of poor balance, unsteady gait, motion sickness, blurred vision, nausea, fatigue, and "fogginess." PT trained in vestibular rehabilitation can conduct a thorough examination to determine the potential source of the dizziness and implement the appropriate treatment. Vestibular rehabilitation strategies include canalith repositioning maneuvers (i.e., the Epley Maneuver) to treat Benign Paroxysmal Positional Vertigo, adaptation exercises aimed at improving gaze stability via the vestibular ocular reflex, habituation strategies to reduce dizziness associated with specific movements, progression of balance and/or gait training, and gradual exposure to visual motion environments.[57,58]

In addition to symptoms arising directly from the vestibular system, individuals who experience trauma to their cervical spine may also experience dizziness. Due to the mechanical forces involved in producing most mTBIs, the cervical spine is often injured as well. While the mechanism is not fully understood, it is believed that disruption of afferent pathways in the cervical spine may result in altered position sense, impaired balance, and the sensation of dizziness. Several evaluation techniques have been suggested for determining dysfunction in the cervical spine related to dizziness including measuring Joint Position Sense Error (JPSE) as described by Feipel et al. in 2006.[59] While the validity of this test has not been fully established, there are no other readily available assessment tools to measure cervical proprioception. Some sites have attempted to develop simple technology to measure JPSE with a standard computer and webcam.[60]

The effectiveness of VRT for mTBI has not been thoroughly studied, though a systematic review published in 2017 concluded that the use of VRT to treat dizziness and balance dysfunction show promise.[61] However, the literature is mostly populated by studies with relatively weak methodology. However, the Murray et al.[61] review noted that no adverse effects were found in any of the studies included. The only randomized control trial included in the review was published by Schnieder et al. in 2014.[62] The results of this study were promising, with a significantly larger percentage of the treatment group (73%) receiving medical clearance at 8 weeks compared to the control group (7%). Unfortunately, because the treatment group received both VRT and treatment for cervical spine dysfunction, the results cannot be attributed to either treatment modality alone.

While the majority of studies on VRT included only participants with chronic symptoms, Reneker et al. described the implementation of VRT as soon as 10 days post-injury.[63] The treatment group participated in cervical manual techniques, as well as progressive vestibular rehabilitation, oculomotor, and neuromotor retraining. The exercises were designed to be challenging and mild symptom exacerbation was expected and monitored throughout the sessions. In this particular cohort of patients, those who participated in the progressive treatment group received medical clearance a median of 10.5 days sooner than the control group, suggesting a positive effect of VRT intervention in symptomatic patients.

Muscular and Neck Pain Management

Due to the acceleration–deceleration forces involved in mTBI, it can be anticipated that some patients may also sustain sprains and/or strains of the cervical spine. Neck pain and headaches, as a result of these whiplash-like forces, can complicate diagnosis and treatment of patients who have sustained traumatic injuries. If left untreated, symptoms arising from the cervical spine could contribute to a more prolonged recovery for the patient. Care should be taken to evaluate the cervical spine of any patient who has sustained a blow to the head, neck or body. Physical therapy interventions for neck pain may include spinal manipulation or mobilizations, soft tissue massage, and exercises to improve cervical spine, scapulothoracic, and shoulder muscular strength, endurance, flexibility and motor control. While evidence for treatment of the cervical spine in mTBI is limited, data are available to suggest that joint mobilization and specific exercises, help alleviate acute neck pain and symptoms related to whiplash-associated disorder.[64] General exercises may not be as effective as specific neck exercises[65,66] and the addition of spinal mobilization seems to have a greater effect than exercise alone[67,68] at decreasing pain and disability. There is not sufficient evidence to support the use of passive modalities such as heat, cold, diathermy and ultrasound.[69]

Neuromuscular Control

In addition to symptom-based management of patients with mTBI, evidence is emerging in sports-related concussion (SRC), that athletes who have returned to play after a concussion are more likely to sustain a secondary orthopedic injury when compared to non-concussed athletes.[70,71] While this phenomenon is not fully understood, it is theorized that neurocognitive deficits in such domains as reaction time and dual task processing may result in decreased neuromuscular control and faulty movement patterns when athletes are faced with the complex demands of their sport.[71,72] It can, therefore, be hypothesized that, prior to returning to competition, athletes should undergo more comprehensive testing and rehabilitation to address potential deficits in neurocognition and neuromuscular control. Training may include biomechanics analysis and progression of visual and cognitive demands. There are currently no published studies to indicate that providing such interventions in athletes with SRC is effective, however, the implementation of neuromuscular control interventions as a means of preventing lower extremity injury has be extensively studied with promising results in favor of regular implementation of such programs.[73,74]

Occupational Therapy Interventions After TBI

The constellation of symptoms experienced after mTBI can disrupt the resumption of an individual's pre-injury roles and occupations. Returning a patient to prior function is the primary objective of OT and occupational therapists utilize a variety of modalities in the rehabilitation process to achieve this goal.

Planning a treatment intervention is influenced by many patient factors including, but not limited to, stage of recovery, age, social supports, comorbidities and preexisting conditions, all of which contribute in part to the formation of the patient's occupational profile. Constructing an occupational profile is an important aspect of the evaluation process, which also assists in developing treatment plans. In the creation of an occupational profile, "the client, with the assistance of the OT practitioner, identifies priorities and desired targeted outcomes that will lead to the client's engagement in occupations that support participation in life."[75] In this section, we describe other commonly utilized modalities by occupational therapists in the treatment of mTBI:

Therapeutic Activity

Therapeutic use of activity is a function-based modality, which utilizes graded tasks and environmentally specific activities that are relevant to the patient's prior or projected level of function. Via these task specific interventions, occupational therapists are able to address deficits in academic, social, vocational, self-care and physical performance. By creating interventions that replicate ecological task demands, therapeutic activity provides practice opportunities to implement and learn compensatory strategies, to develop endurance/activity tolerance, and to return an individual to their most meaningful roles. Therapists can facilitate behavioral plasticity by ensuring the correct level of environmental demand at the correct times in the recovery process of mTBI.[76] Therapists can use these task specific interventions to more thoroughly evaluate a patient's ability to return to work or school and to provide recommendations for appropriate accommodations given the symptoms or deficits. The provision of adequate accommodations will allow a safe return to activities and environments most specific to their pre-injury roles, which is the most functional use of therapeutic activity.

Activity as a modality to aid recovery after mTBI is supported by Majerski et al.[51] in their work with students following an mTBI. They found that participants who reported moderate levels of physical and cognitive exertion from participation in both school and light exercise had better neuropsychological outcomes than those with very little or very high levels of activity. The fact that too little or too much activity can negatively influence recovery highlights the value of monitoring and guiding patients through a graded return to activity. While many patients are hesitant to return to activity for fear of exacerbating symptoms, occupational therapists can help gauge appropriate activity, and can help the patient address fears or anxieties preventing participation.

While facilitating a gradual return to activity is beneficial to recovery, it is important to consider deficits that may affect a person's ability to complete tasks in a safe manner. Driving is one such activity of daily living that carries an increased risk and may be impaired due to perceptual and/or cognitive symptoms following mTBI.[77] Although no single comprehensive assessment tool exists for measuring fitness to drive post-mTBI, occupational therapists can assess relevant predriving skills such as motor function, vision and utilize driving simulators or on road assessments.[78] Given the associated risks of some pre-injury roles and activities, as well as the understanding that overexertion can impede recovery, activity restriction is an equally important consideration within the use of therapeutic activity.

In clinical settings, self-reporting systems to track symptom changes allow therapists to prevent overexertion or a significant exacerbation of symptoms by monitoring changes in pre- and postactivity symptom ratings. This feedback mechanism also enables the patient to safely continue use of therapeutic activity in their rehabilitation routines outside the clinic. Other treatment modalities for symptom management can be incorporated into therapeutic activity, as symptoms such as headache, eye strain, pain, dizziness, or fatigue will often limit activity tolerance.[79]

Vision and Oculomotor Therapy

Visual disturbances are commonly reported after mTBI, ranging from oculomotor dysfunction, decreased acuity, convergence insufficiency, diplopia, and photophobia to fixation and accommodation dysfunction.[80] In a retrospective analysis of ambulatory outpatients with mild TBI, over 90% were found to have one or more symptoms of oculomotor dysfunction.[81] In practice, visual deficits can prove to be a significant limiting factor for participation in pre-injury roles and activities after mTBI. The significance of vision therapy as a treatment modality is evident in another study by Ciuffreda et al.,[82] in which 90% of adult patients with mTBI using conventional vision therapy to address oculomotor subsystems, vergence and accommodation, showed complete or marked improvement in one or more of their primary symptoms. The high prevalence of visual disturbances and their propensity to impair function, coupled with the effectiveness of vison therapy make it a commonly utilized modality in OT for the treatment of mTBI.

Vision therapy can be delivered by a number of practitioners such as optometrists and occupational therapists, not necessarily working independently of one another. Vision therapy for mTBI often includes treatments to improve fusional ranges and convergence abilities via strengthening and teaming of ocular motor muscles. Improved functional outcomes can be achieved with ocular motor-based vision exercises targeting deficient eye movements and muscles, technology and computer-based programs that replicate similar demands or a combination thereof.[83] Improvements in fusional ranges and convergence abilities can, in turn, benefit binocular eye function as well as accommodative abilities of the eye.[84]

Compensatory strategies to assist in symptom management represent another useful aspect of vision therapy. Strategies assisting in the resumption of pre-injury life roles often coincide with remediation-based treatments. Some examples of these compensatory strategies include the use of light filters and tinted lenses in the management of photophobia.[85] Line readers to minimize sensory input during reading to improve attention and increase endurance for near point reading are also useful. Selective occlusion for the management of diplopia to increase activity tolerance has been used clinically and is often self-initiated by patients. While the overarching goal is to remediate visual disturbances, compensatory strategies are important to consider for patient populations that have persistent symptoms outside the acute recovery phase.[78]

Cognitive Rehabilitation

Cognitive complaints after mTBI are another commonly reported symptom, most consistently including deficits in attention, concentration, information processing speed and memory.[86] The effectiveness of cognitive rehabilitation as a modality in the treatment of mTBI is well-supported in the literature, most notably with interventions targeting attention, memory, social communication skills, and executive function.[86]

As a modality, cognitive rehabilitation approaches incorporate remediation techniques, compensatory strategies and often includes variants of cognitive-behavioral therapy to support skill development. Cognitive rehabilitation, like previously discussed modalities within OT, is patient centered with a focus on the resumption of pre-injury roles. In addition to Occupational Therapists, cognitive rehabilitation is sometimes performed by trained psychologists or neuropsychologists. Given the many ways cognitive issues can influence function after mTBI, cognitive rehabilitation efforts for patients with closed head injuries rely on combinations of education, social support, practice, and process training.[87]

Cognitive-behavioral psychotherapy and cognitive remediation appear to diminish psychological distress and improve cognitive functioning among community-living persons with mild and moderate TBI.[88] Remedial intervention programs have demonstrated clinical validity in the treatment of patients with TBI, with limited but growing evidence for efficacy in mTBI[89]; Research in this area is (fortunately) limited by the fact that the majority of those who sustain an mTBI resume normal functioning fairly quickly. There is, however, a considerable subset of patients, approximately 5%−15%, who report persistent cognitive symptoms lasting well beyond the initial 3-month "acute" phase.[88] For these patients, Attention Process Training (ATP-3) and N-Back Exercises[89,90] are two remediation-focused interventions used by OT's to address persistent attentional problems after the acute phase is over. Other interventions are available to address difficulties with memory or executive dysfunction.[91,92]

Given that the majority of patients resume normal cognitive function quickly, compensatory strategies will often be more useful during the acute recovery period to ensure safety and assist with resumption of pre-injury roles. Rees et al.[93] found strong evidence supporting the use of external memory supports to compensate for functional memory problems, though these interventions may not necessarily improve underlying abilities since they do not require the patient to exercise the deficient cognitive skill. Rees et al. also found strong support for the use of internal strategies to improve recall performance for people with mild impairments. Compensatory cognitive strategies can be described as cognitive energy saving techniques (e.g., using a planner rather than remembering a list of tasks) that buoy everyday functioning as the symptoms of mTBI continue to resolve.

CONCLUSION

While the majority of mTBI patients are expected to achieve full symptom recovery within 3 months of injury, treatment to promote effective symptom resolution and a graded return to pre-injury activities can be helpful in reducing the development of chronic symptoms. Owing to the complexity of symptoms experienced following mTBI, often including headache, changes in sleep, balance and dizziness, orthopedic pain, visual disturbances, and changes in cognition and mood, multiple treatment modalities are needed to alleviate acute symptom onset, to prevent the development of chronic disability, and to treat chronic or protracted symptoms. Because treatment often requires specialized care and knowledge about both the nature of mTBI and the subset of experienced symptoms, an interdisciplinary team is best equipped to manage patient care. Such a team reduces redundancy in treatment, and works together to determine an individualized treatment plan for each patient. These treatment plans may include pharmacological intervention, behavioral therapy targeting cognitive functioning, mood symptoms and sleep dysfunction, and specialized therapies to reduce dizziness, orthopedic pain, visual disturbances and addressing barriers to carrying out activities of daily living.

In mTBI, there is no "gold standard" treatment for all patients. Given the significant individual differences in symptom presentation and recovery trajectories, paired with premorbid complications and environmental factors, care must be taken to develop an individualized treatment approach, taking into account each patient's unique circumstances. In terms of assisting the patient's understanding of their injury and their likelihood for recovery, an interdisciplinary team offers the advantage of managing expectations for recovery and determining treatment goals as one unified message, rather than in a mixed or contradicting manner across providers. Bringing together the expertise of multiple different providers who are skilled in the treatment of mTBI, patients may recover to pre-injury functioning more effectively with reduced experience of chronic symptomatology.[48,94,95]

The coordination and collaboration of the interdisciplinary team is critically important and must itself receive attention as a way of providing an integrated treatment approach. Interdisciplinary evaluation allows for individual tailoring of management plans targeted to the symptoms that are impairing to each patient. The neurobiopsychosocial approach allows, not only full formulation and understanding of symptoms, but can also be used to guide management and treatment planning. In the next decade of concussion care, attention should be devoted to evaluating best practices within the interdisciplinary team approach to concussion evaluation and management in order to achieve the best outcomes for the patients we serve.

References

1. McCrea M, Broshek DK, Barth JT. Sports concussion assessment and management: future research directions. *Brain Inj* 2015;**29**(2):276–82.
2. Makdissi M, Schneider KJ, Feddermann-Demont N, Guskiewicz KM, Hinds S, Leddy JJ, et al. Approach to investigation and treatment of persistent symptoms following sport-related concussion: a systematic review. *Br J Sports Med* 2017;**51**(12):958–68.
3. Larson EB, Zollman FS. The effect of sleep medications on cognitive recovery from traumatic brain injury. *J Head Trauma Rehabilit* 2010;**25**(1):61–7.
4. Garza I, Schwedt TJ. Diagnosis and management of chronic daily headache. *Semin Neurol* 2010;**30**(2):154–66.
5. Young WB, Silberstein SD, Nahas SJ, Marmura MJ. Migraine: treating the acute attack. In: Young WB, Silberstein SD, Nahas SJ, Marmura MJ, editors. *Jefferson headache manual*. New York: Demos Medical Publishing; 2011. p. 39–56.
6. Bell KR, Kraus EE, Zasler ND. Medical management of posttraumatic headaches: pharmacological and physical treatment. *J Head Trauma Rehabilit* 1999;**14**(1):34–48.

7. Zasler N, Martelli M. Post-traumatic headache: practical approaches to diagnosis and treatment. In: Weiner RB, editor. *Pain management: a practical guide for clinicians.* 6th ed. Boca Raton, FL: St. Lucie Press; 2002. p. 313—44.

8. Tepper D. Stimulators for the treatment of headache. *Headache: J Head Face Pain.* 2014;**54**(3):593—4.

9. Chou DE, Gross GJ, Casadei CH, Yugrakh MS. External trigeminal nerve stimulation for the acute treatment of migraine: open-label trial on safety and efficacy. *Neuromod J Intern Neuromod Soc* 2017. Epub 2017/06/06.

10. Schoenen J, Vandersmissen B, Jeangette S, Herroelen L, Vandenheede M, Gerard P, et al. Migraine prevention with a supraorbital transcutaneous stimulator: a randomized controlled trial. *Neurology* 2013;**80**(8):697—704.

11. Barker AT, Shields K. Transcranial magnetic stimulation: basic principles and clinical aApplications in migraine. *Headache* 2017;**57**(3):517—24 Epub 2016/12/29.

12. Lipton RB, Dodick DW, Silberstein SD, Saper JR, Aurora SK, Pearlman SH, et al. Single-pulse transcranial magnetic stimulation for acute treatment of migraine with aura: a randomised, double-blind, parallel-group, sham-controlled trial. *Lancet Neurol* 2010;**9**(4):373—80.

13. Cortese F, Coppola G, Di Lenola D, Serrao M, Di Lorenzo C, Parisi V, et al. Excitability of the motor cortex in patients with migraine changes with the time elapsed from the last attack. *J Headache Pain* 2017;**18**(1).

14. Goadsby PJ, Grosberg BM, Mauskop A, Cady R, Simmons KA. Effect of noninvasive vagus nerve stimulation on acute migraine: an open-label pilot study. Cephalalgia : an international. *J Headache.* 2014;**34**(12):986—93 Epub 2014/03/13.

15. Gaul C, Magis D, Liebler E, Straube A. Effects of non-invasive vagus nerve stimulation on attack frequency over time and expanded response rates in patients with chronic cluster headache: a post hoc analysis of the randomised, controlled PREVA study. *J Headache Pain* 2017;**18**(1).

16. Silberstein SD, Mechtler LL, Kudrow DB, Calhoun AH, McClure C, Saper JR, et al. Non-Invasive Vagus Nerve Stimulation for the acute treatment of cluster headache: findings from the randomized, double-blind, sham-controlled ACT1 study. *Headache: J Head Face Pain.* 2016;**56**(8):1317—32.

17. Bikson M, Grossman P, Thomas C, Zannou AL, Jiang J, Adnan T, et al. Safety of transcranial direct current stimulation: evidence based update 2016. *Brain Stimul* 2016;**9**(5):641—61 Epub 2016/07/04.

18. Cappon D, Jahanshahi M, Bisiacchi P. Value and efficacy of transcranial direct current stimulation in the cognitive rehabilitation: a critical review since 2000. *Front Neurosci* 2016;**10**:157 Epub 2016/05/06.

19. Woods AJ. Combating cognitive aging and dementia with tDCS: the Phase III ACT trial. *Brain Stimul* 2017;**10** (2):411.

20. Nemeroff CB, Mayberg HS, Krahl SE, McNamara J, Frazer A, Henry TR, et al. VNS Therapy in treatment-resistant depression: clinical evidence and putative neurobiological mechanisms. *Neuropsychopharmacology* 2006;**31**(7):1345—55.

21. Kar SK, Sarkar S. Neuro-stimulation techniques for the management of anxiety disorders: an update. *Clin Psychopharmacol Neurosci* 2016;**14**(4):330—7.

22. Black RD, Rogers LL, Ade KK, Nicoletto HA, Adkins HD, Laskowitz DT. Non-invasive neuromodulation using time-varying caloric vestibular stimulation. *IEEE J Transl Eng Health Med* 2016;**4**:1—10.

23. Lishman WA. Physiogenesis and psychogenesis in the 'post-concussional syndrome'. *Brit J Psych J Mental Sci* 1988;**153**:460—9.

24. Mittenberg W, Tremont G, Zielinski RE, Fichera S, Rayls KR. Cognitive-behavioral prevention of postconcussion syndrome. *Arch Clin Neuropsychol* 1996;**11**(2):139—45.

25. Gertler P, Tate RL, Cameron ID. *Non-pharmacological interventions for depression in adults and children with traumatic brain injury. Cochrane Database of systematic reviews.* New York: John Wiley & Sons, Ltd; 2015.

26. Al Sayegh A, Sandford D, Carson AJ. Psychological approaches to treatment of postconcussion syndrome: a systematic review. *J Neurol Neurosurg Psychiatry* 2010;**81**(10):1128—34 Epub 2010/08/31.

27. Butler AC, Chapman JE, Forman EM, Beck AT. The empirical status of cognitive-behavioral therapy: a review of meta-analyses. *Clin Psychol Rev* 2006;**26**(1):17—31.

28. Potter S, Brown RG. Cognitive behavioural therapy and persistent post-concussion symptoms: integrating conceptual issues and practical aspects in treatment. *Neuropsychol Rehabil* 2012;**22**(1):1—25.

29. Kay T. Neuropsychological treatment of mild traumatic brain injury. *J Head Trauma Rehabil* 1993;**8**(3):74—85.

30. Silverberg ND, Hallam BJ, Rose A, Underwood H, Whitfield K, Thornton AE, et al. Cognitive-behavioral prevention of postconcussion syndrome in at-risk patients: a pilot randomized controlled trial. *J Head Trauma Rehabil* 2013;**28**(4):313—22.

31. Kabat-Zinn J. *Wherever you go, there you are: mindfulness meditation in everyday life.* New York: Hyperion; 1994.
32. Chiesa A, Calati R, Serretti A. Does mindfulness training improve cognitive abilities? A systematic review of neuropsychological findings. *Clin Psychol Rev* 2011;**31**(3):449−64.
33. Immink MA. Fatigue in neurological disorders: a review of self-regulation and mindfulness-based interventions. *Fatigue: Biomed Health Behav* 2014;**2**(4):202−18.
34. Azulay J, Smart CM, Mott T, Cicerone KD. A pilot study examining the effect of mindfulness-based stress reduction on symptoms of chronic mild traumatic brain injury/postconcussive syndrome. *J Head Trauma Rehabil* 2013;**28**(4):323−31.
35. Ulrichsen KM, Kaufmann T, Dørum ES, Kolskår KK, Richard G, Alnæs D, et al. Clinical utility of mindfulness training in the treatment of fatigue after stroke, traumatic brain injury and multiple sclerosis: a systematic literature review and meta-analysis. *Front Psychol* 2016;7.
36. Perlis ML, Junquist C, Smith MT, Posner D. *Cognitive behavioral treatment of insomnia: a session-by-session guide.* New York: Springer; 2008.
37. Morin CM. Cognitive-behavioral therapy of insomnia. *Sleep Med Clin* 2006;**1**(3):375−86.
38. Ouellet M-C, Morin CM. Efficacy of cognitive-behavioral therapy for insomnia associated with traumatic brain injury: a single-case experimental design. *Arch Phys Med Rehabil* 2007;**88**(12):1581−92.
39. Wu JQ, Appleman ER, Salazar RD, Ong JC. Cognitive behavioral therapy for insomnia comorbid with psychiatric and medical conditions: a meta-analysis. *JAMA Internal Med* 2015;**175**:1461−72.
40. Taylor DJ, Pruiksma KE. Cognitive and behavioural therapy for insomnia (CBT-I) in psychiatric populations: a systematic review. *Intern Rev Psych (Abingdon, England)* 2014;**26**(2):205−13 Epub 2014/06/04.
41. Talbot LS, Maguen S, Metzler TJ, Schmitz M, McCaslin SE, Richards A, et al. Cognitive behavioral therapy for insomnia in posttraumatic stress disorder: a randomized controlled trial. *Sleep* 2014;**37**(2):327−41.
42. Jaffee MS, Winter WC, Jones CC, Ling G. Sleep disturbances in athletic concussion. *Brain Inj* 2015;**29**(2):221−7 Epub 2015/01/15.
43. Rao V, McCann U, Han D, Bergey A, Smith MT. Does acute TBI-related sleep disturbance predict subsequent neuropsychiatric disturbances? *Brain Inj* 2014;**28**(1):20−6 Epub 2013/12/18.
44. Ponsford JL, Ziino C, Parcell DL, Shekleton JA, Roper M, Redman JR, et al. Fatigue and sleep disturbance following traumatic brain injury—their nature, causes, and potential treatments. *J Head Trauma Rehabil* 2012;**27**:3.
45. Aurora RN, Zak RS, Auerbach SH, Casey KR, Chowdhuri S, Karippot A, et al. Best practice guide for treatment of nightmare disorder in adults. *J Clin Sleep Med* 2010;**6**(4):389−401.
46. Seyffert M, Lagisetty P, Landgraf J, Chopra V, Pfeiffer PN, Conte ML, et al. Internet-delivered cognitive behavior therapy to treat insomnia: a systematic review and meta-analysis. *PLoS One* 2016;**11**(2):e0149139.
47. Lal A, Kolakowsky-Hayner SA, Ghajar J, Balamane M. The effect of physical exercise after a concussion: a systematic review and meta-analysis. *Am J Sports Med* 2017. 363546517706137. Epub 2017/06/02.
48. McCrory P, Meeuwisse W, Dvorak J, Aubry M, Bailes J, Broglio S, et al. Consensus statement on concussion in sport—the 5th international conference on concussion in sport held in Berlin, October 2016. *Br J Sports Med* 2017. Epub 2017/04/28.
49. Schneider KJ. Early return to physical activity post-concussion associated with reduced persistent symptoms. *J Pediatr* 2017;**184**:235−8.
50. Grool AM, Aglipay M, Momoli F, Meehan WP, Freedman SB, Yeates KO, et al. Association between early participation in physical activity following acute concussion and persistent postconcussive symptoms in children and adolescents. *JAMA* 2016;**316**(23):2504.
51. Majerske CW, Mihalik JP, Ren D, Collins MW, Reddy CC, Lovell MR, et al. Concussion in sports: postconcussive activity levels, symptoms, and neurocognitive performance. *J Athl Train* 2008;**43**(3):265−74.
52. Leddy JJ, Kozlowski K, Donnelly JP, Pendergast DR, Epstein LH, Willer B. A Preliminary study of subsymptom threshold exercise training for refractory post-concussion syndrome. *Clin J Sport Med* 2010;**20**(1):21−7.
53. Gagnon I, Galli C, Friedman D, Grilli L, Iverson GL. Active rehabilitation for children who are slow to recover following sport-related concussion. *Brain Inj* 2009;**23**(12):956−64.
54. Anzalone AJ, Blueitt D, Case T, McGuffin T, Pollard K, Garrison JC, et al. A positive vestibular/ocular motor screening (VOMS) is associated with increased recovery time after sports-related concussion in youth and adolescent athletes. *Am J Sports Med* 2016;**45**(2):474−9.
55. Corwin DJ, Zonfrillo MR, Master CL, Arbogast KB, Grady MF, Robinson RL, et al. Characteristics of prolonged concussion recovery in a pediatric subspecialty referral population. *J Pediatr* 2014;**165**(6):1207−15.

56. Henry LC, Elbin RJ, Collins MW, Marchetti G, Kontos AP. Examining recovery trajectories after sport-related concussion with a multimodal clinical assessment approach. *Neurosurgery* 2016;**78**(2):232–41.

57. Pavlou M. The use of optokinetic stimulation in vestibular rehabilitation. *J Neurol Phys Therapy* 2010;**34**(2):105–10.

58. Whitney SL, Alghwiri A, Alghadir A. Physical therapy for persons with vestibular disorders. *Curr Opin Neurol* 2015;**28**(1):61–8.

59. Feipel V, Salvia P, Klein H, Rooze M. Head repositioning accuracy in patients with whiplash-associated disorders. *Spine* 2006;**31**(2):E51–8.

60. Basteris A, Pedler A, Sterling M. Evaluating the neck joint position sense error with a standard computer and a webcam. *Man Ther* 2016;**26**:231–4.

61. Murray DA, Meldrum D, Lennon O. Can vestibular rehabilitation exercises help patients with concussion? A systematic review of efficacy, prescription and progression patterns. *Br J Sports Med* 2016;**51**(5):442–51.

62. Schneider KJ, Meeuwisse WH, Nettel-Aguirre A, Barlow K, Boyd L, Kang J, et al. Cervicovestibular rehabilitation in sport-related concussion: a randomised controlled trial. *Br J Sports Med* 2014;**48**(17):1294–8.

63. Reneker JC, Hassen A, Phillips RS, Moughiman MC, Donaldson M, Moughiman J. Feasibility of early physical therapy for dizziness after a sports-related concussion: a randomized clinical trial. *Scandin J Med Sci Sports* 2017. Epub 2017/02/18.

64. Wiangkham T, Duda J, Haque S, Madi M, Rushton A. The effectiveness of conservative management for acute whiplash associated disorder (WAD) II: a systematic review and meta-analysis of randomised controlled trials. *PLoS One* 2015;**10**(7):e0133415.

65. Griffin A, Leaver A, Moloney N. General exercise does not improve long-term pain and disability in individuals with whiplash-associated disorders: a systematic review. *J Orthop Sports Phys Therapy.* 2017;**47**(7):472–80.

66. Ludvigsson ML, Peterson G, O'Leary S, Dedering Å, Peolsson A. The effect of neck-specific exercise with, or without a behavioral approach, on pain, disability, and self-efficacy in chronic whiplash-associated disorders. *Clin J Pain* 2015;**31**(4):294–303.

67. Celenay ST, Akbayrak T, Kaya DO. A comparison of the effects of stabilization exercises plus manual therapy to those of stabilization exercises alone in patients with nonspecific mechanical neck pain: a randomized clinical trial. *J Orthop Sports Phys Therapy.* 2016;**46**(2):44–55.

68. Jull G, Trott P, Potter H, Zito G, Niere K, Shirley D, et al. A randomized controlled trial of exercise and manipulative therapy for cervicogenic headache. *Spine* 2002;**27**(17):1835–43.

69. Wong JJ, Shearer HM, Mior S, Jacobs C, Côté P, Randhawa K, et al. Are manual therapies, passive physical modalities, or acupuncture effective for the management of patients with whiplash-associated disorders or neck pain and associated disorders? An update of the Bone and Joint Decade Task Force on Neck Pain and Its Associated Disorders by the OPTIMa collaboration. *Spine J* 2016;**16**(12):1598–630.

70. Brooks MA, Peterson K, Biese K, Sanfilippo J, Heiderscheit BC, Bell DR. Concussion increases odds of sustaining a lower extremity musculoskeletal injury after return to play among collegiate athletes. *Am J Sports Med* 2016;**44**(3):742–7.

71. Herman DC, Jones D, Harrison A, Moser M, Tillman S, Farmer K, et al. Concussion may increase the risk of subsequent lower extremity musculoskeletal injury in collegiate athletes. *Sports Med* 2016;**47**(5):1003–10.

72. Swanik CB, Covassin T, Stearne DJ, Schatz P. The relationship between neurocognitive function and noncontact anterior cruciate ligament injuries. *Am J Sports Med* 2007;**35**(6):943–8.

73. Michaelidis M, Koumantakis GA. Effects of knee injury primary prevention programs on anterior cruciate ligament injury rates in female athletes in different sports: a systematic review. *Phys Therapy Sport.* 2014;**15**(3):200–10.

74. Taylor JB, Waxman JP, Richter SJ, Shultz SJ. Evaluation of the effectiveness of anterior cruciate ligament injury prevention programme training components: a systematic review and meta-analysis. *Br J Sports Med* 2013;**49**(2):79–87.

75. *American Associatio of Occupational Therapy. Occupational Therapy Practice Framework.* Pittsburgh, PA: AOTA Press; 2014.

76. Ashley MJ. Repairing the injured brain; Why proper rehabilitation is essential to recovering function. *Cerebrum: Dana Forum Brain Sci* 2012;8.

77. Preece MHW, Horswill MS, Geffen GM. Driving after concussion: the acute effect of mild traumatic brain injury on drivers' hazard perception. *Neuropsychology* 2010;**24**(4):493–503.
78. Radomski MV, Davidson L, Voydetich D, Erickson MW. Occupational therapy for service members with mild traumatic brain injury. *Am J Occupat Therapy* 2009;**63**(5):646–55.
79. Michel JA. Attention rehabilitation following stroke and traumatic brain injury: a review. *Eura Medicophys* 2006;**42**(1):59–67.
80. Freed S, Fishman Hellerstein L. Visual electrodiagnostic findings in mild traumatic brain injury. *Brain Inj* 1997;**11**(1):25–36.
81. Ciuffreda KJ, Kapoor N, Rutner D, Suchoff IB, Han ME, Craig S. Occurrence of oculomotor dysfunctions in acquired brain injury: a retrospective analysis. *Optometry* 2007;**78**(4):155–61.
82. Ciuffreda KJ, Rutner D, Kapoor N, Suchoff IB, Craig S, Han ME. Vision therapy for oculomotor dysfunctions in acquired brain injury: a retrospective analysis. *Optometry* 2008;**79**(1):18–22.
83. Thiagarajan P, Ciuffreda KJ. Versional eye tracking in mild traumatic brain injury (mTBI): effects of oculomotor training (OMT). *Brain Inj* 2014;**28**(7):930–43.
84. Zoltan B. *Vision, perception, and cognition: a manual for the evaluation and treatment of the adult with acquired brain injury*. Thorofare, NJ: Slack Incorporated; 2008.
85. Fimreite V, Willeford KT, Ciuffreda KJ. Effect of chromatic filters on visual performance in individuals with mild traumatic brain injury (mTBI): a pilot study. *J Optom* 2016;**9**(4):231–9.
86. Cicerone KP, Langebahn DM, Braden C, Malec JF, Kalmar K, Fraas M, et al. Evidence-based cognitive rehabilitation: updated review of the literature from 2003 through 2008. *Arch Phys Med Rehabil* 2011;519–30.
87. Sohlberg MM, McLaughlin KA, Pavese A, Heidrich A, Posner MI. Evaluation of attention process training and brain injury education in persons with acquired brain injury. *J Clin Exp Neurpsychol* 2000;**22**(5):656–76.
88. Tiersky LA, Anselmi V, Johnston MV, Kurtyka J. A trial of neuropsychologic rehabilitation in mild-spectrum traumatic brain injury. *Arch Phys Med Rehabil* 2005;**86**(8):1565–74.
89. Cicerone KD. Remediation of 'working attention' in mild traumatic brain injury. *Brain Inj* 2002;**16**(3):185–95.
90. Ashley MJ, Ashley J, Kreber L. Remediation of information processing following traumatic brain injury: a community-based rehabilitation approach. *NeuroRehabilitation* 2012;**31**(1):31–9 Epub 2012/04/24.
91. Levine B, Robertson IH, Clare L, Carter G, Hong J, Wilson BA, et al. Rehabilitation of executive functioning: an experimental-clinical validation of goal management training. *J Int Neuropsychol Soc* 2000;**6**(3):299–312 Epub 2000/05/29.
92. Stringer AY. Ecologically-oriented neurorehabilitation of memory: robustness of outcome across diqgnosis and severity. *Brain Inj* 2011;**25**:169–78.
93. Rees L, Marshall S, Hartridge C, Mackie D, Weiser M. Cognitive interventions post acquired brain injury. *Brain Inj* 2007;**21**(2):161–200.
94. Marbury D. TBI treatment will rely heavily on interdisciplinary teams: research for traumatic brain injury has been at a standstill for years. *Behav Healthcare* 2015;**35**(4):32.
95. Pabian PS, Oliveira L, Tucker J, Beato M, Gual C. Interprofessional management of concussion in sport. *Phys Therapy Sport* 2017;**23**:123–32.

Vestibular Rehabilitation for Mild Traumatic Brain Injury (mTBI)

Kim R. Gottshall, PhD, PT[1] and Susan L. Whitney, DPT, PhD[2]

[1]Naval Health Research Center, San Diego, CA, United States [2]Department of Physical Therapy and Otolaryngology, University of Pittsburgh, Pittsburgh, PA, United States

VESTIBULAR CONSEQUENCES OF CONCUSSION

Introduction

The vestibular organs are crucial for motion sensation and maintenance of balance. Imbedded in the temporal bones, they are well-protected, and yet ultimately are vulnerable to concussive shock from abrupt force applied to the head through blunt trauma or over-pressure from explosive blasts. A variety of injuries can occur to the vestibular organ with traumatic brain injury (TBI), both acute and chronic. Dysfunction of the vestibular organs results in continuous or intermittent vertigo and reduction of balance, including increasing the risk of falls. In addition, injury can occur in a number of places in the central vestibular pathway which can also cause impairment in balance function and equilibrium.

It is our opinion that vestibular dysfunction is often unrecognized after TBI, due to the attention paid to primary injuries to the scalp, skull, and brain. Rapid recognition of the possibility of vestibular disorders after TBI should lead to screening for these problems and their prompt treatment. The great advantage of such screening and recognition is that appropriate treatment can often be immediately rendered. For example, lack of recognition of the presence of benign positional vertigo (BPV), one consequence of TBI, can mean that as a head injury patient tries to mobilize, they are struck with terrible vertigo. This vertigo can result in falls and drastic exacerbation of patients' other symptoms such as headache and memory loss. The patient is, thus, bed-ridden or mobility impaired for a long period, even months. Fortunately, a simple treatment, the canalith repositioning maneuver (CRM)[1] can immediately cure BPPV and hugely improve mobilization and even mental status. Other vestibular disorders can also be detected and managed expeditiously to improve recovery. For example, a study of blast-injured subjects in Operation Iraqi Freedom demonstrated improvement if their blast-triggered, migraine-related vertigo was diagnosed and treated.[2]

For the purposes of this chapter we will confine our discussion to mild traumatic brain injury (mTBI). mTBI is the most common disorder military troops experienced during the wars in Southwest Asia and is increasingly becoming a more important topic due to the number of sports-related episodes of concussion, a form of mTBI.[2,3] The symptoms of mTBI are myriad, but one of the most common is dizziness. One of the common effects of sports-related concussion is also dizziness. Assessment for vestibular disorders should be part of the standard clinical doctrine for acute and chronic management of head-injured patients.[3] In this chapter, we will review this assessment from an anatomic and physiologic point of view and for the appropriate clinical approach. We will briefly outline treatment approaches to the various disorders.

VESTIBULAR ANATOMY AND PHYSIOLOGY

The vestibular organs are simply accelerometers that provide information to the brain about the motion of the head. Inside the utricle and the macula are the otolith organs. The otoliths are calcium carbonate crystals fixed in a gelatinous matrix that rests on hair cells. The otoliths are detectors of linear acceleration, either motion in a straight line or slow tilting of the head relative to gravity. In contrast, the semicircular canals (SCC) are rotational or angular accelerometers. They are hollow and fluid-filled. Inertia of fluid in the canals as the head turns results in the deviation of the cupula, the acceleration sensor in each canal. Signals from the hair cells in the otoliths and the SCCs are transmitted along the auditory nerve, in parallel with the signals from the cochlea that encode sound stimuli. In the brainstem, vestibular signals are combined and are modulated and adapted by cerebellar circuits. Disruption of the otoliths, SCCs, auditory nerves, and brainstem circuits are all potential sites of dysfunction of the vestibular system. Active disturbance of these systems results in vertigo and damage to the systems means loss of acceleration information to the brain and loss of balance. Understanding the pathophysiology, loss of function, and neural adaptation of the vestibular system is key to the management of TBI-induced disorders.

mTBI FROM BLUNT VERSUS EXPLOSIVE BLAST TRAUMA

In this discussion we will examine two types of mTBI. We will first look at mTBI secondary to blunt head injury (closed head injury); then we will examine the vestibular disorders associated with mTBI seen after an explosive blast.

Blunt head injury is by far the most common cause of mTBI in the civilian world and is receiving increased attention due to sports-related etiologies, commonly termed "concussion." Such sports-related injuries can occur in high-profile professional athletes as well as the young soccer prodigy playing at the local park on a Saturday morning. Work in our laboratory over the past decade has allowed us to characterize the vestibular disorders seen after closed head injury.[4,5] Table 20.1 shows the characteristics of the four classes of

TABLE 20.1 Vestibular Disorders After Closed Head Injury

Entity	History	Physical Exam	Vestibular Tests
Positional vertigo (PTBPPV)	Positional vertigo	Nystagmus on Dix-Hallpike test or modified Dix-Hallpike test	No other abnormalities
Exertional dizziness (PTEID)	Dizziness during and right after exercise	Abnormalities in challenged gait testing	No other abnormalities
Migraine associated dizziness (PTMAD)	Episodic Vertigo with periods of unsteadiness	Abnormalities in challenged gait testing	VOR gain, phase, or symmetry abnormalitiesHigh frequency VOR abnormalities
	Headaches	±Abnormalities on head impulse testing Normal static posture tests	Normal posturography
Spatial disorientation (PTSpD)	Constant feeling of unsteadiness worsened by standing but still present when sitting or lying down	Abnormalities on standard gait tests	VOR gain, phase, or symmetry abnormalities High frequency VOR abnormalities
		±Abnormalities on head impulse testing	Abnormal posturography
	Drifting to one side while walking Shifting weight when standing still	Abnormalities on static posture tests	Central findings on rotation chair testing

balance disorders seen after blunt trauma. Posttraumatic benign positional vertigo (PTBPPV) is identical to idiopathic BPPV. It is characterized by short episodes of vertigo that occur when changing the head or body position (e.g., rolling over in bed or looking up).[1] The episodes last for only a few seconds. PTBPPV is discussed in more detail in the next section. Posttraumatic exercise-induced dizziness (PTEID) is dizziness that occurs after the completion of physical activity. These individuals complain of unsteadiness or feeling off balance after they finish exercising. They do not generally complain of vertigo. The third class of dizziness seen is posttraumatic migraine-associated dizziness (PTMAD). In this classification, which has received increasing attention over the past few years, individuals complain of a variety of transient types of dizziness. Individuals can have vertigo, unsteadiness, or visual abnormalities. The episodes are intermittent and can last from seconds to hours. Most individuals have more than one type of dizziness episode. In this disorder, migraine headache (either coincident with, or distinct from, the dizziness) is one of the hallmark symptoms. PTMAD is discussed in more detail in the next section.

The final class of dizziness seen after blunt head trauma is posttraumatic spatial disorientation (PTSpD). In this symptom complex individuals complain of unsteadiness when standing still or moving quickly. They also have unsteadiness on uneven surfaces or when walking in poor-light conditions. Like migraine-associated dizziness, patients this group of individuals may have headaches, but unlike that group, headaches are rarely one

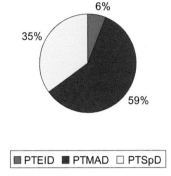

FIGURE 20.1   Comparisons of dizziness; blunt head trauma.

of the dominant symptoms. The hallmark of this condition is the need to use light touch when standing still to avoid from wobbling. We have been able to describe the frequency of these disorders and this data is shown in Fig. 20.1. It should be noted that the frequency of PTBPPV is likely underestimated in this group since many of these individuals may have resolved the BPPV prior to presenting to our clinic.

While blast-related mTBI may seem less relevant, it is becoming an increasingly important etiology of mTBI. Well over 80% of all war injuries are blast-related mTBI in isolation. In the civilian world airbags, compressors, pneumatic tools, and a number of other job site risks have resulted in a sharp rise in the number of blast-related mTBI cases. Dizziness is the number one symptom of blast-related mTBI.[2] Blast-induced mTBI differs from blunt mTBI in a number of ways.[4] The classes of dizziness are in agreement with this finding. Table 20.2 shows the classes of dizziness seen after blast-induced mTBI. The postblast BPV (PBBPV) is identical to the PTBPV with transient positional-induced vertigo episodes. Postblast exertional dizziness (PBED) which was formerly termed postblast exercise-induced dizziness is dramatically different from the PTEID in that postblast individuals get unsteady upon starting to exercise (rather than at the completion of the episode). The symptoms of unsteadiness and disequilibrium as well as headaches are the same but the temporal relationship of these symptoms to exercise is much different and, hence, more troubling to the patient.

The final two classes, postblast dizziness and postblast dizziness with vertigo (PBD and PBDV), are characterized by the following two symptoms: (1) constant unsteadiness which is made worse by more challenging balance environments (uneven surfaces, poor-light conditions, moving quickly, etc.); and (2) constant headaches which fluctuate in severity. The presence of additional episodic vertigo separates the two disorders. The relative frequency of these dizziness types is shown in Fig. 20.2. Unlike after blunt head injury, the frequency of PBBPV, while likely slightly higher than zero, is very small. The classification systems have proved helpful in a variety of ways. They can be understood and are essential to guide treatment and rehabilitation. They also provide prognostic details which help in patient management. Equally as important are that they provide a diagnosis for patients who too often have been told that the dizziness is "something they got from the head injury" and "give it time, it will go away."

TABLE 20.2   Balance Disorders Seen After Blast Exposure

Entity	History	Physical Exam	Vestibular Tests
Positional vertigo (PBBPV)	Positional Vertigo	Nystagmus on Dix-Hallpike test or modified Dix-Hallpike test	No other abnormalities
Exertional dizziness (PBED)	Dizziness during exercise	Abnormalities in challenged gait test	No other abnormalities
Blast-induced disequilibrium (PBD)	Constant feeling of unsteadiness when standing and walking worse with challenging environments	Abnormalities in challenged gait	Abnormal posturography
	Constant headache	Abnormalities in tandem Romberg	Abnormal target acquisition, dynamic visual acuity, and gaze stabilization
		Abnormalities with quick head motion	±VOR gain, phase, or symmetry abnormalities
Blast-induced disequilibrium with vertigo (PBDV)	Constant feeling of unsteadiness when standing and walking worse with challenging environments	Abnormalities in challenged gait	Abnormal posturography
	Constant headache	Abnormalities in tandem Romberg	Abnormal target acquisition, dynamic visual acuity, and gaze stabilization
	Episodic vertigo	Abnormalities with quick head motion	VOR gain, phase, or symmetry abnormalities

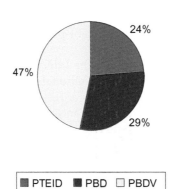

PTEID   PBD   PBDV

FIGURE 20.2   Comparisons of dizziness; blast injury.

POSTTRAUMATIC BENIGN POSITIONAL VERTIGO

BPPV is the most common condition causing vertigo.[1] BPPV is simply the result of calcium carbonate crystals broken loose from the otolith organ ending up in the SCC. Clinicians involved in the diagnosis or treatment of patients that present with vertigo or imbalance should know how to elicit a history of BPV and carry out the Dix-Hallpike test for the diagnosis. The CRM (or as it is commonly known, the Epley Maneuver) is a simple, safe procedure that can immediately cure BPPV. If one is familiar with the diagnosis of BPPV, the CRM is a powerful addition to one's clinical armamentarium.

A full description of the Dix-Hallpike test and the CRM is given in Viirre.[6] In summary, one looks for a history of brief vertigo attacks that are provoked by head movements, such as rolling over in bed, bending over, or reaching up. The vertigo lasts seconds and should stop as the patient lies still. Note that motion sickness and imbalance from a spell of vertigo can last minutes or hours after the actual vertigo episode. The Dix-Hallpike test is carried out with a patient on an examining bench. While being held securely by the examiner, the patient's head is turned 45 degrees to the right or left. The patient is then moved backward with their head hanging 20–30 degrees over the edge of the surface. Onset of a vertigo sensation accompanied by torsional nystagmus (a clockwise or anticlockwise rotation of the eyes as the patient looks straight ahead) is diagnostic.

The CRM is a simple continuation of movements once a positive Dix-Hallpike test is elicited. With the head extended back so it is below the horizontal plane, a sequence of turns of the head and body will remove the offending calcium carbonate crystals from the SCC.

POSTTRAUMATIC MIGRAINE-ASSOCIATED DIZZINESS

Migraine is one of the most common genetic disorders, present in approximately 1 in 6 women and 1 in 10 men. Migraine is a disease complex of which headache is the most common symptom. Migraine aura is well-recognized and its presence is diagnostic of migraine and almost half of migraineurs have dizziness and vertigo episodes.[7] The high incidence of migraine in the general population suggests that a high percentage of people with TBI will have concomitant migraine, even if they were not symptomatic prior to their injury. The posttraumatic headache, dizziness, cognitive difficulties, and symptoms not localized to the head may well be present in TBI patients as the result of onset of migraine headaches.

Migraine headache is diagnosed by using the International Headache Society criteria for headache.[8] The third beta edition of the International Classification of Headache disorders now had criteria for vestibular migraine. In a recent report, 10% of 631 persons with migraine were given a diagnosis of vestibular migraine.[9] Lempert et al. developed a consensus document related to the diagnostic criteria for vestibular migraine that is helpful in determining the diagnosis.[10] Because of the variable penetrance of the condition, review for a family history of recurrent headaches, dizziness, and/or motion sensitivity may be fruitful, even if a formal diagnosis of migraine is not reported in the family.

Treatment of migraine can be effectively carried out by lifestyle and medical management. In TBI patients, particular attention must be paid to provision of adequate regular sleep, regular meals and a well-designed activity program. Medical management includes use of calcium channel blockers (Verapamil), possible use of beta blockers (Inderal), and carbonic anhydrase inhibitors (Topirimate). Topirimate, in particular, has been studied in the TBI dizziness population and has been found to be effective, not only for the dizziness and vertigo, but also for headache control in patients.[11]

SCREENING

The Vestibular/Ocular Motor Screening Tool

The vestibular/ocular motor screening (VOMS) tool was developed to attempt to assist health provider's screen for vestibular and visual problems postconcussion in persons between the ages of 9 and 40.[12] The only equipment required includes a tape measure (cm), a metronome app, and a 14-point font print target. Typical concussion screening prior to the development of the VOMS has included examination of balance, cognition, questionnaires about symptoms and functioning, clinical interviews, and also physical examinations.[13] All of the previous testing has value for the person postconcussion in the diagnosis and management of concussion, but the addition of the vestibular and ocular testing may have added value.[14] The military in the United States in 2012 recognized that people postconcussion have difficulty with vergence and that service members may have dizziness or ocular deficits after concussion.[15]

Henry et al.[16] recently discussed subtypes of concussion including anxiety/mood, vestibular, ocular, cognitive/fatigue, posttraumatic migraine, and cervical. Their theory of best recovery is that each of the six subtypes need to be treated differently and may require a different set of health-care providers depending on their expertise, including clinical psychologists, physicians, physical therapists, and/or athletic trainers. The VOMS was developed to assist health-care providers (physicians, physical therapists, neuropsychologists, and athletic trainers) identify vestibular and/or ocular disorders in person's postconcussion and scores may be associated with recovery.[12,14] Healthy Division I athletes can have VOMS scores above "0," even without concussion.[17] Healthy athletes with a history of motion sickness and those who were female were more likely to have abnormal VOMS scores prior to concussion with 89% of the athletes scoring below the cut score.[17]

The VOMS (Table 20.3) consists of five tests including saccades (up/down, right/left), smooth pursuits, the horizontal and vertical vestibular ocular reflex (VOR) test, visual motion sensitivity (sometimes called VOR cancellation), and vergence.[12] The VOMS has good internal consistency (Cronbach's α of 0.92).[12] Scoring of the VOMS is fairly simple as persons with suspected concussion were asked to rate their symptoms on a 0−10 point scale with 0 indicating no symptoms and 10 indicating the worst possible symptoms. The queried symptoms included nausea, fogginess, headache, and dizziness. Patients are asked to report the intensity of their symptoms (e.g., nausea, headache, fogginess, and dizziness) for each of the tests after they are performed. A cut score ≥ 2 out of 10 on any VOMS item suggests that the person had a concussion. The near point convergence score is not included in the VOMS score since vergence is measured in centimeters from the tip of the person's nose to the point where the target doubles. The average of the three values is recorded. Generally, it takes between 5 and 10 minutes to perform the VOMS.

The VOR items caused the greatest symptoms in the Mucha et al. paper[12] plus the VOR items had the highest total symptom scores. No control subjects had a total individual symptom score of greater than 2 on any individual item tested. It is not clear whether scores on the original VOMS can predict outcome. Ellis et al.[18] used a tool similar to the VOMS in a retrospective study of children postconcussion. The Ellis et al. findings

TABLE 20.3   Vestibular/Ocular-Motor Screening (VOMS) for Concussion[12]

Vestibular/Ocular Motor Test:	Not Tested	Headache 0–10	Dizziness 0–10	Nausea 0–10	Fogginess 0–10	Comments
Baseline symptoms:						
Smooth pursuits						
Saccades—horizontal						
Saccades—vertical						
Convergence (near point)						(Near point in cm): Measure 1: _____ Measure 2: _____ Measure 3: _____
VOR—horizontal						
VOR—vertical						
Visual motion sensitivity test						

Used with permission of Dr. Anne Mucha.

suggested that children who had vestibular and/or ocular symptoms at the onset of their concussion took longer to recover from their concussion. Yorke et al.[19] have reported that the VOMS is not related to the Balance Error Scoring test (BESS)[20,21] or the King–Devick test,[22–24] which are used to test postural control (BESS) and saccadic eye movements and reaction times. The VOMS appears to test different constructs. The VOMS may have value beyond identifying whether the person has had a concussion or not. Recently, Anazalone et al.[14] reported that patient symptoms while performing the VOMS were related to protracted recovery in high-school athletes after having sport-related concussion.

TREATMENT

The vestibular physical therapy (VPT) rehabilitation strategy employs specific exercises designed to decrease dizziness, increase balance function, and increase general activity levels. Exercises to decrease dizziness focus on exposure to specific stimuli for habituation or attenuation of the dizziness response in the brain. Balance retraining involves exercises designed to improve organization of sensory information for balance control and coordination of muscle responses. General activity exercise involves a daily aerobic exercise program of progressive walking, cycling, or swimming.[25]

A VPT program for mTBI patients consists of exercise procedures that target the VOR, cervico-ocular reflex (COR), depth perception (DP), somatosensory retraining (SS), dynamic gait, and aerobic function.[26,27] The VOR, COR, and DP exercises are graded in difficulty, based on velocity of head and object motion, and progression of body positioning from sitting to standing to walking. The SS exercises are graded in difficulty by narrowing the base of support, making the surface uneven, or changing the surface from firm to soft.

Large amplitude head and trunk movements are also employed to increase somatosensory input. These exercises included the Proprioceptive Neuromuscular Facilitation (PNF) techniques of slow reversal head and neck patterns, modified chopping, and lifting for head and trunk in progression from supine, to sitting, and to standing postures and total body mass rolling activities.

Varied walking exercises are graded in difficulty by changing direction, performing with the eyes closed, increasing speed of ambulation, walking on soft surfaces, or navigating stairs.[27] An aerobic home exercise program progressively increases the time, speed, or distance that the patient can tolerate. All patients are encouraged to work at their maximum tolerance while performing the VPT and are instructed to perform the exercises twice daily at home. Patients are monitored by the physical therapist, although treatment frequency varies depending on the setting and the patients symptoms. In the youngest athletes, they may be seen less frequently because of the demands on parents with other children who need transportation to activities after school and work demands. Compliance to the home exercise program is surveyed by the physical therapist during patient visits.

An objective assessment is performed for all mTBI patients by the vestibular physical therapist. A functional test battery consisting of the head impulse test, Romberg test, tandem Romberg test, Dynamic Gait Index (DGI), and the Functional Gait Assessment is administered to each patient.[28] In addition, the Dizziness Handicap Inventory (DHI), of which there is a new pediatric version[29,30] and the Activities-Specific Balance Confidence (ABC) Scale [31] surveys are often administered. The above measurements are obtained pretreatment, during treatment, and after treatment. Subjective patient reports of degree and length of imbalance perception are documented throughout treatment. The length of time required for patients to return to work or play after the initiation of physical therapy is monitored.

As we have noted, vestibular complaints are the most frequent sequelae of blast-induced mTBI.[2] VPT has been established as the most important treatment modality for this group of patients. In 2016, it was included as one of the recommended interventions from the 5th International Concussion Consensus Conference in Berlin.[3] Nevertheless there is little work objectively documenting the impact of VPT on this group of patients. Studies have been completed in the past examining clinical measures like the Glasgow Coma Scale (GCS) on overall recovery pattern after TBI, but outcome measures specifically aimed at examining the adequacy of vestibular tests to track vestibular recovery have been lacking.

Scherer and Schubert reinforced the need for best practice vestibular assessment for formulation of appropriate VPT treatment strategies.[32] Now the application of vestibular testing and rehabilitation in this patient population is needed to provide information on objective outcome measures. VPT is most effective when applied in a customized fashion, tailored to individual patient deficits and needs.[33] While we and others have developed VPT procedures that are applied in "best practices" for blast-induced mTBI vestibular patients,[4] these therapies must be customized for the patient entry level of function and expectation level of recovery.

Knowledge of the patient's disability and diagnosis is critical to building the foundation for return to activity, work, or participation in sports. There has been documentation on the reliability of CDP as a diagnostic tool and on the reliability of the DGI as an outcome tool,[34–37] but those studies have not examined the head injury population which tends to have a different type of vestibular profile than those tested in previous studies. The head injury population is also a younger population than the previous studies represent. Similarly, over the past 5 years, there have been several studies[38–41] examining the gaze stabilization test (GST) as an outcome measure correlated with postural stability. In these studies, the patient groups were small and again the populations were far different from head-injured blast patients, in terms of vestibular dysfunction and age.

What might be considered normal for an older vestibular patient (e.g., poststroke) would still be wholly unacceptable in the young military population intent on returning to active duty. Vestibular clinical centers will establish their own normative values for tests on patients of similar age and activity level. The standard results of these tests can be used to determine return to duty/work status as well as return to physical activity status. While the entire suite of tests provides valuable information, our data indicates that the vertical GST is the most sensitive outcome predictor for the young, military population. This likely indicates that recovery of vestibular function is frequency and velocity dependent. This observation agrees with the work of Paige[42] in which linearity and symmetry of the VOR were examined.

Management of Traumatic Brain Injury Related Dizziness: An Algorithm

Based on these disorders, a simple algorithm has been derived to aid in the management of dizziness post-TBI. In Fig. 20.3, branch points are based on historical or physical findings. Diagnostic categories are indicated in separate shaded boxes. The simplest, and perhaps the most important item is the first: the Dix-Hallpike test. The test should be done on all patients with any complaint of dizziness. This simple procedure and its readily observable sign of torsional nystagmus is the definitive test of BPPV, and leads to the definitive treatment, the CRM. Once BPPV has been tested for and treated, further complaints of dizziness depend on whether the injury is blunt or blast-related.

On the blunt trauma-related arm of disorders, PTEID is defined by dizziness *after* exercise and is treated with appropriate VPT. If there are interspersed episodes of headaches, PTMAD is suspected. A combination of traditional migraine prophylaxis pharmaceuticals and VPT is most effective. Finally, in the blunt trauma-related area, if there is persistent unsteadiness during low effort walking or even during standing, PTSpD is present, and it requires a differently configured program of VPT.

After blast-related trauma, there may be dizziness (PBED) at the onset of exercise. VPT is effective here. Postblast there may be a complaint of constant dizziness. PBD may be reduced with migraine medications. If there are interspersed episodes of vertigo, then PBD + Vertigo is present and in addition to migraine prophylaxis, diuretics such as hydrochlorothiazide or acetazolamide can be effective in reducing the vertigo episodes. As can be seen, a knowledgeable physical therapist is essential for management of this group of patients as well as a diagnostician familiar with the acute posttrauma categories.

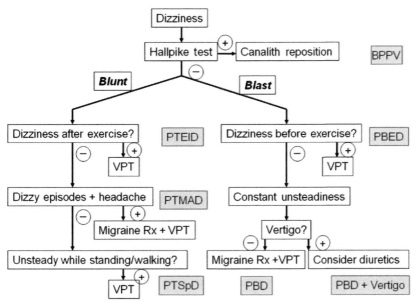

FIGURE 20.3 Algorithm for management of TBI-related dizziness.

Advanced Concepts in Vestibular Consequences of Traumatic Brain Injury

Blunt and blast mTBI have been demonstrated to result in a variety of medical conditions and syndromes. These vary from simple in diagnosis and management, such as BPV to the more complex, such as PTSpD. Fortunately, observers can be readily trained to recognize these various conditions and initiate management. Since dizziness is the leading complaint post-TBI, deployment of formalized protocols and training programs should be implemented in both military and civilian environments such as football, where mTBI is frequent. Medical personnel should be trained to recognize and treat such conditions as migraine-related TBI syndromes.

Despite recent work in the area, there is still a great deal of research with respect to mTBI that is needed. Critical among these are deploying known countermeasures for mTBI, determining the pathophysiology of mTBI so even more specific countermeasures can be developed, studying the effects of multiple blasts and head impacts, and developing diagnostic and therapeutic tools that are mobile, rugged, and easy to use.

Illustrative Case Study of a Person With Sport Concussion

A 25-year-old National Football league player sustained a helmet to helmet hit while playing early in a game during the first part of the second quarter of play. He immediately felt dizzy, had a headache, photophobia, phonophobia, nausea, and experienced fogginess. Nevertheless, he continued to play. Later in the game he sustained a less forceful hit to his head which worsened his symptoms. Only then did he report his symptoms to the medical staff and was removed from the game.

From this case so far, what we know is that he made a poor decision to not remove himself from the game when his symptoms started. It is ideal to remove an athlete from the game if concussion is suspected.[3] Previously it was thought that high impact hits could be identified with the use of technology and then one can predict that the person might have experienced a concussion. High impact hits may not result in concussion for one person, yet for others much lower impacts can result in long-term sequelae postconcussion.[43,44] It is optimal for the athlete to understand that removal from play with a concussion is important for their own health and wellness. Also of note is the fact that the footballer had an onset of dizziness on the field. Lau et al.[45] reported that dizziness on the field is a negative prognostic factor for quick recovery from a concussion. Headache is the most commonly reported symptom postconcussion.[46–48] Fogginess has also been reported previously as a negative prognostic factor related to recovery.[49]

The footballer's past medical history consisted of an old clavicular fracture from childhood and two prior incidents of concussion in high-school and college. It took him about 3 weeks to recover from his previous concussions.

When first seen in physical therapy, he had been told to limit exertion/physical activity and he tried amitriptyline but could not tolerate the side effects and stopped taking the medication. He was put on injured reserve (which means that he was not allowed to go to work to play in the premier league). He does not live near the clinic and must have someone drive him because he gets headaches and photophobia when driving, especially when the sun is very bright. He is married and has an infant at home.

There is not strong evidence for the use of drugs postconcussion in young athletes.[48] In a recent report, 245 children were prescribed medication postconcussion.[50] The factors linked to drug prescription were gender, with girls being prescribed more medications, and those with high (worse) postconcussion symptom scores (PCSSs).[50] Amitriptyline is a tricyclic antidepressant that has been shown to prevent migraine headaches, which is why this medication was prescribed.

The footballer's sensitivity to light might suggest posttraumatic migraine.[51] It would have been optimal if the patient had been asked whether he had a history of migraine or a family history of migraine.[52] Migraine headache development after a concussion is more commonly reported. Persons who develop migraine-like symptoms (e.g., sensitivity to light, sound, and even smell) appear to take longer to get better.[52] It is not clear whether treatment of headaches improves recovery time, but expert experience confirms that persons with persistent head/neck pain and other migraine-like symptoms take longer to recover and are more difficult to treat. It is common for persons with headaches to also have symptoms with VOR cancellation.

Care must be exercised in providing VOR cancellation exercises early in persons with significant motion-sensitivity intolerance. Motion-sensitivity intolerance is defined as experiencing symptom provocation with environments such as grocery stores, being a passenger in a car, optokinetic stimulation (disco ball movement around the person), or being in crowds with motion or noise.

The footballer reported that his headaches were between 1 and 7/10. His symptoms were worse with bending, busy environments, and when "thinking." He also said that he had blurred vision and was unable to drive for 2 weeks after the concussion. His dizziness became worse with head movement, watching television, and during airplane flights. It took 2 hours to get to sleep at night and he appeared to be anxious. His ImPACT scores ranged from 3% on the verbal memory composite to 20% on the reaction time composite. His PCSS[53,54] was 50 (0 is normal and 132 is the worst symptoms score).

Headaches may contribute to prolonged recovery postconcussion by increasing trigeminal nerve sensitivity.[55] When a patient presents with a headache of 7 out of 10, the patient should avoid head/eye movements as these will increase the headache symptom score above 7 very rapidly. If patients have balance deficits, we would work on optimizing balance on any day when the headache is excessive, as balance exercises are less likely to increase symptoms but VOR exercises may be too difficult depending on their baseline symptoms.

"Blurred" vision needs to be investigated via the dynamic visual acuity test to determine whether the patient is within the normal range for loss of visual acuity with head movements. The dynamic visual acuity test consists of the subject with concussion reading optotypes on a chart with no head movement and then reading the visual chart again while their head is moved at 2 Hz by the examiner.[35,56,57]

Also, persons who do not sleep well take longer to get better. Lack of sleep, or insomnia, is a common problem in persons with sport concussion.[58] The concept of "brain rest" is important and if the patient cannot sleep, it is very difficult for them to recover quickly.

The footballer's ImPACT scores (a common neurocognitive test) were very low and below his baseline scores. The PCSS scores are very helpful as they are easy to score and can be collected in a clinic. Change over time can easily be documented. Poor PCSS scores at 10 days have been shown to be a good predictor of children who have not recovered at 30 days.[59]

The footballer's DHI score was 52 and his Activities-specific balance scale score was 83%. During his oculomotor exam, he had normal smooth pursuits and saccades. His near point convergence as 32 cm. His VOMS score was 6.

Normal scores are 0 and the worst score is 100 on the DHI. The scale was developed for persons with dizziness and overall the scale relates to perceived handicap from dizziness. It has been utilized in studies with children and adults with concussion.[26] Higher scores (>60) have been reported in persons with vestibular disorders who are at higher risk of falling. In persons with vestibular disorders, mild disability was suggested for persons who scored 1–30, the moderate range is 31–60, and for severe disability it is 61–100.[60]

Smooth pursuits is the ability to follow a target at 60 Hz or less without saccadic intrusions. Saccades are the ability to move the eyes quickly to acquire a target such as looking quickly to the right and left of a specific target.

The footballer's near-point convergence score of 35 cm was abnormal. Generally, 5 cm or less is considered to be normal. His VOMS score indicated that it would take him longer to get better, although no baseline score was available for comparison.[12]

If his smooth pursuits and saccadic eye movements were grossly abnormal, it would indicate that he had serious central pathology. Smooth pursuit is the ability to follow a target at 60 Hz or less without saccadic intrusions. Saccades are the ability to move the eyes quickly and accurately to a target.

Convergence spasm was seen during testing of gaze holding and during testing for BPPV. During the left Dix-Hallpike, convergence spasm was noted. During VOR x 1 testing, he complained of dizziness and visual blurring. He also had an exophoria that was noted.

His balance was tested and, as expected, it was normal during the single-leg stance, tandem standing and standing on a foam pad with his eyes open. He had increased sway, but no falls, when standing on the foam pad with his eyes closed. Balance difficulties generally resolve quickly after concussion. On the Sensory Organization Test, however, his score was 60. Scores of 70 and above are considered normal for his age. As a professional athlete, a score of 60 is very low.

His functional deficits included dizziness with head movements, sleep problems, headaches, cognitive impairments, convergence insufficiency, and balance deficits.

Several recommendations were made to try to decrease his symptoms, including eye/head exercises for his home program and trying melatonin in order to improve this sleep. For the headaches and cognitive issues, amanatadine was tried which is a neurostimulant that in small trials has been shown to be effective at decreasing symptoms of headaches and improving cognition. He was also provided with vergence exercises and exercises to improve his postural control. He was told to limit his exposure to video games and to try not to increase this heart rate as his symptoms increased more than 5/10 postexertion. Driving and traveling were suggested in moderation so as not to increase his symptoms. Since he was a professional athlete and the goal was to get him back to in the game as soon as possible, a neuro-optometry specialist was also consulted. It is not normal practice to consult with a neuro-optometry specialist that early in the rehab process.

It was difficult to modify his exercise program since he was out of state, although a local physical therapist had been identified. He was given pencil push-ups, exercises with a Brocks string, and combined vergence exercises with saccades. Migraine education was provided for him to try to avoid dietary triggers and to try to get regular sleep 7 days a week.

At 11 weeks postconcussion, he was asymptomatic at rest plus after full workouts. His ImPACT scores had improved to his baseline level, even after exertion. Symptoms were no longer reported with eye/head movements and his balance had returned to normal on the SOT (score was 83). His DHI score was 0 and his ABC Scale score was 100%.

At discharge, he continued to demonstrate an exophoria with the Maddox rod testing and his near point convergence was 5 cm (which is a normal score). He took unusually long to get better as a professional athlete, but he did recover. It is unclear if his recovery would be extended should he have another concussion. He returned to playing professional football aware of the consequences of repeated concussion and was taught to recognize early signs of concussion.

Sport concussion is common and most people recovery quickly. Those people with protracted recovery can be a challenge to care for as they can be symptomatic with movement and exposure to visual stimuli. Overall team management with a physician, physical therapist, athletic trainer, neuropsychologist, and a neuro-optometrist (as needed) appears to optimize care; although not all athletes need the services of the entire medical team, it is ideal to have these members available for support. Collins et al. reported that there may be various forms of concussion subtypes including anxiety/mood, cervical, posttraumatic migraine, ocular, vestibular, and cognitive fatigue.[61] Few persons with concussion have symptoms in all of the above subtypes.

SUMMARY

Concussion is a worldwide concern that results in significant functional limitations and creates difficulty with both work and leisure activities. There is strong evidence that persons postconcussion and postblast injury experience vestibular symptoms with emerging evidence that vestibular rehabilitation is helpful in persons with mTBI. Every person with postblunt head/blast trauma or concussion must be assessed to determine their functional limitations and impairments to optimize their care. As knowledge of concussion advances, we may be able to determine prognosis based on the individuals' presenting signs and symptoms and comorbid factors.

References

1. Bhattacharyya N, Gubbels SP, Schwartz SR, et al. Clinical practice guideline: benign paroxysmal positional vertigo (update). *Otolaryngol Head Neck Surg* 2017;**156**:S1−47.
2. Hoffer ME, Balaban C, Gottshall K, Balough BJ, Maddox MR, Penta JR. Blast exposure: vestibular consequences and associated characteristics. *Otol Neurotol* 2010;**31**:232−6.
3. McCrory P, Meeuwisse W, Dvorak J, et al. Consensus statement on concussion in sport the 5th international conference on concussion in sport held in Berlin, October 2016. *Br J Sports Med* 2017;**51**(11):838−847.
4. Hoffer ME, Donaldson C, Gottshall KR, Balaban C, Balough BJ. Blunt and blast head trauma: different entities. *Int Tinnitus J* 2009;**15**:115−18.
5. Hoffer ME, Gottshall KR, Moore R, Balough BJ, Wester D. Characterizing and treating dizziness after mild head trauma. *Otol Neurotol* 2004;**25**:135−8.
6. Viirre E, Purcell I, Baloh RW. The Dix-Hallpike test and the canalith repositioning maneuver. *Laryngoscope* 2005;**115**:184−7.
7. Vukovic V, Plavec D, Galinovic I, Lovrencic-Huzjan A, Budisic M, Demarin V. Prevalence of vertigo, dizziness, and migrainous vertigo in patients with migraine. *Headache* 2007;**47**:1427−35.
8. Society IH. *International Headache Society Classificaiton: ICHD-3-beta website.* <http://www.ihs-headache.org/ichd-guidelines>; 2017.
9. Cho SJ, Kim BK, Kim BS, et al. Vestibular migraine in multicenter neurology clinics according to the appendix criteria in the third beta edition of the International Classification of Headache Disorders. *Cephalalgia* 2016;**36**:454−62.
10. Lempert T, Olesen J, Furman J, et al. Vestibular migraine: diagnostic criteria. *J Vestib Res* 2012;**22**:167−72.
11. Gode S, Celebisoy N, Kirazli T, et al. Clinical assessment of topiramate therapy in patients with migrainous vertigo. *Headache* 2010;**50**:77−84.
12. Mucha A, Collins MW, Elbin RJ, et al. A Brief Vestibular/Ocular Motor Screening (VOMS) assessment to evaluate concussions: preliminary findings. *Am J Sports Med* 2014;**42**:2479−86.
13. McCrory P, Meeuwisse WH, Aubry M, et al. Consensus statement on concussion in sport—the 4th International Conference on Concussion in Sport held in Zurich, November 2012. *Phys Med Rehabil* 2013;**5**:255−79.
14. Anzalone AJ, Blueitt D, Case T, et al. A positive vestibular/ocular motor screening (VOMS) is associated with increased recovery time after sports-related concussion in youth and adolescent athletes. *Am J Sports Med* 2017;**45**:474−9.
15. Capo-Aponte JE, Urosevich TG, Temme LA, Tarbett AK, Sanghera NK. Visual dysfunctions and symptoms during the subacute stage of blast-induced mild traumatic brain injury. *Mil Med* 2012;**177**:804−13.

16. Henry LC, Elbin RJ, Collins MW, Marchetti G, Kontos AP. Examining recovery trajectories after sport-related concussion with a multimodal clinical assessment approach. *Neurosurgery* 2016;**78**:232–41.

17. Kontos AP, Sufrinko A, Elbin RJ, Puskar A, Collins MW. Reliability and associated risk factors for performance on the vestibular/ocular motor screening (VOMS) tool in healthy collegiate athletes. *Am J Sports Med* 2016;**44**:1400–6.

18. Ellis MJ, Cordingley DM, Vis S, Reimer KM, Leiter J, Russell K. Clinical predictors of vestibulo-ocular dysfunction in pediatric sports-related concussion. *J Neurosurg Pediatr* 2017;**19**:38–45.

19. Yorke AM, Smith L, Babcock M, Alsalaheen B. Validity and reliability of the vestibular/ocular motor screening and associations with common concussion screening tools. *Sports Health* 2017;**9**:174–80.

20. Guskiewicz KM, Ross SE, Marshall SW. Postural stability and neuropsychological deficits after concussion in collegiate athletes. *J Athl Train* 2001;**36**:263–73.

21. Riemann BL, Guskiewicz KM. Effects of mild head injury on postural stability as measured through clinical balance testing. *J Athl Train* 2000;**35**:19–25.

22. Alsalaheen B, Haines J, Yorke A, Diebold J. King-Devick Test reference values and associations with balance measures in high school American football players. *Scand J Med Sci Sports* 2016;**26**:235–9.

23. King D, Brughelli M, Hume P, Gissane C. Assessment, management and knowledge of sport-related concussion: systematic review. *Sports Med* 2014;**44**:449–71.

24. Oride MK, Marutani JK, Rouse MW, DeLand PN. Reliability study of the Pierce and King-Devick saccade tests. *Am J Optom Physiol Opt* 1986;**63**:419–24.

25. Conder RL, Conder AA. Heart rate variability interventions for concussion and rehabilitation. *Front Psychol* 2014;**5**:890.

26. Alsalaheen BA, Mucha A, Morris LO, et al. Vestibular rehabilitation for dizziness and balance disorders after concussion. *J Neurol Phys Ther* 2010;**34**:87–93.

27. Alsalaheen BA, Whitney SL, Mucha A, Morris LO, Furman JM, Sparto PJ. Exercise prescription patterns in patients treated with vestibular rehabilitation after concussion. *Physiother Res Int* 2013;**18**:100–8.

28. Alsalaheen BA, Whitney SL, Marchetti GF, et al. Performance of high school adolescents on functional gait and balance measures. *Pediatr Phys Ther* 2014;**26**:191–9.

29. Jacobson GP, Newman CW. The development of the Dizziness Handicap Inventory. *Arch Otolaryngol Head Neck Surg* 1990;**116**:424–7.

30. McCaslin DL, Jacobson GP, Lambert W, English LN, Kemph AJ. The development of the vanderbilt pediatric dizziness handicap inventory for patient caregivers (DHI-PC). *Int J Pediatr Otorhinolaryngol* 2015;**79**:1662–6.

31. Powell LE, Myers AM. The Activities-specific Balance Confidence (ABC) scale. *J Gerontol A Biol Sci Med Sci* 1995;**50A**:M28–34.

32. Scherer MR, Schubert MC. Traumatic brain injury and vestibular pathology as a comorbidity after blast exposure. *Phys Ther* 2009;**89**:980–92.

33. Hall CD, Herdman SJ, Whitney SL, et al. Vestibular rehabilitation for peripheral vestibular hypofunction: an evidence-based clinical practice guideline: from the american physical therapy association neurology section. *J Neurol Phys Ther* 2016;**40**:124–55.

34. Herman T, Inbar-Borovsky N, Brozgol M, Giladi N, Hausdorff JM. The Dynamic Gait Index in healthy older adults: the role of stair climbing, fear of falling and gender. *Gait Post* 2009;**29**:237–41.

35. Gottshall K, Drake A, Gray N, McDonald E, Hoffer ME. Objective vestibular tests as outcome measures in head injury patients. *Laryngoscope* 2003;**113**:1746–50.

36. Mishra A, Davis S, Speers R, Shepard NT. Head shake computerized dynamic posturography in peripheral vestibular lesions. *Am J Audiol* 2009;**18**:53–9.

37. Nashner LM, Peters JF. Dynamic posturography in the diagnosis and management of dizziness and balance disorders. *Neurol Clin* 1990;**8**:331–49.

38. Pritcher MR, Whitney SL, Marchetti GF, Furman JM. The influence of age and vestibular disorders on gaze stabilization: a pilot study. *Otol Neurotol* 2008;**29**:982–8.

39. Whitney SL, Marchetti GF, Pritcher M, Furman JM. Gaze stabilization and gait performance in vestibular dysfunction. *Gait Post* 2009;**29**:194–8.

40. Goebel JA, Tungsiripat N, Sinks B, Carmody J. Gaze stabilization test: a new clinical test of unilateral vestibular dysfunction. *Otol Neurotol* 2007;**28**:68–73.

41. Badaracco C, Labini FS, Meli A, De Angelis E, Tufarelli D. Vestibular rehabilitation outcomes in chronic vertiginous patients through computerized dynamic visual acuity and Gaze stabilization test. *Otol Neurotol* 2007;**28**:809−13.

42. Paige GD. Nonlinearity and asymmetry in the human vestibulo-ocular reflex. *Acta Otolaryngol* 1989;**108**:1−8.

43. Broglio SP, Eckner JT, Martini D, Sosnoff JJ, Kutcher JS, Randolph C. Cumulative head impact burden in high school football. *J Neurotrauma* 2011;**28**:2069−78.

44. Eckner JT, Sabin M, Kutcher JS, Broglio SP. No evidence for a cumulative impact effect on concussion injury threshold. *J Neurotrauma* 2011;**28**:2079−90.

45. Lau BC, Kontos AP, Collins MW, Mucha A, Lovell MR. Which on-field signs/symptoms predict protracted recovery from sport-related concussion among high school football players? *Am J Sports Med* 2011;**39**:2311−18.

46. Eisenberg MA, Meehan 3rd WP, Mannix R. Duration and course of post-concussive symptoms. *Pediatrics* 2014;**133**:999−1006.

47. Seifert TD. Sports concussion and associated post-traumatic headache. *Headache* 2013;**53**:726−36.

48. Zasler ND. Sports concussion headache. *Brain Inj* 2015;**29**:207−20.

49. Iverson GL, Gaetz M, Lovell MR, Collins MW. Relation between subjective fogginess and neuropsychological testing following concussion. *J Int Neuropsychol Soc* 2004;**10**:904−6.

50. Pinto SM, Twichell MF, Henry LC. Predictors of pharmacological intervention in adolescents with protracted symptoms after sports-related concussion. *Phys Med Rehabil* 2017;**9**(9):847−55.

51. Sufrinko A, McAllister-Deitrick J, Elbin RJ, Collins MW, Kontos AP. Family history of migraine associated with posttraumatic migraine symptoms following sport-related concussion. *J Head Trauma Rehabil* 2018;**33**(1):7−14.

52. Morgan CD, Zuckerman SL, Lee YM, et al. Predictors of postconcussion syndrome after sports-related concussion in young athletes: a matched case-control study. *J Neurosurg Pediatr* 2015;**15**:589−98.

53. Chen JK, Johnston KM, Collie A, McCrory P, Ptito A. A validation of the post concussion symptom scale in the assessment of complex concussion using cognitive testing and functional MRI. *J Neurol Neurosurg Psychiatry* 2007;**78**:1231−8.

54. Merritt VC, Bradson ML, Meyer JE, Arnett PA. Evaluating the test-retest reliability of symptom indices associated with the ImPACT post-concussion symptom scale (PCSS). *J Clin Exp Neuropsychol* 2018;**40**(4):377−88.

55. Tyburski AL, Cheng L, Assari S, Darvish K, Elliott MB. Frequent mild head injury promotes trigeminal sensitivity concomitant with microglial proliferation, astrocytosis, and increased neuropeptide levels in the trigeminal pain system. *J Headache Pain* 2017;**18**:16.

56. Marquez C, Lininger M, Raab S. Establishing normative change values in visual acuity loss during the dynamic visual acuity test. *Int J Sports Phys Ther* 2017;**12**:227−32.

57. Zhou G, Brodsky JR. Objective vestibular testing of children with dizziness and balance complaints following sports-related concussions. *Otolaryngol Head Neck Surg* 2015;**152**:1133−9.

58. Jaffee MS, Winter WC, Jones CC, Ling G. Sleep disturbances in athletic concussion. *Brain Inj* 2015;**29**:221−7.

59. Corbin-Berrigan LA, Gagnon I. Postconcussion symptoms as a marker of delayed recovery in children and youth who recently sustained a concussion: a brief report. *Clin J Sport Med* 2017;**27**:325−7.

60. Whitney SL, Wrisley DM, Brown KE, Furman JM. Is perception of handicap related to functional performance in persons with vestibular dysfunction? *Otol Neurotol* 2004;**25**:139−43.

61. Reynolds E, Collins MW, Mucha A, Troutman-Ensecki C. Establishing a clinical service for the management of sports-related concussions. *Neurosurgery* 2014;**75**(Suppl 4):S71−81.

21

Cognitive Rehabilitation for Mild Traumatic Brain Injury (mTBI)

Justine J. Allen, M.S., CCC-SLP

Division of Speech Pathology, Department of Otolaryngology, University of Miami, Miller School of Medicine, Miami, FL, United States

INTRODUCTION

The majority of experts define cognition in terms of how we attend to, process, reason, and respond to the world around us. Cognition is influenced by each individual's unique human experience and perhaps is our most critical attribute.[1,2]

In light of the dramatic increase in the incidence of mild traumatic brain injury (mTBI), it has been reinforced that brain injury, regardless of etiology and severity, can result in cognitive impairments. Individuals with mTBI experience cognitive deficits and chronic postconcussive symptoms after injury (e.g., headaches, balance problems, dizziness, fatigue, anxiety, concentration issues, psychological and memory difficulties). Capturing the complexity of chronic mTBI and the comorbid disorders that may result in, exacerbate, overlap with, and mimic cognitive impairment is both challenging and essential. It enables differentiation of the presence of true cognitive dysfunction verse individual barriers to cognitive access. Furthermore, it aims to address and refine what can be done to preserve and/or improve cognitive functioning in patients with brain injury, while establishing a multidisciplinary and patient-centric plan of care.[3–7]

One of the primary methods used to achieve this objective is neurorehabilitation. In the past, most experts focused on how neurorehabilitative methods applied to more severe brain injury secondary to trauma or stroke. However, the recent attention being given to mTBI has resulted in increased recognition of the disorder and an increasing body of evidenced-based literature, supporting the use of rehabilitation for this patient group.[5] This chapter will explore the primary and underlying principles of cognitive intervention by focusing on historical perspectives, fundamentals understood by specialists assessing and treating cognitive symptoms, and the current standards of care as it relates to evidence-based practice.

HISTORICAL PERSPECTIVES

The mortality rate of Service Member's (SMs) with acquired brain injury dramatically shifted during and after World War I. With improved survival from head injury during this time frame, it serves as the catalyst that initiated the demand for cognitive rehabilitation.[8]

With the progression to World War II, rehabilitative units with multiple disciplines developed. With some of the first programs for rehabilitation established in Germany, units continued to mobilize and grow across the Soviet Union, Great Britain, and the United States. The continued progression of landmark wars (e.g., Korean War, Vietnam War, etc.) with their corresponding impact on mortality and the subsequent rehabilitative needs is well outlined by the Defense and Veterans Brain Injury Center (DVBIC).[9]

It is important to appreciate that across these time frames, the trailblazers of these institutions and their treatment protocols varied. A constellation of neurosurgeons, clinical neurologists, neuropsychologists, psychologists, physical therapists, occupational therapists, speech language pathologists, psychotherapists, educators, and linguists all participated heavily in instating the foundations of this rehabilitative work.[8,10] For the purposes of this chapter, all members of this group will be referred to as specialists and/or clinicians.

Notably, it was during the 1970s that protocols and guidelines for therapy were established within acute and chronic care at institutions like Rancho Los Amigos Hospital in California and the New York University Institute of Rehabilitation Medicine. Additionally, it was when multiple acute and post-acute cognitive rehabilitation centers came to fruition. This is of historical significance as treatment during this time frame began to evolve; transitioning therapy focuses not only on sensorimotor stimulation in the acute phases, but to the domains of treating cognitive and behavioral dysfunctions in later stages.[8] Additionally, in the 1980s the sports medicine world began to become a platform for many of the advances in mTBI, creating a laboratory for the study of mTBI and informing the broader neurosciences of its implications.[11] Furthermore, the number of brain injury rehabilitation programs in the United States grew from 10 to over 500.[6]

Overall, these critical periods brought together influences from special education, neuropsychology, and cognitive psychology. These perspectives and disciplines frame the solid theoretical framework for systematic instruction, which we now use as the cornerstone for cognitive rehabilitation in mTBI.[3] Along with this framework, came an increased sense of urgency to provide care for our now senior generations of veterans and civilians with acquired brain injury. In 1992, Congress established the Defense of Veterans Head Injury Program (DVHIP), currently known as the DVBIC.[9]

A significant challenge began in the early 21st century when approximately 2 million military personnel deployed to Southwest Asia and a new cohort of SMs with TBI quickly accrued.[10] An increased prevalence of mTBI has been noted since 2001 with the launch of Operation Enduring Freedom and Operation of Iraqi Freedom (OEF/OIF). According to the International Classification of Diseases as of October 2015, over 350,000 individuals have been diagnosed with TBI and approximately 82% of these were determined to be mild in nature.[12–14] It has often been referred to as the "signature wound" of the conflict.[10]

With these rising numbers of injuries there was an increased need for rehabilitative services. However, there was a paucity of literature available regarding the efficacy of cognitive rehabilitation in mTBI and the injury itself was either not recognized or viewed as reversible. Therefore in many circumstances, cognitive treatment was reserved for those with moderate-severe brain injuries alone.[15]

The staggering number of affected individuals eventually created awareness that the neurological cognitive sequelae of mTBI can in fact be very disabling.[5,15,16] With over 30,000 SMs of OIF/OEF returning with nonfatal injuries, the US Department of Veterans Affairs along with the Department of Defense (DOD) began to promote and facilitate funded research efforts and the establishment of research consortia's for these issues.[17]

As of July 2007, the DOD has provided $150 million in funding for research on TBI, a portion of which is allocated to assess rehabilitative care. In September 2007, the Office for Rehabilitation and Reintegration Division (R2D) and the TBI Program of the Surgeon General's Office charged a team of rehabilitation specialists to develop landmark clinical guidelines for state of the art care.[5] The National Defense Authorization Act for Fiscal Year 2010, Section 273 of House Resolution 2647 called for a clinical trial to assess the efficacy of cognitive rehabilitative therapy in TBI and to inform recommendations for mTBI.[18] In December 2016, continued funding provided the support for consensus meetings comprised of speech-language pathologists, neuropsychologists, and occupational therapists to expand upon clinical guidelines.[7]

Given federal support to improve clinical care and an incredible and concerted effort from clinicians and researchers to provide evidenced-based practice for cognitive rehabilitation in mTBI, a new critical period and the spread of emerging literature and therapeutic practices for patients with mild acquired brain injury is at its inception.

FUNDAMENTALS

Before moving forward, several important fundamentals need to be understood. These fundamental principles include neuroplasticity, the influence of comorbidities, and a recognition of the shifting landscape of neurorehabilitation as applied to mTBI.

Neuroplasticity

Neuroplasticity, may be defined as the functional reorganization and compensation within residual neural tissue, mediated by changes in neural circuitry.[19] The growing understanding of the brains capacity for change via learning in the typical brain and relearning in the damaged brain, raises confidence in the ability to enhance functional outcomes and improve the rehabilitative mechanisms that drive recovery.[20] Furthermore, understanding the nature of neuroplasticity is critical to improving rehabilitative strategies and optimizing functional outcomes.[21]

Research suggests that the central nervous system can be modified well after initial neurological insult. Functional adaptions in underlying neural networks have been cited in brain imaging studies of cognitive and behavioral performance.[22] Within the last decade, emergence of improved technology for imaging the central nervous system (CNS) (e.g., fMRI, positron emission tomography, etc.) has led to an increased use of imaging modalities as a primary outcome measure for neurorehabilitative research and the analysis of cortical change over time. Correlating these structural changes with positive cognitive and behavioral measures continues to improve our understanding of the effectiveness of rehabilitative care and the neurological recovery mechanisms response to stimulation.[3,22] Additionally, the developments of practice-dependent and experience-dependent variations in the brain are used to inform cognitive rehabilitation in efforts to lead to optimal cortical plasticity.[22] Principles of experience-dependent neural plasticity after brain damage align with contemporary practices for mTBI. These include descriptions and implications for specificity, interference, salience, time, age, use, repetition, intensity, and transference, which are well outlined by Kleim and Jones in 2008.[3,5,20]

Considering Complexities and Comorbidities

Many individuals with mTBI experience cognitive deficits and postconcussive symptoms immediately after injury. Although the majority of individuals make an excellent recovery, a variety of studies reveal that a range of 15%−30% of individuals continue to report chronic symptoms (i.e., those that last longer than three months post onset).[7] These diffuse symptom patterns commonly include, but are not limited to, headaches, balance problems, dizziness, fatigue, bodily aches and pains, anxiety, irritability, concentration issues and memory difficulties.[7] Of note, there have been numerous studies revealing that a multitude of post-concussive symptoms are largely explained by posttraumatic stress disorder (PTSD) and depression.[23]

As capturing the complexity of chronic mTBI and the comorbid disorders that may cause, intensify, overlap with, or imitate cognitive impairment is challenging, it is critical to leverage positive contextual factors and mitigate comorbidities in order to improve rehabilitative outcomes.[3] It must be informed by medical and neuropsychological diagnosis and take into account the individuals ever-evolving environmental and personal factors.[3,6] Furthermore, obtaining detailed and objective data surrounding this symptomatology is crucial, as some symptoms derived from comorbidities may undermine cognitive abilities and complicate treatment. Additionally, some patients may respond better to particular therapeutic interventions than others.[5,18]

Given the multifactorial nature of post-concussive cognitive symptoms in mTBI, it is critical that clinicians recognize and embrace opportunities to refer patients with the outlined complexities to the appropriate specialists. Team-based cognitive rehabilitation provides the benefit of identifying problems and recognizing opportunities to enhance care through a variety of skilled services.[6] Clinicians should capitalize on multidisciplinary treatment methods to better address all of the patient's needs, provide access to specialized methodologies and optimize cognitive rehabilitation.[5,7] For example, when 257 active duty patients with a history of mTBI participated in multidisciplinary treatment at Brooke Army Medical Center TBI Clinic, results were associated with reduced self-reported persistent postconcussive and PTSD symptoms.[23]

Paradigm Shift

In the context of mTBI, it is critical to acknowledge that a paradigm shift in cognitive rehabilitation has taken place.[21] It is with increasing credibility that direct training of cognitive processes should be carried out in conjunction with other therapeutic interventions. Literature targeting direct training for cognitive domains such as sustained attention, working memory, and executive functions such as problem solving continue to be used effectively with success.[7] This body of work is particularly pertinent as it is aimed to stimulate distinct neural networks. It relies heavily on basic principles of neuroplasticity and the suggestion that neurons possess the remarkable proficiency to change their structure and utility in response to behavioral training.[20] However, treatment methods also benefit from the expansion of this school of thought and has transitioned from utilizing decontextualized drill training exercises to encompass a broader range of cognitive processes and techniques. Cognitive rehabilitation must be tailored to functional recovery goals and the consistent application of therapeutic skill sets within real-life situations.[2,21] When utilized in combination, this contemporary method is patient-centric. It takes the individual into account based on their cognitive complaints, regardless of etiologic correlates.[7]

Evaluating this union is essential as much of cognitive rehabilitation practices are based on the broader research available on interventions for persons with moderate-severe TBI.[5] Although clinicians must remain skeptical in assessing how rehabilitative studies for moderate-severe populations may transfer to care for mild TBI, the neural mechanisms surrounding learning and the therapeutic process as a whole acknowledge that they are applicable to the broader population.[6] Both in the typical and atypical brain, enhanced neurobehavioral function and synaptic plasticity is associated with appropriate structuring of one's environment and experiences.[6] Notably, bridging the gap in available literature for cognitive rehabilitation in mTBI continues to be addressed. In the landmark Study of Cognitive Rehabilitation Effectiveness, a randomized controlled treatment trial validated that clinician directed cognitive rehabilitation was deemed to significantly improve functional cognitive outcomes for individuals in the chronic stage after mTBI.[18]

Landscape of Cognitive Rehabilitation in Mild Traumatic Brain Injury

A limitation in evaluating and describing the landscape of cognitive rehabilitation may be attributed to the lack of a universal and operative definition for cognitive intervention.[13] Cognitive rehabilitation has been described as a broad and diverse group of services, treating a wide array of symptoms and levels of severity. The heterogeneity of the interventions and how they are applied further confound our ability to provide a concrete definition[24]; it does not refer to any one specific approach to treatment.[11] However, according to the Brain Injury Association of America, the largest US advocacy group for individuals with acquired brain injury, cognitive rehabilitation may be summarized as a "systematically applied set of medical and therapeutic services designed to improve cognitive functioning and participation in activities that may be affected by difficulties in one or more cognitive domains."[25]

Despite the multitude of approaches available for cognitive treatment, it is widely accepted within the literature that two key attributes create a binary quantification of cognitive rehabilitation treatment and are traditionally utilized within this population. The Institute of Medicine (IOM)'s 2011 report categorizes these attributes as restorative and compensatory treatments.[24] Restorative and/or rehabilitative approaches, are aimed to decrease impairments in cognitive function (e.g., drill oriented therapy). In contrast, compensatory treatments seek to provide alternatives for carrying out Activities of Daily Living by developing strategies to maximize function, with or without provision of changes to the underlying cognitive impairments (e.g., external memory aids).[3,24] In more recent years, a third domain has been established. Metacognition or "thinking about thinking" refers to the method of assessing, identifying and self-calibrating one's own cognitive and behavioral skills.[3] In culmination, the use of rehabilitative, compensatory and metacognitive approaches in the setting of mTBI will be addressed in this chapter. However, in light of the complexities and comorbidities that may impact cognitive issues in mTBI, multidisciplinary and individualized treatment is recommended to enhance outcomes and reduce risk for complicating and interfering factors. Therefore, clinicians are responsible for analyzing the appropriateness of these three categorical approaches. Clinicians remain liable for recruiting allied disciplines to collaborate and provide alternate treatment methods, to be aware of the growing evidence-based literature over time, and modify therapy in a patient-centered fashion.[7]

Commentary on Cognitive Reserve

Generally, the cognitive reserve (CR) hypothesis suggests that patients with high CR may be able to process tasks in a manner that allows them to better cope with brain damage and/or can sustain greater degrees of brain damage before demonstrating functional deficits. Neural implantation of CR can be noted in either *reserve* (i.e., preexisting differences in neural efficiency and the capacity of brain networks that predate any brain damage, which potentially function at a level that mitigates the risk for disruption) and *compensation* (i.e., ability to develop new responses to pathology via the use of brain networks otherwise not typically used by healthy brains).[22] Markers for CR include levels of intelligence, literacy, educational, and occupational attainment.[22] Research on adults with acquired TBI with varying levels of severity, suggest that larger premorbid brain volume and higher education levels may decrease degree of vulnerability following TBI.[26] Additionally, children and adolescents with high cognitive ability may be somewhat protected from the effects of mild TBI, while those with lower levels of ability demonstrate g6reater vulnerability.[27] Although the impact of CR on rehabilitation practices has not been extensively studied in the mild TBI literature, CR has been acknowledged as an applicable concept to any impact on brain function.[22] Therefore, with trace anecdotal reports of cognitive difficulty, clinicians may consider capitalizing on and encouraging continuation of skills and strategies the patient with high CR may have already self-established and began to utilize.

Commentary on Environmental Modifications

Environmental management is the alteration, restructuring, and exploration of new ways in which an individual can tailor their surroundings to decrease the impact of cognitive dysfunction on everyday life. For example, eliminating distractors (e.g., noise, lighting, crowds) can positively influence cognitive performance.[5–7] Alternatively, a patient's surroundings can be used to implement environmental anchors, external aides, or strategic planning (e.g., shopping during quieter hours). It can also be used to provide just-right challenges, as therapists may be able to tailor the environment in order to increase degree of complexity and/or the level of cognitive demand necessary for patients to achieve specific goals.[5,7] Perhaps secondary to the mild nature of their cognitive deficits, a common clinical oversight in the care of patients with mTBI is the lack of explicit-training for environmental modification. Evaluations and recommendations surrounding environmental alterations should be completed collaboratively with the patient, facilitate context-sensitive needs for a naturalistic setting and consider the patients ability to implement therapeutic tools.[7]

COMPREHENSIVE ASSESSMENT OF COGNITION IN MILD TRAUMATIC BRAIN INJURY

According to the VA/DoD Clinical Practice Guideline for Management of Concussion in mTBI, there is insufficient evidence for recommending routine comprehensive cognitive evaluations in the acute and postacute period.[28] Despite this, cognitive screening activities and patient education within the first 90 days of mTBI have been shown to inhibit or reduce the development of persistent symptoms. They may be used to validate self-perceived and/or caregiver-perceived observations of cognitive changes, to interact with the injured individual, provide patient education and outline the positive expectation for recovery.[5] With persistent cognitive symptoms and associated symptoms that have been refractory to treatment, comprehensive cognitive or neuropsychological assessment is suggested within 30–90 days postonset.[29] However, as most acute cognitive changes resolve or stabilize within 90 days following trauma, comprehensive evaluation is typically deferred to that time.[5] It should be reinforced that prior to considering referral for cognitive evaluation and rehabilitation, preventing and/or managing conditions that may decrease cognitive function (e.g., depression, PTSD, insomnia, substance abuse, and behavioral difficulties, etc.) should be addressed by primary care and/or appropriate providers as much as possible.[5,28,29] Additionally, in practice, the professionals responsible for coordinating these details and evaluating cognition will vary by site, clinical expertise, availability of members of the rehabilitation team, access to resources, structure and size of facility, and the nature of the setting.[5,6]

In providing comprehensive evaluation for mTBI, a variety of reliable and valid tools should be utilized in tandem with self-report and ecologically relevant measures aimed to simulate cognitive demands similar to those experienced in the everyday environment of the individual.[29] Primary goals for comprehensive assessment include developing an accurate portrayal of an individual's level of functioning (e.g., cognitive, emotional, and interpersonal), variables which may influence levels of adaptive function (e.g., situational demands, current living or working environment, beliefs and expectations, etc.), spared neurocognitive abilities, capacity to participate in activities of daily living and rehabilitation, and probable effective methods for cognitive intervention.[6] For example, the International Classification of Functioning, Disability and Health (ICF) published by the World Health Organization, demonstrates clinical utility as it conceptualizes a person's level of functioning and risk for disability as a dynamic interaction between multidimensional conditions. It accounts for both social and medical models of disability. The ICF framework considers the domains of *impairment* (i.e., specific bodily functions or structures that are altered), *disability* (i.e., impact on activities or specific functional abilities), *handicap* (i.e., alterations in social and role function; participation), and *context* (i.e., environmental and personal factors which affect these experiences; whether these are facilitators or barriers).[6,30] Addressing these domains may enable clinicians to achieve the goals of comprehensive assessment.

It is widely acknowledged in the literature that there are two principal modalities for cognitive evaluation. These include both standardized and functional assessment approaches, commonly referred to as nonstandardized measures. In using psychometric or standardized measures, one utilizes norm-referenced tests with clearly defined sets of procedures in order to assess cognitive processes and make inferences about cognitive functioning.[5,31] Nonstandardized or flexible, process-oriented approaches to assessment include more naturalistic, quasi-experimental methods which are particularly useful as they provide a depth analysis of cognition and are likely to help gauge functional performance outside of the clinical setting.[5,6] The ultimate choice for assessment is guided by clinical judgment, experience, the needs of the patient and acquisition of relevant information to evaluate current functioning and plan future treatment.[5]

The general consensus from experts in the field is that standardized tests should be used with caution and as only one component of the evaluation process secondary to the discordance between standardized tests and real-life impairment outside of the clinical setting.[31] Many also acknowledge the multiple psychometric problems related to standardized tests, including the caveat that the majority of cognitive tests have not been designed or validated on individuals with mTBI.[5] However, panels of experts have identified the fundamental components necessary surrounding psychometric properties of cognitive tests. These aim to allow clinicians to better identify appropriate norm-referenced standardized tests with the optimal levels of scientific integrity. Key criteria includes consideration of appropriateness of the standardization sample, reliability, validity, and level of responsiveness.[6,31]

As a supplement to standardized batteries of this caliber, nonstandardized assessment procedures enhance evaluations as they capture more functional perspectives and utilize tasks that more closely approximate natural day-to-day and real-life activities.[6] Use of real-world assessment procedures (e.g., discourse analysis) help identify real-world disability.[32] Of note, the importance of nonstandardized, context-sensitive, situational assessment is supported by extensive research revealing the shortcomings of office bound tests for patients with TBI in addition to the weak correlations between measures of everyday assessment and standardized scores.[32] In culmination, it is recommended that these assessments be used in conjunction with one another with consideration of the broader framework of the person's pre-injury status, development, current and anticipated cognitive demands, and with prioritization of return to meaningful daily activity and participation.[31]

COGNITIVE INTERVENTION

Readers are reminded that this is not an exhaustive review, rather an introduction to the realm of content and are encouraged to refer to Appendix A: Suggested Supplements and Rehabilitative Resources for the larger breadth of this scope of practice. Notably, these resources are critical for content related to step-by-step training and establishing the essential clinical skills necessary prior to patient contact.

Stages of Therapy

Cognitive rehabilitation occurs across the continuum of care. Patients may be seen as they progress through the acute, subacute and postacute stages of their injury.[33] Service delivery also occurs in multiple modalities: individual, group, day treatment programs, intensive inpatient rehabilitation, daily outpatient, or weekly treatment sessions.[11] Beginning in the hospital environment, acute rehabilitation methods are primarily psychoeducational in nature.[34] However, a major role of cognitive therapy is assisting patients to reintegrate back into their community and back into their daily lives effectively.[33] This sporadic generalization of the skills necessary to achieve reintegration into the real-world should not be expected, but *programmed for*. Multiple steps can facilitate maintenance and ensure the generalization of therapeutic skills upon the culmination of therapy; a major staple of this includes being explicit in training.[6]

The research evidence globally supports methodologies such as systematic instruction to plan and sequence treatment, given additional consideration of the patients previously evaluated multifactorial and/or unique needs. Clinicians utilize explicit therapy models and deliberate techniques to scaffold the acquisition, application and adaptation of skills and strategies. Use of this staged learning process (i.e., Phase 1—acquisition, Phase 2—application) enables and encourages the likeliness that patients will apply their therapeutic techniques from simple to complex levels of processing and retrieval, until the ultimate consolidation of their skills.[3,35] Additionally, clinicians may recruit underlying mechanisms of declarative, procedural and contextual knowledge for specific strategy training (i.e., "what to do" being declarative, "how to do it" being procedural, and "when to use it" being contextual).[5]

Of note, throughout treatment consistent consideration of the three phases of "PIE" (i.e., plan, implement, evaluate) can be critical for implementing different types of therapies, facilitating evidence-based decision making and acquiring the necessary data for needs-based modifications.[3] Furthermore, treatment plans should be cognizant of the overall time frame available, maintain realistic discharge standards and be considerate of the patients access to resources and current aptitudes they present with at the onset of treatment.[5]

Guiding Treatment Principles and Common Practices

From the moment of first clinical contact, guiding treatment principles are utilized to foster patient-centered care and guide the clinical decision-making process.[7] In order to optimize the therapeutic process, the cognitive specialists armamentarium is equipped with a variety of principles and methodologies that are applicable even at the acute stages and within comprehensive assessment.

According to the Clinicians Guide to Cognitive Rehabilitation in Mild Traumatic Brain Injury, six key guiding principles are emphasized:

- Recruit Resilience (i.e., maintaining a patient-centered approach, being sensitive to the patients cultural, sociolinguistic and spiritual core beliefs, and incorporating these individualized sources of strength into therapy).
- Cultivate Therapeutic Alliance (i.e., establishing a partnership that reinforces a sincere commitment to helping the patient achieve their goals, one that is based upon trust and reciprocal respect which then serves as the primary foundation for the therapeutic process).
- Acknowledge Multifactorial Complexities (i.e., accurate identification of cooccurring symptoms that may attribute to cognitive symptoms and implementing clinical judgment for therapy-based, referral-based, and team-based approaches to mitigating these factors).
- Build a Team (i.e., reduce comorbid symptoms and risk for competing messages by empowering the patient through a diverse team of health-care providers and specialists, family members, and/or leading figures in their lives to provide support through the recovery process).
- Focus on Function (i.e., deliver intervention through the context of creating effective change in the patient's ability to perform daily life tasks, roles, and participation in society; tailoring treatment to achievement of functional goals over proficiency with isolated cognitive drills).
- Promote Realistic Expectations for Recovery (i.e., emphasis of the positive expectation of recovery and use of strategies to enhance development of self-efficacy and overall therapy outcomes; providing education that this may be achieved with time, effort, and consistent participation in treatment in a collaborative manner).[7]

Early Intervention and Education

Historically, a number of physicians within acute care held the belief that it was best to reassure patients of a complete recovery after concussion. Often, the conversations surrounding the adverse symptoms patients may experience were mitigated in order to reduce the risk for iatrogenic symptom development. In the 1970s this belief began to be challenged with a surge of research analyzing the positive impact of early intervention and education at the acute stages of mTBI.[6]

Currently, a large body of research supports the benefit of psychoeducational interventions during the acute stages of mTBI as efficacious in reducing the severity and duration of postconcussion symptoms.[34] In fact, psychoeducation represents the only treatment for mTBI supported by the highest-level of evidence within VA/DOD Clinical Practice Guidelines for Management of mTBI/Concussion.[13,29] According to Mittenberg et al.,[36] treatment group participants in the acute stage of mTBI who received a printed manual, *Recovering From Head Injury: A Guide for Patients*, and met with a therapist for 1 hour prior to discharge experienced significantly fewer symptomatic days (33 vs 51) and significantly lower average symptom severity levels at 6-month follow-ups as opposed to their matched controls who received only routine hospital care.

Increasing a patient's understanding of the complexities surrounding mTBI is a staple in every therapy program. Providing psychoeducational information validates and normalizes symptomology while simultaneously highlighting appropriate strategies to alleviate issues.[7] In order to enable patients to understand their symptoms, reduce the misattribution of them to significant brain injury, and avoid deterioration of self-efficacy, experts continue to recommend the provision of verbal and written educational material on the neurological sequelae of mTBI and on the positive expectation of recovery.[5]

Motivational Interviewing

According to Miller and Rollnick (2013), "Motivational interviewing is a collaborative, goal-oriented style of communication with particular attention to the language of change. It is designed to strengthen personal motivation for and commitment to a specific goal by eliciting and exploring the person's own reasons for change within an atmosphere of acceptance and compassion."[37]

Importantly and in the context of working with patients with acquired brain injury, motivational interviewing contributes to the therapeutic alliance, facilitates acceptance of deficits, establishes realistic goals, and promotes constructive engagement in the rehabilitative process.[38] It is a method of engaging patients in a manner that helps patients build self-efficacy and self-identify their own strengths and challenges.[7] Use of reflective-listening and open-ended questions facilities a joint decision-making process that enables the patient to assume responsibility in the behavior change process.[3,5]

Motivational interviewing lies between the continuum of "directing" and "following," serving as a "guiding" communication style with sequential phases (i.e., engaging, focusing, evoking, and planning). Above all, motivational interviewing is patient-centered as it is done "for" or "with" the patient, it is not done by an expert "to" a passive recipient.[37] According to experts, when working with patients with mTBI and utilizing motivational interviewing, the "FRAMES" acronym may be applied (i.e., Feedback, Responsibility, Advice, Menus, Empathy, and Self-Efficacy).[5]

Goal Attainment Scaling

In many ways, the use of guiding principles to facilitate achievement in rehabilitation targets creates multiple abstract goals. Goal Attainment Scaling (GAS) demonstrates clinical utility as it offers the patient a concrete, quantifiable, and individualized system to monitor progress and ensure the creation of highly customized goals.[2] This scaling of goals is typically done by identifying, developing and weighing specific goals that are meaningful in nature. Establishing meaningful, functional goals is essential as they are more likely to generate patient engagement and the attainment of targets.[6,7] Additionally, use of a scale allows patients to observe and externalize behaviors by applying a corresponding percentage of time which they effectively implement therapeutic skills and strategies.[6] It is valuable as a biofeedback tool, allowing patients to increase their self-awareness and provide insight into the problems being addressed through concrete feedback about major rehabilitative milestones. GAS provides additional clinical utility as it also facilitates patient care by enhancing collaboration within a multidisciplinary team and providing a resource to gauge readiness for transition through the continuum of care.[2]

Domain Specific Rehabilitation Methods

According to guidelines in mTBI, clinician directed interventions are suggested over self-directed cognitive computer-based programs and exercises.[28,29] A reoccurring and central theme in the literature emphasizes that there is little data to support the use of isolated cognitive drills and exercises via workbooks and/or computer programs which aim to treat domain-specific impairments, as these practices very rarely translate into meaningful improvement in everyday activities and the real-world context.[7]

Traditional rehabilitation procedures have focused on training repetitive decontextualized drills in clinic to improve memory, problem solving, attention, and/or judgment.[21] The lack of efficacy of this type of training is particularly relevant to direct training of memory, problem-solving, and social function.[7] Despite this information, there is a degree of room for appropriately selected methods to be incorporated into cognitive treatment. For example, preliminary data suggests that therapist directed use of computer-based programs combined with instructional support might be beneficial in treating cognition for individuals with mTBI.[23,39]

Upon selection of these modalities, it is critical to reinforce that direct training of cognitive processes must be carried out concurrently with other function specific therapeutic interventions and strategies.[7] According to the evidence-based reviews conducted by the Brain Injury Interdisciplinary Special Interest Group of the American Congress of Rehabilitation Medicine, domain specific treatments should be completed in conjunction with external, internal, compensatory, and metacognitive training.[5] Outlined below are domain-specific cognitive difficulties that are typically found upon comprehensive cognitive assessment in mTBI and brief descriptions of current practice standards and/or treatment methods.

Attention Deficits and Reduced Processing Speed

After mTBI, many patients report attention difficulties.[5] The importance of attention functioning is well established as it is necessary to maintain nearly all aspects of daily life. Even mild attention symptoms can contribute to long-term dysfunction in the patient with acquired brain injury.[6] Interestingly, issues paying attention may be associated with slowed information processing speed, which may be derived from diffuse axonal injury.[5]

Attention is divided into a hierarchy of subsystems, which can simultaneously be very vulnerable to disruption and amendable to treatment. These constructs include focused, sustained, selective, alternating, and divided attention systems.[6] Studies have revealed that patients with attention deficits after mTBI have significantly slowed processing speed in comparison to matched controls, particularly when placed under conditions requiring higher levels of attention control (e.g., dual-task demands).[40] Speed of information processing is our ability to attend to, organize, integrate, manipulate, and apply information in an efficient and timely manner. When this is impacted, an overarching clinical goal is to enable patients to increase their self-awareness of attentional skills and apply strategies or modifications to improve their efficiency within the real world.[5]

It is critical to acknowledge that a number of studies have shown the positive effects of Attention Process Training (APT) in individuals with mTBI. This restorative impairment-based program utilizes frequent and intensive rehearsal of tasks that require high levels of self-monitoring and use of working memory. APT stands apart from traditional domain-specific treatment modalities as it has been shown to improve attention performance on both practiced and nonpracticed tasks of similar cognitive demand.[3,6]

It is appreciated that a number of studies support the notion that *strategies* devoted to attending to solving a problem are more effective than drill training aimed at improving attention in isolation.[7] This is in alignment with Cicerone et al.,[41] whom indicates that the practice standard for the remediation of attention deficits after acquired brain injury should include both direct attention training and metacognitive training. For example, direct attention training with computer-based interventions may be considered as an adjunct to treatment when there is therapist involvement and contribution.[41]

Memory Deficits

Memory problems following acquired brain damage are common.[42] Memory can be quantified as the ability to absorb, store, and retrieve information through a complex set of processes and/or the inclusion of multiple subsystems.[5] These different types of memories (e.g., short-term, working, long-term, retrospective, prospective, etc.) are distinct in nature. However, the distinction between declarative (explicit or conscious recall) and nondeclarative (implicit or automatic recall) memory are particularly relevant to cognitive rehabilitation.[5,6] As declarative memory is conscious, it is encoded and retrieved using working memory and thereby enhanced by learning strategies. Nondeclarative memory alternatively, does not require conscious awareness of learning.[3]

In terms of mTBI, there is no research that supports domain-specific drill training (e.g., exercises to recall lists) to enhance memory.[7] Rather, practice-standards for mild memory impairments suggest the use of internalized strategies (e.g., imagery), external memory compensations (e.g., notebook, dairy), and cognitive assistive technologies (e.g., smart applications) to enhance retrieval.[28,41,43] Training the use of these types of memory compensations and aids within activities of daily living continues to be efficacious and consistently supported by empirical evidence.[5,42]

Executive Function Impairments

Many patients after mTBI report difficulty with high-level executive function, which significantly impacts their ability to participate in both the social and occupational demands of their activities of daily living.[5] Executive function refers to a group of top-down mental processes. Three core executive functions include inhibition (e.g., self-control, interference control), working memory and cognitive flexibility, which serve as the catalysts for higher-order executive functions such as problem solving, reasoning, and planning.[44] Executive function is essential for success and facilitates purposeful behavior in nearly every aspect of daily life.[5,44]

In terms of mTBI, there is a robust body of literature that supports the use of instructional procedures for training individuals to regulate their behavior and thinking, otherwise known as metacognitive strategy training, which serves as the practice standard.[3,41,43] Cognitive remediation strategies that positively impact executive function outcomes in this population is further characterized by the implementation of problem identification, strategic thinking, weighing pros and cons of solutions, monitoring performance, and improving self-regulation.[5]

Social-Communication Issues

Social-communication involves a multifaceted and complex interaction of cognitive domains, an awareness of social constructs and boundaries, and emotional regulation. After acquired brain injury, changes in social-communication and pragmatic skills are one of the most frequent and disabling consequences. They often lead to decreased participation in social activities and overall life satisfaction. In the context of mTBI, these social communication deficits are likely a multifactorial consequence of changes in cognition, behavior, and comorbid psychiatric issues (e.g., PTSD).[3,5,45]

Although there is minimal evidence that discrete social-skills training (e.g., eye-contact drills) generalizes to real-world socialization,[3] there are emerging studies to validate implementation of social-communication strategies with mTBI patients when these deficits do occur. Specific interventions for functional communication including pragmatic conversational training is recommended as a practice standard.[41] Additionally, social skills training in the group setting has shown effectiveness.[43] According to Dahlberg et al.,[45] a randomized control trial revealed that implementation of specific group interventions to improve social communication skills in patients with TBI were efficacious and that treatment effects were maintained at follow up. However, experts caution that the available evidence of social skills intervention is in its infancy and predominantly supports approaches that are context-sensitive to the individual's communication, integrates executive function interventions, situational training and personalized counseling.[46]

Differentiating External, Internal, and Metacognitive Strategies

External and internal cognitive strategies are applied in order to enhance learning, recall of target information and teach functional skills.[3] Training these cognitive strategies refers to both *internal* thinking processes which require conscious thought by the user and *external* strategies that attempt to lessen cognitive demands and accommodate for new changes. These strategies, both internal and external, can be executed across tasks, contexts, and environments.[3,7] In general, internal memory strategies help patients encode incoming information (e.g., via elaboration, visualization, mnemonics, etc.) and external memory aids help patients manage information (e.g., physical aids such as notebooks, planners, smart applications, alarms, etc.)[3,5]

On the other hand, metacognition or "thinking about thinking" includes one's ability to view, observe and assess more basic cognitive processes as they are applied to cognitive subsystems. It includes ones self-awareness, self-monitoring and self-control of cognition while executing an activity.[47] Cognitive strategies and metacognitive strategies are closely intertwined and contingent upon one another. However, the major distinction between them lies in their overarching goal and how the information is used.[48]

Implementing metacognitive strategies provides systematic instruction for when, where and why to use a strategy and determine its success, throughout the phases of learning. This may be achieved by training ordered sequences of self-questioning, self-monitoring, and problem-solving.[3,47] A patient must have sufficient metacognitive ability to *independently* utilize internal and external strategies,[3] as it involves overseeing whether a cognitive goal has been met.[48] Simply stated, while internal and external strategies provide the method to carry out and potentially achieve desired targets, use of metacognitive strategies involves the self-regulation of their success.

External Strategies

External aids are typically tools or devices that allow patients to compensate for cognitive limitations via an alternative method while simultaneously reinforcing residual cognitive skills. External, compensatory aids provide high levels of clinical utility as they can be implanted into natural settings, within Activities of Daily Living, increase independence, and promote participation. There are multiple external aids that should be customized via needs-based assessment and training across contexts.[3,49,50]

According to Sohlberg et al.,[51] a meta-analysis of the literature regarding the use of external cognitive aids revealed that all studies assessed described improved functioning on memory-related activities. Furthermore, positive outcomes were reported in regards to increased independence, functional daily tasks such as arriving to appointments on time, improved navigation, reduced amount of repetitive or perseverative questioning, and enhanced performance on vocational activites.[51] Of note, of the 21 studies reviewed the following external aids were utilized, in order of highest to lowest frequency:

- notebook, diary, or daily planner;
- hand-held calendar devices;
- voice organizers;
- pagers; and
- mobile phones.[51]

According to Sohlberg and Turkstra,[3] selection of external aids may also be further quantified and tailored to patients needs based upon assessment of the following key characteristics:

- target task (e.g., multifunctional vs specialized);
- device complexity (e.g., high tech vs low tech);
- availability (e.g., commercial vs clinical);
- target population (e.g., degree of cognitive function); and
- cognitive compensation (e.g., memory vs problem solving).

Overall, use of external cognitive aids and memory compensation strategies have been substantiated by empirical evidence, particularly for patients with mTBI and mild memory impairment.[21] However, experts warn that there is a critical gap in the research in addressing factors that lead to long-term generalization and maintenance of these aids, such as consistent and descriptive training procedures.[51]

Internal Strategies

Internal, remediation-oriented strategies aim to facilitate access to stored semantic networks, assist with storage and retrieval, and help with encoding of new information via a deeper level of processing.[3,50] Traditionally, the training of internal or restorative strategies is not recommended for individuals with acquired brain injury secondary to their high level of abstraction and demands on awareness. However, patients with mTBI typically benefit from use of internal strategies as the majority of their cognitive skills are preserved. Internal strategies are often helpful for small, concise, domain-specific bodies of information that remain consistent or do not change.[6] For example, evidence suggests that expanding and elaborating on information via imagery training may improve delayed recall of everyday relevant verbal materials (e.g., appointments).[21,52] Internal memory strategies with supporting research include:

- visual imagery (e.g., structured imagery training, method of loci);
- verbal elaboration (e.g., first-letter mnemonics and rhymes, elaborative encoding);
- visual and verbal elaboration (e.g., story method); and
- retrieval techniques (e.g., alphabetic searching, mental retracing).[3]

Metacognitive Strategies

Metacognition or "thinking about thinking" is a set of processes, which plan, monitor and assess performance.[53] It includes both monitoring one's own thoughts and behaviors and then utilizing that data to apply changes, which subsequently improve one's own thoughts and behaviors.[3] This is suited as the prefix "meta" is defined as "involving change."[54]

Metacognitive strategies involve step-by-step procedures that place emphasis on goal formulation, self-monitoring, comparative performance assessment between target goals and current status, strategic decision-making, feedback-based modifications, and implementation of behavior change.[5] According to members of the DCoE and DVBIC consensus conference, "robust literature supports the use of metacognitive strategy training as an intervention for executive function impairments due to TBI."[55] Additionally, metacognitive strategy training has been recommended as a practice standard for impairments including executive function, emotional self-regulation, deficits of attention, neglect, and memory impairments.[41]

Procedures for systematic metacognitive strategy instruction may include forming goals that are relevant to everyday needs, strategy planning to initiate goals, self-monitoring of performance, revising and tailoring methodology as needed, reformulating decisions and/plans, and reviewing effective and ineffective moments.[21] For example Levine et al.,[56] utilized self-instruction and/or metacognitive strategy training for patients with TBI by implementing the following five-step training:

- Asking, "What am I doing" → "STOP!"
- Defining the "main task" → "DEFINE"
- Listing the steps → "LIST"
- Asking, "Do I know the steps?" → "LEARN"
- Asking, "Am I doing what I planned to do?" → "CHECK"[6,56]

Of note, given the complex nature and overlap of multiple cognitive systems when addressing metacognition, it is not clear whether metacognitive strategies are rehabilitative or compensatory in nature. Despite debate regarding underlying mechanisms, evidence points to meaningful brain changes in response to this systematic experience.[3]

Assistive Technology for Cognition

Assistive Technology for Cognition (ATC) can be defined as any assistive technology (AT) that facilitates independence, increases participation, and improves the daily functional capabilities of persons with cognitive impairments. According to the Assistive Technology Act of 2004, the term assistive technology encompasses "any item, piece of equipment, or product system, whether acquired commercially, modified, or customized, that is used to increase, maintain, or improve functional capabilities of individuals with disabilities."[57–59]

There are a plethora of tools and devices ranging from low tech to high tech, that fall under this definition. This includes the external aids (under the section on *External Strategies*) and those that are highly technical such as specialized computer devices/software.[7] However, with the rise of an increasingly dependent and ever-evolving technological society, the use and definition of ATC and AT should be monitored and clinicians are encouraged to remain up-to-date on the practical and logistic implications of potential changes. This is particularly pertinent with the rise of literature on ATC.

Emerging evidence suggests that ATC may be useful to support memory, attention, executive-function, initiation, organization, visual-spatial skills, and language comprehension.[7,58] Additionally, a number of devices have been designed specifically to address deficits in these areas.[21,58] Preliminary research on smartphones demonstrate promising potential for improving functional independence following TBI.[60] This is further appreciated as the US Department of Veteran Affairs recently released their "Concussion Coach" application, which is aimed to educate users about concussion, screen and track symptoms, implement management tools, and provide community-based resources and supports.[61]

In considering the use of ATC for cognitive rehabilitation, experts recommend a variety of principles to ensure appropriate selection and training. These include thoughtful and systematic selection, high frequency training in naturalistic contexts, and reinforcement of patient knowledge, impact, and use of the device.[7]

Generalization and Maintenance

It is widely acknowledged in the literature that mastery and generalization of cognitive skills is typically facilitated through fading learning supports, incorporating and increasing use of targets in variable contexts, and maximizing patient engagement.[3] However, a major strength of the cognitive rehabilitative plan for patients with mTBI is that the generalization of skills which indicate readiness for discharge, is an integral and deeply embedded principal of the therapeutic process from the onset of treatment.[7]

This is evident within structured domain-specific protocols, such as APT, which provides a generalization component.[6] It is also apparent with application of Functional Outcome Measures and GAS. Even in the early stages of treatment, patients and clinicians are working toward generalization and are cultivating a system collaboratively to reflect on the positive outcomes of treatment.[7]

As patients increase their self-management skills, it is appropriate to taper off therapy gradually and/or schedule follow-up at a later date in order to ensure maintenance of skills.[7] Of note, prior to discharge, a discussion which identifies barriers to maintenance, plans for recovery in instances of set-backs, and plans for high-risk situations can foster and promote the long-term maintenance of skills.[6]

CONCLUSION AND RECOMMENDATIONS

The rehabilitative management of the cognitive sequelae associated with mTBI is a quickly evolving, complex and rewarding field. It is equipped with a wide range of intervention approaches and a steadily rising base of evidence-based literature, which clinicians have an ethical obligation to monitor over time.

Reflections on the fundamentals of rehabilitative science, the evolution of cognitive rehabilitation practices as they pertain to mTBI, and up-to-date descriptions of current methodology further emphasizes the need for consistent investigation and consideration of the multifactorial nature of cognitive issues in mTBI. Critical thinking within comprehensive cognitive assessment and for selection of intervention methods must be applied in order to provide effective and meaningful care. Furthermore, domain-specific rehabilitative, compensatory and metacognitive methods as they pertain to attention, memory, executive function, and communication skills should be cultivated in a collaborative and patient-centric manner in order to optimize outcomes.

In culmination, it is recommended that readers review the multiple tools for clinical practice that are provided in Appendix A: Suggested Supplements and Rehabilitative Resources. These resources are compiled by leading experts in the field of cognition and mTBI and include in depth details regarding treatment recommendations, clinical guidelines, and instructive and supportive forms for both clinicians and patients. It is acknowledged that this chapter is limited by its aim to provide a concise understanding of cognitive rehabilitation as it pertains to mTBI. Therefore, clinicians remain responsible for evaluating its use not only in isolation, but also in conjunction with alternative and extensive guides.

APPENDIX A: SUGGESTED SUPPLEMENTS AND REHABILITATIVE RESOURCES

To assist readers, multiple tools for clinical practice are provided on Appendix A, Suggested Supplements and Rehabilitative Resources, which include treatment recommendations, clinical guidelines and "how-to" information, in addition to supportive forms for both clinicians and patients.

VA/DoD Guidance Documents for Cognitive Rehabilitation:

- DoD/VA mTBI Clinical Practice Guideline (Feb 2016).
- Clinicians Guide to Cognitive Rehabilitation in Mild Traumatic Brain Injury: Application for Military Service Members and Veterans (December 2016).
- Cognitive Rehabilitation for Military Personnel with Mild Traumatic Brain Injury and Chronic Post-Concussional Disorder: Results of April 2009 Consensus Conference (Helmick et al., 2010, NeuroRehabilitation, 26, 239−255).
- Mild Traumatic Brain Injury Rehabilitation Toolkit (Borden Institute, 2015):
     Chapter 7—Cognition Assessment and Intervention (Radomski et al.)
     Chapter 9—Performance and Self-Management, Work, Social and School Roles (Davidson et al.)
     Chapter 11—Health Related Quality of Life/Participation Assessment (Weightman et al.)
- Speech-Language Pathology Clinical Management Guidance: Cognitive−Communication Rehabilitation for Combat-Related Concussion/Mild Traumatic Brain Injury. (SLP Working Group, 2012). Borden Institute, 2015.
- Cognitive-Communication Rehabilitation for Combat-Related Mild Traumatic Brain Injury (Cornis-Pop et al., Sep 2012, J. Rehabil. Res. Develop., 49(7), xi−xxxi).
- Clinical Management Guidance: Occupational Therapy and Physical Therapy for Mild Traumatic Brain Injury. (OT/OT Work Team, 2012). Borden Institute, 2015.
- Occupational Therapy for Service Members with Mild Traumatic Brain Injury (Radomski et al., Sep−Oct 2009, American Journal of Occupational Therapy, 64, 646−655).
- SCORE Manuals (SCORE Study Team, 2015)
     http://dvbic.dcoe.mil/research/study-manuals
- Social Cognition Rehabilitation for Veterans with TBI and PTSD: A Treatment Workbook (McCarron, Dasgupta, Campbell, & Adams. 2014). Washington, DC: DVA.
     Available from authors: Kelly. McCarron@va.gov, Megan. Dasgupta@va. gov
- CogSMART (Twamley et al., 2008) http://www.cogsmart.com/
Page 17 of 107 12/2016.

Cognitive Rehabilitation in the Civilian Sector (including moderate TBI):

- Coaching College Students with Executive Function Problems (Kennedy, M. R. T., 2017). NY: Guilford Publishing. (available June, 2017).
- Cognitive Rehabilitation Manual: Translating Evidence-Based Recommendations into Practice (American Congress of Rehabilitation Medicine; Haskins et al., 2012). ACRM Publishing.
- Optimizing Cognitive Rehabilitation: Effective Instructional Methods (Sohlberg, M. M., & Turkstra, L. S., 2011). NY: The Guilford Press.
- Cognitive Rehabilitation: An Integrative Neuropsychological Approach (Sohlberg M.M, Mateer).
- Practice Guidelines for TBI from the Academy of Neurologic Communication Disorders and Sciences (ANCDS):
     http://www.ancds.org/evidence-based-clinical-research

- Evidence-based practice guidelines for instructing individuals with acquired memory impairments: What have we learned in the past 20 years? [Elhardt, L., Sohlberg, M. M., Kennedy, M. R. T., Coelho, C., Turkstra, L., Ylvisaker, M., & Yorkston, K. (2008). Neuropsychological Rehabilitation,18(3), 300–342].
- Self-regulation after traumatic brain injury: A framework for intervention of memory and problem solving [Kennedy, M. R. T., & Coelho, C. (2005). Seminars in Speech and Language,26, 242–255].
- Intervention for executive functions after traumatic brain injury: A systematic review, meta-analysis and clinical recommendations [Kennedy, M. R. T., Coelho, C., Turkstra, L., Ylvisaker, M., Sohlberg, M. M., Yorkston, K., Chiou, H. H. & Kan, P. F. (2008). Neuropsychological Rehabilitation, 18(3), 257–299].
- Practice guidelines for direct attention training [Sohlberg, M., Avery, J., Kennedy, M.R. T., Coelho, C., Ylvisaker, M., Turkstra, L., & Yorkston, K. (2003). J Med Speech-Language Pathol, 11(3), xix–xxxix].
- Evidence based practice for the use of external aids as a memory rehabilitation technique [Sohlberg, M. M., Kennedy, M. R. T., Avery, J., Coelho, C., Turkstra, L., Ylvisaker, M., & Yorkston, K. (2007). J Med Speech Pathol, 15(1)].
- Reflections on evidence-based practice and rational clinical decision making. [Ylvisaker, M., Coelho, C., Kennedy, M., Sohlberg, M., Turkstra, M., Avery, J., & Yorkston, K. (2002). J Med Speech-Language Pathol., 10(3), xxv–xxxiii].
- The Concussion Coach app for Veterans

  https://mobile.va.gov/app/concussion-coach

References

1. Sloman SA. Opening editorial: the changing face of cognition. *Cognition.* 2015;**135**:1–3.
2. Malec JF, Smigielski J, DePompolo R. Goal attainment scaling and outcome measurement in post-acute brain injury rehabilitation. *Phys Med Rehabil* 1991;**72**(2):138–43.
3. Sohlberg MM, Turkstra LS. *Optimizing cognitive rehabilitation: effective instructional methods.* New York: The Guilford Press; 2011.
4. Center DaVBI. *DoD worldwide numbers for TBI;* 2017 [updated 3/12/2017]. Available from: <http://dvbic.dcoe.mil/dod-worldwide-numbers-tbi>.
5. Weightman M, Radomski M, Mashima P, Roth C. *Mild traumatic brain injury rehabilitation toolkit.* Fort Sam Houston, TX: Texas Borden Institute; 2015.
6. Sohlberg MM, Mateer C. *Cognitive rehabilitation: an integrative neuropsychological approach.* New York: Guilford Press; 2001.
7. *Clinician's guide to cognitive rehabilitation in mild traumatic brain injury: application for military service members and veterans;* 2016. 4/21/17. Available from: http://www.asha.org/uploadedFiles/ASHA/Practice_Portal/Clinical_Topics/Traumatic_Brain_Injury_in_Adults/Clinicians-Guide-to-Cognitive-Rehabilitation-in-Mild-Traumatic-Brain-Injury.pdf.
8. Boake C. A history of cognitive rehabilitation of head-injured patients, 1950 to 1980. *Head Trauma Rehabil* 1989;**4**(3):1–8.
9. Center DaVBI. *History.* 3/12/17. Available from: http://dvbic.dcoe.mil/history.
10. Cifu D, Cohen S, Lew H, Jaffee M, Sigford B. The history and evolution of traumatic brain injury rehabilitation in military service members and veterans. *J Phys Med Rehabil* 2010;**89**(8):688–94.
11. Brown J. What about cognitive rehabilitation therapy? 2012. 12/21/17. Available from: http://www.cs.amedd.army.mil/FileDownloadpublic.aspx?docid=814f3bd5-8c7b-4da3-bf40-051dfb813350.

12. Hoge C, McGurk D, Thomas J, Cox A, Engel C, Castro C. Mild traumatic brain injury in U.S. soldiers returning from Iraq. *N Engl J Med* 2008;**358**(5):453–63.

13. Cooper DB, Bunner AE, Kennedy JE, Balldin V, Tate DF, Eapen BC, et al. Treatment of persistent post-concussive symptoms after mild traumatic brain injury: a systematic review of cognitive rehabilitation and behavioral health interventions in military service members and veterans. *Brain Imag Behav* 2015;**9**(3):403–20.

14. Veterans WH. *Afghanistan and Iraq (OEF & OIF)* 12/28/17. Available from: http://www.wehonorveterans. org/veterans-their-needs/needs-war-or-trauma/afghanistan-and-iraq-oef-oif.

15. Roth C, Srarch S. *ANCDS newsletter. Special interview.* 2009. 5/2/2017. Available from: <http://www.ancds. org/assets/docs/Newsletter/ancds fall_2009_1.pdf>.

16. Institute of Medicine. *Cognitive rehabilitation therapy for traumatic brain injury: evaluating the evidence.* Washington, DC: The National Academies Press; 2011. Available from: http://nationalacademies.org/ hmd/~/media/Files/Report%20Files/2011/Cognitive-Rehabilitation-Therapy-for-Traumatic-Brain-Injury-Evaluating-the-Evidence/CRTforTBIreportbrief2.pdf.

17. *Affairs USDoV. VA research on traumaticbrain injury.* 4/12/17. Available from: <http://www.research.va.gov/ topics/tbi.cfm > —intro.

18. Team SS Chapter 1: Study of cognitive rehabilitaiton effectivenesstrial: overview. 2015. 1/21/17. http://dvbic. dcoe.mil/files/DVBIC_SCORE-Study-Manual_Chapter1_Study-of-Cognitive-Rehabilitation-Effectiveness-Clinical-Trial-Overview.pdf.

19. Gonzalez Rothi LJ, Musson N, Rosenbek JC, Sapienza CM. Neuroplasticity and rehabilitation research for speech, language, and swallowing disorders. *J Speech Lang Hear Res* 2008;**51**(1):S222.

20. Kleim JA, Jones TA. Principles of experience-dependent neural plasticity: implications for rehabilitation after brain damage. *J Speech Lang Hear Res* 2008;**51**:S225–39.

21. Cornis-Pop M, Mashima P, Roth C, MacLennan D, Picon L, Hammond C. Cognitive-communication rehabilitation for combat-related mild traumatic brain injury. *J Rehabil Res Dev* 2012;**49**(7). xi–xxxii.

22. Raskin Aea. *Neuroplasticity and rehabilitation.* New York: Guilford Press; 2011.

23. Janak JC, Cooper DB, Bowles AO, Alamgir AH, Cooper SP, Gabriel KP, et al. Completion of multidisciplinary treatment for persistent postconcussive symptoms is associated with reduced symptom burden. *J Head Trauma Rehabil* 2017;**32**(1):1–15.

24. Koehler R, Wilhelm E, Shoulson I. *Committee on cognitive reahbilitation therapy for traumatic brain injury IoM. Cognitive rehabilitation therapy for traumatic brain injury: evaluating the evidence.* Washington, DC: National Academies Press; 2011.

25. *Cognitive rehabilitation: the evidence, funding and case for advocacy in brain injury* [Internet]. Brain Injury Association of America. 2006. http://www.brainline.org/content/2012/06/what-about-cognitive-rehabilitation-therapy.html

26. Kesler SR, Adams HF, Blasey CM, Bigler ED. Premorbid intellectual functioning, education and brain size in traumatic brain injury: an investigation of the cognitive reserve hypothesis. *Appl Neuropsychol* 2003;**10**(3):153–62.

27. Fay TB, Yeates KO, Taylor HG, Bangert B, Dietrich A, Nuss KE, et al. Cognitive reserve as a moderator of postconcussive symptoms in children with complicated and uncomplicated mild traumatic brain injury. *J Int Neuropsychol Soc* 2010;**16**(1):94–105.

28. Defense DoVADo. *VA/DoD clinical practice guideline for Management of Concussion/Mild Traumatic Brain Injury.* Clinician Summary. 2015.

29. Defense DoVADo. *VA/DoD clinical practice guideline for Management of Concussion/Mild Traumatic Brain Injury.* Full Guideline. 2016.

30. Prevention CfDCa. *TheICF: an overview.* 4/28/2017. Available from: <http://www.cdc.gov/nchs/data/icd/ icfoverview_finalforwho10sept.pdf >.

31. Turkstra LS, Coehlo C, Ylvisaker M. The use of standardized tests for individuals with cognitive-communication disorders. *Semin Speech Lang* 2005;**26**(4):215–22.

32. Coehlo C, Ylvisaker M, Turkstra LS. Nonstandardized assessment approaches for individuals with traumatic brain injuries. *Semin Speech Lang* 2005;**26**(4):223–41.

33. The American Occupational Therapy Association I. *Community reintegration of persons with brain injury.* 5/1/ 17. Available from: <http://www.aota.org/-/media/Corporate/Files/AboutOT/Professionals/WhatIsOT/ RDP/Facts/Community > Reintegration fact sheet.ashx.

IV. DIAGNOSIS AND TREATMENT

34. Team S.S. *Chapter 2: Study of cognitive rehabilitation effectiveness clinical trial: pyschoeducational interventions for persistent post-concussion symptoms following combat-related mild traumaticbrain injury;* 2015. 1/21/17.
35. Ehlhardt L, Sohlberg MM, Kennedy M, Coehlo C, Ylvisaker M, Turkstra LS. Evidence-based practice guidelines for instructing individuals with neurogenic memory impairments: what have we learned in the past 20 years? *Neuropsychol Rehabil* 2008;**18**(3):300−42.
36. Mittenberg W, Tremong G, Zielinski R, Rayls K. Cognitive-behavioral prevention of postconcussion syndrome. *Arch Clin Neuropsychol* 1996;**11**(2):139−45.
37. Miller W, Rollnick S. *Motivational interviewing. Helping People Change.* 3rd ed. New York: The Guilford Press; 2013.
38. Medley A, Powell T. Motivational interviewing to promote self-awareness and engagement in rehabilitation following acquired brain injury: a conceptual review. *Neuropsychol Rehabil* 2010;**20**(4):481−508.
39. Team S.S. *Chapter 3: Study of cognitive rehabilitation effectiveness clinical trial: computerized cognitive rehabilitation interventions for persistent symptoms following mild traumatic brain injury.* 2015. 1/21/17. Available from: <http://dvbic.dcoe.mil/files/DVBIC_SCORE-Study-Manual_Chapter3_Computerized-Cognitive-Rehabilitation-Interventions.pdf>.
40. Cicerone K. Attention deficits and dual task demands after mild traumatic brain injury. *Brain Inj* 1996;**10**(2):79−89.
41. Cicerone K, Langenbahn D, Braden C, Malec JF, Kalmar K, Fraas M. Evidence-based cognitive rehabilitation: updated review of the literature from 2003 through 2008. *Arch Phys Med Rehabil* 2011;**92**(4):519−30.
42. Wilson B, Emslie H, Quirk K, Evans J, Watson P. A randomized control trial to evaluate a paging system for people with traumatic brain injury. *Brain Inj* 2005;**19**(11):891−4.
43. Roth C. *Combat-related mild traumatic brain injury (mTBI): the role of speech-language pathologists in working with wounded warriors;* 2009.
44. Diamond A. Executive functions. *Annu Rev Psychol* 2013;**64**:135−68.
45. Dahlberg C, Cusick C, Hawley L, Newman J, Morey C, Harrison-Felix C. Treatment efficacy of social communication skills training after traumatic brain injury: a randomized treatment and deferred treatment controlled trial. *Arch Phys Med Rehabil* 2007;**88**(12):1561−73.
46. Ylvisaker M, Turkstra LS, Coehlo C. Behavioral and social interventions for individuals with traumatic brain injury: a summary of the research with clinical implications. *Semin Speech Lang* 2005;**26**(4):256−67.
47. Kennedy M, Coehlo C. Self-regulation after traumatic brain injury: a framework for intervention of memory and problem solving. *Semin Speech Lang* 2005;**26**(4):242−55.
48. Livingston J. *Metacognition: an overview.* 5/3/17. Available from: http://gse.buffalo.edu/fas/shuell/cep564/metacog.htm.
49. *Using external aids to compensate for memory and organizational problems post-TBI.* 5/4/17. Available from: <http://www.brainline.org/content/2011/04/using-external-aids-to-compensate-for-memory-and-organizational-problems-post-tbi.html>.
50. Perna R, Perkey H. Internal memory rehabilitation strategies in the context of post-acute brain injury: pilot study. *Int J Neurorehabilitation* 3:199. https://doi.org/10.4172/2376-0281.1000199.
51. Sohlberg MM, Kennedy M, Avery J, Coehlo C, Turkstra LS. Evidence-based practice for the use of external aids as a memory compensation technique. *J Speech Lang Pathol* 2007;**15**(1):xv-li.
52. Kaschel R, Della Sala S, Cnagallo A, Falhbock A, Laaksonen R, Kazen M. Imagery mnemonics for the rehabilitation of memory: a randomized group controlled trial. *Neuropsychol Rehabil* 2002;**12**(2):127−53.
53. Chick N. *Metacognition.* 5/7/17. Available from: <http://cft.vanderbilt.edu/guides-sub-pages/metacognition/>.
54. Dictionary C. *Definition of "meta-".* Available from: <http://dictionary.cambridge.org/us/dictionary/english/meta>.
55. Helmick K. Members of consensus C. Cognitive rehabilitation for military personnel with mild traumatic brain injury and chronic post-concussional disorder: results of April 2009 consensus conference. *NeuroRehabilitation* 2010;**26**(3):239−55.
56. Levine B, Robertson I, Clare L, Carter G, Hong J, Wilson B. Rehabilitation of executive functioning: an experimental-clinical validation of goal management training. *J Int Neuropsychol Soc* 2000;**6**(3):299−312.
57. Gillespie A, Best C, O'Neil B. Cognitive function and assistive technology for cognition: a systematic review. *J Int Neuropsychol Soc* 2012;**18**(1):1−19.
58. Leopold A, Lourie A, Petras H, Elias E. The use of assistive technology for cognition to support the performance of daily activities for individuals with cognitive disabilities due to traumatic brain injury: the current state of the research. *NeuroRehabilitation* 2015;**37**(3):359−78.

59. *H.R. 4278 — 108th Congress: Assistive Technology Act of 2004.* 5/24/17. Available from: <http://www.govtrach. us/congress/bills/108/hr4278 >.
60. Wong D, Sinclair K, Seabrook E, Mcay A, Ponsford J. Smartphones as assistive technology following traumatic brain injury: a preliminary study of what helps and what hinders. *Disabil Rehabil* 2016;1–8. Available from: https://doi.org/10.1080/09638288.2016.1226434.
61. *Health. USDoVAVM. Concussion Coach.* 5/26/17. Available from: <http://mobile.va.gov/app/concussion-coach >.

Emerging Technologies for Diagnosing Mild Traumatic Brain Injury

Carey D. Balaban, PhD[1], Kurt D. Yankaskas[2] and Alexander Kiderman[3]

[1]Departments of Otolaryngology, Neurobiology, Communication Sciences & Disorders, and Bioengineering, University of Pittsburgh, Pittsburgh, PA, United States [2]Code 34, Office of Naval Research, Arlington, VA, United States [3]Chief Technology Officer, Neuro Kinetics, Inc., Pittsburgh, PA, United States

OVERVIEW AND INTRODUCTION

Mild traumatic brain injury (mTBI) has proven to be challenging to document objectively.[1] In the presence of a documented traumatic event (blunt trauma, acceleration deceleration, or blast energy exposure), it is defined primarily by the presence and persistence of symptoms that include difficulty thinking clearly, feeling slowed down, difficulty concentrating, difficulty remembering new information, headache, "pressure in the head", neck pain, feeling slowed down or like "in a fog," difficulty concentrating or remembering, confusion and/or drowsiness, fuzzy or blurry vision, nausea or vomiting (acutely), dizziness, sensitivity to light or noise, balance problems, feeling tired or having no energy, irritability, sadness, increased emotional lability, nervousness or anxiety, sleep disruptions (too much or too little), and trouble falling asleep.

By definition, there was, at worst, only a momentary change in conscious and there are no structural imaging findings showing intracranial injury. Emerging technologies, then, are needed to document functional deficits that are associated with the status of symptoms and objective clinical signs during acute, subacute, and chronic periods after injury.

Technologies for objective diagnosis of mTBI face several challenges. A first challenge is a clear differentiation between the empiricist approach of "finding markers" and the neuroscientific, precision-medicine goal of differentially diagnosing the biological bases for

Neurosensory Disorders in Mild Traumatic Brain Injury
DOI: https://doi.org/10.1016/B978-0-12-812344-7.00022-4

the underlying impairments. Even empirical biomarkers for "dinged and not quite right" need to be understood in terms of sites and mechanisms related to the injury and biological attempts to recover. Hence, is also essential that a selective and specific test battery is used to help identify the nature of the injury and track the clinical course in subacute and chronic post-injury periods in what is likely a very heterogeneous group. Are there specific and sensitive findings for injury that are nonlocalizing? Are there specific and sensitive localizing tests to refine a diagnosis? Are there specific and sensitive findings to document resolution of the symptoms and, more importantly, to indicate readiness for partial, or complete, return to normal activities? One incontrovertible consideration, though, is that evidence of delivery of energy to the head remains a necessary contextual criterion for diagnosis of mTBI.

A second challenge is to transcend the temptation to limit testing to familiar contemporary technologies. For example, harmonic sinusoidal oscillation testing of the horizontal vestibulo-ocular reflex or an audiogram may be of limited utility as a specific tool for mTBI testing. Rather, one must consider developing assessment technologies that can illuminate the sources of symptoms and signs that: (1) appear spontaneously; (2) can resolve or transform over time; and (3) can be elicited by dynamic test challenges.

A third challenge is to design technologies that provide rapid, selective, and specific identification of individual patients as having definitive mTBI. This standard requires a test battery to clearly distinguish the affected individuals as outliers from the population termed unaffected, normal, or subclinical. Pragmatically, the test will distinguish affected from unaffected individuals with a history of energy delivery to the head. This level of performance is a persistent "devil in the detail" for emerging technologies; it is a far more rigorous standard than simply showing a significant difference between partially overlapping groups of positive and negative subjects. Adherence to this standard drives the technology development process beyond the mechanical empiricism of enumerating similarities and differences between presentations by markers. Rather, the biologic bases behind specific and sensitive become important clues for making scientific sense of the clinical status of affected individuals.

A fourth challenge is to disentangle the neurosensory consequences of cognition and cognitive effects of neurosensory processing deficits. For example, there are strong interactive comorbidities between balance dysfunction and anxiety,[2,3] and interactions between vestibular dysfunction and cognitive performance.[4] This is manifested more widely in concussion by potential interactions between comorbid sequelae of balance and other neurosensory deficits, psychiatric signs and symptoms, personality features, and cognitive signs and symptoms. This vexing issue was noted more than a decade ago when Moore et al.[5] called for a concerted effort to move concussion from categorical classification to dimensional conceptualization. It was reiterated by Hoge et al.[6] in reference to veterans with mTBI. The prevailing view has been to assess, as independent domains, neurocognitive function, self-reported symptoms, and postural (or balance) control.[7]

The tendency to somaticize appears to be associated with a prolonged recovery from a concussion (defined by symptom reporting).[8,9] Path analysis suggested that somatization has an influence postconcussive recovery by influencing symptom expression.[8] Common sense appears to dictate that controls for propensity to self-report symptoms (and their persistence) need to be considered as part of any new assessment tools.

OBJECTIVE DIAGNOSTIC TECHNOLOGIES

Neurocognitive Tests and Symptom Inventories

The basic instruments for neurocognitive tests and symptom inventories are described in detail in a recent report of the IOM and NRC[10] and were reviewed comprehensively by Arrieux et al.[11] These tests[7,12,13] include the Intermediate Post-Concussion Assessment and Cognitive Test (ImPACT®), King–Devick Test, Automated Neuropsychological Assessment Metrics (ANAM), Sport Concussion Assessment Tool (currently fifth edition, or SCAT5) and new products such as BrainCheck.[14] They can be administered automatically on electronic devices (computer, tablet, or personal digital device). The neurocognitive or neuropsychological components require baseline testing and typically include timed performance assessments inspired by the classic Trail-Making Tests.[15,16] The anecdotal reports that athletes who "low ball" their baseline performance reveal an inherent problem with operational use of these tests.

The Post-Concussion Symptom Scale (PCSS, 25 items)[17] and the Sport Concussion Assessment Tool (5th edition, 22 items) symptom evaluation scale[18] are validated tools in common use. They elicit the seven-point Likert scale responses to describe the severity of similar lists of symptoms (Table 22.1). The scales are used to generate global symptom scores as a proxy for impairment. Because symptom perceptions can be affected by comorbid psychiatric, emotional, and personality features,[19,20] it is important to focus on instruments that can assess somatization[8,9] and relevant psychological and psychiatric features, such as the Minnesota Multiphasic Personality Inventory®-2 and Beck Depression Inventory.[20,21] Other validated instruments are useful to examine the perceived impact of specific symptoms on activities and quality of life. For example, the Dizziness Handicap Inventory is a validated, 25-item instrument that uses a three-point ordinal scale to express the attribution of symptoms and perceived handicaps to dizziness.[22–27] Hence, it is not surprising that DHI scores (and scores) showed reasonably strong positive correlation with responses to dizziness and mild cognitive impairment related items on the SCAT symptom inventory.[28] Other tests of the functional impact of symptoms, such as the Headache Impact Test (HIT-6™), are worthy of consideration for gauging impairment and improvement. A more general approach is represented by the recent efforts of the Patient-Reported Outcomes Information System (PROMIS) to develop a TBI Quality of Life (TBI-QOL) set of item banks focused on more severe forms of TBI.[29,30] The development of quality-of-life items specifically tailored to acute, subacute, and chronic mTBI could be of considerable value for monitoring therapeutic outcomes and the assessment of readiness to return to normal activities.

Identification of symptom clusters and gender differences in symptom expression is one direction for a concerted effort to move from categorical classification to dimensional conceptualization of concussion, as called for more than a decade ago by Moore et al.[5] Dimensional reduction by principal component or factor analysis of self-reporting symptom questionnaires are an approach for identifying symptom items associated with similar underlying dimensions. Table 22.1 shows published results of reductions from two studies, both utilizing groups of normal subjects and acute mild TBI subjects.[28,31] There are some strong similarities between the results, but also differences that may reflect

TABLE 22.1   Symptom Scales and Initial Identification of Symptom Dimensions or Clusters in mTBI

Symptom (Rated Item)	PCSS Position and (Cluster) From Factor Analysis	SCAT Position and (Cluster) From Principal Component Analysis
Headache	1 **(CogMigFatig)**	1 **(PTHx-M)**
Nausea	2 **(CogMigFatig)** (Somatic)	
Vomiting	3 (Som)	4 (Nauseated)
Balance problems	4 **(CogMigFatig)**/(Somatic)	7 *(Dizzy-MCog)*
Dizziness (spinning or moving sensation)	5 **(CogMigFatig)**/(Somatic)	5 *(Dizzy-MCog)*
Fatigue	7 **(CogMigFatig)**	15 **(PTHx-M)**
Trouble falling asleep	8 (Sleep)	22 *(Emotional Lability)*
Drowsiness	11 **(CogMigFatig)**	17 **(PTHx-M)**
Sensitivity to light	12 **(CogMigFatig)** (Som))	8 **(PTHx-M)**
Sensitivity to noise	13 **(CogMigFatig)**	9 **(PTHx-M)**
Irritability	14 **(CogMigFatig)***(Affect)*	19 *(Emotional Lability)*
Sadness	15 *(Affect)*	20 *(Emotional Lability)*
Nervous/anxious	16 *(Affect)*	21 *(Emotional Lability)*
Feeling more emotional than usual	17 *(Affect)*	18 *(Emotional Lability)*
Feeling slowed down	19 **(CogMigFatig)**	10 **(PTHx-M)**
Feeling like "in a fog"	20 **(CogMigFatig)**	11 (Cervicogenic)
Difficulty concentrating	21 **(CogMigFatig)**	13 *(Dizzy-MCog)*
Difficulty remembering	22 **(CogMigFatig)**	14 *(Dizzy-MCog)*
Visual problems/blurred vision	23 **(CogMigFatig)** (Som)	6 *(Dizzy MCog)*
Other	24	
Lightheadedness	6	—
Sleeping more than usual	9 **(CogMigFatig)** (Sleep)	—
Sleeping less than usual	10 (Sleep)	—
Numbness or tingling	18 (Som)	—
"Pressure in head"	—	2 **(PTHx-M)**
Neck pain	—	3 (Cervicogenic)
"Don't feel right"	—	12 **(PTHx-M)**
Confusion	—	16 *(Dizzy-MCog)*

differences in the items and the orders of common items on the two instruments. Factor analysis of PCSS responses, obtained within 7 days of injury, indicated a four-component solution after mTBI, a cognitive-migraine-fatigue (CogMigFatig) factor, an affective (Affect) factor, a somatic (Somatic) factor a sleep-related (Sleep) factor.[31] A principal component analysis of SCAT questionnaire within 6 days of injury, on the other hand, identified a posttraumatic headache/migraine (PTHx-M) cluster, a dizzy with mild cognitive impairment (Dizzy-MCog) cluster, an emotional lability cluster, a cervicogenic cluster and nausea.[28] Despite similar objective findings, female participants with mTBI showed higher scores than their male counterparts on the PTHx-M cluster, while males with mTBI reported higher scores on the Dizzy-MCog complex. These data motivate a deeper exploration of symptom dimensions in acute, subacute and chronic mTBI.

Resting Brain Network Activity

Structural imaging, including tractography,[32–34] is expected to yield negative findings for mTBI. However, network science and network functional imaging[35,36] have been proposed as promising approaches to measure objective changes in brain activity that underlie the signs and symptoms of mTBI. A first step has been examination of resting network activity from fMRI,[37] MEG,[38,39] and EEG[40–42] recordings from patients with mTBI. These studies suggest that there may be modifications in activity between the default mode network (posterior cingulate cortex, inferior parietal cortex, inferolateral temporal cortex, and ventral anterior cingulate cortex) and frontal cortex,[43] which overlaps with the executive network (dorsolateral prefrontal and anterior cingulate cortex). A more recent study indicates that there are frequency specific differences in regional amplitude coupling in mTBI patients as well as augmented slow wave activity.[44] However, the correlational evidence linking these resting activity measures to the degree of cognitive impairment,[43] changes in emotional regulation and the persistence of posttraumatic complaints[45] is not strong.

Tests of Sensory Evoked Brain Activity in Specific Networks

Stimulus-evoked EEG activity has been used standardly for clinical evaluation of neurosensory processing. Commonly used diagnostic tests include evaluation of visual and auditory evoked potentials, which are conducted in conjunction with perceptual tests (e.g., perimetry and audiograms) to provide a more comprehensive clinical picture. Specialized visual and auditory sensory evoked potentials studies have shown some promise in documenting mTBI.

Auditory Processing

Metrics associated with central auditory processing are a very promising emerging area for assessment of mTBI. A proportion of Individuals with chronic blast mTBI[46] and concussions from blunt trauma show abnormal results on tests of central auditory processing, which includes speech comprehension in noise.[46,47] A very interesting study has shown alterations in speech-evoked frequency-following responses (also called the auditory brainstem response to complex sounds, or cABR) in children who were tested during the subacute stage mTBI.[48] These findings motivate further development of objective metrics associated with processing and interpreting complex auditory information.

Visual Evoked Potentials

Chronic mTBI may show P100 latency delays (>15%) or amplitude reductions, but normal ERPs.[49] Luminance affects latency and amplitude differentially in chronic mTBI patients versus controls.[50] It has also been shown that binasal occlusion and base-in prisms induce altered changes in patients with chronic mTBI (1−27 years prior to testing).[51] These findings motivate further development of objective measures of the effects of mTBI on brain activity associated with complex visual information processing.

Quantitative Neurologic, Neurotologic, and Neurophthalmologic Diagnosis

The documentation of abnormal versional (conjugate) and vergence eye movements after mTBI has been a focus of a considerable research interest for more than a decade.[52−61] Technologies that incorporate some of these published results are available commercially. Here, the focus is on considerations for further test development, including oculomotor tests that incorporate cognitive tasks.

The temporal resolution, spatial resolution, and processing algorithms for eye tracking are essential technical considerations for precise and reproducible eye movement assessment. For video−oculographic methods, sampling at a rate of at least 500 Hz appears to be necessary to assess rapid eye movement timing and trajectories[62−64]; eye position resolution and precision should be ≪1 degree of arc for horizontal, vertical and torsional deviations. For slower eye movements, lower sampling rates (e.g., 100 Hz) are adequate.

Commercially available, advanced, video-based binocular eye tracking with infrared illumination systems currently provide independent, real time measurements for each eye at rates up to 250 Hz for horizontal and vertical movements and at rates up to 100 Hz for torsional eye movements. Video techniques generally use dark pupil tracking with detection algorithms for either the pupil centroid or an assumption of the pupil as an ellipse. Advanced eye tracking software uses a symmetric mass center algorithm that is designed to provide more accurate measurements when the pupil area is partially occluded.

Anti-saccade and predictive saccade tasks are examples of oculomotor tests with an embedded task that have proven to be useful in detecting mTBI objectively.[52,54,65,66] Antisaccade task performance can be regarded as a core executive function of response inhibition.[67] An enhanced prosaccadic error rate in subjects with acute mTBI may suggest disruption of inhibitory networks that are critical for suppressing the prosaccade. The inhibitory contributions likely involve the frontal cortex, as well as output from substantia nigra and pars reticulata to the superior colliculus and thalamus.[67] Like other saccades, an antisaccade is thought to be programmed in the frontal cortex. The predictive saccade task, on the other hand, is related to networks controlling timing of movements guided by short-term memory cues, including crus I of the cerebellum, medal prefrontal cortex, posterior cingulate cortex, posterior insula, and parahippocampal gyrus.[68] Because reactive saccades differentially engage a network that is related to oculomotor execution,[68] reactive and predictive saccade performance has differential diagnostic value for objective detection of damaged cortical pathways.

Anomalous convergence eye movements have been described in TBI patients on the basis of qualitative and semiquantitative observations and quantitative oculographic metrics.[55,57,58,61] Demonstrations of convergence insufficiency have typically focused on the range of effective responses to static endpoints (near and far targets).[55,57,58] The results of analyses of convergence performance with oculographic methods in a diverse group of TBI patients[61] suggest that dynamic assessment is a promising line of investigation for differential diagnosis.

Inspection of the consensual pupillary light reflex is a component of standard neurologic exams. Standard commercially available pupillometers can record the time course of the pupillary constriction and subsequent dilation (relaxation) objectively. Metrics for performance have included the onset latency and dynamic assessments of the velocity and magnitude of the response. A recent review[69] provides a comprehensive characterization of the current state-of-the-art. It is suggested that a more parsimonious and mechanistically insightful analyses could emerge by estimating parameters of formal models of the dynamics of these responses[70–75] in mTBI patients and matched control groups.

The near response is a coordinated motor program of disconjugate eye movements, pupil size changes, and lens accommodation. The near triad movement[76] is a coordinated execution of convergent eye movements, pupillary constriction (miosis), and increased lens curvature to track an approaching object. Divergent eye movement, pupillary dilation, and decreased lens curvature occur while tracking a receding object. On-going studies suggest that mTBI can be detected through an examination of the coordination of eye and pupil movements during a binocular disparity tracking task.

Static and dynamic posturography have become standard tools in the assessment of balance disorders. Hence, they have been used for assessing postural control disorders in mTBI (see, e.g.,[77–79]). The method has been useful to document objectively acute, subacute, and chronic emergent and/or a persistent sign of mTBI is responses to step or sinusoidal perturbations of the substrate or visual surround. Notable areas for development are the expanded use of measures such as approximate or Shannon entropy[80–82] to characterize system performance and applying ternary pseudorandom perturbations[83] to rapidly measure the transfer function for postural control.

Gait analysis has also been applied to assess anomalous locomotion after mTBI. Earlier studies in patients with moderate TBI (grade II concussion) demonstrated the utility of dual task cognitive paradigms for revealing gait disorders,[84] which was consistent with the emerging picture of the utility of multiple task challenges for gait assessment in other neurological disorders.[85] Based upon this earlier literature, more recent studies show promising results with applying dual task paradigms in patients with mTBI.[86,87]

Autonomic Function

The exacerbation of symptoms of mTBI by exercise has motivated examination of changes in autonomic motor control after injury. The high frequency relative power of heart rate variability was reported to be reduced during physical exertion in patients with chronic mTBI.[88] In a small sample of athletes, approximate entropy (a measure of complexity of beat-to-beat variability) was depressed transiently in the acute period after mTBI.[89] It is of further interest that altered patterns of heart rate variability may be a component of (developing) comorbid conditions such as anxiety.[90]

Olfactory System Function

Olfactory dysfunction has been documented for some patients with mTBI after either blast-wave exposure[91,92] or blunt-trauma exposures.[93–95] The olfactory system is, in fact, positioned strategically as a sentinel for head injury. The direct exposure of the olfactory epithelium and nerves to ambient air within the nasal cavity confers vulnerability to blast waves, particulate debris, and aerosols from explosions. Bone transmission of energy from impact to the ethmoid bone is another source of potential trauma to the nerves. The olfactory bulb and nerves also play and important role in glymphatic drainage into the lymphatic system.[96] The relatively superficial location of the olfactory bulb, tracts, and piriform cortex also may confer vulnerability for impact to the skull.

Olfactory testing approaches include threshold or suprathreshold Identification tests with a standardized set of odorant stimuli (e.g., Sniffin' Sticks™ or the Alberta Smell Test).[97] Results from limited studies suggested efficacy in detecting acute mTBI,[93] and that olfactory test results may have some prognostic capability for detection of residual brain dysfunction in longer term, follow-up neurological examinations.[91] Similarly, it was reported that acute olfactory dysfunction may be associated with an elevated likelihood of adverse cognitive, neuropsychiatric, and functional outcomes during longer term follow-ups.[95] The current technologies have the advantage of simplicity, but the test–retest reliability is lower than for standard oculomotor and vestibular testing.[97] Further studies are clearly needed to explore the roles of olfactory tests in screening batteries.

Biochemical Markers

Considerable effort has been invested in identifying reliable blood or cerebrospinal biochemical markers for mTBI from among markers for moderate and severe injury, with no definitive outcomes.[98–100] To date, the most definitive finding may be that some biomarkers help acutely in detecting the potentially CT-positive individuals among those who appear to be mild clinically. For example, Sharma et al.[101] reported that blood levels of the gelatinase, matrix metalloproteinase-2, C-reactive protein, and creatinine kinase type B can help differentiate CT-positive from CT-negative patients from samples drawn at an average of 7–10 hours post-injury. Prognostic applications seem to be a promising direction for biomarker technology development.

FUTURE DIRECTIONS: TOWARD INTEGRATIVE PRECISION MEDICAL DIAGNOSIS

A review of the emerging technologies for detecting and monitoring the course of mTBI suggests that we are still at a very rudimentary stage for developing comprehensive, rational approaches that illuminate the underlying neurobiology of the condition. However, there are promising indications that a combination of refined symptom inventories, objective tests of higher order neurological and cognitive functions, and sentinel biomarker tests can be both diagnostic in the short-term for the severity of impairment and prognostic for the likelihood of subacute and chronic complications. We can now envision test systems that integrate dual-tasking, virtual/augmented reality and accelerometer technologies for more challenging, and ecologically valid clinical testing. The same advanced test systems will doubtless see wide usage in the rehabilitation sciences, as well. A major caveat, though, is that the development of these precision technologies will require rigorous attention to patient stratification criteria and both temporal and functional milestones that are critical to monitoring the clinical course of the individual.

References

1. Arnold M, Bousser M, Fahrni G, et al. Vertebral artery dissection: presenting findings and predictors of outcome. *Stroke* 2006;**37**:2499−503.
2. Balaban CD, Jacob RG, Furman JM. Neurologic bases for comorbidity of balance disorders, anxiety disorders and migraine: neurotherapeutic implications. *Expert Rev Neurother* 2011;**11**:379−94.
3. Balaban CD, Thayer JF. Neurological bases for balance-anxiety links. *J Anxiety Disorders* 2001;**15**:53−79.
4. Smith PF. The vestibular system and cognition. *Curr Opin Neurol* 2017;**30**:84−9.
5. Moore EL, Terryberry-Spohr L, Hope DA. Mild traumatic brain injury and anxiety sequelae: a review of the literature. *Brain Injury* 2006;**20**:117−32.
6. Hoge CW, Goldberg HM, Castro CA. Care of war veterans with mild traumatic brain injury—flawed perspectives. *N Engl J Med* 2009;**360**:1588−91.
7. Brolio SP, Puetz TW. The effect of sport concussion on neurocognitive function, self-report symptoms and postural control: a meta-analysis. *Sports Med* 2008;**38**:53−67.
8. Nelson LD, Tarima S, LaRoche AA, et al. Preinjury somatization symptoms contribute to cliical recovery after sport-related concussion. *Neurology* 2016;**86**:1856−63.
9. Root JM, Zuckerbraun NS, Wang L, et al. History of somatization is associated with prolonged recovery from concussion. *J Pediatr* 2016;**174**:139−44.
10. Graham R, Rivara FP, Ford MA, Spicer CM. *Sports concussions in youth: improving the science, changing the culture. Council IoMaNR.* Washington, DC: National Academies Press (US); 2014.
11. Arrieux JP, Cole WR, Ahrens AP. A review of the validity of computerized neurocognitive assessment tools in mild traumatic brain injury assessment. *Concussion* 2017;**2**:CNC31.
12. Brolio SP, Macciocchi SN, Ferrara MS. Sensitivity of the concussion assessment battery. *Neurosurgery* 2007;**60**:1050−8.
13. Alsalaheen B, Stockdale K, Pechumer D, Broglio SP. Validity of the immediate post-concussion assessment and cognitive testing. *Sports Med* 2016;**46**:1487−501.
14. Yang S, Flores B, Magal R, et al. Diagnostic accuracy of tablet-based software for the detection of concussion. *PLoS One* 2017;**12**:e0179352.
15. Reitan RM. Validity of the Trail Making Test as an indicator of organic brain damage. *Percept Motor Skills* 1958;**8**:271−6.
16. Tombaugh TN. Trail making test A and B: normative data stratified by age and education. *Arch Clin Neuropsychol* 2004;**19**:203−14.
17. Collins MW, Iverson GL, Lovell MR, McKeag DB, Norwig J, Maroon J. On-field predictors of neuropsychological and symptom deficit following sports-related concussion. *Clin J Sports Med* 2003;**13**:222−9.
18. Echemendia RJ, Meeuwisse WH, McCrory P, et al. The sport concussion assessment tool, 5th edition: Background and rationale. *Br J Sports Med* 2017;**51**:848−50.
19. Ruff RM, Camenzuli L, Mueller J. Miserable minority: emotional risk factors that influence the outcome of a mild traumatic brain injury. *Brain Injury* 1996;**10**:551−66.
20. Mooney G, Speed J. The association between mild traumatic brain injury and psychiatric conditions. *Brain Injury* 2001;**15**:865−77.

21. Mooney G, Speed J, Sheppard S. Factors related to recovery after mild traumatic brain injury. *Brain Injury* 2005;**19**:975–87.
22. Asmundson GJG, Stein MB, Ireland D. A factor analytic study of the dizziness handicap inventory: does it assess phobi avoidance in vestibular referrals? *J Vestibular Res* 1999;**9**:63–8.
23. Jacobson GP, Newman WW. Tne development of the dizziness handicap inventory. *Arch Otolaryngol Head Neck Surg* 1990;**116**:424–7.
24. Perez N, Garmendia I, Garcia-Granero M, Martin E, Garcia-Tapia R. Factor analysis and correlation between Dizziness Handicap Inventory and dizziness characteristics and impact on quality of life scales. *Acta Oto-Laryngol* 2001;**545**(Suppl):145–54.
25. Tamber A-L, Wilhelmsen KT, Strand LI. Measurement properties of Dizziness Handicap Inventory by cross-sectional and longitudinal designs. *Health Quality Life Outcomes* 2009;**7**:101.
26. Vereeck L, Truijen S, Wuyts FL, Van De Heyning PH. Internal consistency and factor analysis of the Dutch version of the Dizziness Handicap Inventory. *Acta Oto-Laryngol* 2007;**127**:788–95.
27. Vereeck L, Truijen S, Wuyts FL, Van De Heyning PH. The Dizziness Handicap Inventory and its relationship with functional balance performance. *Otol Neurotol* 2008;**28**:87–93.
28. Hoffer ME, Szczupak M, Kiderman A, et al. Neurosensory symptom complexes after acute mild traumatic brain injury. *PLoS One* 2016;**11**:e0146039.
29. Sherer M, Poritz JMP, Tulsky DS, Kisala PA, Leon-Novelo L, Ngan E. Conceptual structure of health-related quality of life for persons with traumatic brain injury: confirmatory factor analysis of the TBI-QOL. *Arch Phys Med Rehabil* 2017. Available from: http://dx.doi.org/10.1016/j.apmr.2017.04.016.
30. Tulsky DS, Kisala PA, Victorson D, et al. TBI-QOL: development and calibration of item bankd to measure patient reported outcomes after traumatic brain injury. *J Head Trauma Rehabil* 2016;**31**:40–51.
31. Kontos AP, Elbin RJ, Schatz P, et al. A revised factor structure for the post-concussion symptom scale: baseline and postconcussion factors. *Am J Sports Med* 2012;**40**:2375–84.
32. Narayana PA, Yu X, Hasan KM, et al. Multi-modal MRI of mild traumatic brain injury. *NeuroImage: Clin* 2015;**7**:87–97.
33. Mohammadian M, Roine T, Hirvonen J, et al. High angular resolution diffusion-weighted imaging in mild traumatic brain injury. *NeuroImage: Clin* 2017;**13**:174–80.
34. Aoki Y, Inokuchi R. A voxel-based meta-analysis of diffusion tensor imaging in mild traumatic brain injury. *Neurosci Biobehav Rev* 2016;**66**:119–26.
35. Stam CJ. Modern network science of neurological disorders. *Nat Rev Neurosci* 2014;**15**:683–95.
36. Eierud C, Craddock RC, Fletcher S, et al. Neuroimaging after mild traumatic brain injury: review and meta-analysis. *NeuroImage: Clin* 2014;**4**:283–94.
37. Sharp DJ, Scott G, Leech R. Network dysfunction after traumatic brain injury. *Nat Rev Neurol* 2014;**10**:156–66.
38. Tarapore PE, Findlay AM, LaHue SC, et al. Resting state magnetoencephalography functional connectivity in traumatic brain injury. *J Neurosurg* 2013;**118**:1306–16.
39. Vakorin VA, Doesburg SM, da Costa L, Pang JR, Taylor MJ. Detecting mild traumatic brain injury using resting state magnetoencephalographic connectivity. *PLoS Comput Biol* 2016;**12**:e1004914.
40. Nuwer MR, Hovda DA, Schrader LM, Vespa PM. Routine and quantitative EEG in mild traumatic brain injury. *Clin Neurophysiol* 2005;**116**:2001–25.
41. Arciniegas DB. Clinical electrophysiologic assessments and mild traumatic brain injury: state-of-the-science and implications for clinical practice. *Int J Psychophysiol* 2011;**82**:41–52.
42. Haneef Z, Levin HS, Frost JD, Mizrahi EM. Electroencephalography and quantitative electroencephalography in mild traumatic brain injury. *J Neurotrauma* 2013;**30**:653–6.
43. Mayer AE, Mannell MV, Ling J, Gasparovic C, Yeo RA. Functional connectivity in mild traumatic brain injury. *Human Brain Map* 2011;**32**:1825–35.
44. Dunkley BT, Da Costa L, Bethune A, et al. Low-frequency connectivity is associated with mild traumatic brain injury. *NeuroImage: Clin* 2015;**7**:611–21.
45. van der Horn HJ, Liemburg EJ, Scheenen ME, de Koning ME, Spikman JM, van der Naalt J. Graph analysis of functional brain networks in patients with mild traumatic brain injury. *PLoS One* 2017;**12**:e0171031.
46. Gallun FJ, Diedesch AC, Kubli LR, et al. Performance on tests of central auditory processing by individuals exposed to high-intensity blasts. *J Rehabil Res Develop* 2012;**49**:1005–24.
47. Hoover EC, Souza PE, Gallun FJ. Auditory and cognitive factors associated with speech-in-noise complaints following mild traumatic brain injury. *J Am Acad Audiol* 2017;**28**:325–39.

48. Kraus N, Thompson EC, Krizman J, Cook K, White-Schwoch T, LaBella CR. Auditory biological marker of concussion in children. *Sci Rep* 2016;**6**:39009.
49. Freede S, Hellerstein LF. Visual electrodiagnostic findings in mild traumatic brain injury. *Brain Injury* 1997;**11**:25—36.
50. Fimreite V, Cuiffreda KJ, Yadav NK. Effect of luminance on the visually-evoked potential in visually-normal individuals and in mTBI/concussion. *Brain Injury* 2015;**29**:1199—210.
51. Yadav NK, Ciuffreda KJ. Effect of binasal occlusion (BNO) and base-in prisms on the visual evoked potential (VEP) in mild traumatic brain injury (mTBI). *Brain Injury* 2014;**28**:1568—80.
52. Heitger MH, Anderson TJ, Jones RD, Dalrymple-Alford JC, Frampton CM, Ardagh MW. Eye movement and visuomotor arm movement deficits following mild closed head injury. *Brain* 2004;**127**:575—90.
53. Suh M, Kolster R, Sarkar R, McCandliss R, Ghajar J. Consortium CaNR. Deficits in predictive smooth pursuit after mild traumatic brain injury. *Neurosci Lett* 2006;**401**:108—13.
54. Heitger MH, Jones RD, McLeod AD, Snell DL, Frampton CM, Anderson TJ. Impaired eye movements in post-concussion syndrome indicate suboptimal brain function beyond the influence of depression, malingering or intellectual ability. *Brain* 2009;**132**:2850—70.
55. Thiagarajan P, Cuiffreda KJ, Ludlam DP. Vergence dysfunction in mild traumatic brain injury (mTBI): a review. *Ophthalmic Physiol Opt* 2011;**31**:456—68.
56. Capo-Aponte JE, Urosevich TG, Temme LA, Tarbett A, Sanghera NK. Visual dysfunctions and symptoms during the subacute stage of blast-induced mild traumatic brain injury. *Military Med* 2012;**177**:804—13.
57. Alvarez TL, Kim EH, Vicci VR, Dhar SK, Biswal BB, Barrett AM. Concurrent visual dysfunctions in convergence insufficiency with traumatic brain injury. *Optom Vis Sci* 2012;**89**:1740—51.
58. Mucha A, Collins MW, Elbin RJ, et al. A brief Vestibular/Ocular Motor Screening (VOMS) assessment to evaluate concussions: preliminary findings. *Am J Sports Med* 2014;**42**:2479—86.
59. Cifu DX, Wares JR, Hoke KW, Wetzel PA, Gitchel G, Carne W. Differential eye movements in mild traumatic brain injury versus normal controls. *J Head Trauma Rehabil* 2015;**30**:21—8.
60. Samadani U, Ritlop R, Reyes M, et al. Eye tracking detects disconjugate eye movements associated with structural traumatic brain injury and concussion. *J Neurotrauma* 2015;**32**:548—56.
61. Tyler CW, Likova LT, Mineff KN, Elsaid AM, Nicholas SC. Consequences of traumatic brain injury for human vergence dynamics. *Front Neurol* 2015;**5**:282.
62. McCamy MB, Otero-Millan J, Leigh J, et al. Simultaneous recordings of human microsaccades and drifts with a contemporary video eye tracker and the serach coil technique. *PLoS One* 2015;**10**:e0128428.
63. Houben MMJ, Goumans J, van der Steen J. Recording three dimenional eye movements: scleral search coils versus video oculography. *Invest Ophthalmol Vis Sci* 2006;**47**:179—87.
64. van der Geest JN, Frens MA. Recording eye movements with video-oculography and scleral search coils: a direct comparison of two methods. *J Neuroxcience Methods* 2002;**114**:185—95.
65. Balaban CD, Hoffer ME, Szczupak M, et al. Oculomotor, vestibular, and reaction time tests in mild traumatic brain injury. *PLoS One* 2016;**11**:e162168.
66. Hoffer ME, Balaban CD, Szczupak M, et al. The use of oculomotor, vestibular, and reaction time tests to assess mild traumatic brain injury (mTBI) over time. *Laryngosc Invest Otolaryngol* 2017;**2**:157—65.
67. Munoz DP, Everling S. Look away: the anti-saccade task and the voluntary control of eye movement. *Nat Rev Neurosci* 2004;**5**:218—28.
68. Lee SM, Peltsch A, Kilmade M, et al. Neural correlates of predictive saccades. *J Cognitive Neurosci* 2016;**28**:1210—27.
69. Ciuffreda KJ, Joshi NR, Truong JQ. Understanding the effects of mild traumatic brain injury on the pupillary light reflex. *Concussion* 2017;**2**:CNC36.
70. Stark L, Sherman PM. A servoanalytic study of the consensual pupil reflex to light. *J Neurophysiol* 1957;**20**:17—26.
71. Sun F, Krenz WC, Stark LW. A systems model for pupil size effect. I. Transient data. *Biol Cybern* 1983;**48**:101—8.
72. Sun F, Tauchi P, Stark L. Dynamic pupillary response controlled by the pupil size effect. *Exp Neurol* 1983;**82**:313—24.
73. Krenz WC, Stark L. Systems model for pupil size effect. II. Feedback model. *Biol Cybern* 1985;**51**:391—7.
74. Schor CM. A dynamic model of cross-coupling between accommodation and convergence: simulations of step and frequency responses. *Optom Vis Sci* 1992;**69**:258—69.
75. Privitera CM, Stark LW. A binocular pupil model for simulation of relative afferent pupil defects and the swinging flashlight test. *Biol Cybern* 2006;**94**:215—24.

76. Leigh RJ, Zee DS. *The neurology of eye movements*. 4th ed. New York: Oxford University Press; 2006.
77. Guskiewicz KM, Ross SE, Marshall SW. Postural stability and neuropsychological deficits after concussion in collegiate athletes. *J Athletic Train* 2001;**36**:263–73.
78. Hoffer ME, Balaban CD, Gottschall KR, Balough BJ, Maddox MR, Penta JR. Blast exposure: vestibular consequences and associated characteristics. *Otol Neurotol* 2010;**31**:232–6.
79. Pan T, Liao K, Roenigk K, Daly JJ, Walker MF. Static and dynamic postural stability in veterans with combat-related mild traumatic brain injury. *Gait Post* 2015;**42**:550–7.
80. Buckley TA, Oldham JR, Caccese JB. Postural control deficits identify lingering post-concussion neurological deficits. *J Sport Health Sci* 2016;**5**:61–9.
81. Sosnoff JJ, Brolio SP, Shin S, Ferrara MS. Previous mild traumatic brain injury and postural conrol dynamics. *J Athletic Train* 2011;**46**:85–91.
82. Gao J, Hu J, Buckley TA, White K, Hass C. Shannon and Renyi entropies to classify effects of mild traumatic brain injury on postural sway. *PLoS One* 2011;**6**:e24446.
83. Peterka RJ. Sensorimotor integration in human postural control. *J Neurophysiol* 2002;**88**:1097–118.
84. Catena RD, van Donkelaar P, Chou L-S. Cognitive task effects on gait stability following concussion. *Exp Brain Res* 2007;**176**:23–31.
85. Yogev G, Hausdorff JM, Giladi N. The role of executive function and attention in gait. *Movem Disord* 2008;**23**:329–472.
86. Fino PC. A preliminary study of longitudinal differences in local dynamic stability between recently concussed and healthy athletes during single and dual-task gait. *J Biomech* 2016;**49**:1983–8.
87. Howell DR, Osternig LR, Chou L-S. Single-task and dual-task tandem gait test performance after concussion. *J Sci Med Sport* 2017;**20**:622–6.
88. Abaji JP, Currier D, Moore RD, Ellemberg D. Persisting effects of concussion on heart rate variability during physical exertion. *J Neurotrauma* 2016;**33**:811–17.
89. La Fountaine MF, Hefferman KS, Gossett JD, Bauman WA, De Meersman RE. Transient suppression of heart rate complexity in concussed athletes. *Autonom Neurosci* 2009;**148**:101–3.
90. Liao K-H, Sung C-W, Chu S-F, et al. Reduced power spectra of heart rate variability are correlated with anxiety in patients with mild traumatic brain injury. *Psych Res* 2016;**243**:349–56.
91. Ruff RI, Ruff SS, Wang X-F. Headaches among Operation Iraqi Freedom/Operation Enduring Freedom veterans with mild traumatic brain injury associated with exposures to explosions. *J Rehabil Res Dev* 2008;**45**:941–52.
92. Xydakis MS, Mulligan LP, Smith AB, Chen CH, Lyon DM, Belllucio L. Olfactory impairment and traumatic brain injury in blast-injured combat troops: a cohort study. *Neurology* 2015;**84**:1559–67.
93. De Kruik JR, Leffers P, Menheere PPCA, Meerhoff S, Rutten J, Twijnstra A. Olfactory function after mild traumatic brain injury. *Brain Injury* 2003;**17**:73–8.
94. Proskynitopoulos PJ, Stippler M, Kasper EM. Post-traumatic anosmia in patients with mild traumatic brain injury (mTBI): a systematic and illustrated review. *Surg Neurol Int* 2016;**7**:S263–75.
95. Schofield PW, Moore TM, Gardner A. Traumatic brain injury and olfaction: a systematic review. *Front Neurol* 2014;**5**:5.
96. Jessen NA, Munk ASF, Lundgaard I. Nedergaard. The glymphatic system--a beginner's guide. *Neurochem Res* 2015;**40**:2583–99.
97. Hummel T, Sekinger B, Wolf SR, Pauli E, Kobal G. 'Sniffin' Sticks': olfactory performance assessed by the combined testing of odor identification, odor discrimination and olfactory threshold. *Chem Senses* 1997;**22**:39–52.
98. Zetterberg H, Smith DH, Blennow K. Biomarkers of mild traumatic brain injury in cerebrospinal fluid and blood. *Nat Rev Neurol* 2013;**9**:201–10.
99. Agoston DV, Shutes-David A, Peskind ER. Biofluid markers of traumatic brain injury. *Brain Injury* 2017;**31**:1195–203.
100. Peskind ER, Kraemer B, Zhang J. Biofluid biomarkers of mild traumatic brain injury: whither plasma tau. *AMA Neurol* 2015;**72**:1103–5.
101. Sharma R, Rosenberg A, Bennett ER, Laskowitz DT, Acheson SK. A blood-based biomarker panel to risk-stratify mild traumatic brain injury. *PloS One* 2017;**12**:e0173798.

Emerging Treatment Modalities

Sara Bressler, BS[1], Mikhaylo Szczupak, MD[2] and Michael E. Hoffer, MD, FACS[2]

[1]Department of Otolaryngology, University of Miami, Miller School of Medicine, Miami, FL, United States [2]Department of Otolaryngology, University of Miami, Miami, FL, United States

INTRODUCTION

Traumatic brain injury (TBI) occurs as the result of forceful motion of, or impact to, the head. Although there are different severities of TBI based on the mechanism and extent of injury, this chapter will focus on mild TBI (mTBI). The definition of mTBI and its significance have been described repeatedly in this book.

The injuries sustained in mTBI can be characterized as either primary or secondary. Primary injuries are defined as focal brain damage due to direct physical trauma at the moment of impact. These are usually irreversible, and the best treatment is initial prevention. Secondary injuries develop as a consequence of the primary injury. Following direct tissue damage, a set of pathologic processes are initiated including edema, inflammation, metabolic dysfunction, excitotoxicity, oxidative stress, and apoptosis (Fig. 23.1). These injuries are delayed and can occur for days to months after the primary injury.[1] As such, secondary injuries are often more devastating than the primary injury. Given their delayed effects, secondary injuries are an ideal target for mTBI therapy and can be addressed to improve functional outcomes. The treatment of secondary injuries is an evolving topic and is the focus of this chapter.

Current mTBI treatment modalities take a conservative approach with steroids and mannitol as the mainstays of treatment. Intensive patient education and cognitive rehabilitation have additionally shown modest effectiveness for mTBI.[2] However, the focus of this chapter will be on emerging therapies, many of which involve neuroprotective strategies with the goal to prevent and/or reduce brain damage induced by secondary injury. Since conservative treatments have an optimal administration period and natural recovery eventually reaches a point of maximal return, emerging therapies may serve to prolong the recovery window and the possibility for continued, meaningful improvement in function. The therapies discussed in may supplement, and eventually replace, existing treatment modalities.

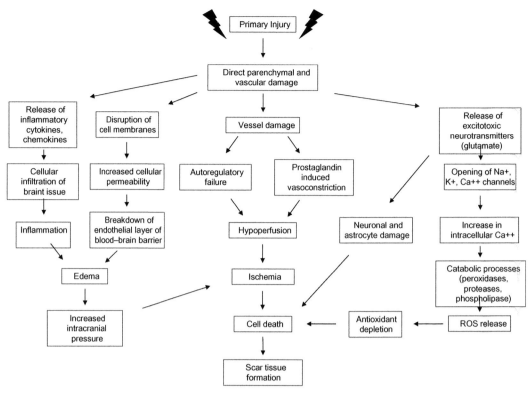

FIGURE 23.1   Pathophysiology of secondary injury following traumatic brain injury.

DEVELOPMENT AND TESTING OF EMERGING TREATMENTS

The development and testing of new agents for TBI and mTBI is a complex process. First, researchers must identify the pathways responsible for injury in TBI. This is followed by the identification of existing agents or development of new agents that affect a given pathway. Researchers may also choose therapies with widespread effects on a variety of pathways. Unfortunately, there is still a great deal of uncertainty about the pathophysiology responsible for secondary injury in TBI, making the development of targeted treatment even more difficult.

Once a candidate agent or technique is identified, the pathway to human use is challenging. A full discussion of this process is well beyond the scope of this chapter, but a brief description of the necessary steps is useful. Before the mechanism of action and efficacy can be demonstrated, a confirmed basic formulation and the safety issues must be examined. After this process, early preclinical trials must be performed to confirm the mechanism of action and efficacy of the agent in animal models with induced TBI. If improved outcomes are demonstrated, dose response work is required to determine how and when to best utilize the agent. After this, drugs and devices must be produced in a special fashion approved for use in humans according to good laboratory practice guidelines. In the case of a drug, the product must be retested in a subset of the prior preclinical work before moving to human use, which usually involves an additional four experimental steps. All of these steps are governed by regulatory bodies such as the US Federal Drug Administration (FDA) and European Medicines Agency (EMA).

A glance at the steps involved in taking a new strategy from concept to the bench to the bedside clearly demonstrates the time, effort, and money involved in this process. As such, it is sobering to realize that the available emerging treatments we will discuss may be limited by whether or not the therapy is protected and whether the owner of the therapy has the capital necessary to support moving the therapy forward. Oftentimes the scientists involved in the research have a vested interest in the outcome and this, unfortunately, must be carefully scrutinized. However, it is vitally important to point out that incorrectly assuming a conflict of interest as a means of discrediting valuable contributions to our therapeutic armamentarium is an equally, if not more, troubling phenomenon and those who engage is this often do so to "protect their turf."

N-ACETYLCYSTEINE/ANTIOXIDANTS/FREE RADICAL SCAVENGERS

The pathophysiology of TBI is complex and multifaceted. Although a variety of pathways are currently being explored, the free radical and oxidative injury pathway, in particular, has garnered special attention as a target in the treatment of TBI. Following mTBI, there is a significant release of excitatory neurotransmitters, such as glutamate, that cause damage to the neurons and astrocytes of the brain (Werner and Engelhard, 2007). These excitatory neurotransmitters overstimulate receptors causing calcium, sodium, and potassium movement across cell membranes and resulting in ion imbalances and uncoupling of electrical processes.[3] Changes in ion gradients, especially calcium, activate several free radical pathways releasing reactive oxygen species (ROS) such as superoxides, hydrogen peroxide, and peroxynitrite. These ROS exhaust the endogenous antioxidant systems of the body causing edema, cell injury, and cell death.[4,5]

Antioxidants and free radical scavengers have demonstrated neuroprotective effects after mTBI. N-Acetyl cysteine (NAC), a commonly used mucolytic and treatment for acetaminophen toxicity, has recently been shown to play a role in mTBI treatment. It is suspected that NAC serves as a precursor for cysteine, a key substrate in the production of the antioxidant glutathione. NAC also acts as an effective scavenger for $\cdot$OH, $\cdot$NO2, CO3$\cdot$ $-$, and thiyl radicals, with slower neutralizing effects on superoxide, hydrogen-peroxide, and peroxynitrite.[6] NAC also reduces levels of the ROS heme-oxygenase 1, and increases levels of antioxidant enzymes such as superoxide dismutase.[3,7] These alterations have been shown to decrease the volume of injury that occurs following mTBI. By maintaining glutathione levels within cells and acting as a scavenger, NAC serves to counter the excitotoxicity and oxidative damage produced by mTBI to ultimately decrease the volume of injury that occurs.

Experimental models in rats have shown that NAC produces significant behavioral recovery after mTBI from blunt-impact trauma. NAC administered in the early post-injury period reduced behavior deficits such as learning and memory in rat and mouse models.[8]

NAC has also been studied in human subjects. In a randomized double blind, placebo-controlled study of active duty service members, administration of NAC following blast exposure mTBI resulted in earlier resolution of symptoms and an increased chance of symptom resolution when compared to a placebo.[9] Other trials of this type are currently underway, but are not mature enough to include in this book. The reader is advised to continue to examine the continuously updating literature for these results.

The effects of NAC on mTBI have also been studied in combination with other drugs. Minocycline is a broad-spectrum tetracycline antibiotic typically used in bacterial infections. When used in conjunction, NAC plus minocycline has been shown to synergize to modulate inflammation, reduce myelin loss, and prevent cognitive and memory deficits in a rat model of mTBI.[10,11] There are ongoing clinical trials for minocycline plus NAC in the treatment of neuropsychiatric conditions such as Bipolar Disorder; however, there are no ongoing trials for mTBI (www.clinicaltrials.gov). The fact that this combination is being tested in humans for other indications speaks to the safety of these drugs and to the potential for the study of minocycline plus NAC for mTBI in human subjects.

Other agents with actions against ROS include polyethylene glycol conjugated superoxide dismutase (PEG-SOD). In PEG-SOD, the superoxide scavenger superoxide dismutase is conjugated to polyethylene glycol to extend its half-life and reduce free radicals. Although PEG-SOD has shown favorable results in animal models and phase II clinical trials have demonstrated an absolute reduction of intracranial pressure in severe TBI patients receiving the study drug, clinical trials failed to show a statistically significant difference in neurologic outcomes or mortality when compared to a placebo.[12,13] In addition, these studies only comment on PEG-SOD use in severe TBI with no existing trials in those with mTBI. However, given that no adverse events were observed in phase II trials, this may be a promising agent for mTBI in future studies.

CANNABINOIDS

The endogenous cannabinoid system is a relatively recent discovery and knowledge about this system and its role in injury continues to expand. Unlike other neurotransmitters that are stored in presynaptic vesicles, cannabinoids are believed to be produced on demand in response to increases in intracellular calcium.[14] As previously described, the release of neurotransmitters such as glutamate causes overstimulation of receptors and ion movement across cell membranes. Calcium influx into cells leads to catabolic intracellular processes including the activation of lipid peroxidases, proteases, and phospholipases causing injury to the tissues[1] (Werner and Engelhard, 2007). The influx of calcium also triggers the production and release of cannabinoids which act to modulate excitotoxicity by binding to CB1 cannabinoid receptors on the presynaptic terminals of glutamatergic synapses and inhibiting further glutamate release.[14,15] It is also believed that cannabinoids play a role in neuroinflammation and vasomodulation, thereby affecting multiple secondary injury pathways in TBI.[16]

Animal models of mTBI and cannabinoids have shown promising results. Administration of 2-arachidonoyl glycerol, an endogenous cannabinoid, after closed head injury in mice resulted in a reduction of edema and better clinical recovery as demonstrated by behavioral function.[17] Although it was previously thought that only CB1 receptors were found in the brain and involved in neuromodulation, subsequent studies have shown that CB2 receptors are also a potential target for TBI treatment. TBI-induced mice treated with a CB2 agonist resulted in attenuated blood brain barrier disruption, decreased edema, reduced number of degenerating neurons, and a reduced number of macrophage and microglia cell counts, indicating decreased inflammation.[18,19]

To date, the only clinical trial evaluating cannabinoid use in TBI has been in patients with severe TBI. Although Dexanabinol (HU 211) showed promising results in animal models, a multicenter, placebo-controlled, phase-III trial with the drug showed that it is safe, but not efficacious, in the treatment of TBI.[20] However, given the promising effects of cannabinoids in animal models of TBI and the increasing availability of cannabinoids as medical therapy, further studies are likely to take place to evaluate the use of cannabinoids in mTBI. Additional studies will also be needed to address the efficacy of plant and synthetic cannabinoids compared to endogenous cannabinoids. Studies in this area are ongoing in our laboratory and in other laboratories around the world.

HYPOTHERMIA

Therapeutic hypothermia is commonly used following cardiac arrest, but has also been shown to be beneficial in the treatment of TBI. Its success in both situations is likely due to its effects on ischemia. In TBI, primary injury leads to damage of vessels, hypotension from autoregulatory failure, and prostaglandin-induced vasoconstriction resulting in cerebral hypoperfusion and ischemia (Werner and Engelhard, 2007). Under normal conditions, the brain is highly metabolically active and produces a large amount of heat that is removed with adequate blood flow. When injury occurs and the brain is under-perfused and generated heat cannot be removed, resulting in further brain damage.[21] Therapeutic hypothermia can reduce brain metabolic rates and demand, thereby reducing heat production and damage. It can also block excitatory neurotramitters, inhibit calcium influx, and decrease edema which are all altered in TBI.[21]

Hypothermia is one of the few emerging therapies discussed in this chapter which has several clinical trials already completed and others ongoing. The benefits of hypothermia have been demonstrated in animal models with experimental brain trauma. In 1994, Dietrich et al. reported that posttraumatic hypothermia initiated 5 minutes after brain injury significantly reduced injury volume and prolonged neuronal survival.[22] Despite several animal models corroborating these findings, hypothermia as a treatment for TBI in human subjects has shown varying results. A review of 13 randomized controlled trials including 1339 patients with severe TBI showed that mortality was reduced in those exposed to hypothermia compared to those treated with standard care, although this is not statistically significant.[23] Furthermore, favorable outcomes were more likely in patients who were initially responsive to standard intracranial pressure lowering therapy and when hypothermia was maintained for more than 48 hours or with longer trials (over 1 year), indicating that hypothermia may be beneficial under specific conditions.[23] Additional studies have also shown reduced mortality rates in those with severe TBI treated with hypothermia; however, these results were more likely to be found in the lower quality trials.[24] Given encouraging results from single center studies, a multicenter trial including 392 patients with severe TBI was initiated, however, mortality rates did not differ between the hypothermia and normothermia groups.[22]

The fact that some trials have shown a benefit in severe TBI indicates the potential use of hypothermia as a treatment for mTBI. The reader should continue to follow the literature as studies on hypothermia and mTBI are ongoing. Additional clinical trials are needed to address optimal temperatures, the time window for initiation, and length of hypothermia, as well as the effects of different cooling methods.[22] While surface cooling and intranasal cooling systems have been tested in humans with TBI, transarterial or transvenous endovascular cooling, extraluminal vascular cooling, and epidural cerebral cooling have only been demonstrated in animal models.[25] These methods may prove beneficial to patients with TBI, including those with mTBI.

STEM CELLS

Stem cells are one of the most innovative advances in medical therapy being investigated worldwide. Although stem cells have been widely used in cancer treatment for years, their use in neurodegeneration and brain injury is a recent development. Primary injury in TBI induces activation of the inflammatory cascade with mobilization of cellular mediators such as inflammatory cytokines and chemokines to the injured tissue. As a result of cellular mediator infiltration, brain tissue undergoes cell death and is eventually turned into scar tissue[1] (Werner and Engelhard, 2007). Stem cells work to counter these immunologic secondary pathways of TBI. Mesenchymal stem cells (MSCs) transplanted into rats 2 hours after TBI resulted in decreased levels of macrophages, infiltrating leukocytes, and proinflammatory cytokines (TNF-a, IL-1, IL-6), as well as increased antiinflammatory cytokines (IL-4, IL-10, TGF-B1).[26] Stem cells may offer additional neuroprotection by their action on angiogenesis, neurogenesis, synaptogenesis, dendritic arborization, and inhibition of apoptosis and via the release of local neurotrophic factors such as BDNF and nerve growth factor.[27,28]

Animal models of stem cell use in mTBI have been promising. Stem cells transplanted into the hippocampus of mTBI-induced rats showed increases in neurotrophic factors, synaptic formations, and functional recovery from learning and memory deficits.[29] These findings were not observed in normal rats or rats with severe TBI injuries.[29] Additional studies have shown that injection of neural stem cells into the ipsilateral or contralateral cortex-hippocampal interface resulted in significant improvement of motor function in mice with controlled cortical impact brain injury.[30] One study, however, determined that single dose intravenous MSC therapy for moderate TBI was not effective, with almost no cells identified in the brain tissue 2 weeks after infusion. No improvements in recovery were noted.[31] These data suggest that intravenous administration is inadequate and localized intracerebral administration is necessary. Further work is necessary to determine the effects of stem cell therapy in those with mTBI, whether intraparenchymal, intraventricular, or intracisternal action is more effective, and to determine the optimal number of injections.

HYPERBARIC OXYGEN

Hyperbaric oxygen (HBO) therapy refers to exposure to a contained environment with 100% oxygen at increased atmospheric pressure. HBO increases oxygen delivery to the tissues of the body by increasing the volume of oxygen dissolved in the blood and is, therefore, a useful treatment in ischemic conditions such as poor wound healing, carbon monoxide poisoning, and burns. TBI shares many similarities with these ischemic conditions. Primary injury leads to vessel damage, hypotension from autoregulatory failure, and prostaglandin-induced vasoconstriction resulting in cerebral hypoperfusion and ischemia (Werner and Engelhard, 2007). The use of HBO following TBI results in relief of hypoxia, reduction in cerebral edema and intracranial pressure via vasoconstriction, and improvement in microcirculation.[32] HBO has also been shown to provide additional antiapoptotic and antiinflammatory effects. Following administration of HBO, animal models demonstrated increased expression of antiapoptotic bcl-2 mRNA with increased ratio of bcl-2 to bax and reduced apoptotic caspase-3 mRNA levels.[32] Matrix metalloproteinases, which are responsible for tissue remodeling and inflammation, were also found in reduced quantities in HBO treated animals.[33]

Clinical trials with HBO in mTBI have shown mixed results. In a study of 56 mTBI patients with prolonged postconcussive syndrome 1–5 years after injury, researchers demonstrated significant improvements in cognitive function following HBO compared to control therapy, indicating that HBO may be a useful treatment even years after trauma.[34] This is a significant finding as this information would substantially increase the window period in which patients may benefit from treatment. In contrast, other studies have shown inconclusive results. In one study of 50 military service members with mTBI, HBO had no effect on postconcussive symptoms.[35] A recently published study by the Department of Defense (DOD) also suggests that HBO is no better than sham air compression treatment. Approximately 72 military service members with persistent postconcussion symptoms were randomized to HBO, sham sessions with room air, or no supplemental chamber procedures, and found that both intervention groups showed improved outcomes compared to standard care and any improvements are likely attributed to placebo effect.[36] A larger confirmatory trial by the DOD is currently underway, although additional military studies have shown similar results.[37] Furthermore, despite some results suggesting that HBO reduces the risk of death and improves GCS, evidence has not shown any improvement in quality of life, resulting in more individuals surviving mTBI, but with greater deficits.[38,39]

There are many aspects of HBO therapy, including a standardized protocol, that must be addressed before it can serve as an effective treatment option for mTBI. In one animal model of TBI, researchers found that HBO given within 3–12 hours reduced neurologic deficits and neuronal loss, but had fewer neuroprotective effects when given at 24–72 hours.[32] Animal models also benefitted from repeated HBO treatments for 3–5 days.[32] Most human studies, however, vary in the time from injury to HBO initiation, as well as in the total treatment time.[38,40] Length of treatment in clinical trials has varied from 35 minutes to 1 hour daily and can last for 3–188 treatments, or until the patient is awake.[41] Studies have also been inconsistent in pressurization used during HBO treatment. Subsequent clinical trials have ranged from 1 to 2.5 atmospheres, possibly contributing to an increased risk for side effects and the conflicting results that have been seen in the literature. These controversies suggest that further work is needed to identify the optimal therapeutic window, frequency, length of treatment, and pressure for HBO in TBI. Although more work needs to be done in this area, there is currently insufficient evidence to support the use of HBO for mTBI.

PROGESTERONE

The effects of progesterone on secondary injury from mTBI are multifaceted. Structural damage from the primary trauma causes breakdown of the endothelial cell layer in the blood brain barrier and damages cell membrane integrity causing vasogenic and cytotoxic edema. These membrane disruptions increase cellular permeability and allow for uncontrolled ion movement and accumulation of water in the brain. When widespread, edema can be associated with increased intracranial pressure and ischemia[1] (Werner and Engelhard, 2007). It is hypothesized that progesterone exerts its neuroprotective effects on these secondary injury processes of cerebral edema, inflammation, and cell death.[42] Animal models of mTBI have confirmed these effects of progesterone by showing reduced edema and subsequent improvement in cognitive and motor impairments.[43]

Progesterone may also have antioxidant effects with reduced levels of lipid peroxidation seen in animal models. This prevents lipid peroxidation induced damage of the blood brain barrier, improving its integrity and preventing edema.[44] Furthermore, studies have demonstrated progesterone to have antiapoptotic properties. Following administration of progesterone and its metabolite allopregnanolone, injured rats showed reduced expression of pro-apoptotic proteins caspase-3 and Bax, and apoptotic DNA fragmentation. These rats also showed improved performance in spatial learning tasks compared to injured rats who did not receive progesterone.[45]

Similar to minocycline with NAC, progesterone has also been demonstrated to work synergistically with other agents. Vitamin D, also a steroid hormone, has been shown to have some neuroprotective properties. It is believed that Vitamin D and progesterone affect similar secondary injury pathways, albeit through different mechanisms. The two drugs, therefore, work synergistically to enhance recovery after TBI.[46] Combination therapy in rat models of TBI showed improved spatial function and memory as well as significantly reduced neuronal loss.[47]

Clinical trials with progesterone have only been conducted in patients with moderate to severe TBI including two phase-II studies that demonstrated decreased mortality and improved functional outcomes without any severe adverse events.[46,48] However, phase-III trials of progesterone in moderate to severe TBI, including Study of a Neuroprotective Agent, Progesterone, in Severe Traumatic Brain Injury (SYNAPSE) and the Progesterone for the Treatment of Traumatic Brain Injury (PROTECT III) trials, have failed. There have been no clinical trials of progesterone after mTBI. However, progesterone is safe for clinical use as demonstrated by its widespread use in endocrine disorders. Given its safety profile and the promising results of phase-II clinical trials in moderate to severe TBI, further investigation is needed to determine its effectiveness in mTBI.

ADDITIONAL PROMISING TREATMENTS

Erythropoietin (EPO) is a glycoprotein that normally plays a role in the differentiation of hematopoietic progenitor cells. EPO receptors are normally expressed in the low quantities in the brain, however injury or ischemia to the brain results in the upregulation of these receptors.[49] When EPO binds to its receptors, it activates the JAK-2 signaling pathway ultimately resulting in neural progenitor cell migration to the site of injury.[50] In animal models, EPO for the treatment of TBI has shown mixed results. While some studies have shown improvement in spatial learning when given 6 or 24 hours after injury, others suggest that EPO is ineffective in improving functional outcomes even at high doses such as 10,000 IU given 15 minutes after injury.[51,52] Some human trials have been performed in moderate and severe TBI demonstrating no benefit of EPO therapy, but further studies are needed to evaluate EPO use in mTBI.[53,54]

Statins are a widely used class of drug for hypercholesterolemia. Their tolerability and safety profile make them as ideal for study in other conditions, such as TBI. Neuroprotective effects of statins may include improvement in endothelial function, antioxidant properties, antiinflammatory properties, and effects on neuronal survival and angiogenesis.[50] Atorvastatin administration in rats with TBI showed significantly reduced functional deficits, increased neuronal survival, and synaptogenesis.[55] In humans, administration of rosuvastatin in patients with moderate TBI improved amnesia test scores however there was no difference in the Disability Rating Scale at 3 months.[56] Further study in patients with mTBI is necessary.

LIMITATIONS OF EMERGING THERAPIES

Many of the clinical trials described in this chapter have failed due to the inability to translate from animal models to human trials. Simple animal models fail to consider the complex clinical scenarios and interplay of numerous factors that occur in human TBI.[57] Although there has been extensive research on oxidative stress and other pathways in animal models, these pathways have not been adequately demonstrated in human TBI and further research is needed to understand the extent of these secondary injury pathways in humans.[58] Furthermore, the interaction of these pathways has not been studied in humans.

The type of injury and animal model used may affect the ability to translate to human use. Although fluid percussion injury is the most widely described mechanism of inducing injury in animals, this mechanism may not accurately mimic the injury that occurs with human TBI.[58] In addition, the pathophysiology of secondary injury in the mouse model may differ from human pathophysiology. The agent under investigation should, therefore, be studied in a variety of different animal models before advancing to clinical trials.[58] Despite promising neuroprotective effects in animal models, many agents are also limited by their narrow therapeutic window, inability to cross the blood brain barrier, and lack of function on specific targets.[59,60] Further study is needed to develop agents with a more targeted function rather than blanket effects.

CONCLUSIONS

mTBI affects thousands of individuals every year. While the primary injury often cannot be treated, the secondary injuries that result are promising targets for treatment. Conservative treatments of mTBI have shown some benefit, but are limited in that they are most effective within a certain time frame. The identification of new agents that target secondary injuries are of great importance in preventing ongoing damage as well as prolonging the window of time in which mTBI survivors can be treated and experience improvement in functional outcomes. Unfortunately, many of the agents discussed in this chapter have shown favorable effects in animal models; however, they have failed to show clear benefit in phase III clinical trials.[58] As a result, continued investigation into these agents, as well as additional therapies for mTBI, is necessary.

References

1. Werner C, Engelhard K. Pathophysiology of traumatic brain injury. *Br J Anaesth* 2007;**99**(1):4–9.
2. Comper P, Bisschop SM, Carnide N, Tricco A. A systematic review of treatments for mild traumatic brain injury. *Brain Inj* 2005;**19**(11):863–80.
3. Yi JH, Hazell AS. Excitotoxic mechanisms and the role of astrocytic glutamate transporters in traumatic brain injury. *Neurochem Int* 2006;**48**(5):394–403.
4. Lewén A, Matz P, Chan PH. Free radical pathways in CNS injury. *J Neurotrauma* 2000;**17**(10):871–90.
5. Arundine M, Tymianski M. Molecular mechanisms of glutamate-dependent neurodegeneration in ischemia and traumatic brain injury. *Cell Mol Life Sci* 2004;**61**(6):657–68.
6. Samuni Y, Goldstein S, Dean OM, Berk M. The chemistry and biological activities of N-acetylcysteine. *Biochim Biophys Acta* 2013;**1830**(8):4117–29.
7. Hicdonmez T, Kanter M, Tiryaki M, Parsak T, Cobanoglu S. Neuroprotective effects of N-acetylcysteine on experimental closed head trauma in rats. *Neurochem Res* 2006;**31**(4):473–81.
8. Eakin K, Baratz-Goldstein R, Pick CG, Zindel O, Balaban CD, et al. Efficacy of N-acetyl cysteine in traumatic brain injury. *PLoS One* 2014;**9**(4):e90617.
9. Hoffer ME, Balaban C, Slade MD, Tsao JW, Hoffer B. Amelioration of acute sequelae of blast induced mild traumatic brain injury by N-acetyl cysteine: a double-blind, placebo controlled study. *PLoS One* 2013;**8**(1): e54163.
10. Abdel Baki SG, Schwab B, Haber M, Fenton AA, Bergold PJ. Minocycline synergizes with N-acetylcysteine and improves cognition and memory following traumatic brain injury in rats. *PLoS One* 2010;**5**(8):e12490.
11. Haber M, Abdel Baki SG, Grin'kina NM, Irizarry R, Ershova A, et al. Minocycline plus N-acetylcysteine synergize to modulate inflammation and prevent cognitive and memory deficits in a rat model of mild traumatic brain injury. *Exp Neurol* 2013;**249**:169–77.
12. Muizelaar JP, Marmarou A, Young HF, Choi SC, Wolf A, et al. Improving the outcome of severe head injury with the oxygen radical scavenger polyethylene glycol-conjugated superoxide dismutase: a phase II trial. *J Neurosurg* 1993;**78**(3):375–82.
13. Young B, Runge JW, Waxman KS, Harrington T, Wilberger J, et al. Effects of pegorgotein on neurologic outcome of patients with severe head injury A multicenter, randomized controlled trial. *J Am Med Assoc* 1996;**276** (7):538–43.
14. Shohami E, Cohen-Yeshurun A, Magid L, Algali M, Mechoulam R. Endocannabinoids and traumatic brain injury. *Br J Pharmacol* 2011;**163**(7):1402–10.
15. Biegon A. Cannabinoids as neuroprotective agents in traumatic brain injury. *Curr Pharm Des* 2004;**10** (18):2177–83.
16. Schurman LD, Lichtman AH. Endocannabinoids: a promising impact for traumatic brain injury. *Front Pharmacol* 2017;**8**:69.

17. Panikashvili D, Simeonidou C, Ben-Shabat S, Hanus L, Breuer A, et al. An endogenous cannabinoid (2-AG) is neuroprotective after brain injury. *Nature* 2001;**413**(6855):527–31.

18. Elliott MB, Tuma RF, Amenta PS, Barbe MF, Jallo JI. Acute effects of a selective cannabinoid-2 receptor agonist on neuroinflammation in a model of traumatic brain injury. *J Neurotrauma* 2011;**28**(6):973–81.

19. Amenta PS, Jallo JI, Tuma RF, Elliott MB. A cannabinoid type 2 receptor agonist attenuates blood-brain barrier damage and neurodegeneration in a murine model of traumatic brain injury. *J Neurosci Res* 2012;**90**(12):2293–305.

20. Maas AI, Murray G, Henney 3rd H, Kassem N, Legrand V, et al. Efficacy and safety of dexanabinol in severe traumatic brain injury: results of a phase III randomised, placebo-controlled, clinical trial. *Lancet Neurol* 2006;**5**(1):38–45.

21. Sahuquillo J, Vilalta A. Cooling the injured brain: how does moderate hypothermia influence the pathophysiology of traumatic brain injury. *Curr Pharm Des* 2007;**13**(22):2310–22.

22. Dietrich WD, Bramlett HM. The evidence for hypothermia as a neuroprotectant in traumatic brain injury. *Neurotherapeutics* 2010;**7**(1):43–50.

23. Peterson K, Carson S, Carney N. Hypothermia treatment for traumatic brain injury: a systematic review and meta-analysis. *J Neurotrauma* 2008;**25**(1):62–71.

24. Sydenham E, Roberts I, Alderson P. Hypothermia for traumatic head injury. *Cochrane Database Syst Rev* 2009;**15**(2). CD001048.

25. Christian E, Zada G, Sung G, Giannotta SL. A review of selective hypothermia in the management of traumatic brain injury. *Neurosurg Focus* 2008;**25**(4):E9.

26. Zhang R, Liu Y, Yan K, Chen L, Chen XR, et al. Anti-inflammatory and immunomodulatory mechanisms of mesenchymal stem cell transplantation in experimental traumatic brain injury. *J Neuroinflam* 2013;**10**:106.

27. Mahmood A, Lu D, Chopp M. Intravenous administration of marrow stromal cells (MSCs) increases the expression of growth factors in rat brain after traumatic brain injury. *J Neurotrauma* 2004;**21**(1):33–9.

28. Parr AM, Tator CH, Keating A. Bone marrow-derived mesenchymal stromal cells for the repair of central nervous system injury. *Bone Marrow Transplant* 2007;**40**(7):609–19.

29. Shindo T, Matsumoto Y, Wang Q, Kawai N, Tamiya T, et al. Differences in the neuronal stem cells survival, neuronal differentiation and neurological improvement after transplantation of neural stem cells between mild and severe experimental traumatic brain injury. *J Med Invest* 2006;**53**(1-2):42–51.

30. Riess P, Zhang C, Saatman KE, Laurer HL, Longhi LG, et al. Transplanted neural stem cells survive, differentiate, and improve neurological motor function after experimental traumatic brain injury. *Neurosurgery* 2002;**51**(4):1043–52.

31. Harting MT, Jimenez F, Xue H, Fischer UM, Baumgartner J, et al. Intravenous mesenchymal stem cell therapy for traumatic brain injury. *J Neurosurg* 2009;**110**(6):1189–97.

32. Wang GH, Zhang XG, Jiang ZL, Li X, Peng LL, et al. Neuroprotective effects of hyperbaric oxygen treatment on traumatic brain injury in the rat. *J Neurotrauma* 2010;**27**(9):1733–43.

33. Vlodavsky E, Palzur E, Soustiel JF. Hyperbaric oxygen therapy reduces neuroinflammation and expression of matrix metalloproteinase-9 in the rat model of traumatic brain injury. *Neuropathol Appl Neurobiol* 2006;**32**(1):40–50.

34. Boussi-Gross R, Golan H, Fishlev G, Bechor Y, Volkov O, et al. Hyperbaric oxygen therapy can improve post concussion syndrome years after mild traumatic brain injury—randomized prospective trial. *PLoS One* 2013;**8**(11):e79995.

35. Wolf G, Cifu D, Baugh L, Carne W, Profenna L. The effect of hyperbaric oxygen on symptoms after mild traumatic brain injury. *J Neurotrauma* 2012;**29**(17):2606–12.

36. Miller RS, Weaver LK, Bahraini N, Churchill S, Price RC, Skiba V, et al. HOPPS trial team. Effects of hyperbaric oxygen on symptoms and quality of life among service members with persistent postconcussion symptoms: a randomized clinical trial. *J Am Med Assoc Intern Med* 2015;**175**(1):43–52.

37. Crawford C, Teo L, Yang E, Isbister C, Berry K. Is hyperbaric oxygen therapy effective for traumatic brain injury? A rapid evidence assessment of the literature and recommendations for the field. *J Head Trauma Rehabil* 2017;**32**(3):E27–37.

38. Bennett MH, Trytko B, Jonker B. Hyperbaric oxygen therapy for the adjunctive treatment of traumatic brain injury. *Cochrane Database Syst Rev* 2012;**12**:CD004609.

IV. DIAGNOSIS AND TREATMENT

39. Rockswold GL, Ford SE, Anderson DC, Bergman TA, Sherman RE. Results of a prospective randomized trial for treatment of severely brain-injured patients with hyperbaric oxygen. *J Neurosurg* 1992;**76**(6):929–34.
40. Huang L, Obenaus A. Hyperbaric oxygen therapy for traumatic brain injury. *Med Gas Res* 2011;**1**(1):21.
41. Hu Q, Manaenko A, Xu T, Guo Z, Tang J, et al. Hyperbaric oxygen therapy for traumatic brain injury: bench-to-bedside. *Med Gas Res* 2016;**6**(2):102–10.
42. Stein DG, Wright DW, Kellermann AL. Does progesterone have neuroprotective properties? *Ann Emerg Med* 2008;**51**(2):164–72.
43. Webster KM, Wright DK, Sun M, Semple BD, Ozturk E, et al. Progesterone treatment reduces neuroinflammation, oxidative stress and brain damage and improves long-term outcomes in a rat model of repeated mild traumatic brain injury. *J Neuroinflam* 2015;**12**:238.
44. Roof RL, Hoffman SW, Stein DG. Progesterone protects against lipid peroxidation following traumatic brain injury in rats. *Mol Chem Neuropathol* 1997;**31**(1):1–11.
45. Djebaili M, Guo Q, Pettus EH, Hoffman SW, Stein DG. The neurosteroids progesterone and allopregnanolone reduce cell death, gliosis, and functional deficits after traumatic brain injury in rats. *J Neurotrauma* 2005;**22**(1):106–18.
46. Cekic M, Sayeed I, Stein DG. Combination treatment with progesterone and vitamin D hormone may be more effective than monotherapy for nervous system injury and disease. *Front Neuroendocrinol* 2009;**30**(2):158–72.
47. Tang H, Hua F, Wang J, Sayeed I, Wang X, et al. Progesterone and vitamin D: improvement after traumatic brain injury in middle-aged rats. *Horm Behav* 2013;**64**(3):527–38.
48. Stein DG. Is progesterone a worthy candidate as a novel therapy for traumatic brain injury? *Dialogues Clin Neurosci* 2011;**13**(3):352–9.
49. Marti HH. Erythropoietin and the hypoxic brain. *J Exp Biol* 2004;**207**(Pt 18):3233–42.
50. Xiong Y, Mahmood A, Chopp M. Emerging treatments for traumatic brain injury. *Expert Opin Emerg Drugs* 2009;**14**(1):67–84.
51. Mahmood A, Lu D, Qu C, Goussev A, Zhang ZG, et al. Treatment of traumatic brain injury in rats with erythropoietin and carbamylated erythropoietin. *J Neurosurg* 2007;**107**(2):392–7.
52. Bramlett HM, Dietrich WD, Dixon CE, Shear DA, Schmid KE, et al. Erythropoietin treatment in traumatic brain injury: operation brain trauma therapy. *J Neurotrauma* 2016;**33**(6):538–52.
53. Nichol A, French C, Little L, Haddad S, Presneill J, et al. Erythropoietin in traumatic brain injury (EPO-TBI): a double-blind randomised controlled trial. *Lancet* 2015;**386**(10012):2499–506.
54. Nirula R, Diaz-Arrastia R, Brasel K, Weigelt JA, Waxman K. Safety and efficacy of erythropoietin in traumatic brain injury patients: a pilot randomized trial. *Crit Care Res Pract* 2010;**2010**:1–5
55. Lu D, Goussev A, Chen J, Pannu P, Li Y, et al. Atorvastatin reduces neurological deficit and increases synaptogenesis, angiogenesis, and neuronal survival in rats subjected to traumatic brain injury. *J Neurotrauma* 2004;**21**(1):21–32.
56. Tapia-Perez J, Sanchez-Aguilar M, Torres-Corzo JG, Gordillo-Moscoso A, Martinez-Perez P, et al. Effect of rosuvastatin on amnesia and disorientation after traumatic brain injury (NCT003229758). *J Neurotrauma* 2008;**25**(8):1011–17.
57. Statler KD, Jenkins LW, Dixon CE, Clark RS, Marion DW, et al. The simple model versus the super model: translating experimental traumatic brain injury research to the bedside. *J Neurotrauma* 2001;**18**(11):1195–206.
58. Doppenberg EM, Choi SC, Bullock R. Clinical trials in traumatic brain injury: lessons for the future. *J Neurosurg Anesthesiol* 2004;**16**(1):87–94.
59. Gilgun-Sherki Y, Rosenbaum Z, Melamed E, Offen D. Antioxidant therapy in acute central nervous system injury: current state. *Pharmacol Rev* 2002;**54**(2):271–84.
60. Kochanek PM, Jackson TC, Ferguson NM, Carlson SW, Simon DW, et al. Emerging therapies in traumatic brain injury. *Semin Neurol* 2015;**35**(1):83–100.

mTBI/Concussion: Assessment and Rehabilitation Strategy and Program Optimization

James K. Buskirk, MS Ed., PT, SCS, AIB-CON

Department of Otolaryngology, Batchelor's Children's Research Institute,
University of Miami, Miller School of Medicine, Miami, FL, United States

BACKGROUND

To provide appropriate assessment and rehabilitative therapies for a specific disorder related to mTBI/Concussion, or its most common component (94% prevalence rate)[1] of vestibular dysfunction (whether peripheral, central, or mixed origins), one must first ascertain and understand the heterogeneity of the commonly multifactorial dysfunction. Establishing a history, including timeline of onset, progression of functional limitations, and associated symptoms is critical for the rehabilitative clinician to establish an effective assessment and subsequent treatment program. A review of prior studies[2] showed effectiveness of various rehabilitation approaches for peripheral vestibular loss with varied outcomes, leading to an individualized approach dependent on objective testing, functional presentation, and symptoms tolerance as most effective, due to progressive, targeted rather than general exercise approach. A lack of understanding of the importance of the multiple components of mTBI, or a lack of understanding of the initial self-limiting compensatory mechanisms and associated timelines may lead the clinician to not fully assess all the components of the disorder and findings relative to the persistent symptoms and functional limitations, and erroneously prescribe an inappropriate rehabilitation program, with less than optimal results obtained. Optimized, or targeted rehabilitation prescription for mTBI with associated vestibular dysfunction component has gained popularity with the advancement of technologies for objectification and quantification of both peripheral and central neurologic sensory and motor dysfunctions, and use of validated scales to quantify the presence and magnitude of common symptoms of mTBI, including (but not limited to): dizziness, vertigo, disequilibrium, sleep disorder, impaired cognition, anxiety and depression, and headache.[3] These are often accompanied by musculoskeletal symptoms and resultant functional activities of daily living (ADL) limitations. Measurement of transmembrane ionic flow and resultant electrical current flow produced at the cellular level, as evidenced by what is elicited by the types I and II hair cells located within the audio-vestibular system, along with mapping of microcircuits linking the vestibular afferents with the cerebellum, hippocampus, and inferior olive has shown a baseline discharge rate inherent to each component anatomic part of the peripheral and central neurologic systems.[4] These rates function in harmony and in real-time, allowing communication among all the component anatomic parts, via the complex network of excitatory and inhibitory synapses inherent to each. The synaptic junctions contain excitatory or inhibitory neurotransmitters which cause action potential modulation with resultant messages sent in the cerebellum via the mossy and climbing fibers, and throughout the central and peripheral systems.[4–7] This baseline engrained pattern of cellular and, therefore, neuron discharges is unique to individuals, and may be altered with injury, surgery, or disease, and positively altered by rehabilitative, specific-task training. Specific motor/movement plans and patterns become engrained over time as a learned pattern, and stored within various parts of the brain and brainstem for basic and advanced cranial nerve functions, and gross motor tasks are initially "learned" within the cerebellum, and then integrated within the basal ganglia. Since some functionality tasks are shared among all individuals, there appears to exist a "common thread" of movement plans and patterns by species, which are further altered by repetitive daily activities. Additional, or refined patterns exist among subsets of individuals pertinent to individual task requirements for ADL, job, or sport related activities. Thus, one could hold to the assumption that this inherent rate of discharge can be altered as an adaptation to environmental changes, or alterations to the discharge rate elicited by external factors (disease, trauma, aging, etc.) or with specific task training, repetitiously. One also can assume also that the impulse patterns can be further modified or altered by training or learning new patterns of behavior and movements, with resultant functional adaptation. This ability for modulation forms the basis for an apparent hierarchy of phases of rehabilitation and recovery from mTBI, vestibular, and balance deficits.[8] Prior studies have also reported a higher incidence of musculoskeletal injury in athletes after sustaining mTBI as compared to control subjects not subjected to head injury.[9,10] This lends itself to the assumption of the second phase of vestibular recovery not being fully completed, with incomplete adaptation to new or relearning prior engrained movement patterns. This may include eye and head motions, as well as postural stability alterations, with learned aberrant auditory and cognitive functions which may also impact physical task performance. The peripheral vestibular system discharges at approximately 90 spikes/second at rest, and increase rapidly with head and body motions.[11] These impulses are carried by both the superior and inferior branches of the vestibular portion of cranial nerve VIII to the vestibular nuclei in the midbrain. The vestibular labyrinths elicit increased unilateral discharges from the side moved toward, and resultant contralateral decreased discharges (inhibition) from the side moved away from. The otolithic system (saccule and utricle) elicit discharges continuously, and increase with translational motions horizontally and/or vertically, in response to changes in alignment with force of gravity. At the vestibular nuclei, various connections or synapses are formed with neurons that connect to the nuclei of cranial nerves III, IV, and VI, the cerebellum, inferior olive, and premotor and motor cortices. The oculomotor cranial nerves activate concentric or eccentric motions of the eyes to maintain focus of the environment onto the ocular fovea. Vergence of the eyes is critical for visual motion detection and spatial perception. Alterations of the necessary pathways for normal eye coordinated motions give rise to aberrant perception and elicits symptoms of disorientation. Movement of the head elicits activation of the semicircular canal mechanisms bilaterally, and concomitant change in orientation with line of gravity of the otolithic system, causing changes in electrical discharge and conduction rates of both. The importance of the oculomotor system, along with the vestibular-ocular reflex (VOR) and coordination of eyes and head motions for rehabilitation processes has been recognized for many years.[12] Absence or dysfunction of such coordination elicits nystagmus and other abnormal eye movements, with resultant retinal slip, or inability to keep a visual target on the retinal fovea. Corrective saccadic eye motions are needed to replace the target back onto the retinal fovea. This extraneous eye movement elicits visual distortion and abnormal spatial perception, or dizziness symptoms. Often a subject with abnormal VOR function will rely solely on oculomotor function for spatial awareness and orientation, opting to avoid head motions entirely. Pathology of the oculomotor system affects both static visual acuity, as well as visual tracking with head and body motions. Further internal feedback loop pathways via the cerebellum, basal ganglia, and motor cortex enable alterations and refining, or "smoothing," functions of excitation and/or inhibition of neuronal pool firing, influencing postural control, and when altered, elicits loss of balance and disequilibrium symptoms. The basal ganglia, additionally, performs centrally similarly to a "switching" mechanism, whereby neural pathways are integrated from, and sent out to, the components of the limbic system, thus modulating emotions and cognitive behaviors associated with the dysfunction. An understanding of this anatomic and physiologic relationship among the component parts allows the rehabilitation clinician to objectify and categorize symptoms reported and, therefore, form the optimized rehabilitative approach for mTBI.

Benign paroxysmal positional vertigo (BPPV) has been described in the literature for many years as the result of otoconia within the otolithic system (saccule and utricle) becoming free floating within the endolymphatic fluid and relocating into one or more of the semicircular canals, causing severe vertigo whenever the subject positions the head in such a manner as to cause the otoconia to move, creating an eddy current. There appears to be a natural turn-over of the otoconia whereby "old," or mature, otoconia are replaced by "new" ones. This process may be regulated by the ionic flow and resultant electrical current produced by the basement membrane and the outer most portion of the cellular membrane of the otoconia. Whether this is an electrical bond or chemical bond, or both, is not fully understood. Therefore, one potential cause of BPPV is alteration of the removal of the "old" otoconia or alteration of the generation of the "new" otoconia. Various external causes of BPPV have also been described, including viral infections, migraine with (or without) accompanying headache, and exposure to trauma such as that sustained which causes central pathologies, like mTBI/concussions. It is thought the otolithic otoconia are held in place on the surfaces/basement membranes of the utricle (more positioned in the horizontal plane) and saccule (more positioned in the vertical plane) by an electrical and/or chemical bond. A disruption of the bond by trauma or by changes in ionic flow and,

IV. DIAGNOSIS AND TREATMENT

thus, electrical current flow at the cellular membrane level may cause loosening of them from the basement membrane and subsequent head motions then position them pathologically into the labyrinths. If the otoconia remain free-floating within the endolymphatic fluid, it is termed canalithiasis. However, if the outermost membranes of the otoconia become "sticky," or adherent to the cupula, and are no longer free-floating within the endolymphatic fluid, it is termed cupulolithiasis.[13] Again, the mechanisms involved in making the otoconia "sticky" are not fully understood, but may be explained by alterations in membrane potentials generated by alterations in ionic flow across the membrane, with resultant chemical and/or electrical effects, causing the affinity or adherence to the innermost lining of the endolymphatic sac within the labyrinth, or directly to the cupula. Several liberatory maneuvers with risks and benefits have been described and compared for efficacy to reposition the otoconia back out of the labyrinths and again into the otolithic organs, thus, relieving the vertigo symptoms.[14] Following performance of the maneuvers, several different exercise programs have been suggested, to continue to resolve the often-present concomitant symptoms of dizziness and disequilibrium, which may last hours or days after the BPPV is resolved,[15] but others have compared follow up exercise program efficacy to no follow up exercise programs to rates of recurrence of symptoms of BPPV and found no significant differences.[16,17] The length of time and number of repetitions per day of the exercise performance varies among opinions, with several variables being involved, including length of time from the onset to the time of clinical intervention. There appears to be a systematic process of recovery from vestibular insult[8] with the initial phase of postural compensation and withdrawal from large body motion to relieve initial symptoms of vertigo and disequilibrium, whereby autogenic compensation or adaptation processes begin shortly after the onset of injury. The clinician sometimes needs to reverse or alter the subject's newly learned restrictive movement patterns, while initializing prescribed exercise programs to reteach and integrate prior engrained movement patterns, or initiate new, novel movements. These include head and eye stabilization, and beginnings of small, simple, body motions for postural control. If not tolerated initially, these may initially be performed laying or sitting, and progressed to upright when tolerated.

The performance of these maneuvers, and follow up rehabilitative exercise programs directly onto the affected vestibular apparatus could be deemed the only true peripheral vestibular system rehabilitation process, since all other forms of rehabilitation, including the follow-up or postmaneuver exercise programs themselves focus on adaptation of the central neurologic processes of motor pattern learning. This phenomenon was described prior with repeated peripheral vestibular insults after undergoing compensatory rehabilitation, whereby similar objective and subjective complaints were elicited.[18]

METHODS

Upon initial assessment, the therapy program begins with the rehabilitation clinician obtaining a thorough history of the etiology of dysfunction. Various questionnaires have been developed to determine the magnitude of functional limitations and causes of and severity of symptoms. It is of utmost importance that the clinician gains an understanding of what has transpired from the time of injury and dysfunction to the time of initial assessment and treatment program. It is presumed there is an alteration almost immediately within the communication processes among all the central neurologic components and, thus, an alteration in the harmonious electrical patterns normally utilized. This alteration is perceived by the brain as an alteration to functionality and a compensatory pattern is begun. This causes a new pattern of afferent and efferent communication pattern, with resultant new feedback loops within the cerebellum, brainstem, premotor cortex, motor cortex, and basal ganglia, and new movement patterns generated. These new patterns are initially learned and stored within the cerebellum, but with repetition and use of the new patterns, they are engrained and stored within the basal ganglia for trunk and limb movements, to be used instead of the old patterns. This process forms the basis for repetitious vestibular rehabilitation exercises, for learning oculomotor, vestibular—ocular, integrated vestibular—visual, vestibular cancelation, and postural and balance functions. An assessment of known, common movement patterns by the clinician may show that newly learned and in-use patterns for functionality may be considered dysfunctional or pathologic in nature, and may place the subject in postural imbalance or at risk of balance loss or fall. For job or sport tasks, these altered movement patterns may cause diminished skills or tasks performance, which could place the subject at risk of further dysfunction or injury. Further studies have shown that following mTBI, the subject becomes more likely to suffer another subsequent head trauma, as well as other multiple orthopedic maladies compared to control subjects who had not previously experienced head injury. These findings may be related to the subject's utilizing maladaptive patterns of head and eye coordinated movements, and/or abnormal postural corrective movement patterns.[10] Spatial orientation and awareness may be altered, contributing also to abnormal adaptation processes. Further, connections between the vestibular components and the frontal lobe components for executive function components of cognition may be affected.

Individualized, optimized, targeted rehabilitation program prescription is the goal of the rehabilitation clinician. To that end, a thorough objective assessment must be performed, which encompasses several domains being assessed. A hands-on, clinical approach is necessary, augmented with tests and measurements, using latest technologies for objectification and quantification of deficits. Sensitivity and specificity of measurement tools must be considered.

CLINICAL EXAM

The clinician should begin with a simple history-taking and questioning involving age, height, weight, orientation, and any prior incidences of similar injury, with mechanism, initial symptoms and perceptions, loss of memory of events leading up to the time of injury (retrograde amnesia), problems forming new memory of events that occurred following the injury (anterograde amnesia), loss of consciousness, and functionality deficits. Details as to how the injury was initially cared for is of interest (transport to a medical facility, tests performed, diagnosis given, recommendations for management, and medications prescribed, etc.). Of particular concern to the examiner is the timeline of when the injury occurred to time of the current exam, and what the subject has been able to tolerate while performing ADL activities since the injury, with symptoms tolerance/limitations of functionality at present. Attention should be paid toward initial phase compensation patterns of restricted head, eyes, and body motions in attempt to limit symptoms production. This information is useful to the clinician when planning/establishing intensity of initial rehabilitative steps toward the goals of the rehabilitative processes to: (1) reduce symptoms; (2) improve static and dynamic balance function; and (3) improve general conditioning and ADL functionality.[12,19] Additional information of contributory past medical history, family history of maladies/illnesses, headache (migraine or other classifications) history, and (if present) method of management, attention and/or learning disabilities, socialization issues, and prior cognitive deficits should be obtained. Changes in cognition or psychologic functionality should be followed by a clinical psychologist. Computerized screenings may be performed to document deficits in mentation. Determination of sleep status, either difficulty falling asleep (sleep onset), or difficulty staying asleep (sleep maintenance), should be performed. Sleep deficits may contribute to symptoms magnification or limit tolerance to cognition or physical activities, and should be managed by a clinical specialist in sleep disorders. Medications for normalizing the sleep cycle without inducing adverse effects of drowsiness or lethargy may be of benefit.

An initial assessment of position changes and gait gives the examiner information as to any mobility limitations. Several validated tests may be employed for objective measures of mobility, such as: Timed Up and Go (TUG), Berg Balance Scale (Berg), Clinical Test of Sensory Interaction and Balance (CTSIB), the Functional Reach Test, Tinetti Balance Test of the Performance-Oriented Assessment of Mobility Problems (Tinetti), the Physical Performance Test (PPT), and the Functional Movement Screen.[20,21] Reflex testing may elicit important hyporeflexia or hyperreflexia as signs of lower- or upper-motor neuron lesion (e.g., clonus, Babinski, etc.). Cerebellar/Coordination signs may be assessed: finger to nose, diadochokinesia, finger/foot tapping, heel-to-shin slide, and VOR cancellation.

Hearing assessment with air and bone conduction auditory capacities may be determined by performing Weber and Rinne tests with a 512 and 1024 Hz tuning fork. The use of both will allow assessment for low- and high-frequency hearing loss to air and bone conduction. Asymmetry or positive findings should be followed with formal audiology testing.

An orthopedic assessment of the cervical spine may follow. The range of motion/mobility deficits or hypermobility should be noted. Strength and mobility assessments should involve the upper and lower segments with active, passive, and segmental accessory motion testing with quadrant testing being performed. Assessment for occipital neuralgia and trigeminal neuralgia should be included. Rotation testing should involve head movements on the cervical spine, head and cervical spine movements on the torso, and torso movements under the stationary cervical spine. Postural deficits may be corrected at this point also. Assessment of cervical-ocular reflex and gaze stability exercises may be assessed at this juncture.

A vision assessment may be performed next, including visual fields assessment, and oculomotor tests: smooth pursuit in horizontal, vertical, and diagonal directions, at varying velocities. Saccadic motions, predictive saccades, and antisaccades in all planes should be assessed. Abnormal spatial perceptions and/or depth perceptual deficits may be assessed with convergence and divergence tests, along with peripheral vision assessment. Sensitivity to motion may be detected with adding OKN stimulation.[22] Assessments of strabismus may be performed with a cover test, and referral for Ophthalmology evaluation if any test appears to be abnormal.

Oculography with augmented infra-red eye tracking technology or Frenzel lenses with Vestibular Electromyogenic Potential (VEMPs), and Video Head Impulse Testing (vHIT) may be helpful in detection of central versus peripheral vestibular dysfunction, evaluating spontaneous nystagmus in light and dark environments, gaze evoked nystagmus, and head shake testing. However, there is conflicting evidence within the literature as to the benefits and sensitivity of these tests.[23-26] Suppression of nystagmus with ocular fixation with Frenzel lenses, Fresnel lens device[27] added may lead the examiner more toward peripheral etiology rather than central origin, but should not be used alone, but in conjunction with other testing methods to be definitive.[28] The results of the testing (detection of nystagmus and direction and performance of the nystagmus) may assist the examiner with decision-making for further testing (e.g., imaging studies, ENG with caloric irrigation, rotational chair, etc., if the patient is seen as being in the acute phase of symptoms onset).

Further testing of Dynamic Visual Acuity (DVAT) in comparison to static acuity and/or a Gaze Stability Test (GST) may assist in detection of velocity limits for gaze stability and target recognition, and Subjective Visual Vertical assessment compared with cVEMP and oVEMP tests may clarify the contribution of the otolithic system (saccule and utricle).[29]

Computerized Dynamic Posturography (CDP) may be used to better determine the various components (vestibular, visual, somatosensory/proprioception) of balance maintenance, and adaptive strategy for compensation for falls prevention, symptoms reduction, and improved functionality.[12] Ideally there exists an optimal relationship among the components for balance maintenance.[30,31] The rehabilitation clinician may use the results of the CDP for planning specific rehabilitative measures to enhance the deficient component(s) and/or implement substitutive strategies. Further integration of the strategies may be achieved with augmented general activity exercise (walking, jogging, cycling, etc.) with the specific task challenges implemented. It should be noted that implementation of a balance rehabilitative program alone, without first initiating visual-based rehabilitative measures, will elicit a less than optimal balance strategy recovery. However, implementation of visual-based strategies has shown improvement of postural stability even without use of postural stability and balance exercises.[32]

The relationship of the executive function component of cognition and functionality must be considered as part of the rehabilitation assessment and treatment program. Several validated psychology scales and assessment tools exist for measurement and quantification of cognition, anxiety, concentration, and memory.[33-37] In sports, the ImPACT® test remains the standard; however, use of it or other similar computerized test measures (e.g., Axon Sports, ANAM) as a standalone measure of magnitude of injury, or readiness for return to participation has been questioned due to invalid baseline test scores due to subjects' intentional manipulation of results, less than optimal testing conditions employed, or variable test–retest results among examiners.[38] However, further research is needed to determine the longitudinal relationship of cognition deficits to task performance and adaptation with vestibular rehabilitation processes. Development of new technologies for quantifying functionality and executive function components of cognition and task performance have been described.[39,40] Use of eye-tracking technologies, and blood/saliva-borne biomarkers, as well as the use of advanced imaging techniques are emerging as potential next-generation measures, due to their not requiring baseline comparative testing, and the limited ability of the subject to intentionally render invalid test results. Use of virtual and augmented reality devices for rehabilitation are also gaining popularity,[41−44] yet further investigation is merited.

PROTOCOL

A comprehensive, team-based approach to assessment and rehabilitation, including targeted, specific vestibular rehabilitation exercise combined with general exercise programs has been shown to elicit positive effects of symptoms limitation and an enhanced speed of functionality recovery after mTBI. Initiation and prescription of rehabilitation protocols is the second of three classically described phases of recovery following vestibular insult[8] and is dependent on the tolerance of the subject, and somewhat determined by the timeline of injury, initiation of symptoms, and up-to-date compensation patterns employed. Recovery from injury is variable among subjects, requiring the astute clinician to formulate a program of recovery specific to the needs of the subject.[30,31,45] The clinician is often first required to reverse first stage patterns of vestibular compensation that self-limit the subject's head, eyes, and body mobilities. Notification of probability of increased symptoms production and use of prophylactic antiemetic medications may limit the subject's anxiety toward initial exercise performance, and enhance compliance. Post-injury increased reflex response times to auditory cues suggests the possibility of enhancing auditory inputs (amplification with aides, etc.) as being helpful for recovery. Initially, exercise may be given with the subject supine or seated, to eliminate confounding somatosensory inputs. Regaining normative mobility of the cervical spine is imperative to allow for the full range of motion of the head and eyes for the vision-based exercises. Vision-based exercises for VOR recovery usually requires 4 weeks duration[46] and requires daily compliance and exercise adherence. Current research efforts toward improved compliance utilizing smartphone technologies and playing video games has shown positive effects. Posture for performing exercises may be progressed from lying to sitting, to standing, to walking, or moving—as tolerated. Frequency and velocity of target acquisition is important, as the VOR is velocity specific. Likened to orthopedic active muscle rehabilitation techniques, velocity of exercises should be varied, and later in the rehabilitation process should be task-specific oriented. Use of timing devices (e.g., metronome) or more advanced computerized DVA and/or GST may be beneficial for measurement of thresholds tolerance.[47,48] Advancement toward balance and proprioceptive exercises requires varied multisensory stimulation, including varied visual inputs limitations and challenging the base of support positions, along with varied surface textures. Progression from static positioning to movement-based exercise should be directed from small movements toward large-arc, segmented, body motions with functional application. Proprioceptive Neuromuscular Facilitation (PNF) exercises may be useful. Postural and balance exercise generally requires longer duration for full recovery, and may take up to 3 months, depending upon the availability of VOR stability and spatial orientation recovery.[49]

During the initial phase of recovery (24−48 hours post-injury), cognitive stress should be avoided, and normalization of the sleep cycle appears to be critical, as protracted recovery appears to result from failure to remove stressors and persistence of abnormal sleep cycles, though this may be age and gender specific. Further research is merited regarding removal of cognitive stressors with sleep pattern modulation, and progression to back to normal daily functions throughout the second and third phases of recovery. Initiation of an appropriate timeline and subsequent immersion into a vestibular and balance rehabilitation programs has shown positive benefits to cognition, even without being involved directly in a cognitive rehabilitative program.

SUMMARY/CONCLUSION

Concussion/mTBI injury continues to gain public and medical professional awareness, as media coverage is heightened and increased medical research efforts give rise to empirical data to support novel objective measures and methods in combination with traditional symptom-based management. While imaging studies and blood/saliva biomarkers tests are emerging for detection, a hierarchal comprehensive assessment and rehabilitative team approach[50] appears to have merit in symptom resolution and progression toward functionality.[8] While efforts are made toward public education of recognition of signs and symptoms of mTBI, education of medical professionals appears merited for appropriate recognition and medical management. The astute medical and rehabilitative clinicians should be aware of the timeline of recovery at the time of assessment, the appropriate steps toward resolution for each of the three recovery stages, and the appropriate initiation and progression of objective testing and rehabilitative methods for each. Since dizziness is the most common symptom following mTBI, vestibular assessment and rehabilitative approaches have shown benefits for head and eye movement stabilization and recovery, and subsequent progressive balance and movement exercises restores static and dynamic balance, gait, and ADL functionality.[51] Compliance and adherence to a prescribed recovery protocol remains a challenge, but new technologies are emerging to address it. This may allow the rehabilitation clinician to assess and monitor subjects remotely, and progress the rehabilitation program when direct access to a professional is limited. The sequelae of mistimed or inappropriate management appear to be a protracted recovery time, limited functionality, and symptoms persistence. Attention to sleep pattern normalization and cognitive recovery processes appear critical at the initial phase of recovery, as these appear to impact headache and accompanying symptoms' persistence. Further research is merited in all aspects of medical/rehabilitative management, particularly the areas of sleep cycle and headache management, dosage and duration of rehabilitative exercise programs, objective measurement protocols to determine when thresholds of recovery steps are met, and thresholds of recovery for the safe return to participation in ADL activities (e.g., driving, sports, etc.). Longitudinal studies of cognition, repetitive trauma effects, and rehabilitative management protocols give the researcher/clinician ample opportunity to advance the science of this malady.

References

1. Gottshall K. Vestibular rehabilitation after mild traumatic brain injury with vestibular pathology. *NeuroRehabilitation* 2011;**29**(2):167—71.
2. Hillier SL, McDonnell M. Vestibular rehabilitation for unilateral peripheral vestibular dysfunction. *Cochrane Database Syst Rev* 2011;**16**:248—9

3. Lei-Rivera L, et al. Special tools for the assessment of balance and dizziness in individuals with mild traumatic brain injury. *NeuroRehabilitation* 2013;**32**(3):463–72.

4. Ito M. Cerebellar long-term depression: characterization, signal transduction, and functional roles. *Physiol Rev* 2001;**81**:1144–95.

5. De Zeeuw CI, Hansel C, Bian F, Koekkoek SKE, van Alphen AM, Linden DJ, et al. Expression of a protein kinase C inhibitor in Purkinje cells blocks cerebellar LTD and adaptation of the vestibulo-ocular reflex. *Neuron* 1998;**20**:495–508.

6. Leitges M, Kovac J, Plomann M, Linden DJ. A unique PDZ ligand in PKCa confers induction of cerebellar long-term synaptic depression. *Neuron* 2004;**44**:585–94.

7. Linden DJ, Connor JA. Long-term synaptic depression. *Annu Rev Neurosci* 1995;**18**:319–57.

8. Balaban CD, et al. Top-down approach to vestibular compensation: translational lessons from vestibular rehabilitation. *Brain Res* 2012;**1482**:101–11.

9. Brooks MA, Peterson K, Biese K, Sanfilippo J, Heiderscheit BC, Bell DR. Concussion increases odds of sustaining a lower extremity musculoskeletal injury after return to play among collegiate athletes. *Am J Sports Med* 2016;**44**(3):742–7.

10. Herman DC, Jones D, Harrison A, Moser M, Tillman S, Farmer K, et al. Concussion may increase the risk of subsequent lower extremity musculoskeletal injury in collegiate athletes. *Sports Med* 2017;**47**(5):1003–10.

11. Fetter M. Acute unilateral loss of vestibular function. *Handb Clin Neurol* 2016;**137**:219–29.

12. Herdman SJ, Whitney SL. Interventions for the patient with vestibular hypofunction. In: Herdman SJ, editor. *Vestibular rehabilitation*. Philadelphia, PA: F.A. Davis; 2007. p. 309–37.

13. Imai T, et al. Classification, diagnostic criteria and management of benign paroxysmal positional vertigo. *Auris Nasus Larynx* 2017;**44**(1):1–6.

14. Zhang, Y.X., et al. Comparison of three types of self-treatments for posterior canal benign paroxysmal positional vertigo: modified Epley maneuver, *Zhonghua Er Bi Yan Hou Tou Jing Wai Ke Za Zhi* 2012;**47**(10):799–803.

15. Beynon GJ. A review of management of benign paroxysmal positional vertigo by exercise therapy and by repositioning manoeuvres. *Br J Audiol* 1997;**31**(1):11–26.

16. Semont maneuver and Brandt-Daroff maneuver. *Zhonghua Er Bi Yan Hou Tou Jing Wai Ke Za Zhi* **2012;47** (10):799–803.

17. Helminski JO, et al. Strategies to prevent recurrence of benign paroxysmal positional vertigo. *Arch Otolaryngol Head Neck Surg* 2005;**131**(4):344–8.

18. Helminski JO, et al. Daily exercise does not prevent recurrence of benign paroxysmal positional vertigo. *Otol Neurotol* 2008;**29**(7):976–81.

19. Magnus, R. Body posture = Korperstellung: experimental-physiological investigations of the reflexes involved in body posture, their cooperation and disturbances; based on a translation by William R. Rosanoff, and on a translation by Franklin Book Programs, Inc., Cairo, for the National Library of Medicine, Amerind, Springfield, VA, USA; 1924 (reprint 1980).

20. Whitney SL, Sparto PJ. Principles of vestibular physical therapy rehabilitation. *Neuro Rehabil* 2011;**29**:157–66.

21. Stanek JM, et al. Active duty firefighters can improve Functional Movement Screen (FMS) scores following an 8-week individualized client workout program. *Work* 2017;**56**(2):213–20.

22. Pavlou M. The use of optokinetic stimulation in vestibular rehabilitation. *J Neurol Phys Ther* 2010;**34**(2):105–10.

23. Cohen HS, et al. Utility of quick oculomotor tests for screening the vestibular system in the subacute and chronic populations. *Acta Otolaryngol* 2017;**138**(4):1–5.

24. Tamas TL, et al. Emergency diagnosis of the acute vestibular syndrome. *Orv Hetil* 2017;**158**(51):2029–40.

25. Lance S, Mossman SS. Misleading signs in acute vertigo. *Pract Neurol*. 2017;**18**(2):162–5

26. van de Berg R, et al. Laboratory examinations for the vestibular system. *Curr Opin Neurol* 2018;**31**(1):111–16.

27. Strupp M, et al. The takeaway Frenzel goggles: a Fresnel-based device. *Neurology* 2014;**83**(14):1241–5.

28. An SY, et al. Clinical roles of fixation suppression failure in dizzy patients in the ENT clinic. *Acta Otolaryngol* 2014;**134**(11):1134–9.

29. Slattery EL, et al. Vestibular tests for rehabilitation: applications and interpretation. *NeuroRehabilitation* 2011;**29** (2):143–51.

30. Collins JJ, De Luca CJ. The effects of visual input on open-loop and closed-loop postural control mechanisms. *Exp Brain Res* 1995;**103**:151–63.

31. Lacour M, Barthelemy J, Borel L, Magnan J, Xerri C, Chays A, et al. Sensory strategies in human postural control before and after unilateral vestibular neurotomy. *Exp Brain Res* 1997;**115**:300–10.
32. Morimoto H, Asai Y, Johnson EG, Lohman EB, Khoo K, Mizutani Y, et al. Effect of oculo-motor and gaze stability exercises on postural stability and dynamic visual acuity in healthy young adults. *Gait Post* 2011;**33**:600–3.
33. Hazlett RL, Tusa RJ, Waranch HR. Development of an inventory for dizziness and related factors. *J Behav Med* 1996;**19**:73–85.
34. Jacobson GP, Newman WW. The development of the dizziness handicap inventory. *Arch Otolaryngol Head Neck Surg* 1990;**116**:424–7.
35. Morris AE, Lutman ME, Yardley L. Measuring outcome from vestibular rehabilitation, part I: quantitative development of a new self-report measure. *Int J Audiol* 2008;**47**:169–77.
36. Morris AE, Lutman ME, Yardley L. Measuring outcome from vestibular rehabilitation, part II: refinement and validation of a new self-report measure. *Int J Audiol* 2009;**48**:24–37.
37. Yardley L, Masson E, Verschuur C, Haacke N, Luxon L. Symptoms, anxiety and handicap in dizziness patients: development of the Vertigo Symptom Scale. *J Psychosom Res* 1992;**36**:731–41.
38. Nelson LD, et al. Rates and predictors of invalid baseline test performance in high school and collegiate athletes for 3 computerized neurocognitive tests: ANAM, Axon Sports, and ImPACT. *Am J Sports Med* 2015;**43**(8):2018–26.
39. Leyva A, Balachandran A, Britton JC, Eltoukhy M, Kuenze C, Myers ND, et al. The development and examination of a new walking executive function test for people over 50 years of age. *Physiol Behav* 2017;**171**:100–9.
40. Perrochon A, Kemoun G, Watelain E, Dugue B, Berthoz A. The "Stroop Walking Task": an innovative dual-task for the early detection of executive function impairment. *Neurophysiol Clin* 2015;**45**(3):181–90.
41. Bergeron M, Lortie CL, Guitton MJ. Use of virtual reality tools for vestibular disorders rehabilitation: a comprehensive analysis. *Adv Med* 2015;**2015**:916735.
42. Chang YJ, Kang YS, Huang PC. An augmented reality (AR)-based vocational task prompting system for people with cognitive impairments. *Res Dev Disabil* 2013;**34**(10):3049–56.
43. Biffi E, Beretta E, Diella E, Panzeri D, Maghini C, Turconi AC, et al. Gait rehabilitation with a high tech platform based on virtual reality conveys improvements in walking ability of children suffering from acquired brain injury. *Conf Proc IEEE Eng Med Biol Soc* 2015;**2015**:7406–9.
44. Khademi M, Hondori HM, Dodakian L, Cramer S, Lopes CV. Comparing "pick and place" task in spatial Augmented Reality versus non-immersive Virtual Reality for rehabilitation setting. *Conf Proc IEEE Eng Med Biol Soc* 2013;**2013**:4613–16.
45. Peterka RJ, Statler KD, Wrisley DM, Horak FB. Postural compensation for unilateral vestibular loss. *Front Neurol* 2011;**57**:1–13; 2011;2:Article.
46. Herdman SJ, Schubert MC, Das VE, Tusa RJ. Recovery of dynamic visual acuity in unilateral vestibular hypofunction. *Arch Otolaryngol Head Neck Surg* 2003;**129**:819–24.
47. Gottshall KR, Hoffer ME. Tracking recovery of vestibular function in Individuals With blast-induced head trauma using vestibular—visual-cognitive interaction tests. *J Neurol Phys Ther* 2010;**34**:94–7.
48. Gottshall K, et al. Objective vestibular tests as outcome measures in head injury patients. *Laryngoscope* 2003;**113**(10):1746–50.
49. Borel L, Harlay F, Magnan J, Chays A, Lacour M. Deficits and recovery of head and trunk orientation and stabilization after unilateral vestibular loss. *Brain* 2002;**125**:880–94.
50. Gottshall KR, Sessoms PH. Improvements in dizziness and imbalance results from using a multi-disciplinary and multi-sensory approach to Vestibular Physical Therapy—a case study. *Front Syst Neurosci* 2015;**9**:106.
51. Alsalaheen BA, et al. Exercise prescription patterns in patients treated with vestibular rehabilitation after concussion. *Physiother Res Int* 2013;**18**(2):100–8.

Index

Note: Page numbers followed by "*f*" and "*t*" refer to figures and tables, respectively.

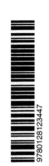